S0-CBI-453

Trichinellosis

Trichinellosis

Proceedings of the
Third International Conference
on Trichinellosis, 3d, Miami Beach, Fla., 1972.

Edited by
Charles W. Kim
State University of New York at Stony Brook

in association with

**M. A. Bier / L. S. Blair / W. C. Campbell / D. D. Despommier /
G. J. Jackson / I. G. Kagan / J. E. Larsh / E. Meerovitch / M. Müller /
E. Sadun / M. G. Schultz / E. J. L. Soulsby**

RC186
T815
I612p
1972
(1974)

Intext Educational Publishers
New York

304736

THIRD INTERNATIONAL CONFERENCE ON TRICHINELLOSIS

Conference Committee

J. E. Larsh, Jr., *Executive Director*
W. C. Campbell, *Secretary-Treasurer*
C. W. Kim, *Program Chairman*
D. D. Despommier, *Coordinator*
L. S. Blair, *Associate Coordinator*

Planning Committee

D. E. Cooperrider
J. DeVore
I. G. Kagan
E. J. L. Soulsby
J. H. Steele
P. Zillman
W. J. Zimmermann
D. E. Zinter

The conference was organized under the sponsorship of
the International Commission on Trichinellosis

Copyright © 1974 by Thomas Y. Crowell Company, Inc.

All rights reserved. No part of this book may be reprinted, reproduced, or utilized in any form or by any electronic, mechanical, or other means, now known or hereafter invented, including photocopying and recording, or in any information storage and retrieval system, without permission in writing from the Publisher.

Library of Congress Cataloging in Publication Data

International Conference on Trichinellosis, 3d, Miami
  Beach, Fla., 1972.
  Trichinellosis; proceedings.

  Includes bibliographies.
  1. Trichina and trichinosis — Congresses.
I. Kim, Charles W., ed. II. Title. [DNLM: 1. Trichi-
nosis — Congresses. W3IN1955p]
RC186.T815I58 1972   616.9′654   74-6357
ISBN 0-7002-2461-0

Intext Educational Publishers
666 Fifth Avenue
New York, New York 10019

Text design by Robert Sugar

Preface

The Third International Conference on Trichinellosis,* held in Miami Beach on November 2–4, 1972, consisted of five symposia covering the following aspects of trichinellosis: morphology and *in vitro* studies; biochemistry and experimental pathology; immunology, clinical and diagnostic aspects; treatment; and epidemiology and control.

This volume, containing 63 papers that were either presented at the conference or submitted afterward, will, we hope, provide a comprehensive understanding of the current knowledge and thinking about the various phases of trichinellosis and will serve to stimulate future research. At the meeting in Miami Beach there were 102 registrants, 25 scientists coming from countries outside the United States. Forty-three papers were presented although 87 abstracts had been submitted. Many of the scientists from abroad who had submitted abstracts were unable to be present in person to deliver their papers; however, they submitted full-length manuscripts for this publication which therefore, constitutes the scientific record of all papers connected with this conference.

There are many individuals without whose generous contributions, interests and efforts the conference and subsequently the publication of these proceedings would not have been possible. The officers and members of the various committees of the Third International Conference on Trichinellosis wish to acknowledge the following patrons: American Association of Veterinary Parasitologists; Elanco Products Co.; Merck & Co.; Smith, Kline and French Laboratories; and National Live Stock and Meat Board; and the following individuals who contributed in the typing and proofing of abstracts and manuscripts for publication: Lorna Aaron, Jacqueline Cacace, June Foy, and Craig Linder. My personal appreciation is also extended to Dr. Larsh, the Executive Director of the conference; to each of the chairmen: Drs. Campbell, Kagan, Meerovitch, Sadun, Schultz, and Soulsby; and to the committee members: Drs. Despommier, Jackson, Müller, and Ms. Blair; who donated their time and effort in making the conference a meaningful scientific experience and the publication of the proceedings of the conference a reality.

* The first two International Conferences were held in Warsaw (1960) and Wroclaw (1969).

We also gratefully acknowledge the following organizations that co-sponsored the conference.

CO-SPONSORS

The American Society of Clinical Pathologists
The Council of the American Society of Parasitologists
American Veterinary Medical Association
Ceskoslovenská Spolocnost Parazitologická pri CSAV
Federación Latinoamericana de Parasitologia
Helminthological Society of Washington
Pan American Association of Anatomy
Polish Parasitological Society
American College of Preventive Medicine
Southern California Parasitologists
Société Belge des Sciences Pharmaceutiques
Société Belge de Parasitologie
Scandinavian Society for Parasitology
International Association of Milk, Food & Environmental Sanitarians, Inc.
Council of the Wildlife Disease Association
World Federation of Parasitologists
College of American Pathologists
Pan American Health Organization
American Veterinary Epidemiology Society
American College of Preventive Medicine
British Pharmacological Society
Council for International Organization of Medical Sciences

Medical Women's International Association
Wildlife Management Institute
The Pharmacological Society of Canada
Hungarian Society of Parasitologists
American Society of Mammalogists
World Association of Pathology Societies
American Medical Association
American Public Health Association
The Conference of State & Provincial Health Authorities of North America
Nederlandse Vereniging voor Parasitologie
Upjohn International Inc.
Society for Experimental Biology
Société Francaise de Parasitologie
Southwestern Association of Parasitologists
New Jersey Society of Parasitologists
Annual Midwestern Conference of Parasitologists
Deutsche Gesellschaft für Parasitologie
Institute of Advanced Sanitation Research, International
International Commission on Trichinellosis
International Congress on Tropical Medicine and Malaria
World Association of Anatomic and Clinical Pathology Societies
Malaysian Society of Parasitology and Tropical Medicine

CHARLES W. KIM
Stony Brook, New York

Contents

Part I: Morphology; *in Vitro* Studies

Part II: Biochemistry; Experimental Pathology

Part III: Immunobiology

Part IV: Clinical and Diagnostic Aspects

Part V: Treatment

Part VI: Epidemiology and Control

List of Contributors

Numbers in parentheses indicate the pages on which the authors' contributions begin.

Patricia C. Allen (145)
Agricultural Research Service, Beltsville, Maryland

John S. Andrews (145)
Agricultural Research Service, Beltsville, Maryland

Omar O. Barriga (421)
School of Veterinary Medicine, University of Pennsylvania

Fernando Beltrán-Hernández (175)
Faculty of Medicine, National University of Mexico

Y. A. Berezantsev (101)
Medical Institute of Sanitation and Hygiene, Leningrad

Allen K. Berntzen (25)
Oregon Zoological Research Center, Portland

A. S. Bessonov (557, 563)
The All-Union K. I. Skryabin Institute of Helminthology, Moscow

Lyndia S. Blair (463)
Merck Institute for Therapeutic Research, Rahway, New Jersey

Malgorzata Blotna (135)
Medical Academy of Poznań

Ernest J. Bowmer (531)
Division of Laboratories, Vancouver, British Columbia

V. A. Britov (567)
Far-Eastern Research Institute of Veterinary Science, Blagoveshchensk-on-Amur

R. G. Bruce (43, 49)
University of Glasgow

Hans Jürgen-Bürger* (367)
Walter Reed Army Institute of Research, Washington, D. C.

William C. Campbell (463)
Merck Institute for Therapeutic Research, Rahway, New Jersey

Leon Chodera (413, 471)
Medical Academy of Poznań

I. Cironeanu (549)
Ministry of Food Industry, Bucharest

J. Čorba (213)
Helminthological Institute of the Slovak Academy of Sciences, Kosice

Catherine A. Crandall (231)
College of Medicine, University of Florida

R. B. Crandall (157)
College of Medicine, University of Florida

Raymond H. Cypess (319)
Graduate School of Public Health, University of Pittsburgh

D. A. Denham (345)
London School of Hygiene and Tropical Medicine

Dickson D. Despommier (7, 239)
College of Physicians & Surgeons, Columbia University

E. E. Efremov (187)
The All-Union K. I. Skryabin Institute of Helminthology, Moscow

G. A. Ermolin (187, 199)
The All-Union K. I. Skryabin Institute of Helminthology, Moscow

Gaétan Faubert (327, 353)
Macdonald College, McGill University

Velia Estela Figueroa-Villalva (175)
Faculty of Medicine, National University of Mexico

J. Carl Fox (597)
Montana State University

* Present Address: Institut für
Parasitologie, Bunteway

Przemysław Gabryel (123, 135)
Medical Academy of Poznań

Zygmunt Gancarz (407)
National Institute of Hygiene, Warsaw

Czesław Gerwel (123, 471)
Medical Academy of Poznań

David Gitlin (319)
School of Public Health, University of Pittsburgh

Alberto Gómez-Priego (175)
Faculty of Medicine, National University of Mexico

Rufus W. Gore (367)
Walter Reed Army Institute of Research, Washington, D. C.

Miroslaw Gorny (221)
Medical Academy of Poznań

Kenneth R. Greer (597)
Montana Fish and Game Department

Leokadia Gustowska (123, 135)
Medical Academy of Poznań

L. D. Hamilton (291, 303)
Brookhaven National Laboratory, Upton, New York

Dale M. Holm (579)
Los Alamos Scientific Laboratory

Robert S. Isenstein (385)
Agricultural Research Service, Beltsville, Maryland

E. R. James (345)
London School of Hygiene and Tropical Medicine

Mahendra P. Jamuar* (291, 303)
Brookhaven National Laboratory, Upton, New York

Krystyna Jarczewska (221)
Medical Academy of Poznań

Dennis Juranek (593)
U. S. Public Health Service, Atlanta, Georgia

Jerzy Kaczmarek (123)
Medical Academy of Poznań

Charles W. Kim (291, 303)
State University of New York at Stony Brook

Wanda Kociecka (123, 471)
Medical Academy of Poznań

M. O. Kolosova (477)
The E. I. Marstynsovsky Institute of Medical Parasitology and Tropical Medicine, Moscow

S. Komandarev (149)
Helminthological Institute of the Slovak Academy of Sciences, Košice and Control Helminthological Laboratories of the Bulgarian Academy of Sciences, Sofia

W. J. Kozek† ,157, 231)
College of Medicine, University of Florida

J. Lamina (483)
Technological University, Munich-Freising

John E. Larsh, Jr. (75)
School of Public Health, University of North Carolina at Chapel Hill

Tsue-Ming Lin (165)
University of Miami School of Medicine

Inger Ljungström (449)
National Bacteriological Laboratory, Stockholm

Donald O. Lyman‡ (571)
Health Services and Mental Health Administration, Berkeley, California

Holger Madsen (615)
University of Copenhagen

James H. Martin (75)
Baylor University Medical Center

Leroy J. Olson (61, 165)
The University of Texas Medical Branch, Galveston

N. N. Ozeretskovskaya (389, 477, 499)
The E. I. Martsynovsky Institute of Medical Parasitology and Tropical Medicine, Moscow

Zbigniew Pawłowski (123, 413, 471)
Medical Academy of Poznań

* Present Address: Department of Zoology, Patna, Bihar

† Present Address: University of California at Davis.

‡ Present Address: State of New York Department of Health, Albany

E. V. Pereverzeva (111, 499)
The E. I. Martsynovsky Institute of Medical Parasitology and Tropical Medicine, Moscow

Wojciech S. Plonka (255, 407)
National Institute of Hygiene, Warsaw

Steven H. Polmar (399)
National Institutes of Health, Bethesda, Maryland

Mabel Purkerson (7)
College of Physicians and Surgeons, Columbia University

George J. Race (75)
Baylor University Medical Center

J. A. Richardson (61)
The University of Texas Medical Branch, Galveston

Albert L. Ritterson (335)
University of Rochester School of Medicine

Eugene B. Rosenberg* (399)
University of Miami School of Medicine

E. J. Ruitenberg (205, 539)
National Institute of Public Health, Bilthoven

Elvio H. Sadun (367)
Walter Reed Army Institute of Research, Washington, D.C.

Myron G. Schultz (593)
National Communicable Disease Center, Atlanta, Georgia

John D. Seagrave (579)
Los Alamos Scientific Laboratory

Diego Segre (421)
College of Veterinary Medicine, University of Illinois

Howard B. Shookhoff (443)
Department of Health, City of New York

J. F. Sluiters (539)
National Institute of Public Health, Bilthoven

R. Spaldonová (149, 213)
Helminthological Institute of the Slovak Academy of Sciences, Košice

Bronisław Stachowski (123)
Medical Academy of Posnań

Miroslaw Stankiewicz† (259, 275)
Veterinary Medical Research Institute, Iowa State University

Charles E. Tanner (327, 353)
Macdonald College, McGill University

V. I. Tarakanov (31, 37, 199)
The Helminthological Laboratory of the Academy of Sciences of U.S.S.R., Moscow

D. Thienpont (515)
Janssen Pharmaceutica, Beerse

E. V. Timonov (3)
The All-Union K.I. Skryabin Institute of Helminthology, Moscow

O. Tomašovičová (149)
Košice and Central Helminthological Laboratories of the Bulgarian Academy of Sciences, Sofia

N. I. Tumolskaya (389)
The E. I. Martsynovsky Institute of Medical Parasitology and Tropical Medicine, Moscow

R. Vandesteene (515)
Janssen Pharmaceutica, Beerse

O. F. Vanparijs (515)
Janssen Pharmaceutica, Beerse

N. L. Veretennikova (111, 499)
The E. I. Martsynovsky Institute of Medical Parasitology and Tropical Medicine, Moscow

Norman F. Weatherly (75)
School of Public Health, University of North Carolina at Chapel Hill

George E. Whalen (399)
Veterans Administration Center, Wood, Wisconsin

John B. Winters (597)
Montana State University

David E. Worley (597)
Montana State University

L. A. Yutkin (563)
Agrophysical Institute, Leningrad

Rolando Zapata (319)
Graduate School of Public Health, University of Pittsburgh

* Present Address: Mount Sinai Hospital, Miami Beach, Florida.

† Present Address: University of Warsaw

Bozenna Zawadzka-Jedrzejewska (407)
National Institute of Hygiene, Warsaw

Jan Zeromski (221)
Medical Academy of Poznań

W. J. Zimmermann (603, 611)
Veterinary Medical Research Institute, Iowa State University

Opening of the Meeting

The meeting was opened by Dr. John E. Larsh, Jr. whose remarks were as follows:

As Executive Director of the conference, and President of the executive committee of the commission, it is my honor and privilege to call to order this the *Third International Conference on Trichinellosis.* I do so with high expectations that the Conference will meet its purposes, namely, (1) to add new knowledge about this important disease of man and other animals, and its etiologic agent, *Trichinella spiralis,* and (2) to emphasize our objective for encouragement of more international coordination of research activities in this and other fields of health.

On the other hand, I open the conference with a heavy heart, because two of our great leaders, Dr. Kozar and Dr. Gould – both excellent scientists and persevering champions of the cause of trichinellosis on a global basis – have been lost by death during the past two years. As you know, both men supported the previous conferences with enthusiasm, and had planned to play leading roles during this meeting. In view of these grievous losses, it is altogether fitting and proper that we should dedicate this conference, the Keynote Address, and the published proceedings of the conference to the memory of Dr. Kozar and Dr. Gould. Therefore, on behalf of the executive committee, the conference officers and planning committee, I sincerely recommend this action to you at this time. Will all those in favor please indicate by standing for a moment of silent tribute to our fallen leaders?

Let the record show that this recommendation for these dedications was accepted unanimously by this assembly.

Dr. Larsh introduced Dr. H. King Stanford, President, University of Miami, who made a warm welcoming address.

Afterward, Dr. Larsh introduced the keynote speaker, Mr. David H. Stroud, President, National Live Stock and Meat Board, Chicago, Illinois, who presented the Kozar-Gould Memorial Lecture on "Trichinosis: Quo Vadimus".

Thanks and appreciation were extended to Dr. King and Mr. Stroud for their contributions to the opening of the Conference, after which Dr. Larsh adjourned the meeting.

In Memoriam

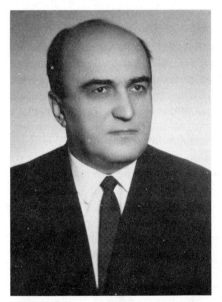

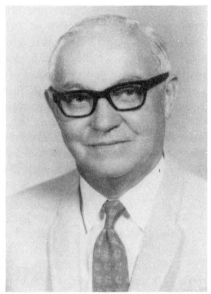

Dr. Zbigniew Kozar   1918–1972   Dr. S. Samuel Gould   1900–1970

They were not similar men; they were stars, to be sure, in the trichinellian galaxy — but not its Gemini. Professor Kozar, tall and powerfully built, was at the height of his powers and as resolute of purpose as he was imposing of physique. More than any other individual he had made Poland an international headquarters of trichinellosis interests and activities. Combining a training in veterinary medicine with an irrepressible academic bent, he and his colleagues in Wroclaw gave the name of that city a special familiarity to trichinellosis workers all over the world. Half a world away, Professor Gould at the age of 70 years was spending his "retirement" years in the Florida sunshine. He was small in stature, and a heart attack had made him physically frail — and yet what boundless enthusiasm was there! He bore his years with grace and gaiety; and when he spoke of trichinellosis he beamed like a happy schoolboy. First and foremost he was a physician and clinical pathologist. Since both the beginning and the end of his career were marked by the appearance of his classic books on trichinellosis, we are inclined to forget that his professional speciality was the pathology of the heart, and that he was responsible for a classic textbook and many articles in that field.

In the context of the Third International Conference on Trichinellosis it is, of course, what Kozar and Gould had in common that is of most importance. Each man had an abiding interest in *Trichinella spiralis* and the disease it causes. Neither of them regarded the infection as a mere research tool for attacking some remote objective; they were interested in trichinellosis itself, in all its aspects. They were captivated by its history. They were concerned about it as a zoonosis and as a clinical conundrum. They confronted the administrative problems of surveillance and control. They were committed to the challenge of trichinellosis research; but it was not laboratory insight that made them leaders in the field—it was the totality of their interest in the subject and their commitment to nurturing that interest in others, be they students, hog raisers, legislators, academicians, or practitioners of human or veterinary medicine. Both men were indefatigable writers and editors. Both had organized trichinellosis conferences in their own countries. Their work on trichinellosis was in part an avocation, something willingly added on top of many other arduous professional duties. [The reader who seeks wider knowledge of the careers of Drs. Gould and Kozar is referred to the *American Journal of Clinical Pathology* **56,** 255–257 (1971), and *Wiadomości Parazytologicne* **18,** 139–141 (1972)].

They seldom met, and did not always see eye to eye, but they had the highest respect for each other. When they dined together in Washington, D.C. just a couple of months before Dr. Gould's death, excited *Trichinella* talk accompanied every course. The exuberance with which Dr. Gould embarked on the conference planning remained undiminished until the day he was stricken with that final heart attack in November, 1970. We who had planned with him and who had learned to expect frequent phone calls and letters packed with suggestions were immediately conscious of the void he had left. One of Dr. Kozar's last editorial pieces was an *in memoriam* report on Dr. Gould as a leader in the field of trichinellosis, and in it he referred to Gould as "the greatest enthusiast of this problem in the United States." How apt that description!—for he was indeed an enthusiast of the most infectious kind. Dr. Kozar himself had been quite ill during his visit to the United States in 1970, but insisted on working assiduously on the planning of the third conference. Back in Wroclaw, he carried on his trichinellosis activities despite the discouragement of chronic illness that persisted into 1972. On February 7, the day he died, I received a letter he had written from his hospital bed a couple of weeks earlier when the gravity of his condition was apparent; typically, he enclosed some conference material and asked for the latest news of the planning.

Dr. Kozar was the moving force of the International Commission on Trichinellosis and its first two international conferences. He was to have been Honorary Chairman of the third Conference in the series. Dr. Gould laid the initial plans for the third conference and was to have presided over it. Its location in the United States was largely a tribute to himself, but he saw it only as an opportunity to achieve a greater international understanding among all who, for reasons of science, medicine, or commerce, are concerned with trichinellosis; his irresistible charm and logic were already being devoted to that end. It is fitting that the conference, and the pages that follow, should be dedicated to the memory of these two men who contributed so much to its inception but who were not spared to be present at its fulfillment.

W. C. C.

Trichinosis: Quo Vadimus

The view of many meat industry nonscientists in the United States and elsewhere is that the presence of trichina in domestic swine is endemic and probably cannot be eliminated. Many persons, including some key federal government officials in a position to reject special project funding, do not believe that the human disease, trichinellosis, is serious enough or that there is sufficient clinical pathology to warrant expenditure of government or industry funds to eliminate the disease. I do not agree with the obvious conclusions to which one is led by these thought processes.

First, if one person in the United States perishes, or any number suffers ill health as a result of consuming commercially marketed trichina-infected pork, then I consider the problem serious. I myself, frequently consume undercooked pork products simply because I have confidence in Zimmerman's figures, which show somewhere around two-tenths of one percent probable infection in the national swine herd (Zimmermann in Part VI, this volume). But the general population and most people in medicine and public health do not have my confidence. The National Live Stock and Meat Board has firmly established through market research that a majority of the consuming public does not believe that fresh pork is necessarily "healthful to eat" or "always safe to eat." There is sufficient evidence to support my belief that the cost of delivering a guaranteed trichina-free product to the consumer is going to be measurably and positively offset by increased opportunity for sales.

Scientists, industries and/or governments of some countries have made successful moves to provide such a trichina-free product. Why not other countries, at least in the places where technology permits? In the United States, obviously, we have the technology. But we also have an annual pig herd of between 80–90 million, spread out over vast geographical territories and processed in more than 2000 factories. This does present problems, but not insurmountable ones. We already have two ideas with excellent potentiality in my opinion. One is the "pooled sample technique," the efficacy of which was established in a midwestern United States meat processing plant which handled and tested about 600,000 hogs over roughly a six-month period. This is a practical method, though not necessarily inexpensive with a cost approximating 6 to 10 cents per animal after simple and inexpensive laboratory setup. The other has not yet been proved outside of the laboratory; a serum innoculation which would immunize the pig, thus preventing it from becoming a trichina carrier. However, its efficacy is proved only in laboratory mice at this time.

There is both hope and opportunity. The National Live Stock and Meat Board will continue to exhort its industry — hog producer, meat packer-processor and retail distributor — to spend necessary funds for research and implementation of elimination programs. We will continue to attempt convincing the public that this is not a serious problem now, but something a home cook or foodservice chef must be aware of as a matter of simple routine. We look forward to the day when a guaranteed trichina-free product is forthcoming and is available in every food store in the United States. This will unfetter pork as an eminently merchandisable protein food. Following the first manufactured brand will come its competitors.

DAVID H. STROUD
National Live Stock and Meat Board
Chicago, Illinois

Trichinellosis

Part I
Morphology; *in Vitro* Studies

Fluorescent Microscopy of *Trichinella spiralis* Morphogenesis and Nutrition

E. V. Timonov

The All-Union K.I. Skryabin Institute
of Helminthology
Moscow

This research was carried out at the Department of Zoology of the Kursk Pedagogical Institute in 1968–1971, under the guidance of Professor Heller. In the books available to us we have not come across any reference to the fluorescent microscopic method in studying the problem under discussion. Therefore, other problems dealing with *Trichinella* are not considered; these are described in another publication (Timonov, 1972).

Fluorescent microscopy enables us to observe the multicolored fluorescence of living *Trichinella* organs at all stages of its ontogenesis. In our experiment, either larvae or adults were stained with 0.02% acridine orange and rhodamine C and were studied under the ML-2 microscope. The time of staining ranged from 3 to 40 min, depending upon the age of the worms.

In the egg cell, acridine orange stains the cytoplasm green, the nucleus dark green, and the nucleolus and the plasma granules bright green. At the first stages of division of the egg, there appears one granule on its surface at first and then another, containing RNA. Later the divided portions of the egg become uniformly stained green.

The young larva, 120 μm long and 5–6 μm wide, has a cavity at its anterior end, the contents of which stain pink with acridine orange. In other parts of the larva many bright green nuclei can be seen. Eight-to-10-day muscle larva stichosome becomes orange, and later green. The 10-day midgut is stained red by rhodamine C. The bright green genital primordium is clearly seen in 13-day larvae. The digestive glands of 13- to 20-day larvae, as well as of mature worms, are stained red by acridine orange. In 20-day muscle larvae these glands stain green.

The sex differentiation of 15-day larvae is apparent. By that time the male rectum is 35 μm long and the female one is 20 μm long. In the anterior end of the female worm, the vagina can be seen. In a 20-hr intestinal female the vagina joins with the uterus. In the male of the same age, more than 100 bright red granules containing RNA can be seen in the gonads. Sperm, eggs and larvae, as well as other organs can be observed in growing intestinal *Trichinella.*

The fluorescent microscopic method can help to elucidate the morphological and physiological details of the alimentary tract and to determine the permeability of the *Trichinella* cuticle. The data obtained lead us to the conclusion that *Trichinella* feeds through the cuticle. The stains penetrate into the worms through the cuticle. The fact that the nature of fluorescence depends upon the time of staining proves the point. When studying muscle larvae 15, 30, and 45 min after staining, one can see that the internal organs fluoresce brighter and brighter irrespectively of their position in respect to the alimentary tract. Ligation of the anterior or the posterior ends of the intestinal *Trichinella* does not change the nature and the rate of staining of the internal organs. The penetration of the cuticle of the intestinal *Trichinella* during the first 20 hr of its development is eight times higher than of the muscle larvae. Due to the bright fluorescence of the midgut one can see what is inside it. The midgut of the infective larvae contains no remnants of food. In the intestinal *Trichinella* the droplike contents can be seen in the midgut only during the first 20 hr of its development when the permeability of the cuticle has not reached its optimal level. Otherwise the midgut of the intestinal *Trichinella* contains nothing. We should note that the lumen of the esophagus does not fluoresce. *Trichinella* does not develop in the bowels of starving mice. This shows the important role that the food of the host plays in the nutrition of the worm. *Trichinella* does not develop outside the host's bowels. It can live in all the mammals, and experimentally it can live in reptiles and birds which differ greatly biologically but provide similar ecological factors, viz., the presence of remnants of decomposing food, and suitable pH, temperature, and other factors in host's intestinal wall. Normally intestinal *Trichinella* penetrate with their anterior ends into the bowel wall and are located within the zone of intestinal absorption. Particles of digested food, which are of the same size range as fluorochrome molecules, are able to penetrate through the *Trichinella* cuticle into the body cavity.

Summary

Living *Trichinella* larvae and mature *Trichinella* were stained with 0.02% acridine orange and 0.02% rhodamine C and studied under a fluorescence microscope. The worms were multicolored. The nature of fluorescence of separate organs changed depending on age. It is established that fluorochromes penetrate into *Trichinella* through the cuticle. The penetration through the mature *Trichinella* cuticle is eight times higher than in muscle larvae. The midgut fluoresced bright red with rhodamine C. The mature *Trichinella* does not contain remnants of foodstuffs. It was concluded that *Trichinella* feeds through the cuticle.

Reference

Timonov, E. V. (1972). Fluorescent-microscopical examinations of morphogenesis, nutrition of *Trichinella spiralis. Mater. Dokladov Vses. Konf. Probl. Trikhinelleza Tcheloveka Zhivotnykh* (Vilnius), 66–70.

Fine Structure of the Muscle Phase of *Trichinella spiralis* in the Mouse

Mabel Purkerson and Dickson D. Despommier

Department of Anatomy and
Division of Tropical Medicine, School of Public Health
College of Physicians & Surgeons, Columbia University
New York

Introduction

The muscle phase of *Trichinella spiralis* has been studied at the ultrastructural level by several groups of investigators (Beckett and Boothroyd, 1961; Ribas-Mujal and Rivera-Pomar, 1968; Fasske and Themann, 1961; and Bäckwinkel and Themann, 1972). Although much useful information has been obtained on the ultrastructural changes during the early invasive phase of the infection, little attention has been given to the mature infection in relation to the interfaces between the normal cell and infected cell, and between the infected cell and the parasite. Further, due to inadequate fixation, dehydration, and infiltration of tissue, it was not possible until now to see structures associated with these interfaces as they normally relate to one another.

The present study therefore concentrates mainly on the host–parasite interface, as well as on the infected cell–normal cell interface, since it is at these interfaces that all exchanges of metabolites and excretion products occur between the host cell and the parasite.

Methods and Materials

Infection with *Trichinella spiralis*

Male CFW mice, 2 months old, served as hosts for *T. spiralis* infections. These infections were induced in the following way. Twenty, 200-gm, male

Wistar rats were each orally infected with 8000 infective muscle larvae previously isolated by means of peptic digestion.

After 7 days all rats were killed with ether and the small intestines were removed and split open. The split open intestines were then placed in a thermal migration device (Despommier, 1973) and gravid adult females, as well as males, were collected. Newborn larvae were then collected from these isolated adult females according to the method of Dennis *et al.* (1970). After concentration, 100,000 newborn larvae were then injected intramuscularly (usually into the thigh area) into each of 20 mice.

Electron Microscopy

Two months later, tissue from the injected area was excised and minced in potassium dichromate-buffered (pH 7.2) 1% osmium solution. The infected tissue was allowed to fix for 4 hr at room temperature. Microscopic examination of muscle presses of tissue from this area revealed numerous mature muscle larvae.

After dehydration in a graded series of ethanols of increasing concentrations, the tissue was placed into propylene oxide for 20 min, followed by 1 hr in a 3:1 mixture of propylene oxide and Epon. This was followed by immersion in 1:1 propylene oxide and Epon for 1 hr, and finally overnight immersion in 1:3 propylene oxide and Epon. The tissues remained in this mixture for an additional period of 8–10 hr, after which the propylene oxide was allowed to evaporate for 18 hr. Finally, the infected tissue was embedded in Epon.

Tissues were sectioned with a diamond knife (E. I. Du Pont De Nemours and Co., Inc., Wilmington, Delaware), stained with lead citrate and uranyl acetate and examined with a Philips-300 electron microscope at 80 kV.

Results

While the emphasis of the observations is on the interfaces between normal and infected host cells, and the infected host cell and parasite, other areas of the infected host cell will also be described because of new information obtained due to the superior fixation of the infected tissue with Dalton's fixative. Further, because intramuscularly induced muscle infections are synchronous (Despommier, unpublished data), it was possible for the first time to state unequivocally the exact age of the infection.

The term "nurse" cell will, henceforth, be applied to the cell in which *T. spiralis* lives. This cell has changed dramatically from a normal striated muscle cell into a cell which supports the growth of the developing larva (Ribas-Mujal and Rivera-Pomar, 1968). The concept of the nurse cell will be more fully expanded in the discussion.

Normal Cell–Nurse Cell Interface

The nurse cell (infected cell) is surrounded predominantly by fibro-blasts (Fig. 1) and capillaries (Fig. 2). Few immunocompetent host cells were observed in areas adjacent to nurse cells at this time. A fluffy, acel-lular fibrous matrix (Bruce, 1970) separates these normal host cells from the cellular portion of the nurse cell (Figs. 1 and 2). Fibers in the outer-most region are probably derived from the fibroblasts and represent colla-gen deposition. However, the fibrous zone closest to the cellular portion of the nurse cell (Figs. 2, 3, and 4) is synthesized by the nurse cell during earlier stages of the infection (Teppema *et al.* in press).

There were never any breaks seen in this fibrous zone which may have connected the interstitial spaces to the cellular region of nurse cell cyto-plasm. The nurse cell, therefore, is completely surrounded by fibrous material which persists throughout the intracellular life of the parasite. The demarcation between the acellular and cellular portion of nurse cell cytoplasm is clearly maintained by plasmalemal membrane (Figs. 2, 3, and 4). In some places, the nurse cell membrane interdigitates with the fibrous zone, (Figs. 3 and 4), while in other areas, this membrane appears to be rather linear (Fig. 2).

Mitochondria, Golgi-like complexes, rough endoplasmic reticulum, and polysomes, as well as smooth endoplasmic reticulum, are found close to the membrane on the cellular side of this membrane (Figs. 3 and 4). It is difficult to determine with certainty whether or not these organelles predominate at this interface as they can also be found, as will be shown, in other regions of nurse cell cytoplasm in abundance.

The Cellular Matrix of the Nurse Cell

The cellular matrix of the nurse cell consists, mainly, of smooth endo-plasmic reticulum (SER) (Ribas-Mujal and Rivera-Pomar, 1968; Bäck-winkel and Themann, 1972). Whorls of SER are found in several patterns which are seen in Figs. 3–6.

In the most commonly observed situation whorls of SER surround vesicles and are numerous and evenly distributed throughout the cyto-plasm (Figs. 3 and 5). Mitochondria are associated with the inner portions nearest the vesicles. Whorls of SER also surround vesicles which have no mitochondria associated with them. In this case, numerous polysomes are seen as well as occasional rough endoplasmic reticulum (RER). Finally, whorls of SER can be seen with no other cytoplasmic organelles associated with them (Fig. 4).

Clusters of other cytoplasmic organelles can be seen in the nurse cell matrix. Figure 7 shows a group of mitochondria associated with a Golgi-like complex, and several nuclei can be seen in Fig. 8. Large numbers of

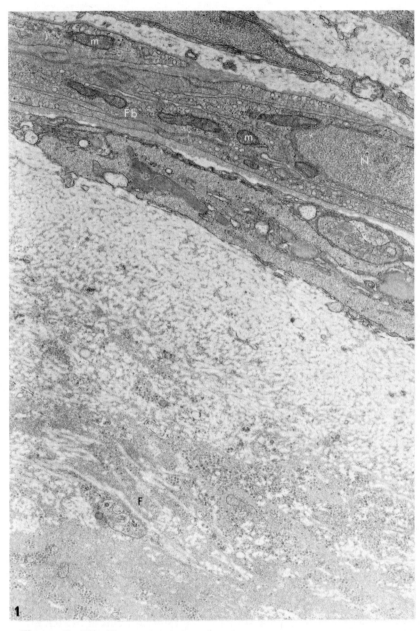

Figure 1 The fibrous, acellular region of the nurse cell seen at higher magnification. Fibers, both longitudinal and cross-sectional views, are seen in the lower half of this region (F). The upper portion of the fibrous zone contains a more scattered distribution of fibers. Several fibroblasts (Fb) are seen adjacent to the outer limits of the fibrous zone. m, Mitochondria; N, nucleus. × 8200.

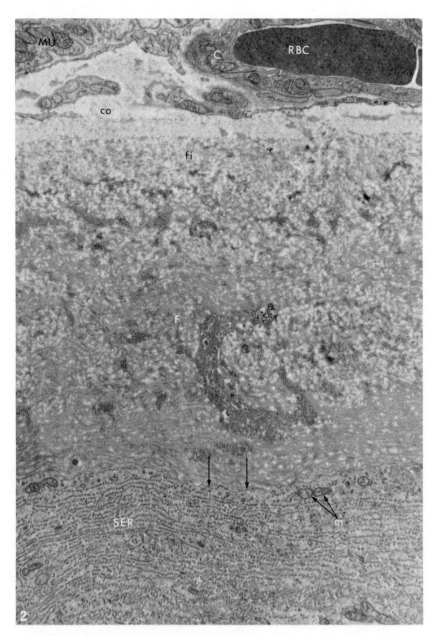

Figure 2 Low magnification view of the periphery of the nurse cell. The acellular fibrous zone (F) extends outward to the adjacent muscle cell (Mu) and capillary (C). The fibrous zone appears to be stratified into layers of fibers which run in at least two directions. The outermost region of the fibrous zone is a mixture of nurse cell-derived amorphous fibers (fi) and fibroblast-derived collagen (co). The cellular portion of nurse cell cytoplasm lies beneath the fibrous zone and contains numerous mitochondria (m), and smooth endoplasmic reticulum (SER). The membrane separating the acellular from the cellular portion of nurse cell cytoplasm is clearly visible (arrows). RBC, red blood cell. × 4000.

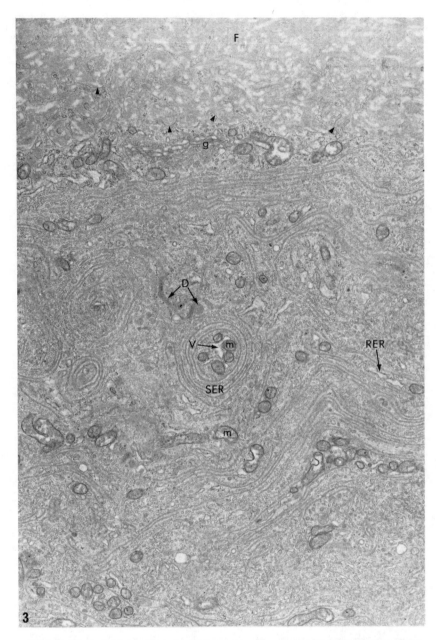

Figure 3 A peripheral region of nurse cell cytoplasm and the beginning of the acellular fibrous zone is seen here. The fibrous zone (F) is clearly separated from the cytoplasm by a membrane (arrowheads). The cytoplasm interdigitates into the fibrous zone and sometimes completely surrounds portions of fibrous material.

The major cellular elements of the nurse cell cytoplasm are also seen in this view. A Golgi-like complex (g) is seen adjacent to the fibrous zone. Whorls of smooth endoplasmic reticulum (SER), seen in both longitudinal and cross-section, predominate. Mitochondria (m) are scattered throughout, and an occasional large vesicle (V) is evident. Some dense bodies (D) are also present. Few areas of rough endoplasmic reticulum (RER) or free ribosomes are seen. $\times$ 11,400.

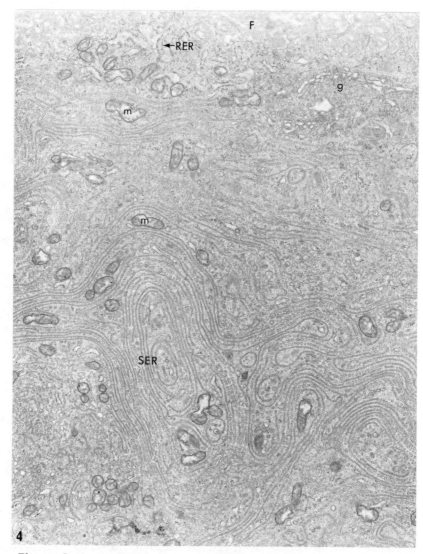

Figure 4 A whorl of SER not associated with clusters of mitochondria (m) or vesicles is shown in this view. Golgi-like complex (g), fibrous zone (F), rough endoplasmic reticulum (RER). ✕ 13,500.

mitochondria and Golgi-like complexes are associated with nurse cell nuclei, but the distribution of nuclei in the matrix apparently is random and cannot be correlated with the location of the larva.

The Nurse Cell–Parasite Interface

The nurse cell cytoplasm closely apposes the cuticular surface of the larva (Figs. 9–11) in properly dehydrated and infiltrated specimens. The interface complex is comprised of the nurse cell inner double unit mem-

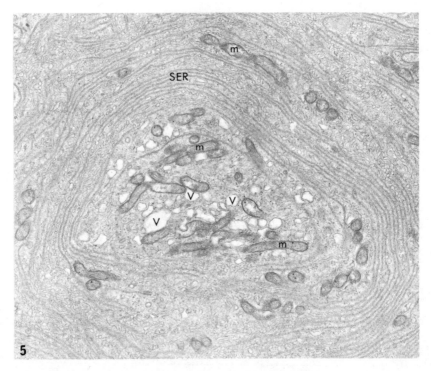

Figure 5 A whorl of SER surrounding a cluster of mitochondria (m) and vesicles (V) is shown in this veiw. × 15,100.

brane, 520 Å thick, a space 400 Å wide, and the outer cuticular surface of the larva.

The membrane–cuticular surface relationship is easily seen in poorly dehydrated specimens where the space between the nurse cell and the larva becomes exaggerated due to shrinkage (Fig. 12). The nurse cell cytoplasm follows closely the outline of the cuticle of the larva, even when the cuticle "wrinkles" (Fig. 11).

The larva was never seen out of contact with the cellular matrix of the nurse cell. Further, no overt cellular necrosis was seen in any portion of nurse cell cytoplasm, confirming observations of Ribas-Mujal and Rivera-Pomar (1968). The nurse cell cytoplasm exhibited no unusual structures in regions adjacent either to the anterior or posterior end of the larva. Nurse cell organelles were not specially arranged near the cuticular surface at 2 months after intramuscular infection.

Discussion

The muscle phase of *Trichinella spiralis* represents a unique intracellular host–parasite relationship. First, it has previously been shown

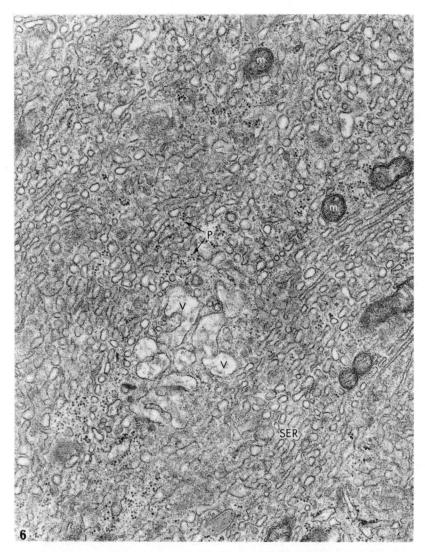

Figure 6 A number of vesicles (V) surrounded by SER and polysomes (P) are evident in this view. Some dense material is seen in the vesicular spaces. (m), Mitochondria. × 35,100.

that the early phases of invasion of skeletal striated muscle by migrating larvae of *T. spiralis* in some way induce morphogenic changes in that muscle cell, resulting in a cell which supports the growth and development of the larva (Ribas-Mujal and Rivera-Pomar, 1968; Fasske and Themann, 1961).

Second, biochemical studies have shown that various metabolites can traverse the infected host cell into the already mature larva and finally become incorporated into parasite protein (Stoner and Hanks, 1955).

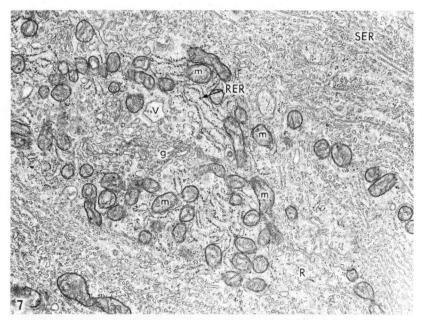

Figure 7 A cluster of mitochondria (m) surround a Golgi-like complex (g). Also visible is RER and numerous cross sections of SER. In addition, a few ribosomes are present (R). (V), Vesicle. $\times$ 11,300.

Third, infections produced by intravenous injection of newborn larvae result in the induction of protection against an oral challenge infection, strongly suggesting that functional antigens from the developing larvae somehow exit from the infected cell and then activate host defense mechanisms (Despommier, 1971).

Finally, studies in rats intravenously injected with ^{125}I-labeled anti-*Trichinella* serum showed that antibodies failed to enter the infected cell cytoplasmic matrix in the mature, i.e., over 30 days old, infection as determined by autoradiography (Ruitenberg, personal communication).

The larva, from the time of penetration to maturity, is always in contact with infected cell cytoplasm (Despommier, unpublished data), and therefore it seems reasonable to suggest that the biological barrier induced by the larva is a selective one which enables the larva to obtain what it needs in order to grow, while excluding host products which may be harmful to this growth process. In essence, this amounts to a "nursing" of the larva. We therefore call the cell a nurse cell.

The nurse cell-cuticle interface has been previously described (Ribas-Mujal and Rivera-Pomar, 1968) as consisting of a rather wide space of variable width. This has been shown to be due to either a too-rapid dehydration through propylene oxide and/or a too-rapid infiltration of infected tissue with Epon.

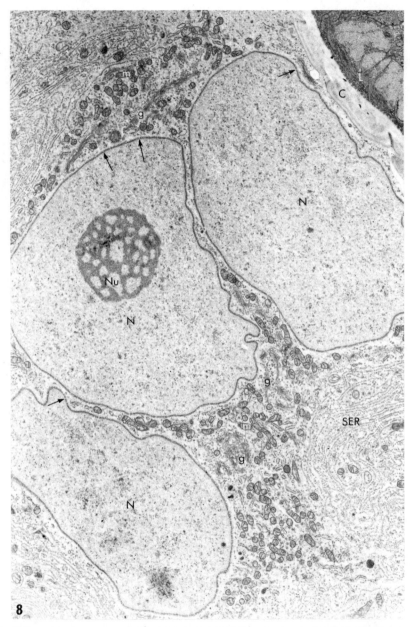

Figure 8   Three nurse cell nuclei (N) are seen in this view. The nucleolus (Nu) is netlike in appearance. Nuclear pores (arrows) are evident in all three nuclei. The chromatin is evenly distributed throughout each nucleus. Large numbers of Golgi-like complex (g) lie adjacent to the nuclei, as well as numerous mitochondria (m). A portion of a larva (L) is seen in the upper right portion of this view. (C), Cuticle; (SER), smooth endoplasmic reticulum. × 4500.

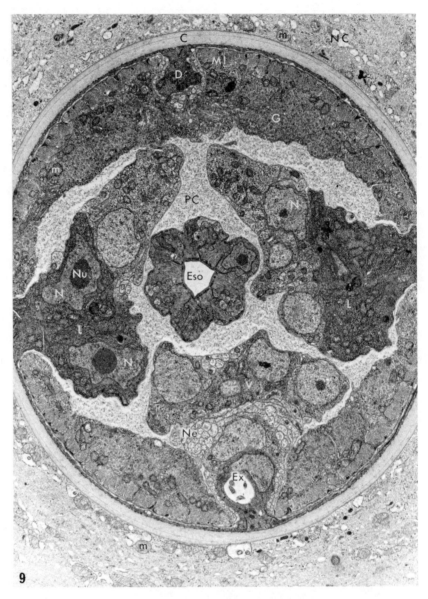

Figure 9 A cross section of the anterior esophageal (Eso) region of the larva is shown. Note the close opposition of the nurse cell (NC) cytoplasm to the entire cuticular (C) surface of the larva. Also shown are lateral lines (L), muscle layer (Ml), glycogen (G), nucleus (N), nucleolus (Nu), dorsal line (D), ventral line (V), nerve (Ne), pseudocoelom (PC), mitochondria (m). × 3000.

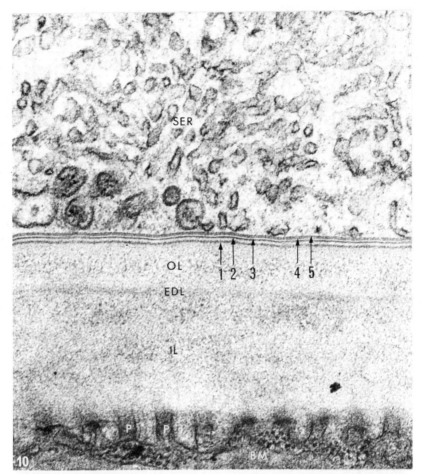

Figure 10 A high magnification view of the nurse cell–cuticular interface. The cuticle consists of an inner layer (IL), an electron dense line (EDL),
and an outer layer (OL). The outermost layer has two additional layers
(arrows 1 and 2). Also evident are subcuticular projections (P) originating
along the basement membrane (BM). There is a space 400 Å wide between
the cuticle and the nurse cell (arrow 3). The nurse cell membrane, 520 Å
wide, is a double unit (arrows 4 and 5). This membrane follows closely the
contour of the larval cuticle. (SER), Smooth endoplasmic reticulum.
× 143,000.

The space between the nurse cell and cuticle was consistently 400 Å
in width. The larva, in live preparations, is able to move about to a limited
degree in the nurse cell. Therefore, it is unlikely that there would be any
connections between the cell membrane and the cuticle, and, indeed, none
was ever observed. The close proximity of host to parasite further suggests
that metabolic exchanges may occur at this interface.

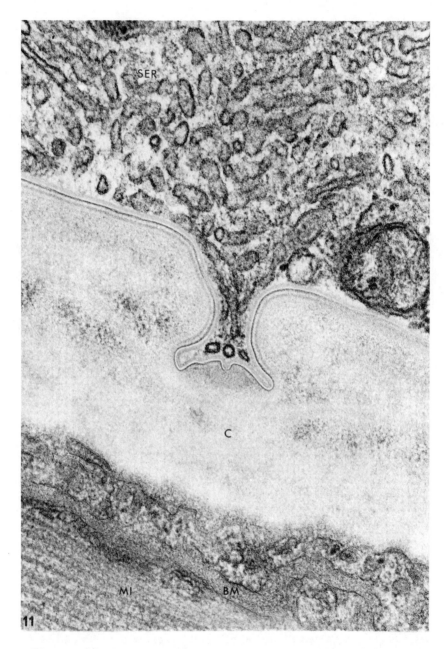

Figure 11 The nurse cell cytoplasm closely adheres to the contour of larval cuticle (C), even when the cuticle "wrinkles," as seen in this view. Also seen are smooth endoplasmic reticulum (SER), basement membrane (BM), and muscle (Ml). $\times$ 143,000.

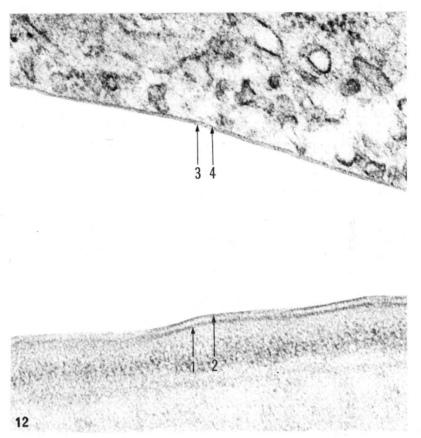

Figure 12 Nurse cell double unit membrane (arrows 1,2) has pulled away from the outer layer of the larval (arrows 3,4) cuticle, allowing the membranes belonging to the host and parasite to be clearly resolved. Membrane separation was seen predominantly in specimens which were dehydrated and infiltrated too rapidly. × 218,800.

The smooth endoplasmic reticulum (SER) component of the nurse cell cytoplasmic matrix has been implicated, on a speculative basis, in obtaining of metabolites for the developing larva (Ribas-Mujal and Rivera-Pomar, 1968).

In the present study, certain structural associations of SER with commonly occurring matrix organelles tend to add support for the above view. Numerous large vesicles usually surrounded by SER were seen throughout the matrix of the nurse cell. These vesicles often contained dense staining material. It is possible that these vesicles help with the function of either bringing metabolites to the larva or carrying secretions and excretions away from the larva. In the present study no attempt was made to trace these vesicles toward or away from the cuticular surface. Vesicles were usually associated with whorls of SER. However, no direct connection was ever seen between these vesicles and SER.

Pronounced accumulations of cell organelles were not seen at the cuticular interface or at the acellular–cellular interface. However, preliminary studies on intramuscularly induced infections in mice at early stages of larval development have shown that large amounts of RER, polysomes, and mitochondria are associated with the nurse cell–cuticular interface. That this local organization is not seen at 2 months after intramuscular infection lends support to the idea that the cuticular surface may be an important absorption or secretion surface during maximum larval growth. By use of radiolabeled substrates coupled with autoradiography at the electron microscope level, it should be possible to begin to correlate some of these structures with a functional role in nutrient uptake.

Large amounts of RER and polysomes were seen near the acellular-cellular interface during the time of maximum synthesis of fibrous material (Teppema *et al.,* in press; Despommier, unpublished observations), further suggesting a local enrichment of nurse cell organelles during worm and nurse cell growth.

The nurse cell, as seen ultrastructurally at 2 months after infection, is essentially the same as seen from day 8 after intramuscular infection. However, profound biochemical, and presumably physiological, changes occur during the ensuing development of the larva that are not wholly attributable to the larval component (Stewart and Read, 1972; in press). These changes include increased synthesis of proteins, RNA, and DNA.

There were no overt signs of cell necrosis in any region of the nurse cell cytoplasm. This confirms the work of Ribas-Mujal and Rivera-Pomar (1968). However, Fasske and Themann (1961) still consider the changes brought about by *T. spiralis* in skeletal muscle as degenerative, but conclude that a balance is somehow achieved which allows both host and parasite to live.

Summary

Mice were given an intramuscular injection of 100,000 live newborn larvae, thereby synchronizing the infection. After 2 months, tissue from the injected area containing numerous mature muscle larvae in the infected cells was prepared for electron microscopy. A superior fixation was obtained using Dalton's fixative for 4 hr at room temperature.

The interfaces between normal and infected host cell and between infected cell and parasite were observed in detail at the ultrastructural level. A major structural feature of the host–parasite relationship was seen at the host cell–parasite interface. In properly dehydrated and infiltrated specimens, a 400-Å wide space was maintained between the host cell and the cuticle over the entire surface of the larva. The concept of the infected host cell as a "nurse" cell is discussed.

Acknowledgments

The authors wish to thank Ms. Lorna Aron and Ms. Hild Kjeldbye for their competent technical assistance and to Dr. Edward Dempsey, Chairman of the Anatomy Department at Columbia University, for allowing us the use of his facilities for ultrastructural research.

This work was supported, in part, by grants 5-RO1-GM-15289, 5-RO1-AI-10627, and RR-05449 from the U.S. National Institutes of Health. M. P. was a U.S. Public Health Service Special Fellow, No. AM-50950. D. D. D. was a recipient of Career Development Award 1-KO4-AI-70255 from the National Institutes of Health.

References

Bäckwinkel, K. P. and Themann, H. (1972). Elektronenmikroskopische Untersuchungen über die Pathomorphologie der Trichinellose. *Beitr. Pathol.* **146,** 259–271.

Beckett, E. B., and Boothroyd, B. (1961). Some observations on the mature larva of the nematode *Trichinella spiralis. Ann. Trop. Med. Parasitol.* **55**, 116–124.

Bruce, R. G. (1970). The structure and development of the capsule of *Trichinella spiralis. J. Parasitol.* **56,** 38–39.

Dennis, D., Despommier, D., and Davis, N. (1970). The infectivity of the newborn larva of *Trichinella spiralis* in the rat. *J. Parasitol.* **56**, 974–977.

Despommier, D. (1971). Immunogenicity of the newborn larva of *Trichinella spiralis. J. Parasitol.* **57**, 531–535.

Despommier, D. (1973). A circular thermal migration device for the rapid collection of large numbers of intestinal helminths. *J. Parasitol.* **59,** 933–935.

Fasske, K., and Themann, H. (1961). Elektronenmikroskopische Befunde an der Muskelfaser nach Trichinenbefall. *Virchows Arch. A* **334**, 459–474.

Ribas-Mujal, D., and Rivera-Pomar, J. M. (1968). Biological significance of the early structural alterations in skeletal muscle fibers infected by *Trichinella spiralis. Virchows Arch. A* **345**, 154–168.

Stewart, G. L., and Read, C. P. (1972). Ribonucleic acid metabolism in mouse trichinosis. *J. Parasitol.* **58**, 252–256.

Stewart, G. L., and Read, C. P. (in press). Deoxyribonucleic acid metabolism in mouse trichinosis. *J. Parasitol.*

Stoner, R. D., and Hankes, L. V. (1955). Incorporation of C^{14}-labeled amino acids by *Trichinella spiralis* larvae. *Exp. Parasitol.* **5**, 435–444.

Teppema, J. S., Robinson, J. E., and Ruitenberg, E. J. (in press). Ultrastructural aspects of capsule formation in *Trichinella spiralis* infection in the rat. *Parasitology.*

Effects of Environment on the Growth and Development of *Trichinella spiralis in Vitro*

Allen K. Berntzen

Department of Parasitology
Oregon Zoological Research Center
Portland, Oregon

Introduction

A large amount of research has been conducted to develop a system for the growth and development of *Trichinella spiralis in vitro*. This work has been summarized by Meerovitch (1965a,b) and Berntzen (1965). Successful culture methods have been developed for growing *T. spiralis* from the encapsulated muscle stage to adults by Meerovitch (1965a) and Berntzen (1965).

With these new tools it was thought possible to devise a system in which excreted and secreted worm metabolic products, as well as the whole worms, could be collected to determine whether or not there is a correlation between these products, from the various stages which may be antigenic to antibody production in the host animal. If a correlation existed, *in vitro* culture could be utilized for collection of antigen materials for other immunological studies.

Prior to the development of the *in vitro* culture system, metabolic antigen collection had been done using a technique of incubation in a simple salt solution. This method has an inherent danger in that the worms are not growing or metabolizing normally and, after a short time, begin to degenerate and eventually die due to improper environmental conditions.

This report is a summary of a study utilizing an *in vitro* culture system for collection of antigenic materials produced by *T. spiralis* during growth from the encapsulated muscle larval stage to mature adults which produced progeny.

Methods and Materials

The strain of *T. spiralis,* obtained from Ely Lilly Co., Indianapolis, Indiana, in 1961, has been maintained in male Sprague-Dawley rats. Stock animals were infected with 1200–1500 larvae/250–300 gm animal by intubation. Larvae for inoculating stock animals were obtained by digestion of 40 gm of ground rat muscle per 1 liter of a 1.0% pepsin (1 : 10,000 Difco) in 0.5% HCl acid solution according to the method of Gursch (1948).

Larvae of *T. spiralis* to be used in *in vitro* culture studies were obtained from rat muscle 60 or more days post-infection, using the methods as previously described (Berntzen, 1965). Sterilization of the larvae and *in vitro* culture methods were as described by Berntzen (1965). The worms were grown *in vitro* in medium 115 (Berntzen and Mueller, 1964) with the exception that serum was replaced with a solution of 10% Ficoll, containing 500 μg/ml α_1, β_1-globulin isolated from human serum (Hansen and Berntzen, 1969). The gas phase was normally 10% CO_2, 10% O_2, 80% N_2 with a bicarbonate buffer system maintained at pH 7.2. At intervals 40% CO_2, 60% N_2 was used for 1-hr periods to stimulate exsheathment of the worms. Medium flow rate was 10 cm^3/hr per culture unit. Incubation temperature was $37°C \pm 0.5°$.

By controlling the culture system gas phase, it was possible to make the cultures synchronous in development; exsheathment was initiated by stimulation for 2 hr with 40% CO_2–60% N_2.

Metabolized medium was continuously collected and samples separated at 4-hr intervals during the 10-day culture period. Worms from culture were collected at four different stages of development: (1) excysted muscle larvae 3 hr after incubation; (2) worms after 12 hr of culture, ready to molt; (3) worms after 20 hr of culture which had molted; and (4) adult males and females with progeny after 8 days of culture.

Preparation of metabolic products for testing their antigenic properties was as follows: protein-containing fractions of the metabolized medium were separated by precipitation with ammonium sulfate. The precipitate was then dialyzed against distilled water for 24 hr, followed by dialysis against 0.1 M phosphate buffer, pH 7.2, for an additional 24 hr at 5°C. The protein was then concentrated using lyphogel (Gelman) until a protein level of 1.2 mg/ml was obtained. This material was then stored at $-20°C$ until used in the various immunological procedures.

Whole worm extracts of the various stages were prepared as follows. Collected worms were lyophilized, ground and extracted with 0.1 M phosphate buffer at 5°C for 24 hr. Particulate material was removed by centrifugation and the supernatant was adjusted by lyphogel concentration to contain 2.0 mg/ml protein as determined by absorption at 280 nm on a Gilford spectrometer. This material was stored at $-20°C$ until used in the immunological procedures.

Antisera were obtained from 30 rats, 350 gm each, 54 days after infection with 1200 muscle larvae. Blood was obtained by cardiac puncture, allowed to coagulate, and centrifuged, and serum was removed by pipette.

The serums were pooled and stored at $-20°C$ until used. Immunoelectrophoresis was performed according to the method proposed by Grabar and Williams (1953) or to the micro modification of this procedure described by Scheidegger (1955).

One percent Difco Noble Agar, containing Veronal buffer pH 8.2, was poured over glass plates or microscope slides 2×3 in. to give a depth of agar of 2 mm on glass plates and 1.5 mm over the microscope slides. After gelling of the agar, wells were cut into the center of the slide plates and filled with the antigen. The preparations were then transferred to an electrophoresis apparatus and an electric potential was applied across them. The glass plates (2×3 in.) were run for 5 hr at 500 V, 40 mA, and the glass slides were run for 2 hr at 80 V, 10 mA. After the electrophoretic segregation had been done, a rectangular trough was cut in the agar parallel to the direction of electrophoretic migration and the trough was filled with antiserum. When the arcs of specific immune precipitation had fully developed, the plates were washed with several changes of saline to remove excess serum from the gel. After washing, the agar gel was dried to a film and the arcs of precipitation were stained with Amidoschwarz 10B, according to the method of Grabar and Williams (1953).

Animals were used to determine whether or not there were protective antigens present in the prepared materials. The procedure was as follows. (1) One milliliter of the antigenic material containing 1.2 mg of protein was mixed with one part Freund's adjuvant. This material was injected subcutaneously and intermuscularly at 10-day intervals to uninfected animals. Thirty days after injection the animals were challenged with an inoculin of 1200 larvae/300 gm rat. (2) Fifty days post-infection the rats were autopsied and the carcasses were digested as in previous procedures and the number of larvae obtained was recorded.

Results and Discussion

Several biological supplements have been found to replace serum for the *in vitro* culture of *T. spiralis*. The two most important supplements are α_1, β_1-globulin (Hansen and Berntzen, 1969) and yeast ribosomes (Buecher and Hansen, 1969). Using these supplements or homologous serum for *in vitro* culture of *T. spiralis,* it is now possible to grow the worms *in vitro* and use the metabolized medium as an antigen source.

The effects of immunizing animals with (1) *in vitro* metabolites; (2) infective muscle larvae; (3) mature male and female worms; and (4) *in vitro* metabolites of undifferentiated larvae obtained after challenge of 1200 larvae/300 gm animal which had prior exposure to the various antigens are shown in Fig. 1.

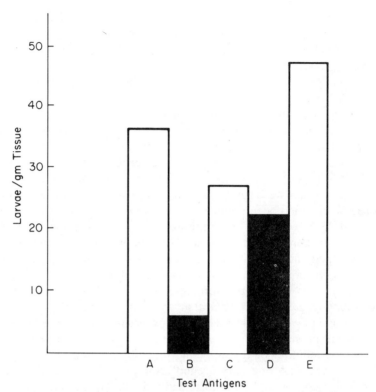

Figure 1 Host response to *Trichinella spiralis* antigens. A. Muscle larvae only; B, metabolized medium, larvae to adult stage; C, adult worms only; D, adult worm metabolites; and E, Freund's adjuvant only (control).

It was found that only the metabolized medium collected from the growth of the muscle larvae to the mature adults produced any protection to the host animal. Using somatic antigens (extracted from worm tissue), little or no protection was observed. Metabolites from adult cultures also gave no protection to the host animal.

Using the electrophoretic and immunogel techniques, we are able to show the host response to the infection of *T. spiralis*. Our results are comparable to those of Tanner (1962, 1965, 1968) with one difference. The difference is with the excretion and secretion of the worms in culture. The results of the immunological response are illustrated in Fig. 1–3.

The use of *in vitro* culture shows promise of a method for developing vaccines against parasitic infection. There is a necessary coordination of *in vivo* to *in vitro* studies to make this possible. Without proper *in vivo* studies, it is difficult to determine at which morphological stage one is working and at which period in the life style.

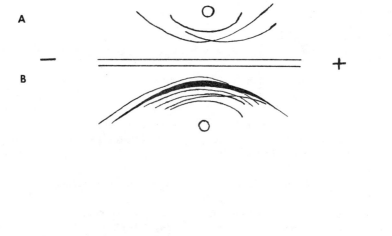

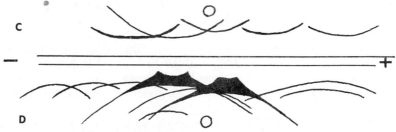

Figure 2 Antigen-antibody response to *T. spiralis* infection. Antiserum rat 54 days post second infection. Antigens used: A, metabolites from *in vitro* culture, stages larval to adult; B, *T. spiralis* adult and second stage from *in vitro* culture; C, *T. spiralis* 4th stage larval metabolites from *in vitro* culture; and D, 4th stage larvae of *T. spiralis*.

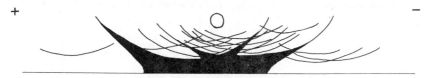

Figure 3 Seventeen precipitating Ab-Ag reactions of complete life cycle of *T. spiralis* in the rat antiserum was 54 days post second infection. Antigen = 1st, 2nd, 3rd, 4th, and 5th stage of *T. spiralis* and metabolites of 4th and 5th stages

Acknowledgments

The author would like to express his appreciation to Ms. Frances Yost for her technical assistance. This work was supported by National Institutes of Health Grant #R01-A109860–03 TMP.

References

Berntzen, A. K. (1965). Comparative growth and development of *Trichinella spiralis in vitro* and *in vivo* with a redescription of the life cycle. *Exp. Parasitol.* **16**, 74–106.

Berntzen, A. K., and Mueller, J. F. (1964). *In vitro* cultivation of *Spirometra mansonoides* (Cestoda) from the procercoid to the early adult stage. *J. Parasitol.* **50**, 705–711.

Buecher, E. J., Jr., and Hansen, E. L. (1969). Yeast extract as a supplement to chemically defined medium for axenic culture of *Caenorhabditis briggsae*. *Separatum Experientia* **25**, 656.

Grabar, P., and Williams, C. (1953). Methode permettant l'étude conjugee des propriétés électophoretiques et immunochimiques d'un mélange de protéines. Application au sérum sanguin. *Biochim. Biophys. Acta* **10**, 193–194.

Gursch, O. F. (1948). Effects of digestion and refrigeration on the ability of *Trichinella spiralis* to infect rats. *J. Parasitol.* **34**, 394–395.

Hansen, E. L., and Berntzen, A. K. (1969). Development of *Caenorhabditis briggsae* and *Hymenolopis nana* in interchanged media. *J. Parasitol.* **55**, 1012–1017.

Meerovitch, E. (1965a). Studies on the *in vitro* axenic development of *Trichinella spiralis*. I. Basic culture techniques, pattern of development, and the effects of the gaseous phase. *Can. J. Zool.* **43**, 69–79.

Meerovitch, E. (1965b). Studies on the *in vitro* axenic development of *Trichinella spiralis*. II. Preliminary experiments on the effects of Farnesol, cholesterol, and an insect extract. *Can. J. Zool.* **43**, 81–85.

Scheidegger, J. J. (1955). Une micro-methode de l'immuno-electrophorese. *Int. Arch. Allergy Appl. Immunol.* **7**, 103–110.

Tanner, C. E. (1962). Immunochemistry of functional precipitating antigens of *Trichinella spiralis* antigens larvae (ab). *J. Parasitol. Suppl.* **48**, 18.

Tanner, C. E. (1965). Identification of host antigen in extracts of *Trichinella spiralis* larvae (ab). *J. Parasitol. Suppl.* **51**, 37.

Tanner, C. E. (1968). Relationship between infecting dose, muscle parasitism, and antibody response in experimental trichinosis in rabbits. *J. Parasitol.* **54**, 98.

The Growth and Development of *Trichinella spiralis* Larvae in a Continuously Changing Liquid Medium and a Constant Gas Phase

V. I. Tarakanov

*The Helmintholgical Laboratory of the
Academy of Sciences of U.S.S.R.
Moscow*

Introduction

The accomplishment of *in vitro* cultivation of helminths enhances the possibilities of studying the nutrition, physiology, biochemistry, and immunochemistry of helminths in man, animals, and plants. Keilty (1914) was the first to report on an increase of the length of *Trichinella* larvae up to 1.5 mm without any signs of organogenesis. McCoy (1936) was able to maintain *Trichinella spiralis in vitro* for 4-5 days. Weller (1943) was able to develop *Trichinella* larvae up to sexual differentiation and the formation of four sheaths. Kim (1961, 1962) observed sexual differentiation and the development of four, rarely five, and even six sheaths. Tarakanov (1963, 1964) demonstrated the 5th larval stage of *Trichinella spiralis* and observed mainly two, rarely three, and very rarely four moltings. Meerovitch (1962, 1965a, 1965b) and Shanta and Meerovitch (1970) reported on the *in vitro* development of *Trichinella spiralis* up to the stage of sexual differentiation with two and rarely three exfoliated sheaths. *Trichinella* larvae did not grow in *in vitro* conditions. Berntzen (1962, 1965) grew adult males and females of *Trichinella spiralis* which produced young larvae in a system of constant change of medium 102B with a gas phase containing 85% nitrogen, 10% oxygen, and 5% CO_2. However, Denham (1967) could not grow *Trichinella* adults by the method of Berntzen (1965) with small modifications. Tarakanov and Krasnova (1970, 1971) demonstrated a partial growth and development of *Trichinella* larvae up to the adult stage in modified medium 102B (Berntzen, 1965) and medium 115 (Berntzen and Mueller, 1964) in a system of continuous change of medium with a gas phase of nitrogen, oxygen, and carbon dioxide. Details of modifications of media and results of *in vitro* cultivation of *Trichinella* larvae are given below.

Materials and Methods

Decapsulated *Trichinella* larvae were isolated by the digestion of white rats infected with *Trichinella spiralis* 3 months previously. The digestion was performed by use of artificial gastric juice for 6 hr at 38° C with constant stirring. The larvae were isolated afterward by means of Baermann's method and then were freed of microorganisms. The bacteriological sterilization was achieved by using a mixture of sodium penicillin, streptomycin sulfate, and Mycostatin at a concentration of 1000 units/ml of Tyrode solution, for 1 hr at 37° C. Before and after sterilization the larvae were washed five times by sedimentation in Tyrode solution. Meat-peptone broth (MPB) and meat-peptone agar (MPA) with sterile larvae in them were checked for the growth of microorganisms.

Eagle's medium was prepared by dilution of the ready-for-use powder "Zellzuchtungs-medium nach Eagle" (AC 15/06/162, produced by Staatliches Institut für Immunpraparate und Nahrmedien, 112, Berlin) in double-distilled water and by the addition of 10% pig serum to the solution. The modification of medium 102B consisted of γ-aminobutyric acid for hydroxybutyric acid and the exclusion of amino-*n*-butyric choline chloride, and preparing extracts from chick embryos in Hanks' solution instead of in distilled water. The modification of medium 115 consisted of using γ-aminobutyric acid instead of DL-β-hydroxybutyric acid; of beef serum without any preservatives instead of A-γ calf serum; and in the exclusion of *d*-ribose, thymidylic acid, α- and β-globulin, Cohn Fraction IV, and γ-amino-*n*-butyric choline chloride. In all media the pH was adjusted to 7.0–7.2 by adding $NaHCO_3$. The sterilization of media was achieved by positive pressure Zeits Filtration. *In vitro* cultivation was carried out by placing aliquots of 2000 *Trichinella* larvae in system of constant flow of medium with a gas phase of 85% nitrogen, 10% oxygen, and 5% carbon dioxide at 37°C, according to Berntzen's method (1965).

Samples of *Trichinella* larvae were taken from cultivation chambers under aseptic conditions 72 hr after cultivation in order to study the growth rates of the worms. All tests were done in triplicate and the values shown in this paper are the means for each medium.

Results

The growth and development of *Trichinella* larvae under the same conditions of cultivation were quite different in different media. In Eagle's medium with a 10% content of pig serum only 2% of *Trichinella* larvae completely underwent molting, increased their length by 79 μm, and reached the 5th developmental stage after 72 hr of cultivation. After 144 hr of cultivation, an additional 1% of *Trichinella* larvae underwent complete molting. The majority of larvae did not complete exsheathing. Fifth-stage larvae preserved their motility for 168 hr. About 7% of larvae with an exfoliated cuticle had poor motility during 17 days, but they did not grow at all.

In the modified medium 102B, *Trichinella* larvae increased in length by 133 μm after completing their molting in 72 hr of cultivation. Under a light microscope about 3% of sheaths were found without larvae, which indicated that exsheathing was complete. Thirty-five percent of larvae did not fully complete their molting, but were very motile when exfoliation was noted at the anterior and posterior ends of larvae. All the larvae which were undergoing the molting process could be differentiated sexually. In males, testes and embryonic phase of copulatory organs were formed; in females, ovary and uterus were formed. After 144 hr of cultivation 18.1% of larvae had completed molting and 56.4% showed incomplete molting. Twenty-one percent of larvae had two exfoliated sheaths but did not increase in length, and some were motile after 17 days of cultivation.

In modified medium 115 the larvae behaved as in modified medium 102B. Some larvae (4.5%) completed their molting, 73% did not complete their molting, and 1.5% had two exfoliated sheaths after 72 hours of cultivation. The remaining larvae did not molt at all. After molting, males and females reached 1.3 mm in length. After 144 hr of cultivation several females measuring 1.39 mm in length and several males measuring 1.3 mm in length were found in the medium. During 12 days of cultivation 5% of larvae preserved their motility.

In the test media neither embryos in the uteri of females, nor sperm in the seminal vesicles of males were found.

Discussion

Our data are in conformity with the results of Berntzen (1965) in that that a small number of *Trichinella* adults with incomplete sexual maturity can be produced in artificial nutrient media under certain optimal conditions. However, the *in vitro* developmental and growth rates were two to three times lower than under *in vivo* conditions.

In contrast to Berntzen's findings (1965) we could not obtain any progeny from *Trichinella spiralis* cultivated *in vitro*. This may be explained by modification procedure in nutrient medium 102B and also by the excluding treatment of larvae in the second digestion solution containing trypsin, pancreatin, and sodium taurocholate before placing them into nutrient medium. We also did not use Berntzen's apparatus (1965) for the acceleration of the exsheathing process in molting larvae. It is possible too that the components of the medium exhibited retarding effect on the growth and development of the worms as the first were purchased from different commercial firms in various countries and not from one commercial firm as in Berntzen's work.

We cannot fully agree with Berntzen's opinion (1965) that *Trichinella* larvae in the intestinal phase undergo only one molt. We think that the problem of the number of molts of *T. spiralis* in the intestinal phase of development has not been finally resolved at present. There are three opinions in regard to this problem at present. A number of workers (Hyman, 1951; Richels, 1955; Wu and Kingscote, 1957; Berntzen, 1965) consider that the encysted *Trichinella* larvae are at the 4th developmental stage and that after their entrance into the alimentary tract they undergo only one molt. Other workers (Hemmert-Halswick and Bugge, 1934; Meerovitch, 1962, 1965a,b; Podhajecky, 1964; Thomas, 1965; Shanta and Meerovitch, 1967a,b; Gridasova, 1969; Timonov, 1970) consider that *Trichinella* larvae undergo two molts in the intestinal phase of development. And a third group of workers (Kreis, 1937; Weller, 1943; Lapage, 1956; Villella, 1958; Kim, 1961, 1962; Tarakanov, 1963, 1964; Ali Khan, 1966) consider that *Trichinella* in the intestinal lumen undergoes four molts. Each opinion was confirmed by data from *in vitro* and *in vivo* experiments.

Our observations showed that *Trichinella* larvae fully completed one molt and rarely showed two incomplete molts. Growth was observed in those *Trichinella* larvae that underwent one complete molt. But since complete sexual maturity was not noted in males and females, copulation did not take place in *in vitro* conditions. We think that it is necessary to provide additional nutrients for the *Trichinella* larvae in *in vitro* conditions, and possibly they have to undergo a second complete molt before copulation can occur. And only then possibly are they able to grow further and mature fully.

Summary

The decapsulated *Trichinella* larvae grew and developed in Eagle's medium with an addition of 10% pig serum, and in modified media 102B and 115 at $37°C$, in a system providing a continuous change of medium with a gas phase containing 85% N_2, 10% O_2, 5% CO_2. *Trichinella* males with a length of 1.3 mm and females with a length of 1.39 mm grew in the modified medium 115. In other media the lengths of nematodes were smaller. *In vitro* multiplication of *Trichinella spiralis* did not take place. The larvae underwent only one complete molt and rarely showed two incomplete molts. The motility of larvae lasted for 17 days.

References

Ali Khan, Z. (1966). The postembryonic development of *Trichinella spiralis* with special reference to ecdysis. *J. Parasitol.* **52**, 248–259.

Berntzen, A. K. (1962). *In vitro* cultivation of *Trichinella spiralis. J. Parasitol.* (Suppl.) **48**, 48.

Berntzen, A. K. (1965). Comparative growth and development of *Trichinella spiralis in vitro* and *in vivo* with a redescription of the life-cycle. *Exp. Parasitol.* **16**, 74–106.

Berntzen, A. K., and Mueller, J. F. (1964). *In vitro* cultivation of *Spirometra mansonoides* (Cestoda) from procercoid to the early adult. *J. Parasitol.* **50**, 705–711.

Denham, D. A. (1967). Applications of the *in vitro* culture of nematodes especially *Trichinella spiralis. Fifth Symp. British Soc. Parasitol. Problems of in vitro culture,* 49–60.

Gridasova, L. F. (1969). Molting of intestinal *Trichinella spiralis. Uch. Zap. Kursk. Gos. Pedagog. Inst.* **59**, 74–82.

Hemmert-Halswick, A., and Bugge, G. (1934). Trichinen und Trichinose. *Ergeb. Allg. Pathol. Pathol. Anat.* **28**, 313–392.

Hyman, Z. H. (1951). "The Invertebrates: Acanthocephala, Aschelminthes and Entoprocta, the Pseudocoelomate Bilateria," Vol. 3. McGraw-Hill, New York.

Keilty, R. A. (1914). Experimental studies of *Trichinella spiralis. Proc. Pathol. Soc. Phila.* **16**, 15–16.

Kim, C. W. (1961). The cultivation of *Trichinella spiralis in vitro. Amer. J. Trop. Med. Hyg.* **10**, 742–747.

Kim, C. W. (1962). Further study of the *in vitro* cultivation of *Trichinella spiralis. Amer. J. Trop. Med. Hyg.* **11**, 419–496.

Kreis, H. A. (1937). Die Entwicklung der Trichinellen zum reifen Geschlechtstier im Darme des Wirtes. *Zentralbl. Bakteriol. Parasitenk. Infektionskr. Hyg. Abt. 1,* **138**, 290–302.

Lapage, G. (1956). "Veterinary Parasitology," Oliver & Boyd, Edinburgh.

McCoy, O. R. (1936). The development of trichinae in abnormal environments. *J. Parasitol.* **22**, 54–59.

Meerovitch, E. (1962). *In vitro* development of *Trichinella spiralis* larvae. *J. Parasitol.* (Suppl.) **48**, 34.

Meerovitch, E. (1965a). Studies on the *in vitro* axenic development of *Trichinella spiralis.* I. Basic culture techniques, pattern of development and the effects of the gaseous phase. *Can. J. Zool.* **43**, 69–79.

Meerovitch, E. (1965b). Studies on the *in vitro* axenic development of *Trichinella spiralis.* II. Preliminary experiments on the effects of farnesol, cholesterol, and an insect extract. *Can. J. Zool.* **43**, 81–85.

Podhajecky, K. (1964). Ecdysis and copulation of *Trichinella spiralis. Stud. Helminthol.* **1**, 175–177.

Richels, I. (1955). Histologische Studien zu den Problemen der Zellkonstans. Untersuchungen zur mikroskopischen Anatomie im Lebenszyklus von *Trichinella spiralis. Zentralbl. Bakteriol. Parasitenk. Infektionskr. Hyg. Abt. 1* **163**, 46–84.

Shanta, C. S., and Meerovitch, E. (1967a). The life cycle of *Trichinella spiralis.* I. The intestinal phase of development. *Can. J. Zool.* **43**, 1255–1260.

Shanta, C. S., and Meerovitch, E. (1967b). The life cycle of *Trichinella spiralis.* II. The muscle phase of development and its possible evolution. *Can. J. Zool.* **45**, 1261–1267.

Shanta, C. S. and Meerovitch, E. (1970). Specific inhibition of morphogenesis in *Trichinella spiralis* by insect juvenile hormone mimics. *Can. J. Zool.* **48**, 617–620.

Tarakanov, V. I. (1963). The *in vitro* cultivation of *Trichinella spiralis,* the agent of trichinellosis. *In* "Gelminty tcheloveka, zhivotnykh, i rastenii i borba s nimi," Moscow, 78–82.

Tarakanov, V. I. (1964). The culture of *Trichinella spiralis* larvae up to the sexually mature stage in artificial nutrient media. *Veterinariya Moscow* (**3**), 43–47.

Tarakanov, V. I. and Krasnova, L. L. (1970). The influence of artificial nutrient media on the *in vitro* development of *Trichinella* larvae. *Tr. Vses. Inst. Gelmintol. Imeni K. I. Skryabina,* **16**, 249–252.

Tarakanov, V. I., and Krasnova, L. L. (1971). The *in vitro* cultivation of decapsulated *Trichinella spiralis* larvae in a system of constant flow of nutrient medium. *Tr. Vses. Inst. Gelmintol. Imeni K. I. Skryabina,* **17**, 229–231.

Thomas, H. (1965). Beiträge zur Biologie und mikroskopischen Anatomie von *Trichinella spiralis* Owen, 1835. *Z. Tropenmed. Parasitol.* **16**, 148–180.

Timonov, E. V. (1970). An *in vivo* study of the morphogenesis of intestinal *Trichinella spiralis* by luminescent methodology. *Parazitologiya* **4**, 237–240.

Villella, J. B. (1958). Observations on the time and number of molts in the intestinal phase of *Trichinella spiralis* in rats. *J. Parasitol.* **44**, 97.

Weller, T. H. (1943). The development of the larvae of *Trichinella spiralis* in roller tube tissue cultures. *Amer. J. Pathol.* **19**, 503–516.

Wu, L. Y., and Kingscote, A. A. (1957). Studies on *Trichinella spiralis*. II. Times of final molt, spermatozoa formation, ovulation and insemination. *Can. J. Zool.* **35**, 207–211.

Freeing Decapsulated *Trichinella spiralis* Larvae from Microorganisms with Antibiotics

V. I. Tarakanov

*The Helminthological Laboratory of the
Academy of Sciences of U.S.S.R.
Moscow*

Introduction

Sterile, decapsulated *Trichinella* larvae are always necessary for their axenic culture in artificial nutrient media. They are needed in large quantities for obtaining exact information of the worms themselves in biochemical and immunological studies. As microbes contain a complex of complete and incomplete antigens, it is desirable to get rid of concomitant microflora for studies of antigenic structure of helminths. This is more necessary if it is taken into account that haptens combining with proteins form complete antigens. Undoubtedly, the freeing of helminths from concomitant microflora has a practical significance in the production of diagnostic substances injected parenterally. Hence, the antigens of helminths free of microbes will be much more specific and will have a smaller number of components.

McCoy (1936) did not describe the method of sterilization of *Trichinella* larvae which he tried to cultivate *in vitro*. The data of Weller (1943) are not convincing as to whether he cultivated sterile *Trichinella* since there was no information on bacteriological control. Kim (1961, 1962) added penicillin and streptomycin to the nutrient media so as to exclude the growth of microbes during the cultivation of *T. spiralis*. Avery (1941) succeeded in obtaining *Trichinella* larvae free from microbes in a modified Baermann's apparatus by allowing them to migrate through sterile sand particles. Meerovitch (1962, 1965a,b) and Shanta and Meerovitch (1970) freed *T. spiralis* from microbes by the method of Avery (1941).

Berntzen (1962, 1965, 1966), Tarakanov (1963, 1964), and Tarakanov and Krasnova (1970, 1971) used a mixture of antibiotics—penicillin, streptomycin, and Mycostatin—for microbiological sterilization of small quantities of decapsulated *Trichinella* larvae with preliminary and subsequent washings of the worms in sterile Tyrode solution by centrifugation. The aim of the present study was to demonstrate the sterilizing action of other antibiotics and to simplify the process of freeing *T. spiralis* from microorganisms.

Materials and Methods

Decapsulated *Trichinella* larvae were recovered by the digestion of white rats infected 3 months earlier. The artificial gastric juice consisted of 3% pepsin used for production of antitoxic sera, 1% concentrated hydrochloric acid, and water. A 100-gm sample of meat was digested in 1 liter of the juice for 6 hr at $37°$ C with constant stirring. The larvae were isolated by Baermann's method, washed to free them from digestion particles, and pooled before sterilization. Then the larvae were washed five times by the sedimentation method through a 15-cm column of sterile Tyrode solution in test tubes (20 × 200 mm). The supernatant liquid was aspirated with a vacuum pump. Sterilization was done by the use of penicillin sodium, streptomycin sulfate, nystatin (Mycostatin), neomycin sulfate, polymyxin B sulfate, and tetracycline hydrochloride, separately or in mixtures, at a concentration 1000 units/ml of Tyrode solution. The method of Berntzen (1965) was also used. Three thousand larvae were placed in each milliliter of the antibiotic solution for 1 hr at $37°$ C. Then the larvae were again washed five times in Tyrode solution in the same manner as before sterilization to free them of the antibiotics. The sterility was checked by introducing 0.2 ml of the worm suspension into meat–peptone broth (MPB) and meat–peptone agar (MPA) with subsequent incubation for 14 days at $37°$ C. In all, two samples were introduced into each medium. If after 14 days of incubation, a slight turbidity in the meat–peptone broth or a single microbe colony on meat-peptone agar was observed, then the worms were considered to be nonsterile. The species of the microorganisms was not determined in these cases. The control test included the *Trichinella* larvae which had undergone all of the above-mentioned treatments, except the antibiotic treatment. The tests were done in triplicate.

Results and Discussion

The results of microbiological sterilization of decapsulated *Trichinella* larvae are shown in Table I. In it one can see that microbes which accompanied *Trichinella* larvae gave growth in MPB 1 day after treatment of *Trichinella* larvae with penicillin sodium or nystatin alone, and on MPA 3 and 5 days after treatment, respectively. The growth of microorganisms in bacteriological media was noticed on the third day after treatment with streptomycin sulfate. Mycostatin, or neomycin sulfate alone and on the fifth day after treatment with polymixin B sulfate. Though complete sterilization was not achieved by these antibiotics, each of them significantly slowed the growth of microorganisms during the incubation period. Tetracycline hydrochloride provided complete microbiological sterilization of decapsulated *Trichinella* larvae during the whole period of our observations. The wide range of its antimicrobial action against gram-positive and gram-negative microbes was fully displayed on the concomitant microflora of *Trichinella* larvae. A mixture of two antibiotics, penicillin sodium and streptomycine sulfate had an incomplete sterilizing effect, as on the third day a growth of new spots of whitish colonies was noted on MPA and a slight cloudiness in MPB. Subsequently the growth of microbes was intensified. The same can be said about the mixture of penicillin, streptomycin, and nystatin. The two other mixtures of antibiotics: (1) penicillin, streptomycin, and neomycin; (2) penicillin, streptomycin, and polymyxin B sulfate, also did not provide complete sterilization as on the seventh day a growth of few spots of microbe colonies was noted in bacteriological media. The mentioned mixtures of antibiotics freed the nematodes from microbes more effectively than when these were used separately. This was seen in the numbers of microbe colonies and in the time of their appearance in media.

The mixtures of antibiotics—(a) penicillin sodium, streptomycin sulfate, and Mycostatin, (b) penicillin sodium, streptomycin sulfate, neomycin sulfate, and polymyxin B sulfate; and (c) Berntzen's (1965) antibiotic mixture—completely freed *Trichinella* larvae from microorganisms during the whole period of our observations.

Sterile *Trichinella* larvae preserved their motility in MPB and MPA at 37° C. In MPA they moved and formed winding tunnels. In MPB many *Trichinella* larvae underwent incomplete molting. On the fourteenth day of incubation in these media only several specimens remained alive. They did not increase in length; on the contrary, they decreased, indicating that the nutrient substances in bacteriological media did not serve for them sources of consumption or nutrition.

In nonsterile media the larvae perished within 2–3 days of incubation. The rapid death of nematodes appeared to be caused by metabolic products of microbes. The introduction of *Trichinella* larvae not treated with antibiotics called forth an abundant growth of various colonies of microorganisms. The procedure, including washing nematodes with sterile Tyrode solution, decreased the bacterial contamination only in a mechanical way and did not provide the freeing from microbes, as the growth of colonies was noted from the first day of incubation in MPB and MPA.

No harmful effects of antibiotics on helminths were noted. Our results were in agreement with Berntzen's studies (1965) in relation to obtaining

TABLE I　Microbiological Sterilization of *Trichinella* Larvae

Antibiotics at a concentration of 1000 units/ml	Growth of microorganisms[a]									
	1		3		5		7		14	
	MPB	MPA	MPB	MPA	MPB	MPA	MPB	MPA	MPB	MPA
Penicillin sodium	+	−	+	+	+	+	+	+	+	+
Streptomycin sulfate	−	−	+	+	+	+	+	+	+	+
Mycostatin	−	−	+	−	+	+	+	+	+	+
Nystatin	+	−	+	−	+	+	+	+	+	+
Neomycin sulfate	−	−	+	+	+	+	+	+	+	+
Polymyxin B sulfate	−	−	−	−	+	−	+	+	+	+
Tetracycline hydrochloride	−	−	−	−	−	−	−	−	−	−
Penicillin sodium + streptomycin sulfate	−	−	+	+	+	+	+	+	+	+
Penicillin sodium + streptomycin sulfate + Mycostatin	−	−	−	−	−	−	−	−	−	−
Penicillin sodium + streptomycin sulfate + nystatin	−	−	−	−	+	+	+	+	+	+
Penicillin sodium + streptomycin sulphate + neomycin sulfate	−	−	−	−	−	−	+	+	+	+
Penicillin sodium + streptomycin sulfate + polymyxin B sulfate	−	−	−	−	−	−	+	−	+	+
Penicillin sodium + streptomycin sulfate + neomycin sulfate + polymyxin B sulfate	−	−	−	−	−	−	−	−	−	−
[Berntzen's method (1965)] Streptomycin 0.5 gm, + penicillin 1,000,000 units + Mycostatin 5000 units in 100 ml of Tyrode solution	−	−	−	−	−	−	−	−	−	−
Control (without antibiotics)	+	+	+	+	+	+	+	+	+	+

[a] Numbers are days after treatment.
+, Growth of microorganisms; −, no growth of microorganisms.

Trichinella larvae free of microbes by using antibiotics. Parallel with Berntzen's method we tested a larger variety of antibiotics in other doses and used another procedure of treatment of *Trichinella* larvae. The method of washing nematodes by sedimenting them through a 15-cm column of a sterile solution, in our opinion, freed better the intestine and cuticle of helminths of microorganisms than the method of centrifugation. Our method of freeing nematodes from microorganisms was easier to accomplish and could be used for production of sterile antigens. Furthermore, it was possible to obtain sterile decapsulated *Trichinella* larvae for their cultivation under axenic conditions and for biochemical studies.

Summary

Trichinella spiralis larvae recovered from infected white rat by digestion in artificial gastric juice were washed in Tyrode solution by the sedimentation method. The freeing of the worms from microorganisms was made by using various antibiotics separately or in combinations at a concentration of 1000 units/ml of Tyrode solution for 1 hr. Tetracycline hydrochloride and the following antibiotic combinations: (a) penicillin sodium, streptomycin sulfate, Mycostatin; (b) penicillin sodium, streptomycin sulfate, neomycin sulfate, polymyxin B sulfate as well as treatment of the worms by the method of Berntzen (1965) provided complete microbiological sterilization of *Trichinella* larvae.

References

Avery, J. L. (1941). A simple method of removing bacteria that adhere to trichina larvae. *Proc. Helminthol. Soc. Wash.* **8,** 6–7.

Berntzen, A. K. (1962). *In vitro* cultivation of *Trichinella spiralis*. *J. Parasitol.* (Suppl.) **48,** 48.

Berntzen, A. K. (1965). Comparative growth and development of *Trichinella spiralis in vitro* and *in vivo,* with a redescription of the life-cycle. *Exp. Parasitol.* **16,** 74–106.

Berntzen, A. K. (1966). A controlled culture environment for axenic growth of parasites. *Ann. N.Y. Acad. Sci.* **139,** 176–189.

Kim, C. W. (1961). The cultivation of *Trichinella spiralis in vitro*. *Amer. J. Trop. Med. Hyg,* **10,** 742–747.

Kim, C. W. (1962). Further study on the *in vitro* cultivation of *Trichinella spiralis*. *Amer. J. Trop. Med. Hyg.* **11,** 491–496.

McCoy, O. R. (1936). The development of trichinae in abnormal environments. *J. Parasitol.* **22,** 54–59.

Meerovitch, E. (1962). *In vitro* development of *Trichinella spiralis* larvae. *J. Parasitol.* (Suppl.) **48,** 34.

Meerovitch E. (1965a). Studies on the *in vitro* axenic development of *Trichinella spiralis*. I. Basic culture techniques, pattern of development and the effects of the gaseous phase. *Can. J. Zool.* **43,** 69–79.

Meerovitch E. (1965b). Studies on the *in vitro* axenic development of *Trichinella spiralis*. 2. Preliminary experiments on the effects of farnesol, cholesterol and an insect extract. *Can. J. Zool.* **43,** 81–85.

Shanta, C. E. and Meerovitch E. (1970). Specific inhibition of morphogenesis in *Trichinella spiralis* by insect juvenile hormone mimics. *Can. J. Zool.* **48,** 617–620.

Tarakanov, V. I. (1963). The *in vitro* development of *Trichinella spiralis* in artificial nutrient media. *Mater. Nautch. Kon. Vses. Obshchestva Gelmintol. AN SSSR* (2), 119–121.

Tarakanov V. I. (1964). The cultivation of *Trichinella spiralis* larvae up to the sexually mature stage in artificial nutrient media. *Veterinariya Moscow* (3), 43–47.

Tarakanov V. I., and Krasnova L. L. (1970). The influence of artificial nutrient media on the *in vitro* development of *Trichinella* larvae. *Tr. Vses. Inst. Gelmintol. Imeni K. I. Skrjabina* **16,** 249–252.

Tarakanov V. I., and Krasnova L. L. (1971). The *in vitro* cultivation of decapsulated *Trichinella spiralis* larvae in a system of constant flow of nutrient medium. *Tr. Vses. Inst. Gelmintol. Imeni K. I. Skrjabina* **17,** 229–231.

Weller, T. H. (1943). The development of the larvae of *Trichinella spiralis* in roller tube cultures. *Amer. J. Pathol.* **19,** 503–516.

Occurrence of Hypodermal Gland Cells in the Bacillary Band of *Trichinella spiralis* during Two Phases of Its Life Cycle

R. G. Bruce

Department of Zoology,
University of Glasgow, Glasgow

Introduction

In a previous paper (Bruce, 1970) the presence of hypodermal gland cells of the bacillary band was demonstrated in adult *Trichinella spiralis,* and thereby linked *Trichinella* more strongly to the other members of the Trichuroidea, in which the ultrastructure of the bacillary band cells had been elucidated in *Trichuris* by Sheffield (1963) and in *Capillaria* by Wright (1963).

Materials and Methods

Preinfective juveniles were obtained by teasing host muscle in balanced salt solution (BSS), infective juveniles by pepsin–HCl digestion; and pre-adults by incubation of host intestine in BSS. The tissue was fixed with buffered glutaraldehyde, postfixed with Millonig's osmium fixative, dehydrated in ethanol, followed by propylene oxide, embedded in araldite, and stained with uranyl acetate–lead citrate.

Results

Preparturition Juveniles

The preparturition juveniles were examined *in situ,* i.e., within the adult female. Hypodermal gland cells have not been observed.

Muscle-Invasive Juvenile

In the muscle-invasive juvenile of days 5–6 postparturition there are cells which are similar in appearance to fully formed hypodermal gland cells present in the later stages with the exception that they do not open through the very thin cuticle (Fig. 1A).

The Preinfective Juvenile

The preinfective juvenile of days 9–10 postparturition does possess fully formed hypodermal gland cells which open through the cuticle (Fig. 1B). The gland cells are situated in both lateral hypodermal cords and occupy most of the area of the cords. A moderate number of cisternae of rough-surfaced endoplasmic reticulum form a network in the basal regions of the cells (Figs. 1B and 2A). Fine strands of material extend from the surface of the pores of the gland cells. These strands of material are probably a precipitate resulting from the fixation process but do indicate the porosity/permeability of the dense cap of the pore surface. In fine structure the outer surface of the pore is quite unlike the membrane surface of the body wall cuticle. The pore area of the gland cells will deposit a small droplet or smear on a glass surface which is metachromatic with toluidene blue. Preliminary experiments to determine the resistance of the gland cell pore to peptic–HCl digestion suggest that it is not capable of withstanding a 1- to 2-hr exposure to a peptic–HCl solution at 37° C. These results have yet to be conclusively confirmed.

The Infective Juvenile

Hypodermal gland cells have not been observed in the infective juvenile. The cells of the lateral hypodermal cords are largely filled with stored glycogen.

The Adult Worm

Gland cells are present in the preadult and adult worm from day 3 postinfection (Fig. 2B). They occupy positions in the lateral hypodermal cords and are distributed along the length of the worm as previously reported (Bruce, 1970).

Discussion

Hypodermal gland cells occur and presumably function at two phases in the life of *T. spiralis,* namely the invasive and early encapsulated phase in the host muscle and secondly virtually throughout the phase of tissue invasion of the host intestine. This association of the gland cells with the periods of tissue invasion, feeding, and major growth of the nematode requires the conclusion that the gland cells play a major role in the physiological relationship between the parasite and the host. The total absence of the hypodermal gland cells in the infective juvenile does not detract from a possible physiological role but merely emphasizes the conclusion,

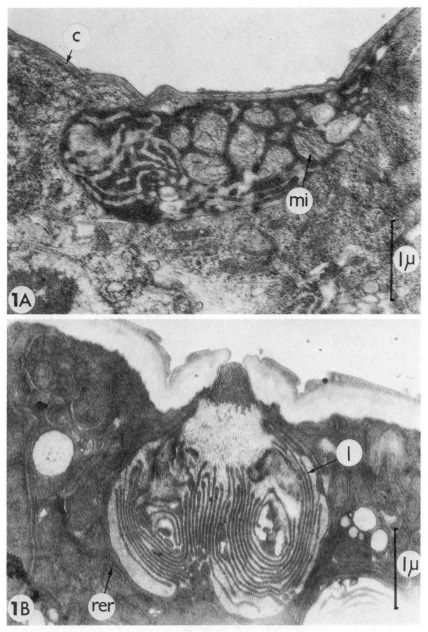

Figure 1 A, An oblique section through a hypodermal cord of a day 5 post-parturition juvenile showing what is believed to be a developing hypodermal gland cell. B, A fully formed hypodermal gland cell of a pre-infective juvenile of day 10 postparturition. Abbreviations: c, cuticle; l, lamella; mi, mitochondrion; rer, rough-surfaced endoplasmic reticulum.

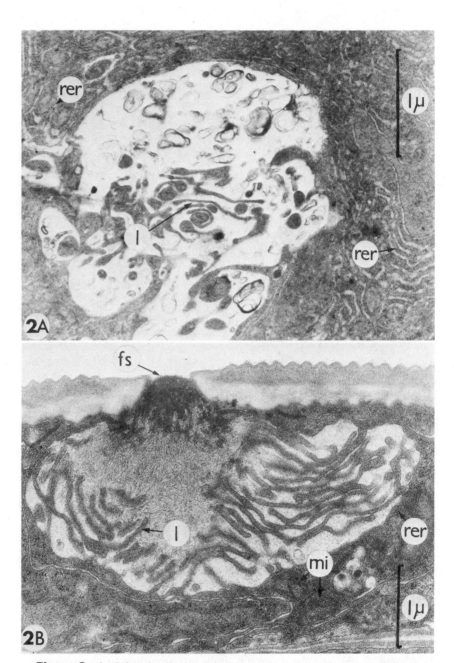

Figure 2 A, A longitudinal section through a hypodermal gland cell to show the concentration of rough-surfaced endoplasmic reticulum in the basal cytoplasm. B, A hypodermal gland cell of an adult. Fine strands of material projecting from the outer surface of the pore can just be seen. Abbreviations: fs, fine strands; l, lamella; mi, mitochondrion; rer, rough-surfaced endoplasmic reticulum.

based on the utilization of the secretory globules of the stichosome, that the infective juvenile is a resting stage.

The transformation, i.e., the elimination of the hypodermal gland cells in the hypodermal cords of *T. spiralis* associated with the onset of infectivity on or about 12 days postparturition is a quite extraordinary event or morphogenesis in a nematode, particularly if not accompanied by a molt as seems to be the case in *T. spiralis*. Bearing in mind the strong probability that the gland cell pore is not resistant to peptic–HCl digestion, the absence of the gland cells in the infective juvenile would enhance the capacity of the infective juvenile to survive the passage through the host stomach.

The actual function of the hypodermal gland cells has not been defined in the present study. However, it can be reasonably deduced from the presence of the considerable amount of rough-surfaced endoplasmic reticulum in the basal part of the cells, the extensive lamellae and the presence of the droplets in an *in vitro* situation that the gland cells do perform a secretory function. Both Wright (1963) in studies of *Capillaria* and Sheffield (1963) in studies on *Trichuris* deduced a possible secretory/osmoregulatory function for the gland cells in these nematodes.

Very recently McLaren (1972) has published evidence of excretory pore cells and anal pore cells in *Dirofilaria* which bear a remarkable similarity in overall form to the bacillary cells of *Trichinella*. McLaren agrees with the previously mentioned authors that an excretory/secretory function for this cell type is quite probable. A similar structural form was shown in the collateral gland cell of the cockroach (Mercer and Brunet, 1959) which is presumed to secrete material for the eggshell in these insects.

The potential antigenicity deriving from the hypodermal gland cells should be considered. At least two possible antigens are present: first, the dense (osmiophilic) surface of the pore which was previously described as a double banded structure (Bruce, 1970), and second, the strands of material which may be observed extending from the outer surface of the pore. If this is secreted material then clearly it may be antigenic. As with the nonutilization of the secretory globules of the stichosome in the infective juvenile (reported elsewhere in this volume), in the case of the gland cell antigens where there is total absence, the potential antigenicity of the infective juvenile *T. spiralis* is markedly reduced in comparison to the earlier juvenile stages in the muscle and the intestinal stages. As a corollary the efficiency of the host's initial defense reaction is probably reduced quite significantly.

Summary

Hypodermal gland cells situated in the lateral hypodermal cords are present in the juvenile nematode during the period of invasion, establishment, and early encapsulation in the host muscle, and in the preadult and adult nematodes parasitic in the tissues of the intestine. They are not present in the "mature" infective encapsulated juvenile.

References

Bruce, R. G. (1970). *Trichinella spiralis:* fine structure of the body wall with special reference to the formation and moulting of cuticle. *Exp. Parasitol.* **28,** 499–511.

Mercer, E. H., and Brunet, P. C. J. (1959). The electron microscopy of the left collaterial gland of the cockroach. *J. Biophys. Biochem. Cytol.* **5,** 257–261.

McLaren, D. J. (1972). Ultrastructural studies on microfilariae (Nematoda: Filarioidea). *Parasitology* **65,** 317–32.

Sheffield, H. G. (1963). Electron microscopy of the bacillary band and stichosome of *Trichuris muris* and *T. vulpis. J. Parasitol.* **49,** 998–1009.

Wright, K. A. (1963). Cytology of the bacillary bands of the nematode *Capillaria hepatica* (Bancroft, 1893). *J. Morphol.* **112,** 233–259.

The Formation and Utilization of Stichosome Secretory Globules in *Trichinella spiralis*

R. G. Bruce

*Department of Zoology,
University of Glasgow, Glasgow*

Introduction

The stichosome and the modified esophagus are two of the morphological features which characterize the Trichuroidea. The specific functions of the stichosome are as yet only partly understood. The observations of Chitwood (1930, 1935) that the stichocytes were linked by ducts to the esophagus in the Trichuroidea was only recently confirmed in *Trichinella* by ultrastructural studies (Bruce, 1970a). This report presents an account of the morphology and function of the stichosome and the esophagus at several stages in the life of *T. spiralis,* namely the preparturition juvenile, the muscle-penetrating juvenile, the preinfective encapsulated juvenile, the infective encapsulated juvenile, the 3–5 day postinfective adult, and the 12–14 day postinfective adult.

Materials and Methods

The early muscle stage juveniles were recovered *in vitro* by gentle teasing of mouse diaphragm, the infective juvenile by peptic–HCl digestion and the adult worm by incubation in balanced salt solution (BSS). The tissue was fixed with buffered glutaraldehyde, postfixed with Millonig's buffered osmium tetroxide fixation, dehydrated with ethanol, embedded in araldite and stained with uranyl acetate–lead citrate.

The *in utero* juvenile, and the preinfective juveniles are well fixed by this method without chopping the worms. The infective juvenile has to be chopped up to achieve good fixation.

Results

The *in Utero* Juvenile 0–12 Hours before Parturition

The esophagus and stichocytes (or stichocyte precursor cells) can be detected in the *in utero* juvenile several hours before parturition. The esophagus is a well-formed triradiate structure with the lumen lined with a cuticular material. The stichocytes even at the very early stage, i.e., about 8–12 hr before birth, contain distinct globules of secretory product (Fig. 1A).

The Muscle-Penetrating Juvenile

In the juvenile worm which is penetrating or has just penetrated a muscle fiber 11–12 days postinfection, or more specifically, 5–6 days postparturition, the stichosome is well developed. In each stichocyte a moderate number of secretory globules are aggregated around a well-formed system of canaliculi which is adjacent to the esophagus.

In this phase of the life cycle, the cytoplasm of the stichocytes is packed with rough-surfaced endoplasmic reticulum but virtually all the secretory globules are closely associated with the well-formed system of canaliculi at the side of the stichocyte adjacent to the esophagus. The stichosome region esophagus shows its characteristic form almost enclosed within its muscle sheath, with one open duct per stichocyte passing through the gap in the muscle sheath of the esophagus.

The Preinfective Encapsulated Juvenile

The juvenile worm younger than 18 days postinfection, i.e., specifically, 11–12 days postparturition, is not infective (Bruce, 1967). In addition, juveniles younger than 12 days postparturition cannot be extracted alive from muscle by peptic–HCl digestion. The preinfective juveniles in this study were taken as the largest worms recovered from a teased muscle preparation of 15–16 days postinfection, i.e., aged 9–10 days postparturition.

The ultrastructure of the stichocytes and the esophagus shows little change in comparison with the day 6 postparturition worm. In each stichocyte the moderate number of secretory globules are closely grouped around the system of canaliculi which lead into the open duct leading from each stichocyte to the esophagus (Fig. 1B).

The globules are not secreted into the esophagus as membrane-bound entities, but as fine particulate matter, presumably semiliquid. The bounding membrane of the globule is broken down and the contents are released in the vesicles which develop and extend from the canaliculi. Residual membrane-containing vesicles may be observed between the open canaliculi (Fig. 2). The fine particulate matter can be seen in the canaliculi, duct, and lumen of the esophagus indicating active export during this phase of the life-cycle. The stichocytes contain very little stored glycogen.

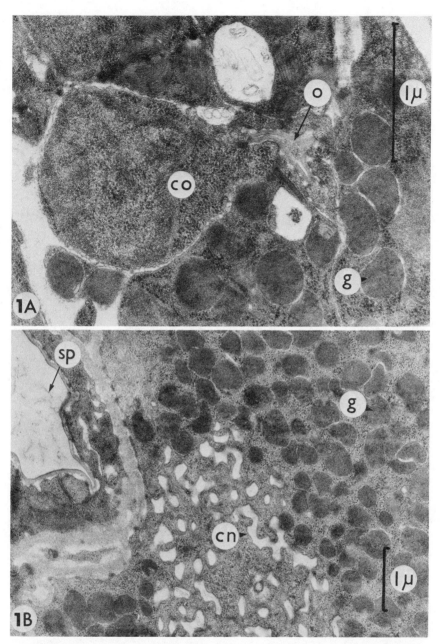

Figure 1 A, Transverse section through the developing esophagus (o) and stichocytes of a preparturition juvenile approximately 8–12 hr before birth. The esophagus is apparently developing within one cell (co) and the cuticle lined triradiate lumen is visible. Note that the stichocytes at this stage are not arranged in a single column. The secretory globules (g) are already present. B, Transverse section of the esophagus and part of a stichocyte of a preinfective juvenile, showing the aggregation of secretory globules (g) around the canaliculi (cn). The stichocyte/esophageal duct is not shown in this micrograph, but traces of the secretory product (sp) are visible in the lumen of the esophagus.

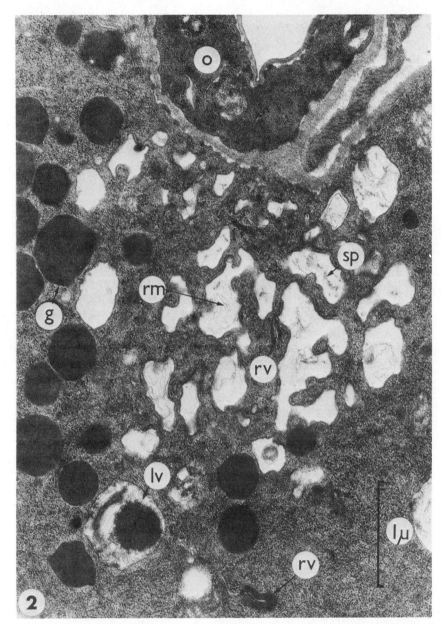

Figure 2 A transverse section through the canaliculi in a stichocyte to show the process of release of the contents of the secretory globules into the canaliculi. One globule is shown in the early stages of breakdown in the liberating vesicle (lv) which is an extension of the canaliculi. In other branches of the canaliculi the remnants of the globule (rm) and vesicle (rv) membranes may be seen. o, Esophagus; g, globule; sp, secretory product.

The Infective Juvenile

The infective juveniles in this study were usually harvested from the host between 25–35 days postparturition. The stichocytes fill most of the cross-sectional area within the body wall in the anterior part of the worm. The basic structure of the stichosome and esophagus is unchanged. However, within each stichocyte the very numerous secretory globules are widely dispersed throughout most of the cytoplasm (Fig. 3A). Canaliculi adjacent to the esophagus are not well organized, although a few can be observed in the stichocytes. An open duct into the esophagus has not been observed. In addition to the well-formed, although widely dispersed, cisternae of rough-surfaced endoplasmic reticulum, each stichocyte contains a considerable amount of stored glycogen. The mitochondria are smaller and more electron-dense than hitherto (Fig. 3B).

The Preadult and Adult 3–5 Days Postinfection

In the 3–5 day postinfection female preadult and adult worms, a well-developed system of canaliculi is present in each stichocyte in the same position as in the preinfective juvenile. The secretory globules are closely grouped around the system of canaliculi, the rough-surfaced endoplasmic reticulum has increased in amount to the extent of occupying most of the space in the cells, and the stored glycogen has decreased (Fig. 4A). The mitochondria in the stichocytes are larger and less electron-dense than in the infective juveniles, and are found mainly in the peripheral regions of the stichocytes. An open exporting duct from each system of canaliculi into the esophagus is present.

The Adult 12–14 Days Postinfection

In the late-stage female adult the basic structure is as before. A small number of secretory globules are grouped around the system of canaliculi. Rough-surfaced endoplasmic reticulum is abundant and very little stored glycogen remains in the stichocytes. Export of fine particulate matter continues through the open stichocyte-esophagus duct (Fig. 4B).

Discussion

There can be little doubt that the secretory globules of the stichosome of *T. spiralis* perform an important function for the nematode. With the evidence that ducts exist between the stichocytes and the esophagus, the route by which these globules could be passed on from the stichocytes, and quite probably to the exterior, has been clarified. The presence of these secretory globules in the stichocytes of preparturition juveniles emphasizes the importance of these globules.

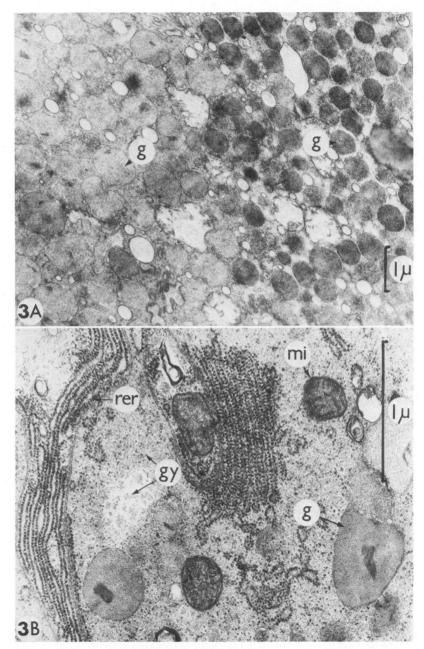

Figure 3   A, A section through part of a stichocyte of an infective juvenile
showing the widespread dispersion of the secretory globules (g). B, A part
of a stichocyte of an infective juvenile near the periphery of two stichocytes
which shows the well-formed although sparse rough-surfaced endoplasmic
reticulum (rer), the small dense mitochondria (mi) and the considerable
amount of glycogen (gy). g, Secretory globule.

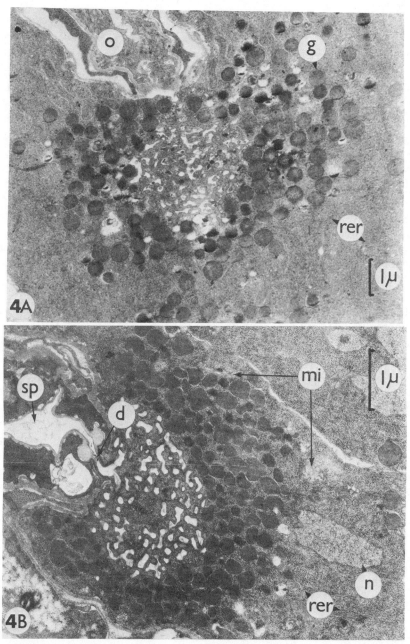

Figure 4 A, A section through a stichocyte of a young adult which shows the aggregation of the secretory globules (g) around the canaliculi, the absence of glycogen and the regeneration of a large amount of rough-surfaced endoplasmic reticulum (rer). o, Esophagus. B, A late stage adult showing an open duct (d) and secretory product (sp) in the lumen of the esophagus. The distribution of the secretory globules and the amount of rough-surfaced endoplasmic reticulum (rer) are similar to that of the young adult. mi, Mitochondria; n, nucleus.

55

The present study also demonstrates that the secretory globules are actively exported from the stichocytes at two distinct periods in the life cycle: during the muscle penetration and early encapsulated phase and during the life of the preadult and the adult worm in the intestine. The secretory globules present in large numbers in the infective juvenile appear to be stored and are not being actively exported.

The periods of maximal production of the secretory globules in the stichosome are associated with the two main periods of growth in the life cycle: the early stages of muscle parasitism by the juvenile worm days 6–12 postparturition, and for virtually the whole of the life of the worm in the host intestine. The criteria for measuring the production of the globules are the amount and organization of the cisternae of rough-surfaced endoplasmic reticulum, and the size and electron opacity of the mitochondria, including the organization of the cristae within the mitochondria and the localization of the mitochondria in the peripheral regions of the stichocytes.

The association of the maximum production and export of the secretory globules to the two periods of the life cycle which are both tissue penetrating and major growth phases cannot be coincidental. Although the exact nature of the lesion around the anterior end of the invading adult worm has not been determined with the electron microscope, the ultrastructure (Bruce, 1970b) and histochemical nature (Bullock, 1953; Zarzycki, 1963; Bruce, 1970b) of the transformation of the muscle cell parasitized by the juvenile worm is well documented and postulates enzymatic digestion by the invading worm, and additionally the induction, and probably to some degree, the control of the development of the capsule and nutrient matrix.

The potential antigenicity of the secretory globules of the stichosome has been established by Despommier and Müller (1970) who gave evidence of 80–90% immunity in animals sensitized with extracted secretory globules. From the current evidence, therefore, it is probable that such an immunity is likely to be initiated by either the preadult and adult worms in the intestine or by the muscle-invasive and early encapsulated stages of the juvenile, but not significantly by the "mature" infective encapsulated juvenile.

Summary

In *Trichinella spiralis* secretory globules in the stichocytes are present at all stages of the life cycle from preparturition juvenile to adult worm. It is shown that the globules are actively exported only at two distinct phases in the life of the worm, namely in the muscle invasive and early encapsulated stage of the juvenile and during intestinal wall invasion by the preadult and adult worms.

References

Bruce, R. G. (1967). The morphology and physiology of *Trichinella spiralis* (Nematoda). Ph.D. dissertation, University of Cambridge.

Bruce, R. G. (1970a). Structure of the esophagus of the infective juvenile and adult *Trichinella spiralis*. *J. Parasitol.* **56,** 540–549.

Bruce, R. G. (1970b). The structure and composition of the capsule of *Trichinella spiralis* in host muscle. *Parasitology* **60,** 223–227.

Bullock, W. L. (1953). Phosphatases in experimental *Trichinella spiralis* infections in the rat. *Exp. Parasitol.* **2,** 150–162.

Chitwood, B. G. (1930). The structure of the esophagus in the Trichuroidea. *J. Parasitol.* **17,** 35–42.

Chitwood, B. G. (1935). The nature of the 'cell body' of *Trichuris* and 'stichosome' of *Agamermis*. *J. Parasitol.* **21,** 225–226.

Despommier, D. D., and Müller, M. (1970). The stichosome of *Trichinella spiralis:* its structure and function. *J. Parasitol.* **56,** *Proc. 2nd Int. Cong. Parasitol.*

Zarzycki, J. (1963). Histochemical studies of capsules of *Trichinella*. *Wiad. Parazytol.* **9,** 453–458.

Part II

Biochemistry; Experimental Pathology

Murine Trichinellosis: Changes in Glucose Absorption and Intestinal Morphology

J. A. Richardson and L. J. Olson

Department of Microbiology
The University of Texas Medical Branch
Galveston, Texas

Introduction

Gastrointestinal nematodes infect millions of humans and animals and must be regarded as important causes of enteric diseases in the world. While these nematodes have received considerable study over the years for various reasons, explanations of how these pathogens cause disease are incomplete or lacking. Based on published reports, surprisingly little attention seems to have been given to the possibility that these nematodes may cause pathophysiological changes of the gut.

Recent experimental evidence has shown that at least three species of gastrointestinal nematodes can cause intestinal malabsorption: *Nippostrongylus brasiliensis* in rats (Symons and Fairbairn, 1962), *Trichinella spiralis* in guinea pigs (Castro *et al.,* 1967) and *Ancylostoma caninum* in dogs (Migasena *et al.,* 1972). The purpose of this study was to confirm and extend our earlier data on absorption from the anterior intestine of mice infected with *Trichinella spiralis*. D-Glucose was used as an indicator of absorptive function. The mouse was selected as the experimental animal because it is a natural host for trichinellosis. An attempt was made to relate data obtained on absorption with data obtained on parasite virulence, worm distribution, and gross and microscopic changes in intestinal morphology. Additionally, the effect of metabolites of cultured larvae and and extracts of these larvae on glucose absorption was given preliminary study.

Materials and Methods

Male albino mice (Webster-Fairfield) were purchased from Euers' Farms, Austin, Texas, and held 5–7 days before use. Animals were housed in air-conditioned quarters and given food and water *ad libitum*. Infective larvae were recovered from mice during a 6- to 12-week postinfection period by pepsin digestion (Olston *et al.*, 1960). Mice under light ether anesthesia were infected by stomach intubation of larvae suspended in nutrient broth gelatin (6.4 gm nutrient broth, 40 gm gelatin, 1 liter distilled H_2O).

Adult worms were recovered by the NaOH digestion technique of Larsh and Kent (1949). In worm distribution studies, the intestine was removed and divided into halves. Each half was slit longitudinally and cut into 5- to 8-cm segments prior to digestion in 40 ml of 0.05% NaOH (w/v). The digest was refrigerated at $6°C$ for 24 hr at which time 1 ml of 40% formalin was added to each jar.

In preparation for morphological studies, the small intestine was removed, washed in Krebs-Ringer bicarbonate (KRB), and divided into first and second quarters and posterior half. These segments were everted on a metal rod. The everted segments were fixed and stored in 10% buffered formalin and examined with a dissecting microscope for gross changes. For histological studies, a 5.5-cm upper jejunal segment was removed as described below for *in vitro* tests, everted, rinsed in cold KRB, and preserved in cold buffered formalin. A 1-cm section was removed from the center of the segment, mounted in paraffin, sectioned (7 μm) and stained with hematoxylin and eosin.

D-Glucose absorption from the upper jejunum was measured by the *in vitro* technique of Crane and Wilson (1958). Mice were anesthetized with ether. The abdomen was opened by a midline incision and the intestine was exposed. Two incisions were made in the small intestine to isolate a jejunal segment of approximately 5.5 cm in length; the first incision was located approximately 10–11 cm distal to the stomach. The segment was rinsed in cold KRB and everted. One end of the segment was cannulated to a rubber catheter and the other end was ligated with silk suture to form a sac. The segment was immersed in 9 ml of KRB containing 1 mg glucose/ml. One-half ml of test solution was placed inside the sac. The test tube was incubated in a water bath at $37°C$ for 1 hr and gassed gently with 5% CO_2 in O_2. The solutions outside and inside the sac were referred to as the mucosal and serosal solutions, respectively. Four to 7 min elapsed between the removal of the segment from its blood supply and the start of the experiment. Following incubation the final glucose concentration of the serosal and mucosal solutions were determined by the glucose oxidase method of the Worthington Biochemical Corporation.

The effect of larval metabolites and sonicate on glucose absorption was also studied using the Crane and Wilson technique. Larvae were collected from mice by pepsin digestion and sonicated (Lin and Olson, 1969) or cultured for 3 days at $37°\,C$ as described by Kagan (1960) with the exception that streptomycin was omitted. A 5.5-cm upper jejunal segment was removed from normal mice, as described above, everted and placed in 5 ml of test solution consisting of 2.5 ml of larval metabolites (supernatant from cultures containing 83,000 larvae) or sonicate (soluble components of 50,000 larvae) and 2.5 ml KRB. Control segments were incubated in 5 ml KRB. The glucose concentration was adjusted to 1 mg/ml. The serosal surface was incubated in 0.5 ml of the respective solution.

Experimental Design and Results

A consistent and easily measured criterion of infection in animals is weight loss. In the first experiment, mice were infected with 100, 150, 200, 250, and 300 larvae per gram body weight (L/gm) and observed for deaths and weight changes. The oral LD_{50} ($\pm SE$) was found to be 192 ± 11, 146 ± 8 and 115 ± 4 L/gm for 7, 14, and 21 days postinfection, respectively. Data on mice infected with 50 L/gm in a later experiment are included for comparison.

Infected animals showed weight loss as early as the second day postinfection (Fig. 1). Weight changes, like survival, were dose dependent. Mice infected with 100 or more L/gm lost weight until day 7 when the weights leveled off and remained low until all the mice died. By contrast, mice infected with 50 L/gm, showed a slight and transient weight loss. By the beginning of the fourth week, these mice began to gain weight at a rate parallel to that of the controls.

In the second experiment 80 mice were infected with 50 L/gm from two lots of larvae and sacrificed in groups of four to six between days 3–28 postinfection to determine the distribution of *T. spiralis* in the small intestine. Differences in infectivity of the two lots were slight; 41% of the inoculum was recovered from lot 1 viability controls killed on day 6 and 45% were recovered from lot 2 controls killed on day 7 postinfection.

Maximum worm burdens were recovered on day 7 with 45% of the infective dose recovered (Fig. 2). Worm burdens fluctuated between 30 and 45% of the infective dose between days 6 through 14 postinfection at which time worm elimination began. A small number of worms (4%) was still present 28 days following challenge.

In a third experiment to study the effects of infection on intestinal morphology, 166 mice were divided into three groups and infected with 42 L/gm (Group A) 100 L/gm (Group B) and 150 L/gm (Group C); 22 mice were uninfected controls. Mice were killed in groups of five over

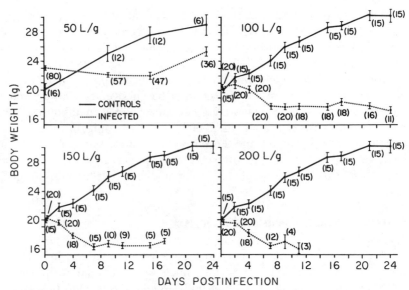

Figure 1 Body weight changes (mean ±SE) of mice following infection with 50, 100, 150, or 200 larvae per gram body weight (L/gm). Numbers of live mice are in parentheses. Decreasing numbers in the 50 L/gm experiment reflect experimental use and not deaths from infection as in other groups.

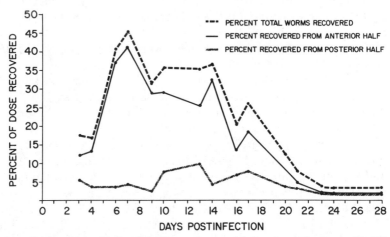

Figure 2 Percent of infective dose recovered following infection with 50 L/gm over a 28-day postinfection period.

a 4- to 28-day postinfection period. Five mice from each group were killed 5 days postinfection as controls on worm viability and harbored 32, 35, and 33% of the inoculum from groups A, B, and C, respectively. The first and second quarters of the small intestine were examined and classified as having one of the following appearances:

Normal: villi are long, slender and fingerlike (Fig. 3).

Hobnail: villi are shortened and blunted.

Convoluted-mosaic: villi are severely atrophied with fused bases and abnormal patterns.

The segments were subsequently graded as follows:

0: normal;

1+: hobnail villi covering less than one-half the surface area of the segment;

2+: hobnail villi covering one-half or more of the surface area of the segment;

3+: convoluted-mosaic villi covering less than one-half the surface area of the segment;

4+: convoluted-mosaic villi covering one-half or more of the surface area of the segment.

The results showed that convoluted-mosaic changes occurred in all groups with the first quarter most severely involved (Fig. 4). The onset and severity of these changes were dose dependent since on day 4 the changes were most severe in Group C and least severe in Group A. Convoluted-mosaic changes were seen in both quarters of Group C by day 4, in the first quarter of Group B by day 8, and in both quarters of Group A by day 7. On day 10 the convoluted-mosaic changes were most severe in the first quarter of Group A; thereafter, these changes diminished in severity, but persted until the end of the experiment. Convoluted-mosaic changes in the first quarter of Group B persisted until the end of the experiment; however, no convoluted-mosaic changes were seen in the second quarter. Convoluted-mosaic changes were seen in the second quarter of

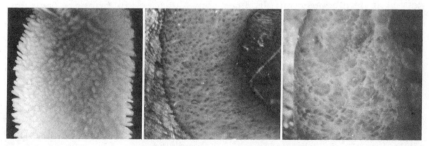

Figure 3 Everted small intestine showing normal villi (left), hobnail (middle), and convoluted-mosaic (right).

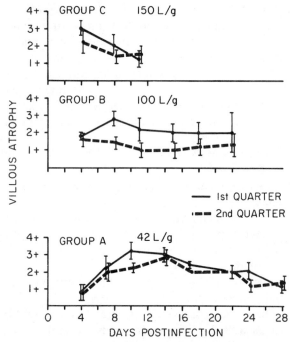

Figure 4   Villous atrophy following doses of 42, 100, and 150 L/gm.

Group A and C, but these changes were not as severe as in the first quarter and did not persist until the end of the experiment.

Hobnail changes occurred in both quarters of all groups by day 4 and persisted to some extent in each group throughout the experiment. The first and second quarters had equal degrees of hobnail changes. Neither convoluted-mosaic nor hobnail changes were seen on the intestinal segments from 22 normal control mice.

In a fifth experiment microscopic changes in the jejunum following infection were studied. Twenty mice were infected with 50 L/gm and 15 served as uninfected controls. They were sacrificed in groups of 5 on days 1, 5, and 12 postinfection to obtain jejunal segments. Stained sections of these segments were examined for villous length, crypt depth, and thickness of the muscularis externa. The data reported are the averages of numerous measurements of villi and crypts from each group of mice (Table I). The data for the uninfected controls are overall mean values, since no differences were noted between these groups.

Villous length was significantly decreased and crypt depth was significantly increased as soon as day 1 postinfection and remained abnormal throughout the study. Likewise villous length:crypt depth ratios were significantly altered throughout. The muscularis externa became significantly thickened over control values by day 12 (Table I).

Table I Comparison of villous length, crypt depth, muscularis externa thickness, and villous:crypt ratios of intestinal segments from infected (I) and uninfected control mice (U)

Group	Villous length (μm)	Group	Crypt depth (μm)	Group	Muscularis thickness (μm)	Group	Ratios
U	489[a]	I-day 5	210|	I-day 12	114	U	3.41
I-day 1	400|	I-day 1	199|	I-day 1	81	I-day 1	2.13
I-day 5	384|	I-day 12	186	I-day 5	69|	I-day 5	1.90|
I-day 12	288	U	149	U	69|	I-day 12	1.68|
	SE ±9.3		SE ±4.4		SE ±2.8		SE ±0.10

[a] Means compared by Duncan multiple range test at 5% probability level. Values not spanned by same line are significantly different.

We have completed several experiments in which mice were given different doses of larvae ranging from 50 to 180 L/gm and killed at various intervals for recovery of segments and *in vitro* tests on glucose absorption. These data have demonstrated a dose-dependent effect on absorption, i.e., severity of malabsorption increased with dose. However, dose had little effect on time of onset of malabsorption which was within 2–4 days after infection in the various dose groups. But, as expected from our LD_{50} data, doses in excess of 100 L/gm were sufficiently lethal to leave few or no survivors for absorption tests beyond week 3. Hence, we decided in the sixth experiment to infect mice with a dose that was sublethal but adequate to cause signs of this disease, e.g., weight loss, villous atrophy.

Sixty mice were infected with 50 L/gm from two lots of larvae and 12 mice were tested as uninfected controls. Infected animals were sacrificed over a 48-day postinfection period for *in vitro* tests on glucose absorption. Control animals were tested near the beginning, middle, and termination of the experiment. Ten viability control mice, five for each lot of larvae used to infect the mice, were sacrificed on day 6 postinfection and yielded 21% and 40% of the infective dose.

Serosal to mucosal (S/M) ratios for infected mice were significantly below that of controls as early as day 3 (Fig. 5). These ratios dropped again on day 6 and remained at this level for the next 10 days. A recovery phase toward normal absorption was apparent on days 20 and 24. With the exception of day 31, ratios for days 27 to 41 did not differ significantly from the normal ratio. The S/M ratio for day 48 unexplainedly dipped significantly below normal values.

Mean S/M ratios for uninfected mice were constant throughout this experiment and in the range obtained repeatedly for such animals in our other absorption experiments.

Serosal and mucosal glucose concentrations demonstrated that both levels were altered in the infected animals (Fig. 6). Serosal concentrations on days 31, 34, and 41 were significantly higher than control values, and

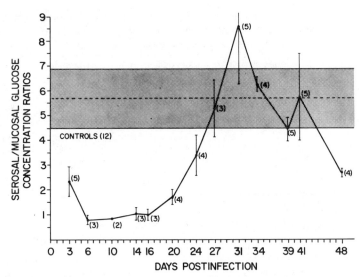

Figure 5   Mean S/M ratios (±SE) following infection with 50 L/gm.

serosal values on days 3 to 24 and on day 48 were significantly lower than the normal mean of 177 mg/100 ml. The mucosal concentration on day 31 was the only value significantly lower than the control mean of 36 mg/100 ml, and the values from the infected mice for days 3 to 16 and 34 to 48 were significantly higher than the normal mean.

In the seventh and eighth experiments, intestinal segments were incubated in larval metabolites or larval sonicate. No malabsorption was detected on the basis of S/M ratios following incubation of intestinal seg-

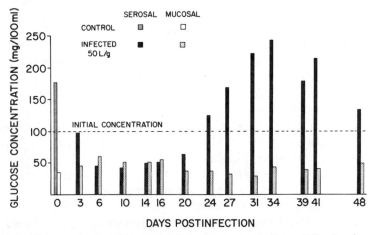

Figure 6   Mean serosal and mucosal glucose concentrations following infection with 50 L/gm.

Table II Effect of larval metabolites on S/M ratios of intestinal segments from normal mice

Group	No. animals	Ratios
KRB	6	6.74[a]
Incubation Medium	10	7.57
Metabolites	7	8.49
		SE ± 0.76

[a] Means compared by Duncan multiple range test at the 5% probability level.

ments in metabolites (Table II). However, the S/M ratio for the sonicate treated group at the end of the 1-hr test period was significantly reduced as compared to that of the control. This difference was due to the decrease in the glucose absorbed from the mucosal solution (Table III).

Discussion

Analysis of data on mice infected with approximately 50 L/gm yields some interesting correlations between changes in glucose absorption, villous structure, body weight, and worm burdens. Weight loss, villous atrophy, and malabsorption become increasingly severe during the first week of infection and remained severe throughout the second week of infection (Figs. 1, 4, 5, respectively). In the third week it became apparent that a recovery phase was in effect, since the mice had commenced to gain weight, villi were becoming more normal in structure and glucose absorption was increasing toward normal. Chronologically these third-week changes coincided with the onset of decreasing worm burdens (Fig. 2).

More data are needed before cause–effect relationships for these changes can be identified, although we have repeatedly demonstrated that this infection somehow can cause these changes. We are of the opinion that malabsorption is initiated because of direct effects of these nematodes on the mucosa, i.e., traumatic and toxic. The onset of malabsorption after

Table III Comparison of S/M ratios and serosal and muscosal glucose concentrations following incubation of segments in sonicate and KRB test solutions.

Treatment	No. Animals	Ratio	Serosal[a]	Mucosal[a]
KRB	12	7.93 ±2.12	96 ±12	19 ±3[b]
Sonicate	15	3.35 ±0.82	99 ±8	40 ±4[b]

[a] Results given as milligram per 100 ml of solution.
[b] Means compared by Student's t-test; P < .001.

infection (2–4 days) in several experiments in this study seems too early to be due to an allergic reaction by the gut to these nematodes, although we do not rule out the possibility that immune reactions may contribute to these changes in the period after onset and during recovery. Since no study has been made of changes in the bacterial population of the mouse small intestine following *T. spiralis* infection, the possibility that bacteria play a role in the malabsorption of these mice cannot be excluded. However, the prompt (within 1 hr) induction of malabsorption obtained in the experiment with *Trichinella* sonicate is evidence that components of these worms can directly initiate malabsorption.

It seems reasonable that the recovery phase of absorption was causally related to the loss of worms which occurred at this time; however, strict proof that worm elimination, per se, results in a return to normal absorption remains to be obtained. A useful experiment in this regard would be to monitor glucose absorption after prematurely terminating the intestinal phase of trichinellosis by an appropriate anthelmintic, or during an extension of this phase by corticosteroids.

The lag period between infection and onset of malabsorption approximates the time required by infective larvae, upon entering the gut, to mature into adult worms. Possibly adults secrete materials that are quantitatively and or qualitatively different from those of larvae, and directly toxic to epithelial cells. In this connection our preliminary data showed that larval metabolites did not affect glucose absorption, although sonicate from larvae did reduce absorption. Another point to consider is the effect on absorption of premuscle larvae, deposited in large numbers by adult worms in gut tissue. Since deposition of these larvae has been reported to begin at approximately 5 days postinfection (Harley and Gallicchio, 1971; Villella, 1970; Berntzen, 1965; Gould *et al.,* 1955), it seems unlikely that these larvae play a role in explaining the lag between infection and the onset of malabsorption.

Another and more attractive explanation for the lag between infection and onset of malabsorption is based on the turnover rate of intestinal epithelial cells in mice. While the turnover rate of this strain of mice is not known, other strains have been shown to replace their small intestinal epithelium every 2–3 days (Creamer, 1967). Therefore the lag above may represent the time required to replace existing normal cells, after infection, with biochemically defective or immature cells. On this basis, one can hypothesize that *T. spiralis* (infective larvae and adults) following invasion of mucosa, secrete or, in dying, release substances that are damaging to the intestinal epithelial cells causing premature shedding of these cells from the villus. The crypts respond by increasing the rate of production of epithelial cells and hence immature cells move out of the crypts and up the villi at a rate too rapid to permit maturation to a full enzymatic load. Within a few days, these cells have replaced existing functionally mature cells and malabsorption can be detected. On the basis of this explanation, the lag between onset of worm elimination and the recovery phase of absorption may reflect the time needed to return to a normal turnover rate of mucosal cells. It has been suggested that the gut responses as described above are nonspecific and are the responses of intestinal mucosa to a number of noxious substances, various enteric infections (Sprinz, 1962), or various diet deficiency states (Sprinz, 1962; Nelson *et al.,* 1962).

Further studies are needed to test the theory that immature cells are responsible for the malabsorption in these mice by comparing turnover rates and enzymatic patterns of cells in infected and normal mice. In this connection Castro and Gentner (1972) have shown that the activity of intestinal disaccharidases is greatly reduced in guinea pigs on days 4 and 5 after infection with *T. spiralis.* The present study did provide some evidence that *T. spiralis* infection does alter crypt activity in that crypt lengths had increased. We also noted that goblet cell thecae were increased in number. According to Creamer (1967) when intestinal epithelial cells are lost at an increased rate, the crypts lengthen and the mitotic rate may also increase.

Symons (1960, 1961) found that although malabsorption occurred in the jejunum of the rat infected with *Nippostrongylus brasiliensis,* there was evidence that absorption by the ileum compensated for the jejunal defect and hence the overall absorption by the small intestine was essentially normal. This aspect of absorption has not been tested in murine trichinellosis.

Data on worm distribution in the small intestine showed that the majority of worms localize in the anterior half. During the third week of infection, the percentage of worms in the anterior half of the intestine began to decrease and the percentage of worms in the posterior half began to increase. This shift in distribution was accompanied by a reduction in total worm burden, i.e., an explusion of worms from the small intestine. The distribution of worms in this study agrees quite well with that reported earlier (Olson and Richardson, 1968) for mice infected with 3000 larvae. Other studies on worm distribution in the mouse have been done with relatively low infective doses. Most investigators agree that the majority of adults are located in the anterior half of mouse small intestine at least through days 11 to 14 postinfection (Larsh and Hendricks, 1949; Larsh *et al.,* 1952; Podhajecky, 1962).

Summary

During the first week of infection, mice infected with 50 *Trichella spiralis* larvae per gram body weight, developed villous atrophy and other morphological changes of the mucosa. *In vitro* D-glucose malabsorption began and weight loss also occurred during the first week. These changes remained severe during the second week, but in the third week postinfection a "recovery phase" began. Chronologically the recovery phase coincided with the onset of decreasing worm burdens, weight gain, and normalization of intestinal morphology and absorption. In addition normal gut segments incubated in supernatant of *T. spiralis* larval sonicate were unable to absorb glucose normally, whereas gut segments incubated in supernatant from cultured larvae absorbed glucose normally as compared to controls.

Acknowledgment

Supported in part by the James W. McLaughlin Fellowship Fund for the Study of Infection and Immunity.

References

Berntzen, A. K. (1965). Comparative growth and development of *Trichinella spiralis in vitro* and *in vivo*, with redescription of the life cycle. *Exp. Parasitol.* **16,** 74–106.

Castro, G. A., and Gentner, H. (1972). Disaccharidase deficiency associated with the intestinal phase of trichinosis in guinea pigs. *Proc. Soc. Exp. Biol. Med.* **140,** 342–345.

Castro, G. A., Olson, L. J., and Baker, R. D. (1967). Glucose malabsorption and intestinal histopathology in *Trichinella spiralis* infected guinea pigs. *J. Parasitol.* **53,** 595–612.

Crane, R. K., and Wilson, T. H. (1958). *In vitro* method for the study of the rate of intestinal absorption of sugars. *J. Appl. Physiol.* **12,** 145–146.

Creamer, B. (1967). The turnover of the epithelium of the small intestine. *Brit. Med. Bull.* **23,** 226–230.

Gould, S. E., Gomberg, H. J., Bethell, F. H., Villella, J. B., and Hertz, C. S. (1955). Studies on *Trichinella spiralis.* II. Time of initial recovery of larvae of *Trichinella spiralis* from blood of experimental animals. *Amer. J. Pathol.* **31,** 936–942.

Harley, J. P., and Gallicchio, V. (1971). *Trichinella spiralis:* migration of larvae in the rat. *Exp. Parasitol.* **30,** 11–21.

Kagan, I. G. (1960). Trichinosis: A review of biologic, serologic and immunologic aspects. *J. Infec. Dis.* **107,** 65–93

Larsh, J. E., Jr., and Hendricks, J. R. (1949). The probable explanation for the difference in the localization of adult *Trichinella spiralis* in young and old mice. *J. Parasitol.* **35,** 101–106.

Larsh, J. E., Jr., and Kent, D. E. (1949). The effect of alcohol on natural and acquired immunity of mice to infection with *Trichinella spiralis. J. Parasitol.* **35,** 45–53.

Larsh, Jr., J. E., Gilchrist, H. B., and Greenberg, B. G. (1952). A study of the distribution and longevity of adult *Trichinella spiralis* in immunized and non-immunized mice. *J. Elisha Mitchell Sci. Soc.* **68**, 1–11.

Lin, T. M., and Olson, L. J. (1969). Prolonged toxic effect of *Trichinella spiralis* larval sonicate on the absorption of glucose by guinea pig intestine. *J. Parasitol.* **55**, 223–224.

Migasena, S., Gilles, H. M., and Maegraith, B. G. (1972). Studies in *Ancylostoma caninum* infection in dogs. I. Absorbtion from the small intestine of amino acids, carbohydrates and fat. *Ann. Trop. Med. Parasitol.* **66**, 107-127.

Nelson, R. A., Code, C. F. and Brown, A. L., Jr., (1962). Sorption of water and electrolytes, and mucosal structure in niacin deficiency. *Gastroenterology* **42**, 26–35.

Olson, L. J., and Richardson, J. A. (1968). Intestinal malabsorption of D-glucose in mice infected with *Trichinella spiralis. J. Parasitol.* **54**, 445–451.

Olson, L. J., Richards, B., and Ewert, A. (1960). Detection of metabolic antigens from nematode larvae by a microculture-agar gel technique. *Tex. Rep. Biol. Med.* **18**, 254–259.

Podhajecky, K. (1962). Localization of intestinal trichinellae in the small intestine of mice in their intestinal phase. *Wiad. Parazytol.* **8**, 633–636.

Sprinz, H. (1962). Morphological response of intestinal mucosa to enteric bacteria and its implication for sprue and asiatic cholera. *Fed. Proc.* **21**, 57–64.

Symons, L. E. A. (1960). Pathology of infestation of the rat with *Nippostrongylus muris* (Yokogawa), IV. The absorption of glucose and histidine. *Aust. J. Biol. Sci.* **13**, 180–187.

Symons, L. E. A. (1961). Pathology of infestation of the rat with *Nippostrongylus muris* (Yokogawa), VI. Absorption in vivo from the distal ileum. *Aust. J. Biol. Sci.* **14**, 165–171.

Symons, L. E. A., and Fairbairn, D. (1962). Pathology, absorption, transport, and activity of digestive enzymes in the rat jejunum parasitized by the nematode *Nippostrongylus brasiliensis. Fed. Proc.* **21**, 913–918.

Villella, J. B. (1970). Life cycle and morphology. In S. E. Gould (ed.), "Trichinosis in Man and Animals." Charles C. Thomas, Springfield, Illinois, pp. 19-60.

Light and Electron Microscopy of the Intestinal Tissue of Mice Parasitized by *Trichinella spiralis*

George J. Race

Department of Pathology,
Baylor University Medical Center,
Dallas, Texas

John E. Larsh, Jr.

Department of Parasitology and Laboratory Practice,
School of Public Health,
University of North Carolina at Chapel Hill

James H. Martin

Department of Pathology,
Baylor University Medical Center,
Dallas, Texas

Norman F. Weatherly

Department of Parasitology and Laboratory Practice,
School of Public Health,
University of North Carolina at Chapel Hill

Introduction

In our first histopathological study of the anterior small intestine of mice 6 months old when challenged with *Trichinella spiralis* larvae (Larsh and Race, 1954), it was observed that the events were similar in those strongly immunized by four stimulating infections before being challenged and in controls given only the challenging infection. There was in both groups an acute inflammatory response predominated by "polymorpho-nuclear cells" (neutrophils) and a later subsiding subacute or chronic phase characterized by the presence of a mixed mononuclear collection of lymphocytes, plasma cells, and macrophages. These responses differed in the immune and nonimmune mice only in the time of the initiation of the inflammation and the severity of the response as measured, especially, by the numbers of infiltrating cells. In the immunized mice, an inflammatory response was evident at the first period (12 hr) selected for observation, and by 4 days the acute phase had reached a peak. This phase represented a severe panmucosal and submucosal inflammatory reaction. On the other hand, in the nonimmunized mice, inflammation was not evident until 4 days after challenge, and the peak of the acute response (at about 8 days) was much less striking than that noted in the immunized mice. At 7 days after the challenging infection, the immunized mice harbored significantly fewer worms in the small intestine than the previously nonimmunized mice, which had been shown earlier to expel significant numbers between 11 and 14 days (Larsh *et al.,* 1952). Therefore, in both groups, the elimination of significant numbers of adult worms occurred during a period when the inflammation was subsiding. This close association of intestinal inflammation and worm expulsion suggested that the former might be directly responsible for the latter.

In view of this possibility, attempts were made later to determine whether the degree of inflammation after challenge is related to the level of immunity at the time of the challenging infection. These studies provided evidence for a quantitative relation between the inflammation and elimination of adult worms. The least striking degree of inflammation and loss or stunting of worms was noted in mice immunized with larvae irradiated to prevent their development beyond the preadult, or Phase I, stage (Kim, 1957; Larsh *et al.,* 1959). An effect intermediate between this and the striking one noted above after the use of nonirradiated larvae for stimulating infections to involve Phase I, II, and III was observed when these larvae were irradiated to produce sterile adult worms, or Phases I and II (Larsh *et al.,* 1962). In addition, the relation between intestinal inflammation and worm loss was noted in young mice, 5 weeks old, infected with a single dose of *T. spiralis* larvae (Larsh *et al.,* 1956). In this case, inflammation developed between 5 and 7 days, it reached a peak at 11 days, and the worms were expelled between 15 and 17 days. Thus, as would be expected in immature mice that had not reached their full immunological competence, the inflammation developed more slowly and the reactions were much less severe than those noted above in mice 6 months of age when challenged in this way. Finally, it has been apparent in these various earlier histopathological studies that the size of the challenging infection dictates to an important degree the severity of the inflammatory response. Within limits, this would, of course, be expected to play a role in the anamnestic response.

We have used another approach in our laboratory to test the direct association of the inflammation and expulsion of adult worms. These studies were based on the premise that interference with the inflammation, or complete inhibition of it, should on the basis of our hypothesis result in the retention of adult worms. Two earlier studies employed the use of cortisone injections and whole-body, X-irradiation for this purpose. In both cases, the mice had been immunized by stimulating infections before being treated and challenged. After prolonged, daily injections of cortisone, the intestinal inflammation was prevented entirely, and adult worms from the challenging infection were not expelled (Coker, 1956). Likewise, irradiation treatment (450 R given 4 or 8 days before challenge produced similar results (Yarinsky, 1962; Larsh *et al.,* 1962).

With the recent interest in the effects of antilymphocytic serum on certain lymphoid tissues and associated immune responses (Lance, 1970), still another such approach to the study of the direct association of inflammation and worm loss seemed evident. If our hypothesis for the mechanism of immunity to *T. spiralis* in mice is valid (Larsh, 1967; Larsh *et al.,* 1964a, b, 1966, 1969, 1970a, b, 1972), the use of an antiserum, i.e., antithymocyte serum or ATS, to eliminate, or inactivate, the small, long-lived, recirculating lymphocytes (Simpson and Nehlsen, 1971; Lance, 1970) should prevent the specific delayed hypersensitivity response, and thereby the resultant tissue injury that triggers the nonspecific inflammatory response. Therefore, the present study was designed to test the effect of ATS in mice after they had been artificially sensitized by a method and schedule shown repeatedly to result in the expulsion of significant numbers of worms from a challenging infection.

Materials and Methods

Strain of Mouse and Parasite

The strain of Swiss white mice used in this study was one from our colony that has been randomly inbred for more than 30 years. Only males were used. The strain of *T. spiralis* is one that was isolated from a hog in 1936, and, after passages in laboratory rats for 7 years, it has been maintained in our strain of mice for more than 30 years.

Methods for Standardizing Doses and Infecting Mice

These were those recommended by Larsh and Kent (1949) with minor modifications by Weatherly (1970).

Preparation of the "Antigen–Adjuvant" Mixture for Sensitizing the Mice

These procedures have been detailed elsewhere (Larsh *et al.,* 1969, 1972). Each sensitization consisted of 0.08 ml (10 μg *Trichinella* protein) of the mixture (equal volumes of antigen and Freund's complete adjuvant), which was injected in equal amounts into each of the four footpads. The second sensitization was made later with a freshly prepared mixture.

ATS

The antiserum used in this study was obtained from Microbiological Associates, Inc., Bethesda, Maryland. It had been produced in rabbits by the use of mouse thymocytes and Freund's complete adjuvant. Its immunosuppressive power had been tested by skin grafts of DBA to C57BL/6 mice. Mean survival time was reported as 26.3 ±2.5 days, whereas in controls it was 10.4 ± 1.3 days. These preparations are reported to have low toxicity, hence are not absorbed before marketing.

To monitor the effect of the ATS on circulating WBC during the experiment, differential counts were made by conventional means. Eight additional mice were placed in each of the three groups to compare at intervals the average percentages of cell types in the experimentals (sensitized, then suppressed with ATS), sensitized controls (sensitized, not suppressed), and regular controls (not sensitized, not suppressed). Also, similar numbers of untreated, uninfected, mice were included to check the effect of the challenging infection on these measurements. The mice were marked so that they could be alternated for samples to avoid as much as possible the effects of repeated bleedings. Blood samples were first taken 4 days after the daily injections of ATS were begun, and at 3-day intervals until necropsy of the test mice, i.e., for a total span of 22 days.

The most pertinent observation was the effect of ATS on mononuclear cells. After 6 injections of ATS, the percentage of these cells had fallen to 22, compared with 68 for neutrophils. There was little change throughout the remainder of the experiment. The sensitized controls, on the other hand, showed about the reverse during the same period of time, i.e., 55% mononuclear cells versus 35% neutrophils.

Preparation of Tissues

For the reason that the majority of worms in a challenging infection in old mice (3 months and older) establish in the anterior half of the small intestine regardless of the level of immunity at the time of challenge, all of our tissue studies, including the present one, have been confined to this region. The entire anterior half of the small intestine was removed and fixed immediately in paraformaldehyde (Lynn *et al.,* 1966). Later, each sample was cut into links that ranged in size from 3 to 5 mm. Some of these segments were embedded in paraffin for the preparation of H & E sections by routine procedures. Others were cut into blocks about 2 mm long and 1 mm thick, postfixed in osmium tetroxide, and embedded in Epon 812 resin. Samples of these were sectioned with glass knives at 0.5–1.0 μm in thickness and stained with Paragon stain (Martin *et al.,* 1966). Other samples were used for electron microscope preparations. Thin sections from an ultramicrotome were stained with lead citrate and uranyl acetate for viewing under an RCA EMU-3 and a Phillips Model 300 electron microscope.

Method for Evaluating the Tissue Responses

The intestinal samples were collected and coded by one of us (NFW), and after preparation were assigned "blind" to another (GJR) for examinations. Also, some H & E sections were submitted "blind" to a third person (JEL) to allow for additional study and evaluation in the event that agreement was not evident in the two separate reports. It should be emphasized that it was necessary in some cases to examine large numbers of slides, in areas adjacent to and removed from the worms, before drawing conclusions as to the exact nature of the histopathological changes. This is an ever-present problem in such studies, but we believe the use of a small (100 larvae) challenging infection added to it in this instance. In any event, primary consideration in evaluating the tissue responses was given to the kinds and numbers of infiltrating cells. The initiation of acute inflammation and the severity of it were based on the time of the first appearance of infiltrating neutrophils, and, at later periods, on the increasing numbers of these cells. In all cases, efforts were made to select representative sections for photomicrographs that would illustrate the most consistent findings in the large numbers of sections examined.

We used the thin sections and the electron microscope sections to confirm certain pertinent findings, especially cell types, noted in the extensive studies of H & E sections.

Experimental Design

Sixty-six male mice, 12 weeks old, were separated into three groups of 22 each. Group I mice were the experimentals. On days 0 and 10, they were injected into the footpads with the antigen–adjuvant mixture prepared from *T. spiralis* larvae. On the day after the second sensitization, each mouse was injected intraperitoneally with 0.1 ml of ATS. These injections were continued daily for 15 additional days, at which time each mouse was challenged with 100 *T. spiralis* larvae. The daily ATS injections were continued until the mice were killed for study. Four each were killed at 2, 6, and 10 days after infection to obtain intestinal tissue samples, and the remaining 10 were killed at 11 days after challenge to recover and count the numbers of adult worms present in the small intestines.

It should be added that the time periods selected for tissue studies (2, 6, 10 days after challenge) were based on observations made in our earlier tissue work. Thus, the 2-day period was considered a logical one to show the expected earlier initiation of acute inflammation in the sensitized controls than in the regular controls, and the 6- and 10-day periods were considered satisfactory to measure within these limits of time the severity of this response in the two groups. We believed that a comparison of all three groups at these time periods would permit a conclusion either: (1) that the experimentals responded in a manner similar to one of the other groups, or, based on our hypothesis, (2) that they failed to develop acute inflammation during the period between challenge and necropsy.

The 22 Group II mice, the sensitized controls, were handled in the same way, except that ATS injections were not given. The 22 Group III mice were not sensitized or treated with ATS, hence they served as regular (normal) controls given only the challenging infection.

In other words, the experimentals were sensitized and then suppressed with ATS. The sensitized controls received the same two sensitizations, but were not suppressed, and the regular controls were neither sensitized nor suppressed. Comparisons among groups were made by tissue studies at 2, 6, and 10 days after infection, and by counts of adult worms at 11 days after infection. The results of the worm counts were presented elsewhere (Larsh *et al.,* 1972), hence the present report deals only with a comparison among the groups as to the tissue responses in the proximal half of the small intestine, and the serologic responses.

Serologic Tests

For the sake of direct comparison with results from infected donors in an earlier study (Larsh *et al.,* 1966), the same methods, and the same battery of tests and antigens were used, except that the complement-fixation test was added in the present study. Therefore, serum samples in the present experiment were tested by the indirect hemagglutination (IHA) test with Melcher's acid-soluble protein fraction, the bentonite floccula-tion (BF) test both with Melcher's and metabolic (ES) antigens, the screened latex agglutination (LA) test with Melcher's antigen, the indirect fluorescent antibody (IFA) test with cuticles of larvae as antigen, and the CDC laboratory branch complement-fixation (CF) test with Melcher's antigen. Blood for testing was collected from a separate group of experi-mental mice 17 days after the second sensitization when they had received 16 daily injections of ATS, and from another group 11 days after chal-lenge when they had received a total of 27 such injections. Samples from separate groups of the sensitized controls were taken at the same time, viz., 17 days after the second sensitization, and 11 days after challenge. The only sample from the regular controls was taken 11 days after chal-lenge. Of course, normal mouse serum samples, and those from infected mice were included in all tests as negative and positive controls, respec-tively.

Results

Light Microscope Observations of Paraffin Embedded Tissues

Two Days after Challenge   It was obvious by the examination of numer-ous H & E sections from the experimentals (sensitized, suppressed) that the 18 days of ATS treatment had produced striking small lymphocyte deple-tion in the thymus-dependent paracortical areas of lymph nodes (Fig. 1*). The degree of depletion is appreciated more fully by direct comparison

---

* Figures 1-14 are of tissues from the anterior half of the small intestine stained with hema-toxylin and eosin for study and photomicrograph preparation under the light microscope. All of these figures, except Figs. 1 and 2, include sections of adult *T. spiralis.* Figures 15–26 are of similar tissues that were processed for study and preparation of electron micrographs under the electron microscope.

with such tissue from a sensitized, nonsuppressed control at this time period (Fig. 2). Based on observations of sections in areas adjacent to, and removed from, the worms, there was little or no evidence of an inflammatory response in these experimental mice (Figs. 3 and 4). Some lymphocytes were noted, but not in numbers that appeared to be greater than normal.

In the sensitized controls (sensitized, not suppressed), the presence of neutrophils, although not numerous, indicated that the acute inflammatory response had been initiated (Figs. 5 and 6). In various sections, plasma cells also showed an increase over normal numbers.

In the regular controls (not sensitized, not suppressed), the absence of neutrophils indicated that the acute inflammatory response had not yet been initiated (Figs. 7 and 8), but some sections showed many plasma cells and lymphocytes.

Six Days after Challenge In the experimentals, sections of lymph nodes continued to show the depletion of paracortical areas, and there was no evidence of acute inflammation. As expected, the parasites were larger than those noted at 2 days, and an increase in plasma cells was noted around them. In the tissues of the sensitized controls, large numbers of neutrophils around the parasites indicated unquestionably that the acute inflammatory response was in progress. Again, numbers of plasma cells were noted in the surrounding mucosa. Finally, in the tissues of the regular controls, large mononuclear cells and lymphocytes had infiltrated without evidence of a necrotizing reaction, and the presence of a few infiltrating neutrophils indicated that the acute response had been initiated.

Ten Days after Challenge Overall, in the tissues of the experimentals, few infiltrating cells of all types were present (Fig. 9), hence suppression had continued to be effective to a striking degree. However, at higher magnification, some large mononuclear cells and plasma cells were seen (Fig. 10). In the tissues of the sensitized controls, the inflammatory reaction was striking (Fig. 11), and as evidenced by large numbers of neutrophils (Fig. 12), the acute response was recorded as marked in degree. It should be added that many other cell types were seen, including eosinophils. Finally, the tissues of the regular controls showed a moderate inflammatory reaction (Fig. 13) with the presence of infiltrating lymphocytes, plasma cells, and eosinophils. On the basis of the much smaller number of neutrophils present in the sections (Fig. 14), it was evident that the acute phase of the inflammation was considerably less severe at this time than that seen in the sensitized controls (Fig. 12).

Light Microscope Observations of Plastic Embedded Tissues

These Paragon-stained thin sections (0.5–1.0 μm thick) provide for tissue observations intermediate in magnification between those for

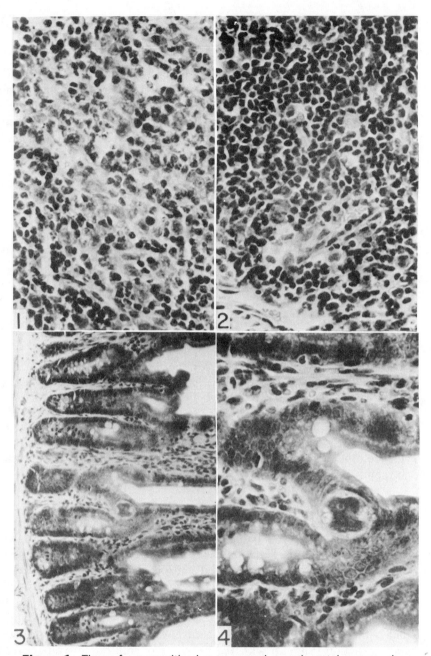

Figure 1 Tissue from sensitized, suppressed experimental mouse, showing striking lymphoid depletion in the thymus-dependent paracortical area of a lymph node. × 450.

Figure 2 Lymphoid tissue without depletion from a sensitized, nonsuppressed control mouse. Note contrast with Fig. 1. × 450.

Figure 3 Tissue from sensitized, suppressed mouse at 2 days, showing little or no evidence of inflammatory response in the intestinal mucosa. × 180.

Figure 4 Enlargement of Fig. 3. × 450.

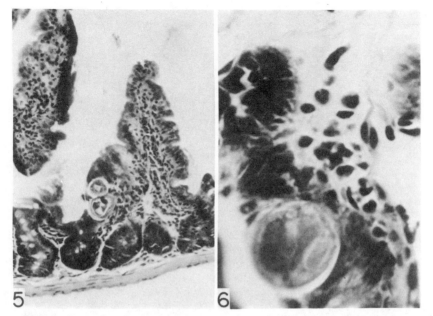

Figure 5 Tissue from sensitized, nonsuppressed control mouse at 2 days, showing presence of infiltrating neutrophils and mononuclear cells. Thus, the acute inflammatory response is under way. In some sections, plasma cells also were increased over normal numbers. × 180.

Figure 6 Higher magnification of tissue from sensitized, nonsuppressed mouse at 2 days. Note neutrophil. × 720.

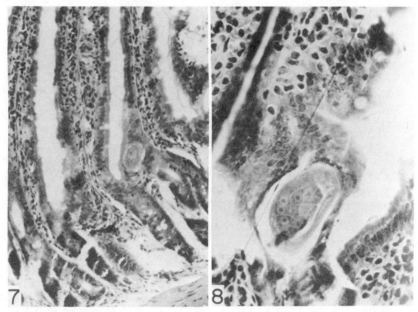

Figure 7 Regular control mouse, not sensitized and not supressed, at 2 days. The absence of neutrophils indicates that the acute inflammatory response has not yet been initiated. Some sections showed an increase in numbers of plasma cells and lymphocytes. × 180.

Figure 8 A higher magnification of tissue from another regular control at 2 days. × 450.

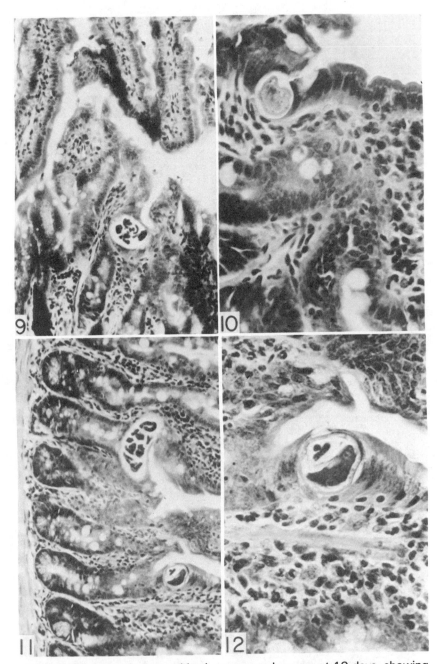

Figure 9 Tissue from sensitized, suppressed mouse at 10 days, showing few infiltrating cells of all types due to continued suppression. × 180.

Figure 10 Tissue from sensitized, suppressed mouse at 10 days at higher magnification, showing large mononuclear cells and plasma cells. × 450.

Figure 11 Tissue from sensitized, nonsuppressed mouse at 10 days, showing a marked, acute inflammatory reaction evidenced by infiltration of large numbers of neutrophils and many other cell types, including eosinophils. × 180.

Figure 12 Same as Fig. 11. Note numerous neutrophils. × 450.

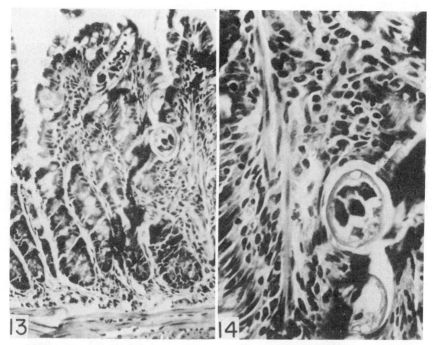

Figure 13 Tissue from a regular control at 10 days, showing a moderate inflammatory reaction with the presence of infiltrating lymphocytes, plasma cells, and eosinophils. Fewer neutrophils were present in these sections than in those from the sensitized, nonsuppressed mice. × 180.

Figure 14 Regular control mouse at 10 days. The acute inflamation was considerably less severe at this time than that noted in the sensitized, non-suppressed mice (Fig. 12). × 450.

routine histological study and studies by electron microscopy. On day 2, the preparations from the experimentals showed a close approximation of the worm cuticle to the surrounding tissue, the columnar absorbing cells, and mononuclear cells in the submucosa. In the sensitized controls, the greatest point of interest was the presence of lymphocytes in the superficial mucosa, and in the regular controls infiltrated mononuclear cells were evident.

On day 10, the noteworthy features were the large parasites and numerous plasma cells in the tissue samples from the sensitized controls, and lymphocytes, plasma cells, and eosinophils in the samples from the regular controls.

Electron Microscope Observations

Two Days after Challenge In sections from the experimentals, there was confirmation of the striking lymphoid depletion noted above in the H&E sections viewed by light microscopy. The columnar absorbing cells were intact. They, as well as the cuticle of the parasite, appeared to be normal in appearance (Fig. 15). Plasma cells were the predominant ones in these sections (Fig. 16). In the case of the sensitized controls, plasma cells also were seen (Fig. 17). However, it is noteworthy that at this early period other mononuclear cells were seen, as well as some neutrophils and eosinophils (Fig. 18). In another section, apparently through the stichosome region of the parasite, the hypodermal gland cell and secretory granules were evident (Fig. 19). As would have been expected from the above observations of H&E sections, decidedly fewer infiltrating cells were noted in tissues from the regular controls (Figs. 20 and 21).

Ten Days after Challenge   Again, in the tissues of the experimentals, plasma cells predominated (Figs. 22 and 23). In tissues from the sensitized controls and the regular controls, confirmation of the above observations of H&E sections was obtained. Neutrophils, eosinophils, and plasma cells were noted in sections of tissue from the sensitized controls (Fig. 24), and in tissues of the regular controls, lymphocytes, plasma cells, and eosinophils were seen (Figs. 25 and 26).

Serologic Results   These results are shown in Table I. At 17 days after the second sensitization, it will be noted that the serums of both the experimentals and sensitized controls were positive in low titers in some tests. For the reason that the IFA test can show reactions with any antibody, perhaps these results are most meaningful. Considering the limits of reproducibility of this test ($\pm$ one fourfold dilution), there was little or no

Table I   Serologic Results at Two Time Periods after Sensitization

	Antibody titers in the various tests					
	BF		LA	IHA	CF	IFA
Group of mice	(ML35)[a]	(LES)[b]	(ML35)[a]	(ML35)[a]	(ML35)[a]	(LCA)[c]
Experimentals						
A. 17 days after sensitization	–	–	–	1:128	1:8	1:4
B. 28 days after sensitization[d]	–	1:5	–	1:128	AC[e]	1:16
Sensitized Controls						
A. 17 days after sensitization	–	1:10	+	1:256	1:16	1:16
B. 28 days after sensitization[d]	1:5	1:10	+	1:256	1:32	1:16
Regular Controls						
11 days after challenge	–	–	–	–	–	1:4

[a] Melcher's larvae acid-soluble fraction antigen, lot 35 (CDC).
[b] Larval excretion-secretion antigen.
[c] Larval cuticular antigen.
[d] Eleven days after challenge.
[e] Anticomplementary.

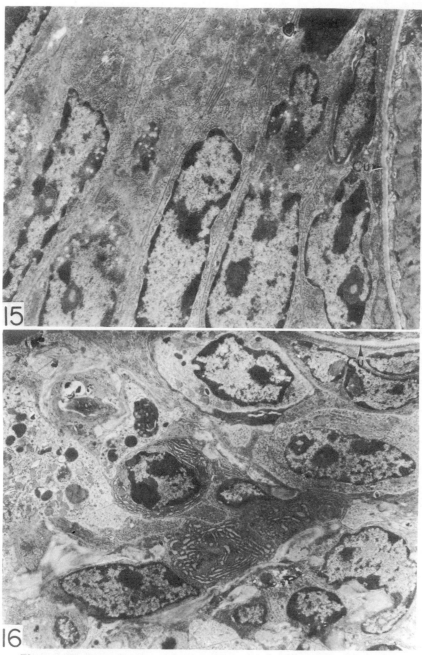

Figure 15 Electron micrograph (EM) of tissue from sensitized, suppressed mouse at 2 days, showing normal columnar epithelium and cuticle (Cu) of parasite. × 7850.

Figure 16 Sensitized, suppressed mouse at 2 days. EM showing presence of plasma cells. Note parasite cuticle (Cu). × 5350.

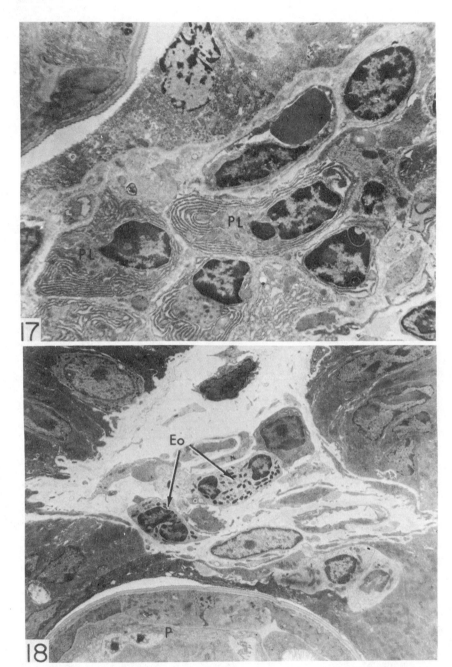

Figure 17 Sensitized, nonsuppressed mouse at 2 days. EM showing multiple plasma cells (PL). × 5850.

Figure 18 Sensitized, nonsuppressed mouse at 2 days. EM showing eosinophils (Eo) and parasite (P). × 3700.

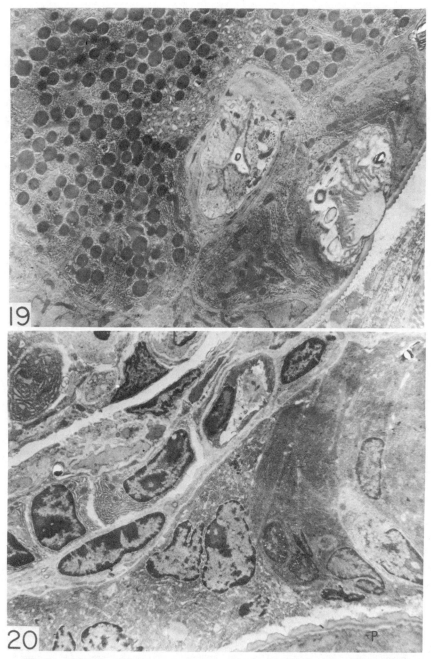

Figure 19 Sensitized, nonsuppressed mouse at 2 days. EM showing parasite with hypodermal gland cell and secretory granules. × 6150.
Figure 20 Regular control mouse at 2 days. EM showing younger plasma cells, columnar cells, and parasite (P). × 5400.

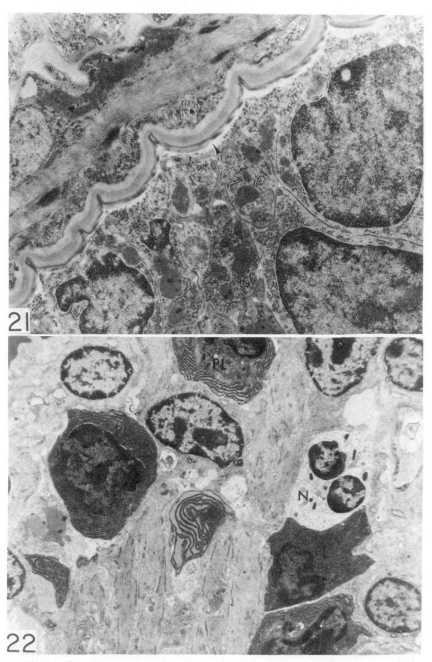

Figure 21 Regular control mouse at 2 days. Note junction of parasite and columnar epithelial cells (arrow). × 14,000.
Figure 22 Sensitized, suppressed mouse at 10 days. EM showing plasma cells (PL) with one neutrophil (N). × 5350.

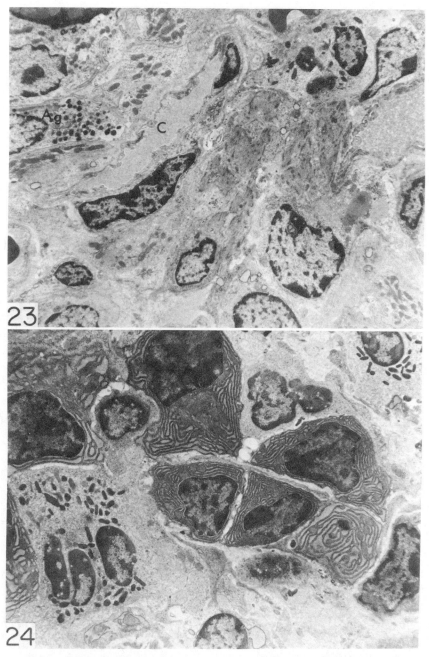

Figure 23 Sensitized, suppressed mouse at 10 days. EM showing eosinophil, smooth muscle, capillary (C), and argentaffine cell with characteristic granules (Ag). × 6500.

Figure 24 Sensitized, nonsuppressed mouse at 10 days. Note multiple large plasma cells and two eosinophils. × 5300.

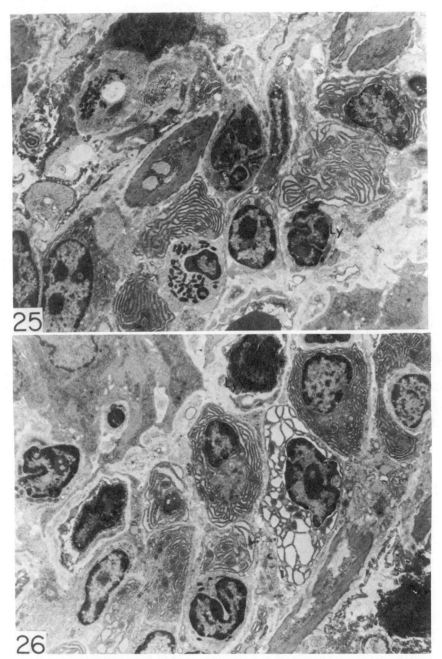

Figure 25 Regular control mouse at 10 days. EM showing multiple plasma cells, eosinophils, and lymphocyte (Ly). × 5400.

Figure 26 Regular control mouse at 10 days. Note neutrophil, plasma cells, and lymphocyte (Ly). × 5400.

difference between titers of the two groups. At 28 days after the second sensitization, the IFA titers were the same in these groups, and little difference was noted in the other positive tests. Therefore, the challenging infection with living larvae produced little, if any, effect on the serologic responses of these mice within 11 days. The serum of the regular controls given only the challenging infection reacted only in the IFA test at low titer. It should be added that normal mouse serum samples were negative in all tests, whereas those from mice infected with 400 larvae 7 weeks earlier were negative in the LA test and positive in the BF test with Melcher's antigen (1:5) and metabolic antigen (1:1280), in the IHA test with Melcher's antigen (1:256), in the CF test with Melcher's antigen (1:16), and in the IFA test with cuticular antigen (1:4).

Discussion

The above observations of tissue responses as revealed in H&E sections of the small intestine of the sensitized, nonsuppressed controls and the regular controls compared favorably with those reported earlier in old mice given a stimulating infection(s) before challenge (Larsh and Race, 1954; Larsh et al., 1959, 1962, 1966) and in their controls, as well as in young mice after an initial infection (Larsh et al., 1956). Previously stimulated mice responded more rapidly after challenge than controls, as evidenced by an earlier initiation of acute intestinal inflammation, and showed a more severe reaction at the peak period. Therefore, the present results with mice artificially sensitized with products from infective larvae would seem to indicate that the provocative allergen(s) is contained within, or released from, these larvae. In any event, the association of the inflammation and later expulsion of significant numbers of adult worms in all of the previous studies also was confirmed in the present one. At 11 days after the challenging infection with 100 larvae, the sensitized controls harbored significantly fewer adult worms than the regular controls (Larsh et al., 1972).

Perhaps due to the use of a comparatively small challenging infection in the present study, early infiltration of mononuclear cells was seen. Although these cells, which are observed characteristically in areas of delayed hypersensitivity (DH) responses, migrate to local areas of DH involvement at about the same time as neutrophils that are thought to be responding to the chemotactic factors released in the areas of tissue injury, the latter move much more rapidly and in larger numbers (Movat, 1971). For this reason, especially in cases of severe local injury, the great abundance of neutrophils can mask the early presence of mononuclear cells, leaving a false impression of their absence. The reason for the predominance of mononuclear cells in the later phase (subacute or chronic) appears to be due mainly to the death of the neutrophils, which have been shown to have a short life span compared with that of the mononuclears (Cronkite and Fliedner, 1964). In any case, our failure to note an early mononuclear infiltration in mice strongly immunized by stimulating infections before being challenged by a large dose (400) of larvae (Larsh and Race, 1954) probably was due to a masking effect of the neutrophils. This is supported by the fact that in a later study with a much smaller challenging dose (100) of larvae such early infiltration was observed (Larsh *et al.*, 1966).

The presence of mononuclear cells in the sensitized, nonsuppressed controls at 2 days after challenge in the present study, as evidenced by observations of paraffin (Figs. 5 and 6) and plastic embedded sections under the light microscope, as well as those made under the electron microscope, would suggest that their migration was in response to a chemotactic factor(s) released by committed small lymphocytes after interaction with the specific allergen (Bloom, 1969). In the actual event of such a specific DH reaction, it would be expected on the basis of an anamnestic response that the sensitized cell-allergen reaction had occurred soon after challenge in these mice that had been strongly sensitized by two prior footpad injections with allergen and Freund's complete adjuvant.

Another early observation in the sensitized, nonsuppressed controls was the presence of eosinophils (Fig. 18). The results of Basten and Beeson (1970) in studies with rats provide strong support for a role of lymphocytes in the mechanism of eosinopoiesis. Most germane to the present discussion was their finding that rabbit antirat ALS injected 24 hours before, and daily for 5 days after, challenge with *T. spiralis* resulted in a significant reduction in the numbers of blood eosinophils compared with those in controls injected with normal rabbit serum. The fact that "sensitized" lymphocytes enclosed in diffusion chambers were still capable of stimulating eosinopoiesis was interpreted by them to mean that a diffusible factor exerted an effect on bone marrow. This suggests to us the possibility that activated lymphocytes, i.e., after interaction with the specific allergen, might release an effector molecule that is specifically chemotactic for eosinophils and thus would explain their presence in the tissue soon after challenge (Fig. 18). On the other hand, it is possible that the diffusible substance of Basten and Beeson requires interaction with a specific immune complex to produce the chemotactic factor for eosinophils as suggested by the work of Cohen and Ward (1971). They found that lymphocytes from lymph nodes of delayed-hypersensitive guinea pigs, when cultured in the presence of specific antigen, released an active soluble substance(s) that reacted *in vitro* with immune complexes formed with the same antigen to produce a potent chemotactic factor for eosinophils. They showed that this specific factor possesses *in vivo* as well as *in vitro* activity and, therefore, it might be important in situations where eosinophils are participants in inflammatory or immunological reactions.

The above observations of tissue responses by these various means in the sensitized experimentals suppressed with ATS bear out the conclusions reached by others after prolonged administration of this potent immuno-suppressant to mice (Simpson and Nehlsen, 1971). In addition to our demonstration of the depletion of small lymphocytes in the thymus-dependent paracortical areas of lymph nodes, these workers also showed that in more than 90% of nodes examined, there was hyperplasia of medullary plasma cells even in mice treated continuously with ATS for many months. In addition, they observed small lymphocyte depletion of the thymus-dependent periarteriolar region of the spleen in most of the mice observed. Considering the putative preferential suppression by ALS of cell-mediated responses as opposed to humoral responses, and in view of the evidence that this immunosuppressant does not have a discernible effect on secondary humoral responses (Medawar, 1969; Lance, 1970), it is especially noteworthy that we observed, as did Simpson and Nehlsen (1971), the persistence of plasma cells at all periods tested.

The sensitized, suppressed experimental mice, despite continued injections of ATS, showed a slight rise in serologic reactivity as measured by two separate tests (BF with metabolic antigen, and the IFA test with larvae cuticular antigen) during the 11 days after the challenging infection until necropsy (Table I). However, because these rises were so slight, and in view of using living larvae for the challenge, no conclusion can be made in this instance as to the effect of the ATS on the secondary humoral response. When the battery of serologic tests used here (minus the CF test) was employed in an earlier study (Larsh et al., 1966), it is of interest that the serum from the donor mice infected with 400 larvae 31 days previously reacted only in the IHA test (1:200). A similar response (1:256) was noted in the positive serum controls used in the present study with serum from mice infected 7 weeks previously, but reactivity also was noted in the BF test with both antigens, and in the CF and IFA tests. These results in mice infected with the same dose of larvae might suggest that the IHA response is comparatively early, whereas the others develop later. In any event, it is clear that our mice, whether stimulated with living larvae or artificially sensitized by larval extract, are poor antibody producers as measured by tests considered to be the best ones available for use in trichinellosis.

As shown earlier in our mice subjected to cortisone or whole-body, X-irradiation, the sensitized experimentals suppressed with ATS harbored at 11 days after the challenging infection significantly more worms than the sensitized, nonsuppressed controls (Larsh et al., 1972). In fact, the suppressed mice harbored about the same number of worms as the regular controls. Therefore, we have now shown by three different treatments that the worms are not expelled in the absence of the acute inflammatory response. In the case of ATS, it is of direct interest that two other laboratories have reported the prolonged persistence of T. spiralis in mice after an initial infection when this immunosuppressant was administered (Kozar *et al.,* 1971; Machnicka, 1972), and that another laboratory has reported the same observation after use of ALS (DiNetta *et al.,* 1972).

In conclusion, the present study has provided additional direct support for our view that the nonspecific inflammatory responses in the small intestine after challenge are the secondary, but direct, cause for the elimination of significant numbers of adult worms. Indirect support for the role of nonspecific intestinal inflammation in the expulsion of adult worms comes from earlier observations in our laboratory after challenging mice with *T. spiralis* 2 days after an oral infection with 800 *Ancylostoma caninum* larvae (Cox 1952; Goulson, 1958), and from observations elsewhere after such challenge of mice infected with *Salmonella typhimurium* (Brewer, 1955). In the *A. caninum* studies, the subsequent initial infection with 200 or 240 *T. spiralis* larvae resulted in a significant reduction in the average numbers of adult *T. spiralis* recovered 7 days later compared with those in controls infected only with *T. spiralis.* Based on studies by Kerr (1936), who reported that neutrophilic infiltration into the intestinal tissue of mice had occurred within 24 hours after oral infection with *A. caninum* and that the cellular response reached a zenith at 48 hours, it would appear that this inflammatory response was in some way responsible for the reduced numbers of adult *T. spiralis* recovered after the dual infections. In the case of *S. typhimurium,* the larvae of *T. spiralis* and the bacterial inoculum were given simultaneously by the oral route and there was a reduction in the average number of adult *T. spiralis* recovered after 7 days as compared with controls. Inflammation produced rapidly by the bacteria was suggested as the most likely cause of this phenomenon (Brewer, 1955).

In all probability, certain of the many chemical changes known to occur as a consequence of acute inflammation create conditions unfavorable for the worms. One example of indirect evidence for this is the change in the distribution of the worms after challenging immunized and nonimmunized mice with 200 larvae (Larsh *et al.,* 1952). In these mice, 5–6 months old at necropsy, regardless of their level of immunity at the time of challenge, the majority of worms established in the anterior half of the small intestine. However, between 3 and 11 days, the immunized mice harbored significantly fewer worms in this region, whereas between 14 and 24 days the numbers were similar. The greatest difference between groups was at 7 days. The numbers of worms in the large intestines of both groups were relatively low for the first 4 days. The peak of worms in this region was noted soon after the sudden loss of worms from the anterior half of the small intestine (between 5–7 days in the immunized mice, and 11–14 days in the nonimmunized mice), and relatively large numbers persisted for many days. Therefore, in view of the fact that there was not a significant difference between the two groups in the numbers of worms in the posterior half of the small intestine for 14 days after challenge, these various observations would suggest that the change in distribution of the worms was due to an unfavorable environment in the upper small intestine.

In any case, a more direct and convincing observation has been made recently in regard to one chemical change associated with inflammation, viz., acidosis, which had a significant detrimental effect on *T. spiralis* (Castro *et al.,* 1973). In the likelihood that such changes due to inflammation are important in the expulsion of this and other tissue parasites, it appears that a fertile field of investigation has been opened for those with the skills to study and assess the physiological and biochemical changes that follow tissue injury produced in response to such agents.

Summary

This study involved the use of three groups of mice: (1) experimentals, sensitized and then suppressed with antithymocyte serum (ATS), (2) sensitized controls, sensitized and not suppressed, and (3) regular controls, not sensitized and not suppressed. At 2 and 10 days after a challenging infection, tissue samples from the anterior small intestine were prepared by routine histological techniques and by the Paragon-stained thin section technique for examination under the light microscope, and by electron microscope techniques for study under the electron microscope. Observations at 6 days after infection were limited to the examination of routine H&E sections.

At all time periods, the H&E sections of tissues from the experimentals showed depletion of the thymus-dependent areas of lymph nodes, and there was no evidence of an acute inflammatory response. On the other hand, the tissues of the sensitized controls and regular controls showed responses similar to those reported in several of our earlier studies. That is, acute inflammation was seen at the 2-day period in the sensitized controls, and it was much more pronounced at the 6-day and, especially, the 10-day period when it was marked in degree. In contrast, inflammation was not evident at the 2-day period in the regular controls, and it was minimal at 6 days and only moderate at 10 days.

The observations of the Paragon-stained thin sections and the electron microscope preparations confirmed certain pertinent findings, especially cell types, noted in the extensive studies of the H&E sections.

The results of this study substantiated the previously reported potent immunosuppressant effect of ATS; they showed that the suppressed mice failed to develop acute intestinal inflammation, and that the initiation of this response was earlier, and at its zenith it was much more severe in the sensitized, nonsuppressed mice than in the nonsensitized, nonsuppressed mice. Serologic findings with various tests were inconclusive.

Acknowledgements

The authors acknowledge with sincere appreciation the assistance in the serologic studies of Miss Dorothy Allain and Dr. Alexander J. Sulzer of CDC. Supported in part by Grant AI-10,671 from the U.S. National Institutes of Health.

References

Basten, A., and Beeson, P. B. (1970). Mechanism of eosinophilia. II. Role of the lymphocycte. *J. Exp. Med.* **131**, 1288–1305.

Bloom, B. R. (1969). Elaboration of effector molecules by activated lymphocytes. In H. S. Lawrence and M. Landy (eds.), "Mediators of Cellular Immunity" Academic Press, New York, pp. 252–256.

Brewer, O. M. (1955). A study of the effects of *Salmonella typhimurium* on the acquired resistance of mice to *Trichinella spiralis*. *J. Elisha Mitchell Sci. Soc.* **71**, 170–171.

Castro, G. A., Cotter, M. V., Ferguson, J. D., and Gorden, C. W. (1973). Trichinosis: physiologic factors possibly altering the course of infection. *J. Parasitol.* **59**, 268–276.

Cohen, S., and Ward, P. A. (1971). *In vitro* and *in vivo* activity of a lymphocyte and immune complex-dependent chemotactic factor for eosinophils. *J. Exp. Med.* **133**, 133–146.

Coker, C. M. (1956). Some effects of cortisone in mice with acquired immunity to *Trichinella spiralis*. *J. Infec. Dis.* **98**, 39–44.

Cox, H. W. (1952). The effect of concurrent infection with the dog hookworm, *Ancylostoma caninum*, on the natural and acquired resistance of mice to *Trichinella spiralis*. *J. Elisha Mitchell Sci. Soc.* **68**, 222–235.

Cronkite, E. P., and Fliedner, T. M. (1964). Granulocytopoiesis. *N. Engl. J. Med.* **270**, 1347 and 1403.

DiNetta, J., Katz, F., and Campbell, W. C. (1972). Effect of heterologous antilymphocyte serum on the spontaneous cure of *Trichinella spiralis* infections in mice. *J. Parasitol.* **58**, 636–637.

Goulson, H. T. (1958). Studies on the influence of a prior infection with *Ancylostoma caninum* on the establishment and maintenance of *Trichinella spiralis* in mice. *J. Elisha Mitchell Sci. Soc.* **74**, 14–23.

Kerr, K. B. (1936). Studies on acquired immunity to the dog hookworm, *Ancylostoma caninum*. *Amer. J. Hyg.* **24**, 381–406.

Kim, C. W. (1957). Immunity to *Trichinella spiralis* in mice infected with irradiated larvae. *J. Elisha Mitchell Sci. Soc.* **73**, 308–317.

Kozar, Z., Karmańska, K., Kotz, J., and Seniuta, R. (1971). The influence of antilymphocytic serum (ALS) on the course of trichinellosis in mice. I. Histological, histochemical and immunohistological changes observed in the intestines. *Wiad. Parazytol.* **17**, 541–548.

Lance, E. M. (1970). The selective action of antilymphocyte serum on recirculating lymphocytes: a review of the evidence and alternatives. *Clin. Exp. Immunol.* **6**, 789–802.

Larsh, J. E., Jr. (1967). The present understanding of the mechanism of immunity to *Trichinella spiralis*. *Amer. J. Trop. Med. Hyg.* **16**, 123–132.

Larsh, J. E., Jr., and Kent, D. E. (1949). The effect of alcohol on natural and acquired immunity of mice to infection with *Trichinella spiralis*. *J. Parasitol.* **35**, 45–53.

Larsh, J. E., Jr., and Race, G. J. (1954). A histopathologic study of the anterior small intestine of immunized and nonimmunized mice infected with *Trichinella spiralis*. *J. Infec. Dis.* **94**, 262–272.

Larsh, J. E., Jr., Gilchrist, H. B., and Greenberg, B. G. (1952). A study of the distribution and longevity of adult *Trichinella spiralis* in immunized and nonimmunized mice. *J. Elisha Mitchell Sci. Soc.* **68**, 1–11.

Larsh, J. E., Jr., Race, G. J., and Jeffries, W. B. (1956). The association in young mice of intestinal inflammation and the loss of adult worms following an initial infection with *Trichinella spiralis*. *J. Infec. Dis.* **99**, 63–71.

Larsh, J. E., Jr., Race, G. J., and Goulson, H. T. (1959). A histopathologic study of mice immunized with irradiated larvae of *Trichinella spiralis*. *J. Infec. Dis.* **104**, 156–163.

Larsh, J. E., Jr., Race, G. J., and Yarinsky, A. (1962). A histopathologic study in mice immunized against *Trichinella spiralis* and exposed to total-body X-irradiation. *Amer. J. Trop. Med. Hyg.* **11**, 633–640.

Larsh, J. E., Jr., Goulson, H. T., Weatherly, N. F. (1964a). Studies on delayed (cellular) hypersensitivity in mice infected with *Trichinella spiralis*. II. Transfer of peritoneal exudate cells. *J. Parasitol.* **50**, 496–498.

Larsh, J. E., Jr., Goulson, H. T., and Weatherly, N. F. (1964b). Studies on delayed (cellular) hypersensitivity in mice infected with *Trichinella spiralis*. I. Transfer of lymph node cells. *J. Elisha Mitchell Sci. Soc.* **80**, 133–135.

Larsh, J. E., Jr., Race, G. J., Goulson, H. T., and Weatherly, N. F. (1966). Studies on delayed (cellular) hypersensitivity in mice infected with *Trichinella spiralis*. III. Serologic and histopathologic findings in recipients given peritoneal exudate cells. *J. Parasitol.* **52**, 146–156.

Larsh., J. E., Jr., Goulson, H. T., Weatherly, N. F., and Chaffee, E. F. (1969). Studies on delayed (cellular) hypersensitivity in mice infected with *Trichinella spiralis*. IV. Artificial sensitization of donors. *J. Parasitol.* **55**, 726–729.

Larsh, J. E., Jr., Goulson, H. T., Weatherly, N. F., and Chaffee, E. F. (1970a). Studies on delayed (cellular) hypersensitivity in mice infected with *Trichinella spiralis*. V. Tests in recipients injected with donor spleen cells 1, 3, 7, 14, or 21 days before infection. *J. Parasitol.* **56**, 978–981.

Larsh, J. E., Jr., Goulson, H. T., Weatherly, N. F., and Chaffee, E. F. (1970b). Studies on delayed (cellular) hypersensitivity in mice infected with *Trichinella spiralis*. VI. Results in recipients injected with antiserum or "freeze-thaw" spleen cells. *J. Parasitol.* **56**, 1206–1209.

Larsh, J. E., Jr., Weatherly, N. F., Goulson, H. T., and Chaffee, E. F. (1972). Studies on delayed (cellular) hypersensitivity in mice infected with *Trichinella spiralis*. VII. The effect of ATS injections on the numbers of adult worms recovered with challenge. *J. Parasitol.* **58**, 1052–1060.

Lynn, J. A., Martin, J. H., and Race, G. J. (1966). Recent improvements of histologic technics for the combined light and electron microscopic examination of surgical specimens. *Amer. J. Clin. Pathol.* **45**, 704–713.

Machnicka, B. (1972). *Trichinella spiralis*: influence of antilymphocytic serum on mouse infections. *Exp. Parasitol.* **31**, 172–177.

Martin J. H., Lynn, J. A., and Nickey, W. M. (1966). A rapid polychrome stain for epoxy-embedded tissue. *Amer. J. Clin. Pathol.* **46**, 250–251.

Medawar, P. B. (1969). Antilymphocytic serum: its properties and potential. *Hosp. Prac.* May issue, 26–33.

Movat, H. Z. (1971). The acute inflammatory reaction. In H. Z. Movat (ed.) "Inflammation, Immunity and Hypersensitivity." Harper & Row, New York, p. 88.

Simpson, E., and Nehlsen, S. L. (1971). Prolonged administration of antithymocyte serum in mice. II. Histopathological investigation. *Clin. Exp. Immunol.* **9,** 79-98.

Weatherly, N. F. (1970). Increased survival of Swiss mice given sublethal infections of *Trichinella spiralis. J. Parasitol.* **56,** 748–752.

Yarinsky, A. (1962). The influence of X-irradiation on the immunity of mice to infection with *Trichinella spiralis. J. Elisha Mitchell Sci. Soc.* **78,** 29–43.

Inhibition and Prevention of Inflammatory Reactions to Helminth Larvae in Host Tissues

Y. A. Berezantsev

Department of Epidemiology and Parasitology
Medical Institute of Sanitation and Hygiene
Leningrad

Introduction

The most intimate host–parasite relations are displayed in intracellular and tissue parasitism. The interrelation of tissue parasites and the host has not yet been sufficiently investigated. Of special interest is the compatibility of these organisms particularly under long-term parasitization. Attention should be drawn to morphological and physiological relations between the larvae of various parasitic worms and the intermediate and reservoir host tissues. Acute inflammation produced in response to such a parasite invasion disappears, and capsules of a peculiar morphological structure, unlike usual cicatricial tissue, are formed around the larvae. In some cases of larval development, the phagocytic reaction is entirely absent from the tissues.

Why then, in spite of different antigenic structures of the two organisms, and the immune response developing in the host against the parasites, do the latter survive in host tissues without provoking any acute inflammatory events? One knows that even in cases of tissue or organ homotransplantation (monozygotic twins excepted) the antigenic incompatibility results in graft rejection or resorption as soon as the antibody titer of the recipient becomes sufficiently high. In the host, on the contrary, capsules of specific structure provide an optimal environment for parasites often for several years. In our view, both suppression of the leukocytic reaction and formation of capsules occur under the influence of parasites, an ability that developed during the process of evolution.

The present article deals with a morphological study on the relations between tissue larvae of some trematode, cestode, and nematode species and the host body; it enabled us to place the problem in new light.

Materials and Methods

Several experimental parasite–host systems were used. These were metacercariae of *Posthodiplostomum cuticula* in fishes; plerocercoids of *Diphyllobothrium latum* in fishes and amphibians; *Spirometra erinacei-europaei* in golden hamsters; strobilocerci of *Hydatigera taeniaeformis* in white mice and rats; *Toxocara canis* larvae in the kidneys of dogs; *Physocephalus sexalatus* (Spirurata) in amphibians, reptiles, birds, and mammals, and *Trichinella spiralis* larvae in white mice and rats. In addition, a great number of cases was studied of spontaneous invasion of fishes by the plerocercoids of *D. latum;* of amphibians and reptiles by plerocercoids of *S. erinacei-europaei;* of various species of rodents by strobilocerci of *H. taeniaeformis;* of the intermediate hosts by *Taenia hydatigena, T. pisiformis, T. solium, T. crabbei, T. parenchimatosa, Taeniarhynchus saginatus;* of ungulate mammals and man by *Echinococcus granulosus;* of various rodents by *E. multilocularis;* of various species of mammals and man by *T. spiralis* larvae; and of moles by *Porrocaecum depressum* (Ascaridata, Anisakidae).

The organs and tissues invaded by helminth larvae were examined hislogically. For the purpose of comparison, the same technique was used to examine the capsules surrounding foreign bodies (pieces of paraffin or celloidin) that were introduced subcutaneously into fishes, amphibians, and mammals.

Results

Trichinella larvae within a muscle fiber should, at first, be thought of as an intracellular parasite. Like a barrier, the sarcolemma, a semipermeable biological membrane, prevents the parasite from being affected by humoral and phagocytic reactions of the host. Although the larva is developing in a muscle fiber, the leukocytes do not penetrate below the sarcolemma. Only later (from day 14) do they begin to destroy at some length the invaded and distrophically altered muscle fiber not involving the area of sarcoplasm adjacent to the larva. During the entire period of parasitization, the parasite is closely associated with this area by metabolic processes. As soon as a bit of sarcoplasm becomes "naked," probably through losing the sarcolemma, it will be encapsulated together with the larva developed within it. The encapsulated sarcoplasm shows reactive alterations; it contains divided nuclei of the muscle cell with large nucleoli (from RNA), increased cytoplasmic glycogen and RNA content, and increased amounts of mitochondria, endoplasmic reticulum. Golgi complexes, etc. (Themann, 1960; Bruce, 1970; and others). An intensive protein synthesis, high activity of succinate dehydrogenase, of alkaline and acid phosphatase as well as of other enzymes is demonstrated (Stoner and Hankes, 1962; Zarzycki, 1963; Stoyanov and Nenov, 1965; Schanzel and Holman, 1966; Kozar *et al.*, 1969; Bruce, 1970; and others).

The thick interior layer of the capsule consists of hyalinized collagen. In due course, it thickens, especially at the poles; later on, calcification occurs and spreads over the entire capsule, which, finally, leads to destruction of the larva (Berezantsev, 1961). Cellular elements, newly formed vessels, preterminal sensory nerve fibers and nerve endings are located in a very thin external layer of the capsule. The supply of nutritional substances from the blood and the removal of metabolic products occurs through the capsule. High molecular weight proteins cannot penetrate through the wall. It protects the parasite from phagocytes and from specific antibodies that may appear in the host's blood. If larvae are placed into immune serum, precipitates are formed around oral openings, and the larvae introduced into muscles or the abdominal cavity are soon destroyed by phagocytosis. Glucose, salt ions, and various substances (including amino acids) pass through the larval capsule and cuticle. Those substances labeled with iodine, phosphorus, carbon, etc., isotopes were demonstrated in the capsule, in the encapsulated sarcoplasm, and in the larva by the autoradiographic method (McCoy *et al.*, 1941; Stoner and Hankes, 1955; Zarzycki *et al.*, 1966; Kasprzak *et al.*, 1971).

We consider the capsule formed around *Trichinella* larvae as a specific inflammatory process that develops in response to certain compounds excreted by the parasite. The capsule acquires an organelle-like structure. Prevention of the protective inflammatory reaction occurs (Berezantsev, 1960, 1962a, 1963). A certain physiological "equilibrium" is established between the parasites and host by the capsules, which provides the larvae a longer life expectancy. Acute inflammation is absent in the developed capsules (Fig. 1). It reappears only if larvae are destroyed, or during their "aging." It depends, to our mind, on reduced physiological activity of the parasite. Hence, the synthesis of substances that induce the capsule-forming reaction of the host appears to be disturbed. This also occurs, for all appearances, by activation of the protective reactions of the host. In such a case, the capsule wall reveals an accumulation of leukocytes, macrophages, and giant cells that destroy the capsule, the encapsulated sarcoplasm, and the larva within it. Such destruction of some part of the encapsulated larvae takes place at different periods of invasion (Fig. 2).

The larvae of many other species of nematodes may also be encapsulated in the tissues of vertebrate reservoir hosts. The specificity of the structure of the capsules of these larvae depends on the extent of their adaptation to tissue parasitism (Berezantsev, 1962b). The larvae, by chance prevented from migration (e.g., *Ascaris suum* in laboratory animals), will be encapsulated as foreign bodies and destroyed. *Toxocara canis* larvae appear to be, to some extent, adapted to tissue parasitism and may be

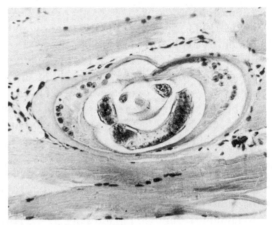

Figure 1 *Trichinella spiralis* larva surrounded by a capsule with a thick hyaline layer under which one may see an area of sarcoplasm with altered muscular nuclei. Muscles of white rat 5.5 months after infection.× 180.

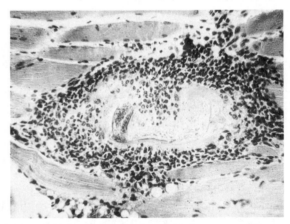

Figure 2 Break of the capsule by leukocytes that had penetrated to a dead *T. spiralis* larva. White mouse 1.5 years after infection. × 180.

encapsulated in tissues of different mammals. Their capsules, although showing signs of inflammation, acquire the features of a specific structure. *Physocephalus sexalatus* larvae are well-adapted tissue parasites, and a relative physiological equilibrium may be achieved between them and their reservoir hosts. Their capsules in the tissue of vertebrates have the same organization. The internal layer of the capsule consists of young fibroblasts in which RNA can be demonstrated. The thick external layer is constructed of concentrically arranged fibroblasts and collagenous fibers provided with blood vessels. The capsules still contain a small amount of inflammatory cells (Fig. 3). An organlike structure is characteristic of the capsules of *P. depressum* larvae. A layer of young uniform fibroblasts, also having a high content of RNA and arranged concentrically, adjoin them directly. Outward they become continuous with a more mature fibrous tissue. The third external layer of the capsule consists of a small-meshed network of collagenous fibers in whose meshes lymphocytes predominate. The layer is rich in lymphatic vessels. The capsule enclosing the larva is covered with a peritoneal sheet and suspended from the stomach surface of the mole (reservoir host) on a thin fibrous pedicle through which large vessels pass to supply the capsule (Fig. 4).

A certain consistent pattern is observed in the capsules of nematode larvae. Close to the parasite there is located a reactively altered tissue: either young fibroblasts or an area of sarcoplasm *(T. spiralis).*

Cestode larvae are adapted tissue parasites, which indicates they are ancient parasites. Plerocercoids of Diphyllobothriidae and Taeniidae are responsible for the formation of specific uniform two-layered connective capsules in different tissues of intermediate hosts (Berezantsev, 1962c). Their internal layer consists of a dense fibrous tissue poor in cellular elements and not infrequently hyalinized *(E. granulosus, T. solium, T. hydatigena).* The external layer of the capsule is of a loose-fibrous structure with a multitude of cellular elements and vessels. Around the *E. granulosus* cysts, there are developing thick capsules; cysticerci of *T. hydatigena* and *T. pisiformis* dangle on a thin fibrous pedicle into the abdominal cavity of the host. In the formed capsules, there are usually no signs of inflammation; cellular infiltrates of polymorphonuclear leukocytes, lymphocytes, and macrophages appear on the surface of the capsule only in case of a disturbed parasite–host equilibrium. Therefore, many authors refer to different numbers of capsule layers, e.g., in *E. granulosus* and *T. solium,* differentiating among the inflammatory infiltrates with various cells.

Plerocercoids of Diphyllobothriidae appear to be less specialized (though more ancient) tissue parasites than those of Taeniidae. They are not provided with membranes; they often change their location and become reencapsulated in the host tissues, and can migrate into the reservoir host to be encapsulated again (Berezantsev, 1962c).

The intermediate hosts of Taeniidae often show age immunity against specific parasites, which is distinctly pronounced in rodents in regard to the strobilocercus of *H. taeniaeformis.* Infection may occur only during a short period in the young host. During the first days of development of the strobilocercus, no reactive changes of connective tissue are observed in the liver around them (Fig. 5). Lack of inflammation gives evidence of the tissue's being actively suppressed by the parasite. Later, a capsule of fibroblasts develops that is induced by the parasite and provided with an ample vascular network (Fig. 6). In the liver of aged rodents, capsules around the parasite are lacking, since the onset of the acute inflammatory process

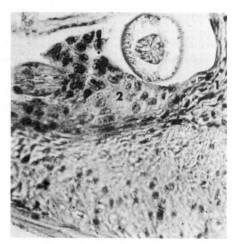

Figure 3 Encapsulated *P. sexalatus* larva in the submucous layer of the stomach of the white mouse 30 days after infection. 1, Fibrous layer of the capsule; 2, internal layer of the capsule consisting of young fibroblasts. × 360.

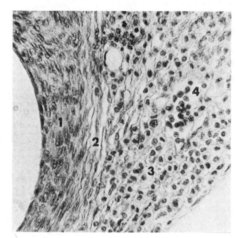

Figure 4 Part of a capsule of *P. depressum* larva on the surface of the stomach of a mole. 1, Internal layer consisting of young fibroblasts; 2, fibrous layer of the capsule, 3, external layer consisting of collagenous fibers and lymphocytes, 4, lymphatic vessels. × 360.

destroys them. Thus, it is solely in the body of a young host lacking the perfectly protecting inflammatory reaction (Poltev, 1947; Zdrodovski, 1955; and others) that strobilocerci are able to suppress the inflammation and induce the formation of capsules of specific structure in the tissues (Berezantsev, 1965).

With metacercariae of *P. cuticula* encapsulated in the muscles of fish,

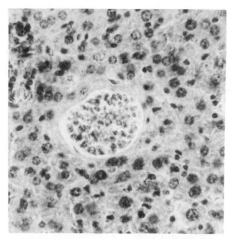

Figure 5 Strobilocercus of *H. taeniaeformis* developed in the liver of the white mouse 4 days after infection. No signs of inflammatory reaction.

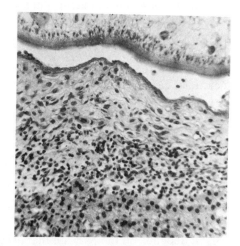

Figure 6 Encapsulated strobilocercus of *H. taeniaeformis* in the liver of the white rat 4.5 months after infection. 1, Strobilocercus; 2, internal fibrous layer of the capsule; 3, external less matured layer of connective tissue with a multitude of cells and vessels.

no signs of inflammation are noticed either. The formation of capsules begins simultaneously with the appearance of young fibroblasts around the invaded parasite. Little by little, the fibrous capsule grows thicker, a multitude of pigment cells (chromatophores) make their appearance, and an ample network of blood vessels develops. The narrow internal layer of the capsule becomes hyalinized (Fig. 7). The structure of the capsule is similar to that of cestode larvae (Berezantsev and Dobrovolski, 1968).

In nonspecific hosts, the parasites are usually not able to encapsulate

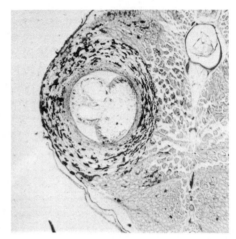

Figure 7 Encapsulated metacercaria of *P. cuticula* in muscles of a young *Rutilus rutilus caspicus.* × 250.

(e.g., *E. multilocularis* in man), since an acute inflammation with necrotic tissue develops around them. The reaction either leads to destruction of the parasite (plerocercoids of *D. latum*) or does not ensure it a normal living process *(E. multilocularis).*

Around foreign bodies (paraffin, celloidin), there were formed the usual cicatricial capsules with scanty blood vessels.

Discussion

In the tissues of specific hosts, nematode, cestode, and trematode larvae give rise to the formation of peculiar capsules different from those of foreign bodies. Sometimes the capsules acquire an organlike structure. Such encapsulation does not result from a mechanical stimulation of tissues; it depends on the parasite that excretes certain substances produced in its evolution as a tissue parasite. The majority of nematode and cestode larvae after invasion induce an ordinary acute inflammation with a leukocytic-lymphoid infiltrate that disappears as soon as a capsule has been formed. In some cases, the formation of cestode or trematode larval capsules is not followed by an acute inflammation. Moreover, the substances excreted by parasites seem to provoke negative chemotaxis in leukocytes. The signs of inflammation appear in capsules only after the destruction of the parasite.

The connective capsules of helminth larvae serve as a barrier or a biological semipermeable membrane between the parasite and the host. In their functional value, the capsules may be compared to the histohematic barriers of mammals (Stern, 1961). The selective permeability of capsules is evidently caused by the function of endothelial cells of capillaries as well as by the basic substance of the connective tissue (hyaluronic acid).

During the process of evolution, selection occurs in parasites along the lines for acquiring a capacity to inhibit and prevent the host protective reactions so as to utilize them for the formation of capsules of special structures, which secure the existence of parasites in tissues. As for adaptations of the host, they proceed in an opposite direction toward improving nonspecific and specific protective mechanisms against parasites.

Summary

Encapsulation of nematode *(Trichinella spiralis, Porrocaecum depressum, Physocephalus sexalatus, Toxocara canis)*, cestode (Diphyllobothriidae and Taeniidae), and trematode *(Posthodiplostomum cuticula)* larvae was studied in the tissues of vertebrates that are intermediate or reservoir hosts. The larvae were found to inhibit, and to prevent the protective inflammatory reaction in host tissues, and to induce (by excreting certain substances) the formation of capsules of a peculiar morphological structure. By carrying out the function of a semipermeable biological membrane, these capsules ensure the nutrition and normal life processes for the larvae in host tissues. The more the helminth larvae have specialized to tissue parasitism during evolution, the more specific their capsule structure, and the rarer are the signs of actual inflammation.

References

Berezantsev, Y. A. (1960). Razvitiye lichinok *Trichinella* v myshtsakh. *Wiad. Parazytol.* **6**, 360–363.

Berezantsev, Y. A. (1961). Protsess obyzvestvleniya lichinok *Trichinella*. *Acta Vet. Hung.* **9**, 357–366.

Berezantsev, Y. A. (1962a). Inkapsulyatsiya lichinok nematod v tkanyakh mlekopitayushchikh. *Vestn. Leningrad. Univ.* **21**, 42–53.

Berezantsev, Y. A. (1962b). Inkapsulyatsiya lichinochnykh stadiy tzestod v tkanyakh promezhutochnykh khozyaev. *Acta Vet. Hung.* **12**, 87–98.

Berezantsev, Y. A. (1962c). O vzaimootnoshenii plerotserkoidov nekotorykh difillobodriid s tkanyami dopolnilte'nykh khozyanov. *Tr. Astrakhan. Zapovednika* **6**, 33–43.

Berezantsev, Y. A. (1963). Advances in the study of migration and encapsulation of *Trichinella* larvae in the host organism (in Russian). *Med. Parazitol. Parazit. Bolez.* **32**, 171–176.

Berezantsev, Y. A. (1965). O prirode vozrastnogo immuniteta pri lichinochnykh teniidozakh. *Mater. Nauch. Konf. Vses. Obshchestva Gelmintol. ANSSSR Moskva* **3**, 36–40.

Berezantsev, Y. A., and Dobrovolsky, A. A. (1968). Processy inkapsulyatsii metacercariy trematod *Posthodiplostomum cuticula* (Normann, 1832), Dubois, 1936 v rybakh. *Tr. Astrakhan. Zapovendika* **11**, 7–11.

Bruce, R. G. (1970). The structure and composition of the capsule of *Trichinella spiralis* in host muscle. *Parasitology* **60**, 223–337.

Hankes, L. V., and Stoner, R. D. (1962). *In vitro* metabolism of tryptophan-2-C^{14} and glycine-2-C^{14} by *Trichinella spiralis* larvae, and chemical fractionation of C^{14}-labeled larvae. *Proc. First Int. Conf. Trichinellosis Warsaw,* 313–318.

Kasprzak, K., Radola, P., Gustowska, L., and Gabryel, P. (1971), Incorporation of glycine-1-C^{14} and 1-lysine-C^{14} into the muscles of rats infected with *Trichinella spiralis* larvae. *Acta Parasitol. Pol.* **19**, 1–7.

Kozar, Z., Zarzycki, J., Czechowicz, K., and Jeppa-Szumowska, E. (1969). Autoradiographic studies on incorporation of amino acids in the muscular phase of trichinellosis. *Wiad. Parazytol.* **15**, 662–666.

McCoy, O. R., Downing, V. F., and Van Voorhis, S. N. (1941). The penetration of radioactive phosphorus into encysted *Trichinella* larvae. *J. Parasitol.* **27**, 53–58.

Poltev, V. J. (1947). Filo-iontogenez osnovnykh faktorov immuniteta. *Usp. Sovrem. Biol.* **23**, 289–296.

Schanzel, H., and Holman J. (1966). Lokalisation der alkalischen Phosphatase in der trichinellabefallenen Muskulatur. *Angew. Parasitol.* **7**, 252–259.

Stern, L. S. (1961). Histo-gematicheskie bar'ery, Moskva.

Stoner, R. D., and Hankes, L. V. (1955). Incorporation of C^{14}-labeled amino acids by *Trichinella spiralis* larvae. *Exp. Parasitol.* **4**, 435–444.

Stoner, R. D., and Hankes, L. V. (1962). Incorporation of tritium-labeled tryptophan by *Trichinella spiralis* larvae and demonstration of nonprecipitating antibody to tritium-labeled *Trichinella* antigen. *Proc. First Int. Conf. Trichinellosis Warsaw,* 306–312.

Stoyanov, D. and Nenov, S. (1965). Nekotorye histokhimicheskie izmeneniya v tkanyakh morskykh svinok, invazirovannykh *Trichinella spiralis. Med. Parazitol. Parazit. Bol.* **34**, 392–396.

Themann, H. (1960). Elektronenmikroskopischer Beitrag zur Entwicklung und zur Aufbau der Trichinenkapsel. *Wiad. Parazytol.* **6**, 352–354.

Zarzycki, J. (1963). Histochemical studies of capsules of trichinellae. *Wiad. Parazytol.* **9**, 453–458.

Zarzycki, J., Kozar, Z., and Czechowicz, K. (1966). An attempt to use the autoradiographic method for studying host-parasite relationship in trichinellosis. *Wiad. Parazytol.* **12**, 553–560.

Zdrodovski, P. F. (1955). Problemy infectsii, immuniteta: allergii. *Moskva.*

Effects of Phytohemagglutinin in Experimental Trichinellosis

E. V. Pereverzeva, N. N. Ozeretskovskaya,
and N. L. Veretennikova

*The E. I. Martsynovsky Institute of Medical
Parasitology and Tropical Medicine
U.S.S.R. Ministry of Public Health
Moscow*

Introduction

The immunological reactions of a predominantly cellular nature are of significance in the process of elimination of adult *Trichinella* and destruction of muscle larvae (Coker, 1956; Larsh, *et al.*, 1964; Larsh, 1967). Different immunosuppressive drugs and antilymphocyte serum change the course of infection markedly (Coker, 1956; Ozeretskovskaya *et al.*, 1966, 1969; Zarzycki *et al.*, 1969; Kozar *et al.*, 1971). The role of lymphoid tissue in the development of intestinal forms of *Trichinella* and in the encystation and resorption of muscle larvae has been demonstrated (Pereverzeva *et al.*, 1971). However, the effect of factors stimulating the immunological activity of the host in trichinellosis has been much less studied. Phytohemagglutinin (PHA) is one of the most active nonspecific stimulants of immunological reactions (Nowell, 1960; Marshall and Roberts, 1963). We studied the effect of PHA on implantation of *Trichinella* larvae in the intestines, survival of adults, duration of the migrating period, development and features of larval encystation, and density and reaction of the lymphoid tissue and peripheral blood.

Materials and Methods

The study was carried out in 400 albino mice on the average weighing 18 to 20 gm, and each mouse was experimentally infected with 80 *Trichinella* larvae (Martsynovsky strain) that were 3½ months of age. The animals were divided into four groups depending on the stage of the worm devel-

111

opment. In group 1 the mice were treated with PHA in the early enteral stage (2 to 4 days after invasion), in group 2 they were treated at the stage of larval migration (6 to 11 days), in group 3 they were treated at the stage of larval encystation (25 to 30 days), and the fourth group served as controls.

PHA in sterile salt solution was injected intramuscularly into the foot pads in a dose of 50 mg/kg. The animals were sacrificed at 7, 15, 21, 35, and 90 days after invasion. Gastrocnemius and masseter muscles were examined. The material was fixed in 10% neutral formalin and Carnoy solution. Celloidine sections of 8–12 μm were stained with hematoxylin-eosin (H & E), picrofuchsin after Van Gieson and Romeis, and Romanovsky-Giemsa. The implantation and survival of the worms in the intestine were determined visually by examining all parts of the intestinal tube. The larval density in the muscles was determined by digesting in acidified pepsin.

Results

In mice treated with PHA the implantation of *Trichinella* larvae in the intestine was changed markedly as compared with the controls (Table I). In the group of mice treated with PHA at 2 to 4 days after invasion no worms were found in the intestines by the seventh day. When PHA was given at 6 to 11 days after invasion, the percent of implanted and maturating *Trichinella* was 21% at 7 days, 14% at 15 days, and 8% at 21 days, while in the controls it was 42%, 30%, and 21%, respectively. Elimination of the adults was observed by 35 days after invasion. In the group of mice treated with PHA at 25 to 30 days after invasion, no adult *Trichinella* was found at 35 days.

Thus, administration of PHA markedly reduced the implantation rate of *Trichinella* larvae and shortened the survival of adults in the intestine. PHA inhibited the production of larvae. This is confirmed by the fact that in mice treated with PHA at 2 to 4 and 6 to 11 days after invasion, *Trichinella* larvae in the diaphragm were found only on the fifteenth day, whereas

Table I   The Percentage of Implanted *Trichinella* in the Intestine of Mice Treated with PHA

Group number	Days of treatment (after invasion)	Implanted larvae as percent of larvae given			
		7 Days	15 Days	21 Days	35 Days
1	2–4	0	0	0	0
2	6–11	21	14	8	0
3	25–30	40	33	26	0
4	Control	42	30	21	0

in controls they were found as early as on the seventh day. Occasional *Trichinella* larvae demonstrable in striated muscle fibers of the experimental animals on the fifteenth day after invasion do not have differentiated structure and contain no glycogen. By the twenty-first day the number of larvae in the muscles increases, and they have a clear-cut structure and much glycogen; however, in comparison to the controls, they measure only 180 to 190 μm in size, have only a cylindrical form, and are far from being encapsulated. In the controls for the same interval all larvae in the muscles are at least 440 μm, and are all spirally twisted.

The affected muscle fibers are destroyed only for a distance of 210–610 μm, whereas in the controls the length of destruction is 900–1300 μm. Along invaded muscle fibers are claviform extensions of the sarcoplasm and its degenerative fragmentation (Fig. 1). In contrast to the controls, the sarcoplasm undergoes no lysis and is compact, with very few nuclei. Instead of being basophilic and fuchsinophilic, it shows affinity for eosin and picric acid. The claviform fragments of the affected muscle fibers are frequently isolated from the surrounding tissues by granulation. At 35 days after invasion, the *Trichinella* larvae in the muscles are encysted but have not formed a tight spiral, and the hyalin layer of the cyst wall is only 1.5–2 μm (Fig. 2).

At all stages of the development of the larvae in the muscles, extensive cellular infiltrations (1000–1500 μm) around the worms and the affected muscle fibers, and the formation of granulomas are observed. These infiltrations contain 45% lymphocytes, 23% fibroblasts, 18% polymorphonuclear leukocytes, 10% monocytes, and 4% histiocytes. In some places accumulations consisting only of lymphocytes and plasma cells are observed with admixtures up to 10% of multinuclear giant cells. Over 50% of the larvae with destroyed internal structures are within the granuloma and undergo lysis (Fig. 3). As a result, at 90 days after invasion, the larval density declines, in the total histological section of the masseter muscle only three to four encapsulated larvae and one to two infiltrates are found at the site of the dead *Trichinella,* whereas in the controls, up to 58–70 larvae are found. Cellular infiltration around the cysts does not subside, encysted sarcoplasm is hyalinized and resorbed, and the loss of the remaining larvae continues.

In contrast to groups 1 and 2, the larval density in group 3 was four times that of the controls at 35 days after invasion (Table II). A majority of the larvae are spiral-shaped and encysted (Fig. 4). Younger spindle-shaped forms are also found. However, as in the other groups, extensive infiltrations of the same cellular composition around the parasites, intramuscular vasculitis, and a mass loss of encysted *Trichinella* larvae are observed. At 90 days after invasion there are no marked histomorphological changes in the muscles. Occasional proliferation of muscle nuclei and small intramuscular lymphohistiocytic infiltrates are found. As compared with findings at

Table II The Density and the Loss of Larvae (Percent) at 35 and 90 Days after Invasion in Mice Treated with PHA at the Different Stages of Infection

The day of sacrifice (after invasion)	Number of larvae per gram	Days of treatment (after invasion)			
		2–4	6–11	25–30	Control
35	Average	11	600	5037	1280
	Percent of control	99	53	+239[a]	0
90	Average	1293	417	1155	3726
	Percent of control	65	89	69	0

[a] The density of larvae increased (percent)

35 days, *Trichinella* larvae are very few: in the masseter muscle only two to three cysts and one to two infiltrates are found at the sites of lysed *Trichinella*. The larvae retain their morphological structure. The hyaline layer of the cyst walls is uniform; it measures $43-50\,\mu$m at the poles, and $13\,\mu$m at the sides. The sarcoplasm tightly surrounds the larvae, but in some cysts it is almost completely hyalinized. As in the other groups, at 90 days after invasion, the cysts are surrounded by extensive cellular infiltrations involving up to 10–15 muscle fibers; and in some places the cysts are completely destroyed by cellular infiltrates (Fig. 5). The continuing mass loss of larvae together with inhibition of production of larvae lead to a marked reduction in the larval density. Thus, as compared with the controls, in mice of group 1 the larval density was reduced at 35 days by 99%, and at 90 days by 65% (Table II). In the group of mice treated with PHA at 6–11 days after invasion the larval density was reduced at 35 days by 53%, and at 90 days by 89%. However, in mice treated at 25–30 days after invasion the larval density at 35 days increased by 239%, but at 90 days it decreased by 69% as compared with the controls (Table II).

Treatment with PHA at 2–4 and 6–11 days after invasion was also accompanied by considerable increase of leukocytosis and marked lymphomonocytic reaction. During the first 4 weeks, up through the thirty-fifth day, the number of leukocytes in these mice was up to 21,000–24,000/ mm^3. A decrease in the number of leukocytes to 11,000/mm^3 was observed by 90 days only. In mice treated with PHA at 25–30 days after invasion, the leukocyte count from the seventh to the twenty-first day of invasion varied from 7,000 to 12,000/mm^3, increased at 35 days to 19,000/mm^3 and decreased to 9000/mm^3 by 90 days after invasion, no significant differences in the leukogram were observed (Fig. 6). In the controls the leukocyte count during the first three weeks was 8000–13,000/mm^3, increased to 16,000/mm^3 by 35 days, and it decreased to 14,000/mm^3 by 90 days after invasion (Fig. 6). The percent of lymphocytes in mice treated with PHA reached 74–82% between the fifteenth day of invasion and 90 days (Fig.7); there were 9% of monocytes. In the controls lymphocytes throughout the

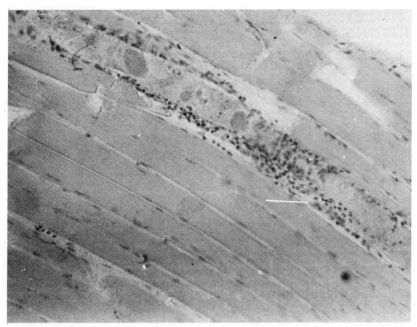

Figure 1 Destructed muscle fiber 21 days after invasion showing eosinophilic fragments of sarcoplasm, and cellular infiltration. H&E, × 80.

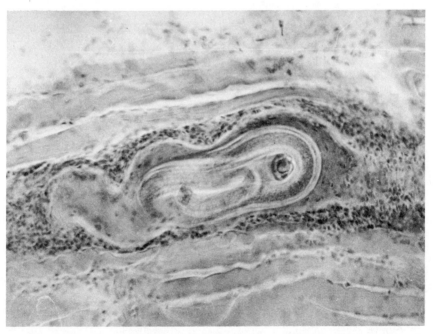

Figure 2 The encapsulated *Trichinella* larvae 35 days after invasion in mouse treated with PHA at 6–11 days. H&E, × 140.

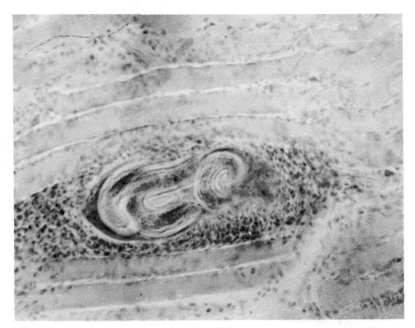

Figure 3 Larva 35 days after invasion undergoing destruction in a granulomatous infiltration (the same group of animals). H&E, × 140.

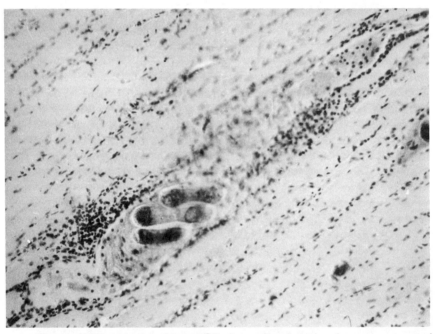

Figure 4 Encapsulated larva 35 days after invasion in mouse treated with PHA at 25–30 days. H&E, × 140.

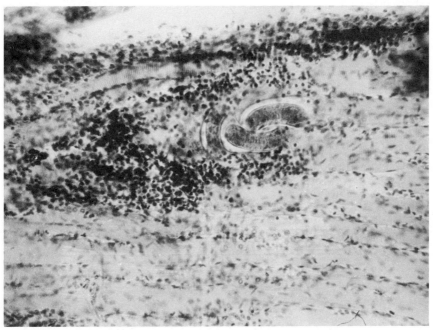

Figure 5 The same group of animals. Massive cellular infiltrations around *Trichinella* larvae. H&E, × 140.

infection were at the level of 55–60% (Fig. 7); the monocytes did not exceed 1–4%.

Discussion

The data obtained indicate that in experimental trichinellosis of mice the treatment with PHA, a stimulator of metabolic activity and of transformation of small lymphocytes (Marshall and Roberts, 1963), leads to a low percentage of implanted enteral worms and their rapid elimination from the intestine. Reduction of invasion of skeletal muscles at early intervals is due mainly to the reduced number of implanted larvae (Table II). Of great interest is the as yet unexplained increase of the larval density by 239% in group 3 (Table II). A similar reduction of the larval density in groups 1 and 3 of experimental animals at 90 days and the results of our morphological studies indicate that the function of the cysts is disturbed and thus a mass loss of larvae ensues. This process is most pronounced in animals treated with PHA 2 weeks after invasion (Table II), that is preceeding the vigorous activation of protective immunologic responses (Oliver-Gonzáles, 1941; Mills and Kent, 1965; Larsh, 1967). Much lower

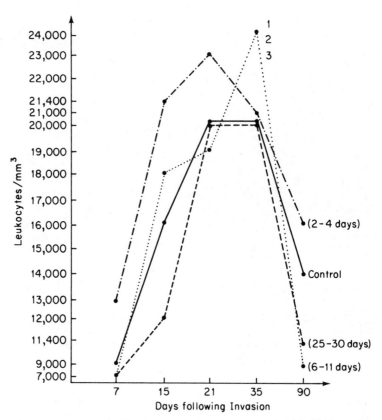

Figure 6 The dynamics of leukocytosis in mice treated with PHA at the different stages of experimental trichinellosis.

intensity of invasion in group 1 at 35 days as compared with that at 90 days is doubtlessly due to the digestion of the larvae at the time of preparation for counting and to the delay in their maturation and encapsulation by PHA.

The stimulating effect of PHA on cellular reactions in the muscle tissue was accompanied by leukocytosis and lymphocytosis which is in agreement with the current data on the effect of PHA on lymphocytes of the peripheral blood (Brody and Soltys, 1969). Our observations correspond to those of Kozar (1969) and Kozar and Kotz (1969) who noted a reduction in the adult count and an increase of the inflammatory reaction in the muscles upon stimulation with bacterial antigens.

Thus, at all stages of experimental trichinellosis PHA causes active cellular reactions in tissues. This leads to a reduction of implantation and survival of mature *Trichinella*. The extensive myositis and even angiomyositis promotes mass loss and resorption of muscle larvae. These pro-

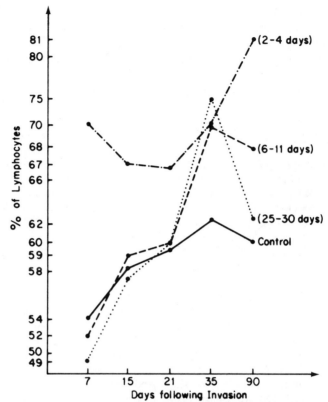

Figure 7 The dynamics of percent of lymphocytes in mice treated with PHA at the different stages of experimental trichinellosis.

cesses develop against the background of increasing leukocytosis of the blood and lymphomonocytic reaction.

Summary

In 400 albino mice each infected with 80 *Trichinella* larvae the effect of phytohemagglutinin (PHA) in a dose of 50 mg/kg given at 2–4 (group 1), 6–11 (group 2) and 25–30 (group 3) days after invasion was studied. In group 1 at 7 days no worms were found in the intestines; in group 2 on the seventh day the percent of implanted worms was reduced from 42% to 21%, on the fifteenth day from 30% to 14%, and on the twenty-first day from 21% to 8%. Larvae in the muscle were found in groups 1 and 2 only on the fifteenth day. On the twenty-first day they were 180–190 μm in size and showed no signs of encystation. At all stages an extensive infiltration with granulomas around larvae in muscles was observed. On the thirty-fifth day the larval density was reduced by 99% (group 1) and 53% (group 2), and on the ninetieth day by 65% and 89%, respectively. In group 3 the larval density on the thirty-fifth day was increased by 239%, and on the ninetieth day it was reduced by 69%. There was leukocytosis up to 35 days in groups 1 and 2—21,000–24,000/mm^3 (74–82% lymphocytes)—as compared to the controls—8000–13,000/mm^3 (55–60% lymphocytes).

References

Brody, J. I., and Soltyis, H. D. (1969). Immunologic memory of phytohemagglutinin-stimulated lymphocytes. *Blood* **34**, 765-773.

Coker, C. M. (1956). Cellular factors in acquired immunity to *Trichinella spiralis* as indicated by cortisone treatment of mice. *J. Infec. Dis.* **98**, 187-197.

Kozar, M. (1969). Effect of stimulation or inhibition of RES in mice on the course of trichinellosis. *Wiad. Parazytol.* **15**, 624-625.

Kozar, Z., and Kotz, J. (1969). Histopathological and histochemical investigations on *Trichinella spiralis* infected mice after RES stimulation. *Wiad. Parazytol.* **15**, 626-627.

Kozar, Z., Karmanska, K., Kotz, J., and Seniuta, R. (1971). The influence of anti-lymphocytic serum (ALS) on the course of trichinellosis in mice III. Histological, histochemical and immunohistological changes observed in striated muscle. *Wiad. Parazytol.* **17**, 503-540.

Larsh, J. E., Jr. (1967). The present understanding of the mechanism of immunity to *Trichinella spiralis*. *Amer. J. Trop. Med. Hyg.* **16**, 123-132.

Larsh, J. E., Jr., Goulson, H. T., and Weatherly, N. F. (1964). Studies on delayed (cellular) hypersensitivity in mice infected with *Trichinella spiralis*. I. Transfer of lymph node cells. *J. Elisha Mitchell Sci. Soc.* **80**, 133-135.

Marshall, W. H., and Roberts, K. B. (1963). The growth and mitosis of human small lymphocytes after incubation with phytohemmagglutinin. *Quart. J. Exp. Physiol. Cog. Med. Sci.* **48**, 146-155.

Mills, C. K., and Kent, N. H. (1965). Excretions and secretions of *Trichinella spiralis* and their role in immunity. *Exp. Parasitol.* **16**, 300-310.

Nowell, P. C. (1960). Phytohemagglutinin an initiator of mitosis in cultures of normal human lymphocytes. *Cancer Res.* **20**, 462-466.

Oliver-González, J. (1941). The dual antibody basis of acquired immunity in trichinosis. *J. Infec. Dis.* **67**, 292-300.

Ozeretskovskaya, N. N., Potyekayeva, M. A., Tumolskaya, N. I., Marguliss, T. D., and Vishnevskii, V. A. (1966). The effect of steroids at the acute phase of trichinellosis and reconvalescence. II. The effect of steroids on the clinical conditions and morphology of muscle lesions in trichinellosis. *Med. Parasitol. Parasit. Biol.* **35**, 164-171.

Ozeretskovskaya, N. N., Kolosova, M. O., Schernyaeva, A. I., Pereverzeva, E. V., Tumolskaya, N. I., and Bekish, O. J. L. (1969). Benzimidazoles and steroid hormones in the therapy of experimental trichinellosis. *Second Int. Conf. Trichinellosis Wroclaw*, June 26-29. 77-80.

Pereverzeva, E. V., Ozeretskowskaya, N. N., and Veretennikova, N. L. (1971). Histomorphological investigations on polar bear strain of *Trichinella*. *Wiad. Parazytol.* **17,** 466–475.

Zarzycki, J., Kozar, Z., Czechowicz, K., and Teppa-Szumowska, E. (1969). Histochemical studies on the effect of imuran R on the muscular phase of trichinellosis in mice. *Wiad. Parazytol.* **15,** 630–633.

Experimental Trichinellosis and Thiabendazole Treatment in *Macaca mulatta:* Clinical and Electromyographic Observations

Wanda Kociecka, Czeslaw Gerwel, Zbigniew Pawłowski
Clinic of Parasitic Diseases
Jerzy Kaczmarek, Bronisław Stachowski
Neurosurgical Clinic
Przemysław Gabryel, and Leokadia Gustowska
Department of Pathological Anatomy,
Medical Academy of Poznań

Introduction

Data on electromyographic changes in human trichinellosis are fragmentary because they represent only single observations on individual patients in advanced stages of the infection (Marcus and Miller, 1955; Waylonis and Johnson, 1964, 1965; Kowalczyk *et al.,* 1969). Electromyographic changes in experimental trichinellosis were studied only in rats and dogs (Waylonis and Johnson, 1964) but not in primates. These animals have rarely been used for experimental trichinellosis (Nelson and Mukundi, 1962; Gretillat and Vassilades, 1968). The idea of this experiment was to observe the dynamics and development of electromyographic changes in trichinellosis of a primate and to evaluate its correlation to the clinical picture, number of muscle larvae, and histopathology of the muscle tissue. The observations were made in a very early period of infectión, in a later one, and after thiabendazole treatment.

Materials and Methods

A 6-year-old male *Macaca mulatta* (Zimmerman, 1780) monkey, 12 kg body weight, was used for the experiment. He had spent most of his life in a zoo. He was kept in a comfortable condition and cared for by a special nurse some weeks before and during the 8.5 months of experimental observation. He was also well trained to tolerate necessary manipulations with a minimal stress. Encapsulated *Trichinella spiralis* larvae (2500) from a rat with an 8-month-old infection were given to the monkey *per os.* The monkey was under daily observation but the manipulations, e.g., electromyography, muscle biopsy, and blood taking, were done all in the same 11 days. Days 26, 14, and 1 before infection and 12, 22, 42, 68, 145, 160, 174, and 190 days after infection were chosen as the optimal checkpoints in this experiment. The thiabendazole, in a daily dose of 300 mg, was done between 145 and 150 days of trichinellosis, so the last three observations were done after therapy.

Electromyographic examination was performed during rest and voluntary and reflectory muscle activity by means of Myocatograph Alvar apparatus. The concentric and polar needle electrodes were inserted in the muscles of forefeet and thighs. The fibrillation and fasciculation, the number, amplitude and duration of motor unit potentials, and needle potentials were analyzed.

Left or right biceps were biopsied aseptically after local anesthesia. A small part of the muscle tissue taken by biopsy was examined histopathologically and about 500 mg was digested following trichinoscopy. About 5 ml of blood taken by venipuncture was used for determining serum proteins, aminotransferases (SGOT, SGPT) level, and the number of leukocytes, including eosinophils. Because of pneumonia the monkey was sacrificed by ether narcosis on day 225 of trichinellosis. The postmortem examination was supplemented with detailed parasitological and histopathological studies of muscle tissue.

Results

Twenty-five hundred *Trichinella spiralis* larvae induced clinically manifest trichinellosis in *Macaca mulatta* monkey. The infection manifested itself on the sixteenth day by swollen mouth and forefeet, periorbital edema, conjunctivitis, apathy, thirst, decreased appetite, and weight loss (Figs. 1 and 2). The acute symptoms disappeared in about 42 days; apathy and weight loss persisted longer but were later replaced by excitement and normalization of the body weight (Chart 1). The serum protein, especially the albumin fraction, decreased to 3.8 gm/100 ml on day 68, then slowly increased. The aminotransferases, especially SGOT, sharply increased and remained at a high level during the infection; the maximal level was found on day 174, i.e., 24 days after thiabendazole therapy. The leukocytes and eosinophil counts in venous blood changed irregularly and were not taken into consideration.

The number of *Trichinella* larvae increased gradually to 474/gm in 68 days. The difference in the number of larvae between 68 and 145 days did

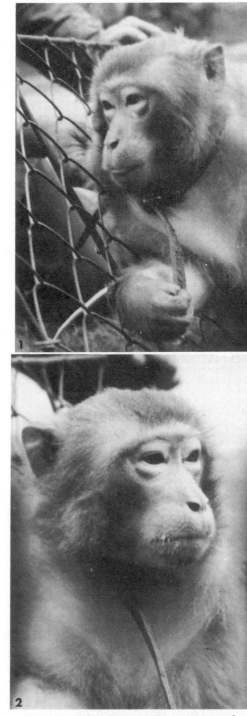

Figure 1 Periorbital edema, mouth and forefeet swollen on day 18 of trichinellosis.

Figure 2 Periorbital edema and swollen mouth still present on day 29 of trichinellosis.

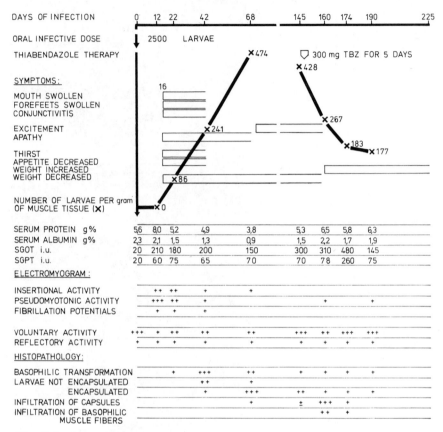

Chart 1

not exceed 10%. After thiabendazole therapy the number of larvae decreased sharply within 24 days down to 183 gm, i.e., 43% of the intensity before thiabendazole treatment.

Electromyogram before infection was normal (Fig. 3). As early as the twelfth day, pathological changes, e.g., insertional activity, pseudomyotonic activity and fibrillation potentials were evident (Figs. 4, 5, and 6), the voluntary activity was decreased (Fig. 7), and the reflectory activity was increased. On days 22 and 42 the changes still persisted, except for pseudomyotonic activity, which disappeared more quickly. On days 68 and 145, a normalization of electromyogram was observed (Fig. 8). After thiabendazole therapy pseudomyotonic activity reappeared (Fig. 9), but the voluntary or reflectory activity was undisturbed (Fig. 10).

There were no histopathological changes in muscle tissue on the twelfth day after infection. Basophilic transformation of muscle fibers was first

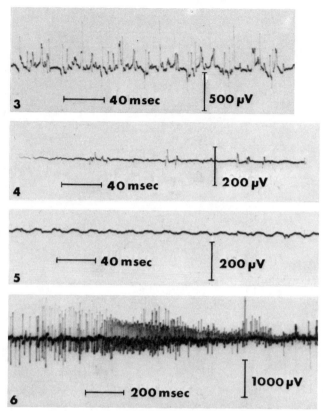

Figure 3 Electromyogram. Voluntary activity before infection (right thigh, biceps muscle).

Figure 4 Insertional activity on twelfth day of trichinellosis (left thigh, biceps muscle).

Figure 5 Fibrillation potentials on twelfth day of trichinellosis (left thigh, biceps muscle).

Figure 6 Pseudomyotonic activity of twelfth day of trichinellosis (right hand, intercostal I muscle).

observed on day 22 (Figs. 11 and 12), and the complete changes typical for trichinellosis by day 42 (Figs. 13–15). After thiabendazole therapy cellular reaction was intensified with infiltration to the basophil-transformed muscle fibers (Fig. 16). The majority of *Trichinella* capsules was surrounded by a cellular infiltration mostly of monocytes. Even 40 days after thiabendazole therapy the infiltration was intense, the disintegration of capsules and larvae was common, and some resorptive granulomas were present in place of infiltrated capsules (Fig. 17).

At the postmortem examination on day 225 of trichinellosis and 75 days after thiabendazole therapy, symptoms of bilateral pneumonia were found. The intensity of the invasion of central parts of the biceps muscle

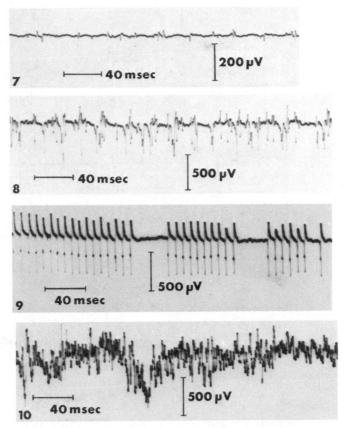

Figure 7 Voluntary activity on twelfth day of trichinellosis (left thigh, biceps muscle).

Figure 8 Voluntary activity on day 145 of trichinellosis (left thigh, quadriceps muscle).

Figure 9 Pseudomyotonic activity on day 190 of trichinellosis and 40 days after thiabendazole therapy (left thigh, quadriceps muscle).

Figure 10 Voluntary activity on day 190 of trichinellosis (left thigh, biceps muscle).

was 177 *Trichinella* larvae per gram of muscle tissue as determined by trichinoscopy and 195 by the digestion method. The highest number (882/gm) of larvae was found in the tongue; more than 300/gm in the diaphragm, pectoral, and intercostal muscles; and less than 100/gm in abdominal rectus, psoas, femoral, and tail muscles. In histopathological examination, capsules surrounded by infiltration as well as free of surrounding cells were found. A slight basophilia of separate uninfected muscle fibers could be detected.

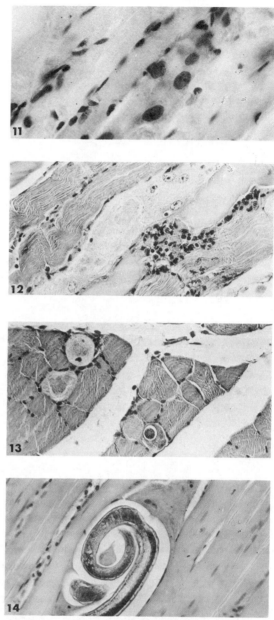

Figure 11 Early basophil changes of the muscle fiber. Balloonlike enlarged nuclei moving from the periphery toward the center of the fiber. Twenty-second day of trichinellosis. H & E, × 80.

Figure 12 Typical basophilia of the muscle fiber. Indistinct cross-striations, granular sarcoplasm, balloonlike nuclei. Twenty-second day of trichinellosis. H & E, × 80.

Figure 13 Basophilic fibers. New encapsulated larva. Forty-second day of trichinellosis. H & E, × 80.

Figure 14 Encapsulated larva. Thin capsule, absence of cellular infiltrate. Forty-second day of trichinellosis. H & E, × 180.

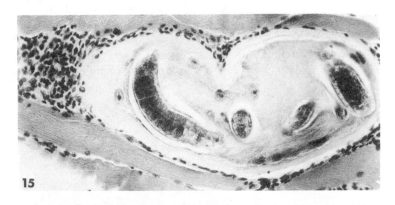

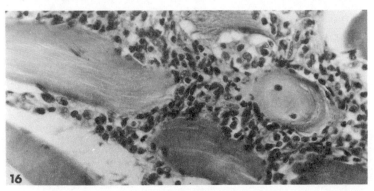

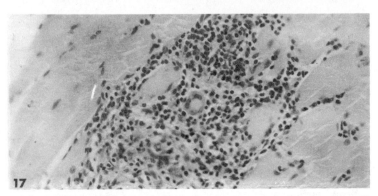

Figure 15 Encapsulated larva surrounded by cellular infiltrate. Day 68 of trichinellosis. H & E, × 160.

Figure 16 Development of inflammatory reaction. Infiltration of cells to basophilic fibers. Day 160 of trichinellosis, 10 days after thiabendazole therapy. H & E, × 160.

Figure 17 Resorptive granuloma in place of infiltrated capsule. Autopsy material. Day 225 of trichinellosis, 75 days after thiabendazole therapy. H & E, × 80.

Discussion

The experiment was performed in a single *Macaca mulatta* monkey, in which the dynamics of electromyographic changes and their correlation with the clinical picture, the number of *Trichinella spiralis* larvae, and the histopathological changes were studied. After this experiment a similar one was performed in a female *M. mulatta,* but she died early because of a gastric malignancy. This was the most likely conclusion considering a very low intensity of invasion (five *Trichinella* larvae per gram). Observations in the second animal confirmed two of the three changes, which are the most important conclusions of the present experiment.

The first conclusion is that the changes in the electromyogram appeared on the twelfth day before the appearance of any clinical symptoms and histopathological changes, including basophilic transformation. This observation agrees with that of Waylonis and Johnson (1965) on the early appearance of electroymyographic changes in *Trichinella*-infected rats and dogs. The second conclusion is that in the later period of trichinellosis the development of electromyographic changes and their normalization corresponds well with the histopathological picture of the muscle tissue and the increasing or stable number of *Trichinella* larvae. The third conclusion is that thiabendazole treatment strongly activated the cellular infiltration of basophilic fibers and *Trichinella* capsules, which resulted in diminished number of muscle larvae. The electromyographic pathological changes and the increased level of aminotransferases were the clinical equivalents of this activation.

The larvicidal effect of thiabendazole on *T. spiralis* has been observed by Campbell and Cuckler (1966), and Kozar and Kozar (1966–1967). In this experiment the effect was demonstrated as late as day 145 of infection. Its clinical and parasitological consequences have not been thoroughly investigated although thiabendazole is widely used in symptomatic human trichinellosis. The use of thiabendazole, which strongly increased the cellular, humoral, and allergic responses of the host, may be contraindicated in severe human trichinellosis (Łapszewicz *et al.,* 1969). On the other hand, the treatment with thiabendazole has to be taken into account in the evaluation of electromyographic changes in human patients, even when the drug has been taken some weeks before. Our experiment showed that the histological sequelae of thiabendazole action are visible up to 40 days after treatment.

The course of trichinellosis in different host species may differ in some aspects. The difference between albino rats and the observed monkeys lies, among other respects, in the appearance of muscle basophilia. In rats it is present on the fifth day after invasion (Gabryel and Gustowska, 1967) but in monkeys it has not been found by the twelfth day. The general impression is that the whole picture of *T. spiralis* infection in *M. mulatta* corresponds better to human trichinellosis than to any other experimental trichinellosis. This is especially true for the time of appearance and development of clinical symptoms and disproteinemia, as well as the action of thiabendazole. These findings justify the use of a primate for complex investigations of those aspects of trichinellosis, e. g., electromyography and histopathology, which could not be traced continuously in human patients, but are of scientific and practical value.

Summary

One *Macaca mulatta* was infected with 2500 encapsulated *Trichinella spiralis* larvae. The monkey was under clinical observation for 8½ months. The thiabendazole treatment was performed between 145 and 150 days after invasion. Laboratory and electromyographic examinations as well as muscle biopsies were done before infection and on 12, 22, 42, 68, 145, 160, 174, and 190 days after onset of trichinellosis. Leukocytosis, eosinophilia, blood protein level, proteinogram and transaminase activity were observed. Electromyographic examination was performed during rest and voluntary or reflectory muscle activity. Five hundred to 700 mg of biceps muscle taken by biopsy was examined histologically and parasitologically. The pathological changes of electromyogram, proteinogram and transaminase activity, found on the twelfth day of invasion, preceeded the appearance of clinical symptoms of trichinellosis (day 16) and muscle fibers basophilia (day 22). The changes in proteinogram and increased transaminase activity were more persistent (up to day 68). On day 68 the intensity of invasion was 474 *Trichinella* larvae per gram of muscle tissue.

Soon after the thiabendazole treatment, some clinical symptoms reappeared, the transaminase activity was again very high, the pathological changes of the electromyogram became evident, and the cellular reaction around the *Trichinella* larvae was reactivated. The number of *Trichinella* larvae dropped gradually to 177/gm of muscle tissue on day 190 of invasion.

Acknowledgements

This study was supported by grant CDC-E-P-2, Center for Disease Control, U.S. Public Health Service.

References

Campbell, W. C., and Cuckler, A. C. (1966). Further studies on the effect of thiabendazole on trichinosis in swine with notes of the biology of the infection. *J. Parasitol.* **52**, 260–279.

Gabryel, P., and Gustowska, L., (1967). Veränderungen der quergestreiften Muskelfasern im fruhen Stadium einer *Trichinella spiralis* Infektion. *Morphol. Jahrb.* **111**, 174–180.

Grétillat, S., and Vassilades, G. (1968). La trichinose experimentale du singe (Souche ouest-africaine de *Trichinella spiralis* Owen, 1835). *Bull. Soc. Pathol. Exot.* **61**, 246–251.

Kowalczyk, M., Poznańska, H., Emeryk-Szajewska, B., and Fidziańska-Dolot, A. (1969). Electromyographic, histologic and enzymatic studies on the muscle system in trichinosis in human patients. *Przegl. Epidemiol.* **23**, 489–499.

Kozar, Z., and Kozar, M. (1966–1967). Experimental studies in mice on the therapy of trichinellosis (Thiabendazole, neguvon, cortisone, azulen, sera). *Acta Parasitol. Pol.* **14–15**, 133–161.

Łapszewicz, A., Pawłowski, Z., and Gabryel, P. (1969). Thiabendazole in human trichinellosis. *Wiad. Parazytol.* **15**, 759–760.

Marcus, S., and Miller, R. W. (1955). An atypical case trichinosis with report of electromyographic findings. *Ann. Intern. Med.* **43**, 615–622.

Nelson, G. S., and Mukundi, J. (1962). The distribution of *Trichinella spiralis* in the muscles of primates. *Wiad. Parazytol.* **8**, 629-632.

Waylonis, G. W. D., and Johnson, E. W. D. (1964). The electromyogram in acute trichinosis: Report of four cases. *Arch. Phys. Med. Rehabil.* **45**, 177–183.

Waylonis, G. W. D., and Johnson, E. W. D. (1965). Electromyographic findings in induced trichinosis. *Archi. Phys. Med. Rehabil.* **46**, 615–625.

Morphology and Histochemistry of Muscle in *Trichinella*-Infected Rats Treated with Thiabendazole

Przemyslaw Gabryel, Leokadia Gustowska,
and Malgorzata Blotna

Department of Pathological Anatomy
Medical Academy of Poznań

Introduction

Application of thiabendazole (Thb) in the intestinal phase of trichinellosis prevents the development of a clinically pronounced disease. This drug kills the worms, inhibits the maturation of the larvae, and sterilizes the female worms (Campbell and Cuckler, 1964; Kozar *et al.,* 1966; Blair and Campbell, 1971). Treatment with Thb in the muscular phase leads to damage of the encysted larvae and to a strong inflammatory reaction with phagocytosis of the remnants of the cysts and parasites.

However, the mechanism by which the drug acts is still obscure. Some observations show direct action of Thb on the *Trichinella spiralis* larvae. The recent investigations of Kozar *et al.* (1967) suggest an indirect action of the host, which may impair the development and survival of the parasite. Our earlier investigations proved that the transformation of the sarcoplasm surrounding the parasite is necessary for the growth and survival of the larvae. The disintegration of the cyst content leads to death of the larva (Gabryel and Gustowska, 1967, 1970; Kasprzak *et al.,* 1971).

Our present investigation attempts to answer the question whether the damage to the *T. spiralis* larva during Thb treatment is not a secondary phenomenon to the primary injury of the basophilic substance in its surrounding.

Materials and Methods

Twenty-five white, male Wistar rats, weighing 200–220 gm, were used in these investigations. The invasive material was obtained by digestion of skeletal rat muscles infected with *T. spiralis* in an artificial gastric juice. The invasion was carried out with a dose of 4000 digested larvae, applied through a tube into the esophagus. This caused an invasion of a high intensity. Thb in suspension was given to animals through the esophagus in daily doses of 30 mg/rat for 5 days.

The control groups included: (1) noninfected animals that obtained Thb in the above-mentioned doses; and (2) infected animals untreated with Thb. Animals of the experimental groups were sacrificed 5 and 15 days after the last dose of Thb. Morphological and histochemical investigations of the tongue, diaphragm, and femoral muscles were performed.

Histochemical determinations were carried out as follows: (1) alkaline and acid phosphatase by Gomori's method; (2) succinate hydrogenase activity according to Pearse; and (3) RNA determination by Brachet's method and by Bertalanffy's method (control with RNase) Hematoxylin and eosin staining was used.

The estimation of biological value of larvae was carried out on the basis of the following criteria: (1) percentage of dead larvae obtained after digestion; and (2) invasiveness of larvae to the new host (mouse) by xenodiagnosis (Kociecka, 1971).

Results

Infected Animals, Untreated with Thb

Four months after infection, 70–150 *T. spiralis* larvae were found in the histological sections of the tongue. The morphological details of the muscles, cysts, and larvae were similar to those given in the literature. In the particular animals few lymphocytes were present surrounding one to five cysts only (Fig. 1).

Twelve months after infection the morphological picture was similar to that in the former group. About 15% of cysts underwent calcification. The histochemical results were the same as those shown in our previous investigations (Figs. 2A, 3A, 4A, 5A).

Noninfected Animals Treated with Thb

No deviation from the normal picture of the muscles were found in the applied morphological and histochemical investigations.

Infected Animals Treated with Thb

Morphological Investigations. Animals were infected 4 months before. About 40% of cysts were surrounded by numerous macrophages, eosino-

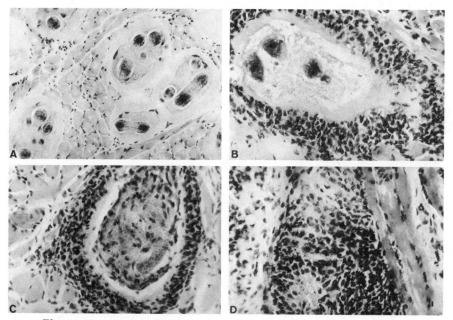

Figure 1 Histological picture in rats at 4 months of infection. A, In control (untreated) rat; B, 5 days after the last dose of Thb; C and D, 20 days after the last dose of Thb.

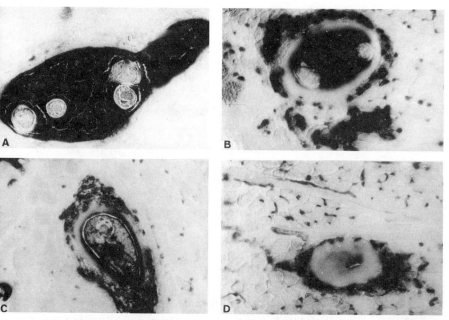

Figure 2 Alkaline phosphatase activity in rats at 4 months of infection. A, In control (untreated) rat; B, 5 days after the last dose of Thb; C and D, 20 days after the last dose of Thb.

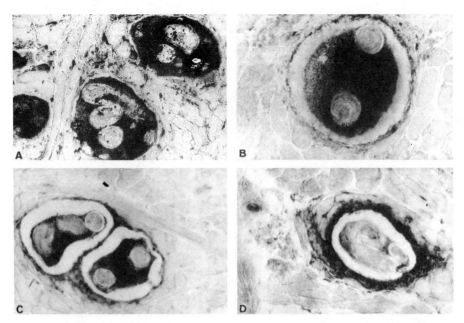

Figure 3 Acid phosphatase activity in rats at 4 months of infection. A, In control (untreated) rat; B, 5 days after the last dose of Thb; C and D, 20 days after the last dose of Thb.

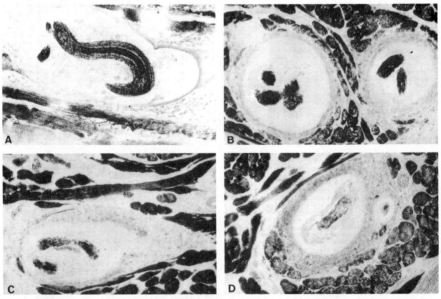

Figure 4 Succinic dehydrogenase activity in rats at 4 months of infection. A, In control (untreated) rat; B, 5 days after the last dose of Thb; C and D, 20 days after the last dose of Thb.

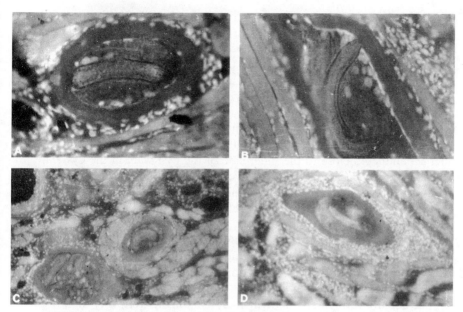

Figure 5 RNA reaction after Bertalanffy in rats at 4 months of infection. A, In control (untreated) rat; B, 5 days after the last dose of Thb; C and D, 20 days after the last dose of Thb.

phils, and lymphocytes in investigated animals 5 days after the last dose of Thb. These cells often infiltrated the cyst wall and invaded the basophilic substance surrounding the larvae. The content of the cysts underwent disintegration and it lost its basophilic character (Fig. 1B). The structure of the larvae was indistinct; some of the larvae were destroyed. Single granulomas with multinuclear giant cells containing remnants of the capsule and larvae were present.

About 60% of cysts were not surrounded by inflammatory cells. The content of these cysts shows a distinct disintegration and lack of basophilia. The nuclei lying in the cysts were either vesicular or pyknotic; the nucleoli were weakly stained. The structure of the larvae was less distinct than in the control material. We found that the number of infiltrated cysts rose to 75% in animals investigated 15 days after the last dose of Thb (Fig. 1C, D). There was also an increase in resorptive granulomas. The picture of the cysts without infiltrations were similar to that seen in the former group.

In rats that had been infected for 12 months, the inflammatory infiltrations were present around 15% of the cysts only: the inflammatory reaction became less intensive than in the former group.

Histochemical Investigations Alkaline Phosphatase. Rats with 4-month infection; 5 days after the last dose of Thb. A very strong activity was found around the noninfiltrated larvae. When inflammatory infiltration was present reaction products appeared in the cytoplasm of the cells and in the content of the cysts, especially close to the inner side of the cyst wall (Fig. 2B). The activity of the alkaline phosphatase varied markedly from slightly positive to negative. In the larval body no activity was present.

Fifteen days from the last dose of Thb the amount of the reaction product in the content of noninfiltrated cysts was smaller than in the control group. An increased activity was present in the cells surrounding the cysts. In the content of such cysts the activity varied greatly; the reaction product accumulated close to the inner side of the cyst wall, in the cyst capsule itself, and occasionally outside the cysts (Fig. 2C, D). Reaction product occurred within the larval body. Alkaline phosphatase activity was very high in the walls of capillaries of both groups of animals both 5 and 15 days following the Thb treatment.

Acid Phosphatase. Rats with 4-month infections showed an increased intensity of reaction in the content of noninfiltrated cysts when compared with the control material. This concerned both groups of animals, 5 and 15 days after the last dose of Thb (Fig. 3B).

The activity varied in the individual cysts, ranging from very high (Fig. 3C) to complete inactivity when the cysts were surrounded by inflammatory cells. This was especially distinct 15 days after the last dose of Thb (Fig. 3D). The activity was very weak or diminished completely in the larval body of such infiltrated cysts. The reaction product was also localized in the inflammatory cells.

In animals with 12-month infections, acid phosphatase activity was similar to that of the control group in most cysts, but in the individual cysts it was either weaker or negative. The results were similar in animals 5 and 15 days after the last dose of Thb.

Succinic Dehydrogenase. The activity was very strong in the muscle fibers and in the larval body in the animals infected 4 months before and 5 days after Thb treatment (Fig. 4B). Fifteen days after the last dose of the drug, the activity disappeared in all the larvae surrounded by inflammatory cells. At the same time the reaction product appeared in the inflammatory cells (Fig. 4C, D).

RNA was present in the larval body, cyst content, and the nucleoli of the nuclei lying inside the cysts in all the animals with 4-month infection and 5 days following the Thb treatment (Fig. 5B).

The amount of RNA was smaller or it disappeared completely if inflammatory infiltrations and destruction of the cysts occurred. RNA was present in the larvae long after it had disappeared from other structures. The amount of cysts and larvae without RNA increased 15 days after the last dose of the drug (Fig. 5C, D). Twelve months after the infection, RNA was present in the larval body, the inflammatory cells, and within the content of the cysts, but its amount was smaller than in the control group. In the individual cysts there was a complete lack of RNA.

Estimation of the Biological Value of T. spiralis *Larvae.* Animals examined 4 months after the infection showed the same amount of dead larvae before and 5 days after treatment with Thb (10–12 larvae/gm). A strong increase in the number of the dead larvae was found in this group of animals 15 days after Thb treatment. The invasiveness of the larvae examined by xenodiagnosis decreased after Thb treatment. The amount of the mature larvae was smaller in the alimentary tract of the mouse. It was already seen 5 days after treatment in animals infected 4 and 12 months before.

Discussion

Thiabendazole effect on the course of *Trichinella* infection in the early muscular phase of the disease was studied by several authors (Campbell and Cuckler, 1966; Kozar *et al.*, 1966, 1967). The early muscular phase of trichinellosis seemed unsuitable for studying the action of the drug because of the presence of metabolic disturbances and acute inflammatory reaction in the muscles. This makes the assessment of a pharmacological effect rather difficult.

Our study concerns rats infected 4 and 12 months previously. In the late muscular phase inflammatory reactions vanish and some sort of equilibrium is created between the parasite and the host. In spite of the fact that larvae are coated with tight capsules, the transport of substances from host blood vessels to the larvae is still operating Kasprzak *et al.* (1971) had shown an incorporation of [1-^{14}C] glycine and [1-^{14}C] lysine to basophilic substance surrounding larvae to a higher degree than to muscle fibers in the period to 5 weeks since the infection. Zarzycki *et al.* (1966, 1968) were able to demonstrate penetration of ^{32}P through the wall of the cyst and its content to the larval body up to 8 weeks, and also human serum albumin-^{131}I up to 11 weeks of infection. Thus, the cyst surrounding the larval body should not be considered as a tight barrier separating the parasite from the host. On the contrary, it facilitates a rapid penetration of substances from the blood vessels of the host to the larval body.

Results of the current study have shown that Thb applied in the fourth and twelfth month after the infection causes larval damage and disintegration. Even though morphological studies do not indicate sure viability of the larvae, specimens examined 15 days following Thb therapy show that 75% of the cysts were infiltrated by inflammatory cells in rats infected 4 months earlier. The remnants of capsules and larvae were also visible between the cells of granulomas.

An estimation of the biological value of the larvae from digested muscles has also confirmed that many parasites die during Thb treatment and the remaining ones lose their invasive properties. The number of dead larvae was especially high 15 days after Thb therapy had been stopped.

Antiparasitic mechanism of Thb action remains still unclear. Campbell and Cuckler (1964, 1966) concluded that this action is larvacidal, while Blair and Campbell (1971) raise the possibility of sterilization of female parasites. Kozar *et al.* (1967) suggested an indirect effect through inhibition of metabolism in muscles. According to these authors the reduction of active transport of ions from blood to the muscle fibers takes place, the oxidative processes slow down, and glycogen synthesis is inhibited. Metabolic disturbances of the host presumably act indirectly on the parasite through creation of unfavorable conditions for its growth. The described disturbances take place rather slowly and it is difficult to explain the rapid and massive disintegration of larvae in this way. In our studies damage of up to 40% of the cysts was already evident 5 days after the completion of Thb treatment.

Our previous work had shown that the growth and survival of the larva in an infected muscle fiber is monitored by the transformation of the sarcoplasm surrounding the larval body. Electron-microscopic studies had demonstrated that in the sarcoplasm surrounding the larva, new protein-synthesizing structures were formed in place of the disintegrated myofibrils (Gabryel and Gustowska, 1967; Blotna, 1967; Gabryel *et al.,* 1969; Bäckwinkel and Themann, 1972). These proteins are apparently necessary for the larva. In the case of a lack of transformation there is no chance for the growth and survival of the parasite. On the other hand, we can suggest that the disintegration of the basophilic substance in the cyst can lead to secondary injury and death of the larva. This conclusion is also justified by the results of our investigations. Most of the cysts already showed morphological and enzymatic disturbances 5 days after the last dose of Thb. At the same time there was a lack of such disturbances in the body of the larvae. The RNA content and succinic dehydrogenase activity did not drop until several days following Thb treatment. The larva died also at a later time.

Forty percent of the cysts were infiltrated and the cyst content was damaged 5 days after Thb treatment. At the same time our biological investigations showed that in this period the amount of dead larvae was the same before and after the treatment.

Our present observations lead us to the conclusion that the basophilic substance is damaged earlier than the larva itself.

The activation of inflammatory cells in the intermuscular tissue was a secondary result of the cysts and larva injury. The inflammatory cells surrounded only the damaged cysts, and the amount of the infiltrated cysts increased up to 15 days from the last Thb dose. The activation of the inflammatory cells is probably caused by disintegration products of the cysts and larvae. They leak out of the inside of the cyst through the damaged cyst wall. Such a leak is possible and we were able to observe it in our analysis of alkaline phosphatase activity.

Summary

Rats infected with *Trichinella spiralis* larvae 4 and 12 months before were given thiabendazole (Thb) in daily doses of 30 mg/rat for 5 days. The animals were sacrificed 5 and 15 days after the last dose of thiabendazole. The muscles were examined morphologically and histochemically.

The obtained results show, that during the treatment the damage of the *Trichinella* larvae is a secondary phenomenon to the primary injury of the basophilic substance surrounding the larvae. The inflammatory and resorptive reactions appear around the injured cysts only. Their intensity lasts even several days after the total excretion of the drug from the body.

Acknowledgments

This study was supported by research grant CDC-E-P-2, Center for Disease Control, U.S. Public Health Service.

References

Bäckwinkel, K. P., and Themann, H. (1972). Elektronenmikroskopische Untersuchungen über die Pathomorphologie der Trichinellose. *Beitr. Pathol.* **146,** 259–271.

Blair, L. S., and Campbell, W. C. (1971). Reversibility of thiabendazole induced sterilization of *Trichinella spiralis. Wiad. Parazytol.* **17,** 641--644.

Blotna, M. (1967). Ultrastructural changes in muscle fibres in Trichinosis. *Acta Med. Pol.* **8,** 402–405.

Campbell, W. C., and Cuckler, A. C. (1964). Effect of thiabendazole upon the enteral and parenteral phases of trichinosis in mice. *J. Parasitol.* **50,** 481–488.

Campbell, W. C., and Cuckler, A. C. (1966). Further studies on the effect of thiabendazole on trichinellosis in swine, with notes on the biology of the infection. *J. Parasitol.* **52,** 260–279.

Gabryel, P., and Gustowska, L. (1967). Veränderungen der quergestreiften Muskelfasern in frühen Stadium einer *Trichinella spiralis* Infection. *Morphol. Jahrb.* **III,** 174–180.

Gabryel, P., and Gustowska, L. (1970). Trichinellosis basophilia of the muscle fibre. *Acta Parasitol. Polon.* **18,** 1–6.

Gabryel, P., Gustowska, L., Blotna, M., Kasprzak, K., and Radola, P. (1969). Pathomorphology of muscular trichinellosis in comparative histological, histochemical, ultrastructural, autoradiographic and immunofluorescent investigations. *Wiad. Parazytol.* **15,** 655–657.

Kasprzak, K., Radola, P., Gustowska, L., and Gabyrel, P. (1971). Incorproation of glycine-1-^{14}C and lysine-1-^{14}C into the muscles of rats infected with *Trichinella spiralis* larvae. *Acta Parasitol. Polon.* **19,** 1–7.

Kociecka, W. (1971). Behavior of *Trichinella spiralis* larvae with animals treated by thiabendazole and hydrocortisone. *Wiad. Parazytol.* **17,** 627–639.

Kozar, Z., Zarzycki, J., and Kozar, M. (1966). Morphologic observations of *Trichinella*-infected muscles in mice treated with thiabendazole and neguvon. *Wiad. Parazytol.* **12,** 589–604.

Kozar, Z., Zarzycki, J., Seniuta, R., and Martynowicz, T. (1967). Histochemical study of drug effects on mice infected with *Trichinella spiralis. Exp. Parasitol.* **21,** 173–185.

Zarzycki, J., Kozar, Z., and Czechowicz K., (1966). An attempt to use the autoradiographic method for studying host–parasite relationships in trichinellosis *Wiad. Parazytol.* **12,** 553–560.

Zarzycki, J., Kozar, Z., and Czechowicz, K., and Teppa-Szumowska E. (1968). Autoradiographic studies with P^{32} of the muscular tissue in *Trichinella spiralis* infected mice. *Wiad. Parazytol.* **14,** 145–154.

Biochemical Studies of Trichinous and Nontrichinôus Pork

John S. Andrews and Patricia C. Allen

Animal Parasitology Institute
Agricultural Research Center
Agricultural Research Service
U.S. Department of Agriculture
Beltsville, Maryland

Introduction

Von Brand *et al.* (1952), Kurylo-Borowska and Kozar (1960), and Castro and Fairbairn (1969) reported that the lipid content of the dry substance of *Trichinella spiralis* larvae was 5.5%, 18.3%, and 9.1%, respectively. Moore (1966) isolated from larval cuticle a pyridine-soluble, immunogenic fraction that may have been a lipid or a mixture of lipids. Castro and Fairbairn (1969) made a detailed chemical fractionation of the total larval lipids which showed that phospholipids and cholesterol accounted for 82%. The total lipids contained at least 37 different acids, ten of them present in major amounts, along with diglycerides, triglycerides, and cholesterol esters.

Because of the relatively high lipid content of *T. spiralis* larvae, and because preliminary experiments suggested that trichinous pork may contain more free sterols than nontrichinous pork, the authors decided to investigate the sterol fraction in their search for a compound unique to *Trichinella* that might be used to detect the presence of *Trichinella* in living swine or in pork meat.

This report describes progress on the methods that have been used at the USDA Animal Parisitology Institute to find and identify sterols of possible diagnostic significance in detecting porcine trichiniasis.

Materials and Methods

Trichinous and nontrichinous diaphragm muscles were obtained from barn-raised hogs at this Institute immediately after slaughter. The meat

145

was frozen by immersion in liquid nitrogen ($-195°$ C), wrapped in aluminum foil, and broken up into smaller pieces with a mallet. The pieces were then pulverized in a mechanical blender and approximately 100 gm of each were lyophilized by standard procedures and stored at $-10°$C.

The lyophilized samples were then brought to room temperature and were forced separately through an 80-mesh screen, thus providing a homogeneous sample for analysis. The particles that went through the screen were caught on a 200-mesh screen, weighed, and transferred to an airtight container for storage at $-10°$ C. The remainder was saved and also stored at $-10°$ C.

Decapsulated *Trichinella* were obtained by artificial digestion from infected rat muscle. *Trichinella* cysts were recovered manually from trichinous hog muscle that had been chopped up with a blender and washed in a 200-mesh screen. The larvae and cysts were then separately washed several times with distilled water and were lyophilized and stored at $-10°$ C.

One-gram portions of each of the lyophilized pork samples were extracted three times with 100 ml anhydrous ether at $4°$ C. The three extracts were combined and evaporated under vacuum until the odor of ether could no longer be detected. The lyophilized larvae and cysts were similarly extracted with proportionately smaller volumes of ether in accordance with the dry weight of the samples, 0.1 and 0.23 gm, respectively.

The ether extracts were chromatographed on 250-μm layers of silica gel using hexane, diethyl ether, and acetic acid (90:10:1 v/v/v) as a solvent (Stahl, 1965). The plates were sprayed with concentrated H_2SO_4 and charred on a hot plate to visualize the various lipids.

Preparative chromatograms were made of the same extracts on 500-μm layers of silica gel and chromatographed in the above-mentioned solvent. Known cholesterol was chromatographed simultaneously with the extracts as a standard. The thin layer plates were sprayed with rhodamine 6G in 90% ethanol and the bands at the same R_f as known cholesterol were scraped from the plates. The silica gel containing the sterols was funneled into Pasteur pipettes plugged with glass wool. The sterols were eluted from the silica gel by percolation of 10 ml of benzene through the pipettes. The benzene eluates were evaporated to dryness under nitrogen.

The sterols from the various sources were chromatographed on paraffin oil-impregnated silica gel layers using acetone-H_2O (4:1 v/v) as a developing solvent as described by de Souza and Nes (1969). Known cholesterol was chromatographed simultaneously with the extracts as a standard. The plates were allowed to dry for 5 min, were sprayed with an acidic solution of *p*-anisaldehyde in ethanol, and then were heated for 5–10 min at $110°$ C for visualization.

Results and Discussion

Thin layer chromatography of the crude ether extracts indicated that free sterols comprised a significant portion of the total lipids of the *T. spiralis* larvae and cysts and further that trichinous pork contained relatively more free sterols than nontrichinous pork. Reversed phase chromatography of the sterols from the various sources indicated the presence in cysts of at least one sterol having an R_f value lower than that of known cholesterol in that chromatographic system. This compound was not detected in nontrichinous pork.

References

von Brand, T., Weinstein, P. P., Mehlman, B., and Weinbach, E. C. (1952). Observations on the metabolism of bacteria-free larvae of *Trichinella spiralis*. *Exp. Parasitol.* **1**, 245–255.

Castro, G. A., and Fairbairn, D. (1969). Carbohydrates and lipids in *Trichinella spiralis* larvae and their utilization *in vivo*. *J. Parasitol.* **55**, 51–58.

Kurylo-Borowska, Z., and Kozar, Z. (1960). The general chemical composition of muscle *Trichinella spiralis* larvae. *Wiad. Parazytol.* **6**, 357–359.

Moore, L. L. A. (1966). Studies on the acquired immunity of white mice to somatic and cuticular antigens of *Trichinella spiralis*. *Dissertation Abstracts* **26**, 4132.

de Souza, N. J. and Nes, W. R. (1969). Improved separation of sterols by reversed-phase thin-layer chromatography. *J. Lipid Res.* **10**, 240–243.

Stahl, E. (1965). "Thin-Layer Chromatography: A Laboratory Handbook." Springer-Verlag, New York, p. 149.

The Effect of Alloxan Diabetes on Intestinal and Muscle Trichinellosis

R. Špaldonová, S. Komandarev, and O. Tomašovičová

Helminthological Institute of the Slovak Academy
of Sciences, Košice, and
Central Helminthological Laboratories of the
Bulgarian Academy of Sciences, Sofia

Introduction

The question of allergic reactions in the mechanism of immunity against helminthic parasites is gaining importance in spite of various experimental results on the direct effect of antibodies. It is difficult to give an unqualified answer to that question, since the physiological and biological properties of the helminths frequently are measured indirectly as immunological or allergic reactions of the host.

For this reason, any method available to eliminate or to inhibit one of the above reactions can be successfully applied to explain the mechanism of immunity against helminths. There is abundant information in the literature on the relation between between glucose levels and hypersensitive reactions, hence this seemed worthy of study.

Uzan and Cohen (1956) saved a guinea pig from histamine shock by the injection of glucose. Also, Goth *et al.* (1957) stated that in rats with alloxan diabetes there was no characteristic edema and no increased histamine level observed in the plasma after intravenously applied dextran or egg albumen; and Thompson (1961) found that a diabetes-producing dose of alloxan (175–200 mg/kg) protected about 50% of horse-serum sensitized rats.

Adamkiewicz (1963) investigated the relation between glycemia and immunological responses. He indicated that hyperglycemia induced by increased doses of sugar, cortisone, or adrenaline, or by diabetes suppressed anaphylactoid reactions, true anaphylaxis, and tuberculin reactions. He hypothesized that hyperglycemia inhibits some antigen–antibody interaction, which results in suppressed hypersensitivity.

Thompson and de Falco (1965) reported an inhibitory effect of alloxan

149

and glucose on general anaphylaxis in rats. In these animals, the protecting effect of alloxan is eliminated by insulin when the adrenal cortex functions normally. Alloxan also prevents histamine shock in mice. Data can be found in the parasitological literature on the relation between the blood sugar levels of the host and the degree of invasion, or the effectiveness of the immunological reaction.

According to Tolbert and McGhee (1960), Heguer and MacDougall produced hyperglycemia in the canary by intraperitoneal application of glucose or by use of feed with a high glucose content. In canaries with high blood sugar levels, *Plasmodium cathemerium* infection was more severe than in the control birds that had not been given glucose.

Tolbert and McGhee (1960) investigated the influence of alloxan diabetes on *Plasmodium berghei* infections in rats and found infections to be inhibited. Parasitemia was considerably lower in diabetic animals than in those that had not been given alloxan, or in cases where the latter had been applied but had not caused diabetes.

Some authors have investigated the glucose level in trichinellosis of man with regard to diagnosis. According to Augustine (1936), McDonald and Waddell found decreased blood levels; and Augustine (1936) added that this decrease is characteristic only during the intestinal stage of trichinellosis.

Other authors have reported the relations between blood sugar levels and the intensity of infection or the clinical course. According to Nitzulescu and Gherman (1959), Lewis fed guinea pigs a glucose-rich diet and he demonstrated that 22 days after the *Trichinella spiralis* invasion the count of muscle larvae in the masseter muscles of the controls was double that found in the experimental animals. In another experiment, the same author induced hypoglycemia with insulin and on day 21 he noted a considerably larger count of muscle larvae than that in the controls.

Nitzulescu and Gherman (1959) described a clinical case of a diabetic patient who did not fall ill with trichinellosis after eating a larger amount of infected meat than his companion who became seriously ill. The authors stated that the immunity in the diabetic patient had been the result of hyperglycemia.

Pawlowski (1967) found a maximum decrease in the blood sugar level on the seventh day after infection with *Trichinella spiralis* in rats. By the end of the intestinal expulsion period (day 14), the blood sugar level rose to or surpassed the normal values. The author acknowledged the fact that the changes in the blood sugar levels induced by glucocorticoid therapy or by adrenalectomy affect intestinal trichinellosis by increasing the caloric values. Alloxan and insulin-induced hyperglycemia led to an increased number of intestinal trichinellae on the seventh day after infection. The results of subsequent experiments indicated to Pawlowski that a glucose-rich diet renders expulsion of adult worms more difficult.

The purpose of the present work was to determine the influence of alloxan diabetes on the number of *T. spiralis* adult worms and muscle larvae after challenging immunized and nonimmunized mice.

Materials and Methods

A total of 681 white male mice of 20–25 gm weight were used in three series of experiments.

Series I (Nonimmunized Mice)

This series of experiments was conducted to examine the effect of hyperglycemia on the number of muscle larvae recovered. Increased glucose levels were achieved by alloxan (Lachema, Brno). The latter is a substance that damages pancreatic β-cells and thus causes so-called alloxan diabetes. Two-hundred-forty white male mice of 20–25 gm weight were used in the experiment. One-hundred-forty mice were given a single dose of 100 mg/kg alloxan into the coccygeal vein one week before experimental infection. In this experiment, animals with a 250 mg/100 ml hyperglycemia were included. Only one experimental group consisted of animals with a 200 mg/100 ml level and evaluation of this group was made separately. One-hundred mice were not given alloxan and served as controls. All animals were infected with 270 $\pm$15 *Trichinella spiralis* larvae through a stomach tube. The glucose levels were measured by the method of Homolka (1969). Blood samples were taken from the retroorbital venous plexus using Nöller's method. Evaluation was carried out on the fortieth day after infection. The mice were killed, the skin and internal organs were removed, and the muscles of the entire animals were digested in an artificial digestive juice consisting of hydrochloric acid, pepsin and water. The isolated larvae were counted in an agar suspension and compared with the controls.

Series II (Nonimmunized Mice)

The experiment was conducted on 236 mice, i.e., 116 experimental animals and 120 controls. The experimental mice were given a single dose of 100 mg/kg alloxan intravenously. On the fifth day after alloxan injection, the blood sugar levels were recorded for each of the mice according to Homolka (1969). Only those animals were included that showed a high blood sugar level of 200–395 mg/100 ml. Both experimental and control animals were infected with 300 larvae. Intestinal trichinellae were counted each day from day 1 to day 21 after infection.

Series III (Immunized Mice)

The experiment was conducted with 205 white mice (99 experimental and 106 control animals). Both experimental and control mice were immunized with three intraperitoneal applications of 1500 muscle larvae at 1-month intervals. The experimental animals were given alloxan on the seventh day after the last immunization, and both experimental and control animals were infected with muscle larvae. The intestinal trichinellae were counted as in Series II.

Results

Series I

It follows from the results of the experiment that mild hyperglycemia did not affect the number of muscle trichinellae as compared to that of the controls (Table 1). However, severe diabetes (300–500 mg/100 ml) increased the number of larvae in the muscles by 49%.

Series II

The dynamics of intestinal trichinellosis in nonimmunized mice revealed a certain parallelism with muscle infections up to day 11 after infection; mice with marked hyperglycemia always had a larger count of intestinal worms as compared with the control group. After day 11, a certain delay in expelling intestinal trichinellae was observed in alloxan mice. As a result of this, the number of intestinal trichinellae in diabetic mice counted every other day corresponded to the number counted in the controls 4 days earlier.

Series III

In immunized mice, hyperglycemia did not produce any substantial difference in the dynamics of intestinal trichinellosis (Fig. 1).

Discussion

The results obtained in our experiments indicate that the alloxan-induced hyperglycemia in the experimental animals led to an increased number of muscle trichinellae as compared with the controls. Mild hyperglycemia (200 mg/100 ml) did not increase the severity of muscle infections. The purpose of the Series II and III experiments was to determine

Table I   Effect of Hyperglycemia on the Intensity of *Trichinella spiralis* Invasion

Blood glucose level (mg/100ml)	Larval count	% Recovery
Normal (120–140)	32,298	100
Mild hyperglycemia (200)	35,820	110
Severe hyperglycemia (300–500)	48,440	149

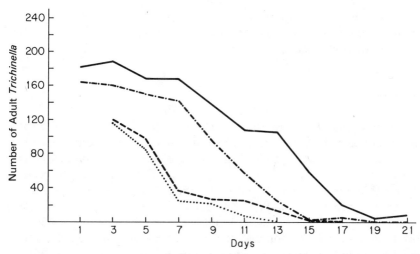

Figure 1 Dynamics of the number of intestinal *Trichinella* in alloxan-treated mice: immunized, nonimmunized, and controls, ———, Alloxan nonimmunized; – · – ·, controls; – – –, alloxan immunized; · · ·, controls.

the reason for the increased numbers of muscle larvae in animals with marked hyperglycemia (Series I). Special attention was devoted to the "critical" periods from the beginning of the intestinal invasion, i.e., days 11 and 12, and days 5 and 6 in nonimmunized and immunized animals, respectively. In the former group, the increased numbers of muscle trichinellae in alloxan-treated mice cannot be explained by a certain positive nutritive effect of hyperglycemia in the animals, since such a difference was not evident in the immunized animals.

The substantial differences in the number of intestinal worms in experimental and control mice form the eleventh day after infection suggest that the effect of hyperglycemia is in relation to the allergic responses of the host. As a result, hyperglycemia prolonged the persistence of the worms.

Our view coincides with that of Goth *et al.* (1957), Thompson (1961), Adamkiewicz (1963), and Thompson and de Falco (1965) regarding the inhibiting effect of alloxan diabetes on various allergic reactions in animals.

Our explanation confirms, although at first sight contrasting, the clinical observations of Nitzulescu and Gherman (1959) when a diabetic patient did not fall ill with trichinellosis in spite of having eaten a larger quantity of infected meat than a companion with severe illness. In this case, we cannot speak about immunity against trichinellosis, since detailed analysis was not possible for understandable reasons; we may speak only about the lack of clinical symptoms of trichinellosis.

With regard to the fact that trichinellosis is connected with allergic reactions it might be suggested that the allergic stimuli of the organism were inhibited by the diabetic state of the patient; as a result, the clinical symptoms of trichinellosis were lacking.

Summary

The authors investigated the effect of alloxan diabetes on *Trichinella spiralis* infections in white mice. They found that a low hyperglycemia did not affect substantially the number of muscle larvae recovered, whereas severe hyperglycemia increased the numbers by an average of 49% as compared with controls. It was found that until 11 days after infection there were greater numbers of adult worms in the intestines of the treated mice and afterward there was a delayed expulsion of worms compared with controls. In immunized mice, on the other hand, hyperglycemia did not affect the numbers or persistence of adult worms.

On the basis of the results, the authors suggest an inhibitory effect of hyperglycemia on the allergic response of the host to the parasite. Consequently, adult worms in large numbers persisted, and this accounted for the greatly increased numbers of muscle larvae.

References

Adamkiewicz, V. W. (1963). Glycemia and immune responses. *Can. Med. Ass. J.* **88** (15), 806–811.

Augustine, D. L. (1936). Blood sugar values and the tolerance for dextrose in trichinosis. *Amer. J. Hyg.* **24** (1), 170–176.

Goth, A., Nash, W. L., Nagler, M., and Holman, J. (1957). Inhibition of histamine release in experimental diabetes. *Amer. J. Physiol.* **191**, 25–28.

Homolka, J. (1969). Klinické biochemické vyšetrovacie metódy. *Statni Zdravotnicke Nakladatelstvi, Praha.*

Nitzulescu, V., and Gherman, I. (1959). Hyperglycemia ca factor de aparare in infectia trichinozica. *Med. Interna* **2**, 269–272.

Pawlowski, Z. (1967). Adrenal cortex hormones in intestinal trichinellosis. III. Effect of adrenalectomy and hydrocortisone, insulin, alloxan and glucose treatment on elimination of *Trichinella spiralis* adult in hooded rats. *Acta Parasitol. Pol.* **15**, 179–189.

Thompson, G. E. (1961). Alloxan and hypersensitivity. *Nature London* **190**, 822.

Thompson G. E., and de Falco, R. 1965. Alloxan and hypersensitivity. II. Effect of alloxan on hypersensitivity reactions in the mouse, rat and guinea pig. *Cornell Vet.* **55** (1), 66–74.

Tolbert, M. G., and McGhee, R. B. (1960). The effect of alloxan diabetes on *Plasmodium bergei* infection in albino rats. *J. Parasitol.* **46** (5) 552–558.

Uzan, M., and Cohen, M. (1956). Effect of hyperglycemia sur le shoc histaminique et anaphylactique chez animal. *Tunisie Med.* **44**, 39.

Part III

Immunobiology

Part III

Immunobiology

Intestinal and Serum Immunoglobulins and Antibodies in Mice Infected with *Trichinella*

W. J. Kozek* and R. B. Crandall

Department of Immunology and Medical Microbiology,
College of Medicine, University of Florida,
Gainesville, Florida

Introduction

In the immunized animal, the small intestine is the site of a host response to infection which results in reproductive inhibition and early expulsion of the helminth. The role of antibody in this immune response is uncertain and the changes in intestinal antibody populations associated with this response have not been well characterized. The purpose of this study was to examine the immunoglobulin and antibody responses after initial *Trichinella* infection and after a challenge infection in immunized animals to determine (1) if the intestinal response involved prominent leakage of serum antibodies into the intestinal tract and (2) if the secretory immunological system of the intestine was stimulated.

Materials and Methods

Animals

Three groups of female, CD mice (Charles River, Wilmington, Massachusetts), 6–8 weeks old were used. The mice were maintained in facilities fully accredited by the American Association for Accreditation of Laboratory Animal Care.

Group 1 contained 30 mice inoculated *per os* with 350 *Trichinella spiralis* larvae. Mice were perfused in groups of four at 3, 8, 14 and 22 days after inoculation. Two additional mice were held in reserve during each perfusion period and substituted for any mouse that died within 2 hr after perfusion was started. Uninfected CD mice of the same age and sex served as controls. Mice in Groups 2 and 3 were inoculated three times with 200

*Present address: California Primate Research Center, University of California, Davis, California.

T. spiralis larvae at 1-month intervals and challenged with 300 *T. spiralis* larvae 12 weeks after the last inoculation. There was one exception to this inoculation schedule: mice in Group 2, which were perfused at 7 and 11 days following challenge inoculation, were inoculated three times with approximately 300 rather than 200 *Trichinella* larvae. In Group 2 the intestines of four mice were perfused at 12 hr, 36 hr, and 7 and 11 days after challenge. In Group 3 the intestinal contents of 4 mice were collected at these same time periods after challenge inoculation. Mice inoculated three times but not challenged served as controls.

Intestinal Perfusion and Contents

Content of the small intestine was obtained and processed as described previously (Crandall and Crandall, 1972). The intestine was flushed out with cold saline, the content was homogenized in a blender and then centrifuged to remove particulate material, and the supernate was pressure dialyzed under vacuum to a small volume.

The technique for perfusion of the small intestine *in situ* was similar to that described by Bazin *et al.* (1971). Briefly, the perfusion apparatus consisted of a saline reservoir, polyethylene delivery and drainage tubes, and a flow regulating clamp. The delivery tube was passed through a water bath which kept the temperature of the perfusion fluid (0.9% sodium chloride irrigation solution, Travenol Laboratories, Morton Grove, Illinois) entering the intestine between 34° and 37°C. Food was removed from mice the evening prior to perfusion to decrease blockage of the draining tube by intestinal content. Mice were anesthetized by intraperitoneal injection of Nembutal and bled prior to perfusion from the suborbital sinus. Anesthesia was maintained by placing 3–5 drops of dilute Nembutal into the peritoneal cavity. The intestine was exposed through an abdominal, midline incision. The pylorus was ligated and the glass-tipped end of the delivery tube was inserted into the lumen through a small incision in the duodenal wall. The tube was held in place by a ligature around the duodenum. In the same manner, the ileocecal junction was ligated and the drainage tube was inserted. The intestine was flushed out rapidly to remove solid contents and then perfused, usually for 6 hr, at a rate of 10–20 ml/hr. The perfusate was collected in tubes held in an ice bath. The perfusates were centrifuged to remove large particles, and those perfusates collected during the first 3 hr were pooled. Pools were concentrated by pressure dialysis against saline to a volume of 0.8–2 ml. The sediment from centrifugation of perfusates was examined for evidence of bleeding during the perfusion. Perfusates and sera were stored at −20°C until used.

Chemical and Immunological Tests

Protein content of perfusates and intestinal contents was determined by the method of Lowry *et al.* (1951). The levels of IgA and IgG$_1$ were measured by radial immunodiffusion. The results were expressed as total protein and immunoglobulin in the intestinal content or 3-hr perfusate. A two-sample rank test was used to compare immunoglobulin levels; a probability value of 0.05% was considered significant. Antibody titers in sera and detection of antibody in perfusates and contents were carried out by the indirect fluorescent antibody (FA) technique in two mice from each time-group examined. All tests were performed as described in a previous study (Crandall and Crandall, 1972).

Results

The protein, immunoglobulin, and antibody measurements from all experiments are summarized in Tables I and II. In the perfusion experiments, only traces of blood (erythrocytes) were detected in the sedimented pellet in most cases; however, in some mice internal bleeding was considerable. These cases are noted below.

Serum Immunoglobulin Levels and Antibody Titers

IgG_1 A significant increase in serum IgG_1 over preinoculation levels was observed at 14 and 22 days after primary infection (Group 1). In both hyperinfected groups (2 and 3) the high levels before challenge, about 5 mg/ml, were further increased after the challenge infection. The higher concentrations of IgG_1 at 7 and 11 days in Group 2 in comparison with Group 3 probably reflects the larger inocula given this group (see Materials and Methods).

To measure antibody titers, all sera were diluted 1:40 to avoid any possibility of nonspecific staining in the indirect FA test. Antibody at a titer of 1:320 was detected at 14 days following primary infection; titers remained at approximately this level in the hyperinfected animals. There was an indication of increased titers during the first week after challenge infection of hyperinfected mice.

IgA The concentrations of serum IgA remained essentially unchanged during primary infection. In the hyperinfected groups, the IgA levels were variable but generally higher than following initial infection.

Serum IgA antibodies were detected at low titers (1:40) 14 days after inoculation; titers remained relatively low in all groups of mice. The higher titers observed at 7 and 11 days in Group 2 again probably reflects the higher inocula administered to these mice.

Immunoglobulin Levels and Antibody Activity in Perfusates and Gut Contents

IgG_1 IgG_1, in the perfusates from initial infection (Group 1), was either not detected or detected at concentrations too low to measure (less than 0.1 mg total Ig). Total protein content of perfusates remained un-

Table I IgA and IgG$_1$ Levels in Serum, Perfusates, and Intestinal Contents of Mice Inoculated with *Trichinella spiralis.*[a]

Days post inoculation	Total protein	IgA Serum (mg/ml)	IgA Perfusate (total mg/3 hr)	IgG$_1$ Serum (mg/ml)	IgG$_1$ Perfusate (total mg/3 hr)
Group 1[b]					
0	1.17 (0.86–1.37)	0.40 (0.26–0.51)	0.14 (0.09–0.17)	1.26 (1.01–1.29)	tr[c]
3	1.18 (0.53–2.65)	0.48 (0.46–0.53)	0.32 (0.04–0.83)	0.95 (0.47–1.41)	tr
8	6.95 (0.56–24.96)	0.75 (0.59–1.01)	0.20 (0.09–0.42)	1.10 (0.76–1.31)	0[d]
14	1.05 (0.59–1.87)	0.59 (0.36–0.75)	0.40 (0.14–0.79)	2.73 (2.01–3.57)	tr
22[e]	1.18 (0.45–1.58)	0.50 (0.46–0.54)	0.39 (0.14–0.69)	4.41 (2.43–7.22)	0

Days post challenge	Total protein	IgA Serum (mg/ml)	IgA Perfusate (total mg/3 hr)	IgG$_1$ Serum (mg/ml)	IgG$_1$ Perfusate (total mg/3 hr)
Group 2[f]					
0	1.31 (0.88–1.76)	0.68 (0.36–1.01)	0.57 (0.16–1.34)	5.08 (2.74–6.38)	0
½	1.35 (0.84–1.98)	1.60 (0.97–1.98)	0.56 (0.18–1.44)	6.40 (4.33–11.40)	tr
1½	1.52 (1.30–1.79)	0.68 (0.36–1.08)	0.47 (0.33–0.62)	4.21 (2.74–5.28)	tr
7	5.5 (2.59–9.6)	1.24 (0.71–1.98)	1.42 (0.70–1.52)	13.7 (6.8–21.4)	0.75 (0.22–2.14)
11	9.0 (1.52–24.2)	1.06 (0.73–1.80)	0.94 (0.59–1.23)	18.5 (17.1–20.3)	1.75 (0.19–5.99)

Days post challenge	Total protein	IgA Serum (mg/ml)	IgA Perfusate (Contents total mg)	IgG$_1$ Serum (mg/ml)	IgG$_1$ Perfusate (Contents total mg)
Group 3[f]					
0	5.8 (5.1–7.2)	1.52 (0.8–3.1)	0.57 (0.43–0.70)	5.6 (2.3–8.1)	0.47 (0.35–0.61)
½	3.5 (3.1–4.1)	2.3 (1.2–3.1)	0.81 (0.26–1.10)	5.9 (3.6–8.1)	0.14 (0.11–0.18)
1½	6.6 (4.7–8.5)	1.7 (0.9–3.5)	0.84 (0.50–1.15)	4.9 (2.1–7.6)	0.29 (0.22–0.37)
7	7.3 (5.6–8.5)	2.8 (1.7–5.0)	1.32 (0.97–1.60)	6.4 (5.5–8.1)	0.45 (0.28–0.53)
11	6.7 (5.0–8.8)	1.4 (1.0–1.7)	1.57 (0.58–1.98)	10.9 (8.4–14.4)	0.48 (0.38–0.60)

[a] Data given as mean of four animals with range in parentheses.
[b] Initial inoculation.
[c] Less than 0.1 mg total.
[d] None detected.
[e] Group consisted of three mice.
[f] Hyperimmune mice.

changed after primary infection with the exception of a single animal perfused at 8 days which gave an unexplained, high concentration. Only trace amounts of IgG_1 were detected in perfusates from the hyperinfected mice (Group 2) until day 7 and 11. Perfusates from most of these animals were obviously bloody and the total protein levels were elevated. It was assumed that the intestinal bleedings was induced by trauma during perfusion rather than by the infection. The IgG_1 in the intestinal contents of hyperinfected mice (Group 3) was easily measured; with the exception of a decrease in total protein and IgG_1 at 12 hr, there was little change following challenge infection.

Antibody was detected in IgG_1 of perfusates at 14 days after initial infection. Antibody activity of varying intensity was detected in perfusates of hyperinfected animals at all time intervals examined. No pattern of antibody response in respect to challenge infection was evident. Antibody in intestinal content of hyperinfected animals was detected first at 12 hr after challenge infection and at low levels at all subsequent times after challenge.

IgA Perfusates, following primary infection (Group 1), contained similar amounts of IgA. In hyperinfected groups (2 and 3) IgA levels were usually higher, and a significant increase in IgA was obvious by the second week after challenge in both groups, although intestinal bleeding in Group 2 made this observation of questionable significance.

Antibody was detected in perfusates at day 8 following initial infection and appeared to be increased by day 14. In hyperinfected groups antibody was detected by 24 hr after challenge infection and usually at all the succeeding periods investigated.

Discussion

The serum immunoglobulin and antibody responses of CD mice to *Trichinella* infection and hyperinfection observed in this study generally agree with the results of a previous study with two other strains of mice (Crandall and Crandall, 1972). In both studies an increase in serum IgG_1 during the second week of infection paralleled antibody detection in this class. Hyperinfected animals maintained elevated serum IgG_1 levels and antibody titers, and gave evidence of an anamnestic response after a challenge infection. In contrast, serum IgA levels were variable; hyperinfected animals had somewhat elevated levels but generally there was comparatively little IgA response to infection or hyperinfection and serum antibody titers remained low.

The purposes of this study were to determine if the intestinal immune response to *Trichinella* infection involved (1) leakage of serum immunoglobulins into the gut and (2) stimulation of the secretory immunological

Table II IgA and IgG$_1$ Antibody Detection in the Serum, Perfusates, and Intestinal Contents of Mice Infected with *Trichinella spiralis*[a]

Days post inoculation Group 1	IgA		IgG$_1$	
	Serum	Perfusate[b]	Serum	Perfusate[b]
0	0	0	0	0
8	0	+	0	0
14	40–80	2–4+	320	1+
22	0–40	2–4+	320	1–2+
Days post challenge Group 2[c]	Serum	Perfusate[b]	Serum	Perfusate[b]
0	0–40	0	160–320	1–2+
½	0	0–2+	320	1–4+
1½	0	2+	320	1+
7	160	3–4+	320–640	4+
11	40–160	2+	160	0–2+
Days post challenge Group 3[c]	Serum	Contents[b]	Serum	Contents[b]
0	40	0	80–160	0
½	0	+	160	0–1+
1½	0	0–1+	160–320	1–2+
7	40	1–2+	320	0–2+
11	0–40	1–2+	320	1+

[a] Two mice tested at each time period.
[b] Indirect FA technique done on undiluted, concentrated perfusates and contents. 0 = undetected antibody, 1+ to 4+ = weak to strong fluorescence.
[c] Hyperimmune mice.

system. Mice given a series of *Trichinella* infections, as in this study, are reported to develop an intense inflammatory response in the mucosa and submucosa of the upper intestine within 1 day after a challenge infection; this accelerated, acute inflammatory response is considered to be immunologically initiated perhaps by a cell-mediated response (Larsh, 1968). Regardless of mediation, this inflammation could be associated with extravasation of serum Ig and antibody; in addition, it has been demonstrated that following *Trichinella* infection mice develop a systemic anaphylactic sensitivity to *Trichinella* antigens (Briggs and DeGiusti, 1966). An intestinal infection in immune animals might be anticipated to produce an intestinal anaphylactic response with increased vascular permeability and leakage of serum immunoglobulins.

This study demonstrated IgG$_1$ antibody in the intestine during *Trichinella* infection, but does not indicate any major leakage of this serum immunoglobulin into the intestine during initial infection or challenge infection of hyperinfected mice. In fact, the concentration of IgG_1 in the intestinal content appeared to be reduced early after challenge infection when an intestinal anaphylactic response would be expected. This study does not exclude the possibility that the intestinal response to *Trichinella* includes a period of increased intestinal permeability and plasma leakage which could be demonstrated with the application of more sensitive techniques and by inclusion of more time intervals after infection.

It is well established that the immunoglobulin-containing cells of the intestinal mucosa are part of the secretory immunological system which can function independently of the systemic immunological system and in which IgA is the principal immunoglobulin class (Heremans, 1968). It is not known if this system has any role in immunity to intestinal helminth infections. The results of this study indicate a secretory, immunological response to *Trichinella* infection, although a direct demonstration of secretory IgA was not attempted. The high concentrations of IgA in the intestinal contents and perfusates in relation to the serum levels is consistent with the described local production and secretion of this immunoglobulin. IgA antibody to *Trichinella* was detected more or less independently of serum titers, suggesting local production and secretion; in contrast, IgG_1 intestinal antibody was always associated with high serum titers. Intestinal IgA antibody was detected after both initial infection and challenge infection of hyperinfected mice; however, it cannot be concluded from the results whether the IgA intestinal response was significantly increased in the hyperinfected animals.

Summary

The intestinal and humoral immunoglobulin and antibody responses to *Trichinella* infection and hyperinfection were compared to determine if the intestinal response involved secretion of immunoglobulins and if leakage of serum immunoglobulins into the intestinal tract was prominent. The small intestines of groups of four mice each were perfused with warm saline *in situ* for 3 hr at 3, 8, 14, and 22 days following oral inoculation of 300 *Trichinella* larvae. Similar perfusions were done on groups of mice immunized by three oral inoculations of larvae; these groups were perfused at 12 and 36 hr, and at 7 and 11 days following a challenge inoculation of 300 larvae. The intestinal contents of mice from groups similar to the immunized and challenged mice were obtained by washing out the small intestine. Concentrations of IgG_1 and IgA were measured in sera and concentrated intestinal perfusates and contents by radial immunodiffusion; the indirect fluorescent antibody technique was used to titer antibody and to determine immunoglobulin class.

Serum IgG_1 levels were increased by the end of week 2 after initial inoculation; high serum levels of IgG$_1$ were maintained in the immunized groups. Serum IgG$_1$ antibody was detected at 14 days after initial inoculation and increases in antibody titers were observed in immunized mice. IgG$_1$ levels in intestinal content or prefusate generally remained at low levels, but antibody was detected when serum antibody titers were high. Serum IgA levels were variable after primary inoculation and hyperinoculation although concentrations were usually higher in the hyperinoculated mice. Serum antibody in IgA was detected with low titers by day 14 after initial inoculation and remained low in immunized mice. Intestinal levels of IgA increased after challenge of immunized animals. Antibody was detected 8 days after initial inoculation and at all times following challenge inoculation of immunized animals.

The results confirm the serum IgG$_1$ and IgA responses to *Trichinella* infection and hyperinfection previously reported. No evidence was obtained of an anaphylactic response with marked increases in intestinal content of serum immunoglobulins. The lack of correlation between antibody content or concentrations in serum and secreted IgA suggested local intestinal synthesis of this immunoglobulin.

Acknowledgments

We wish to thank Ms. Marybruce Dowd for her technical assistance.
Supported in part by Public Health Service Grants AI-03212 and AI-05345 from the NIAID and NIH Training Grant 5TI AI 0128.

References

Bazin, H., Levi, J., and Heremans, J. F. (1971). The metabolism of different immunoglobulin classes in irradiated mice. IV. Fate of circulating IgA of tumor or transfusion origin. *Immunology* **20**, 563–570.

Briggs, N. T., and DeGiusti, D. L. (1966). Generalized allergic reactions in *Trichinella*-infected mice: the temporal association of host immunity and sensitivity to exogenous antigens. *Amer. J. Trop. Med. Hyg.* **15**, 919–929.

Crandall, R. B., and Crandall, C. A. (1972). *Trichinella spiralis:* immunologic response to infection in mice. *Exp. Parasitol.* **31**, 378–398.

Heremans, J. F. (1968). Immunoglobulin formation and function in different tissues. *Curr. Top. Microbiol. Immunol.* **45**, 131–203.

Larsh, J. E., Jr. (1968). Experimental trichiniasis. *Adv. Parasitol.* **6**, 361–372.

Lowry, O. H., Rosebrough, N. J., Farr, A. L., and Randall, R. J. (1951). Protein measurements with the Folin phenol reagent. *J. Biol. Chem.* **193**, 265–275.

Blood Eosinophilia Induced by the Intestinal Stages of *Trichinella spiralis* in Immunized Animals

Tsue-Ming Lin and Leroy J. Olson

University of Miami School of Medicine, Miami, Florida
University of Texas Medical Branch, Galveston, Texas

Introduction

Eosinophilia is a common associate of helminthic infections. Since Brown's observations in 1897 on a patient with trichinellosis, eosinophilia has been known as a prominent sign and aid in the diagnosis of this infection (Gould, 1945). Opie (1904 a,b) reported that, while bacteria caused eosinopenia, *Trichinella* infection induced blood eosinophilia in guinea pigs. The eosinophilia became evident in the second week and reached a peak in the following 2 weeks. His experimental findings have since been repeatedly observed by numerous investigators. Primarily based on the time of onset, this host response is generally believed to be induced by the larvae migrating in the tissues (Gould, 1945; Ismail and Tanner, 1972). The role of the intestinal stage in this response has been difficult to assess in part because of the production of premuscle larvae by adult worms as early as 4–5 days after infection (Villella, 1970; Harley and Gallicchio, 1971).

However, there is some evidence in the literature which indicates that the intestinal stages (preadult and adult) can initiate an eosinophilia, i.e., the observations of blood eosinophilia in experimental animals within 4 days after infection by Pollay *et al.* (1954), Zaiman *et al.* (1963), and Ismail and Tanner (1972).

Zaiman *et al.* (1963) have used irradiated larvae to infect rats in an attempt to assess the role of the intestinal stages in causing an eosinophilia. Conflicting results were obtained, i.e., larvae irradiated with 12,000 or 16,000 R failed to stimulate an eosinophilia, whereas larvae irradiated with 14,000 R did. Zaiman and Villverde (1964) further observed moderate blood eosinophilia in uninfected parabiotic rats which had been separated from their infected partners at 4½–5½ days after infection. However, it is difficult to understand that the uninfected twins showed marked eosinophilia earlier than their infected twins, and also showed a second rise

165

in eosinophils at 3 or 4 weeks after infection. Campbell and Cuckler (1966) observed blood eosinophilia in one rat with this infection which was given anthelminthics and found at sacrifice to have only a very small number of muscle larvae.

Recent studies (Litt, 1961; Cohen and Sapp, 1968; Basten *et al.,* 1970; Boyer *et al.,* 1970; Cohen and Ward, 1971) have shown that an eosinophilia is preceeded by events involving antigen, specific antibody, and/or other reactions. Thus, Campbell (1942) did not observe blood eosinophilia in guinea pigs until 2–4 days after an initial injection with ascaris keratin, and maximum eosinophilia was not reached until 5–10 days. Very similar results were obtained by other investigators using other immunogens (Basten *et al.,* 1970; Spry, 1971; Archer and Binet, 1971). Taking this time factor into consideration, the blood eosinophilia of early infection reported by many investigators could well be induced by the intestinal worms rather than the subsequent migrating larvae. It is also possible that intestinal worms stimulate a further increase in eosinophilia during the remainder of their stay in the gut.

The present study was carried out to demonstrate a blood eosinophil response to the intestinal phase of trichinellosis in guinea pigs, based on the assumption that the onset of an eosinophilia after this infection should be accelerated in immunized or sensitized animals as are other immune reponses (Archer, 1963).

Materials and Methods

Albino guinea pigs were purchased at 200 gm from Albino Farms, New Jersey, were kept in air-conditioned quarters and fed on water and commercial feed *ad libitum.* Blood for eosinophil counts was obtained from the marginal veins of the ear at the same time (9–11 A. M.) each day; duplicate counts of each sample were made with a hemocytometer by the propylene glycol diluent technique (Olson and Schulz, 1963).

Trichinella spiralis was maintained in albino mice purchased from Texas Inbred, Houston, Texas. Infective larvae were recovered by pepsin digestion of infected mice and orally administered to guinea pigs in the afternoon (Castro and Olson, 1967). Larval sonicate was prepared as described by Lin and Olson (1969). Antiserum was obtained by heart puncture of guinea pigs infected with 20,000 larvae 6–10 weeks earlier.

Results

Four experiments each with a different design were carried out. Each experiment included four groups of animals: SC, immunized (sensitized) and challenged; S, immunized only; C, challenged only; N, neither immunized nor challenged.

Experiment 1

Animals were immunized and challenged 32 days later by a single infection with 2500 and 20,000 larvae, respectively. The immunizing infection produced a mild eosinophilia first apparent in the third week. Comparison of means showed that the SC group responded to challenge with a prompt increase in eosinophil counts beginning on day 2; counts continued to rise throughout the remainder of the experiment (Fig. 1A). By contrast, the eosinophil response in challenge controls, group C, was delayed 1 week. Data on individual animals from the SC and S groups, in addition to showing the effect of challenge on cell counts of immunized animals, further showed the variation in this kind of experiment (Fig. 1B).

Experiment 2

Animals were immunized and challenged 30 days later by infection with 2500 and 2000 larvae, respectively. As shown in Fig. 2A, immunization elicited a rather high eosinophilia in group S which reached a peak in 4 weeks and declined rapidly in the fifth week. In SC animals the challenge infection appeared to postpone this decline as a result of a second eosinophil response within 4 days after challenge. This second peak was seen in three out of four SC animals and in none of the control S animals (Fig. 2B).

Experiment 3

Animals were immunized with subcutaneous injections of 0.5 ml of larval sonicate given daily on days 0 through 5 and again on day 12. A challenge infection of 20,000 larvae was given on day 28. Saline injections were similarly given to nonimmunized animals. The eosinophilia due to immunization had largely disappeared 1 week after the last injection (Fig. 3). Beginning on day 2 post-challenge a second rise in counts was noted for the SC group; counts for other groups remained low.

Experiment 4

A single intraperitoneal injection of 4 ml antiserum was given to each SC and S animal. A similar injection of normal guinea pig serum was given to each C and N animal. A challenge infection of 20,000 larvae was given to each SC and C animal one day after the injection of antiserum. The eosinophil counts for SC animals were increased on day 4 and clearly elevated on day 7 (Fig. 4). Animals in Group C showed a similar, but lesser response.

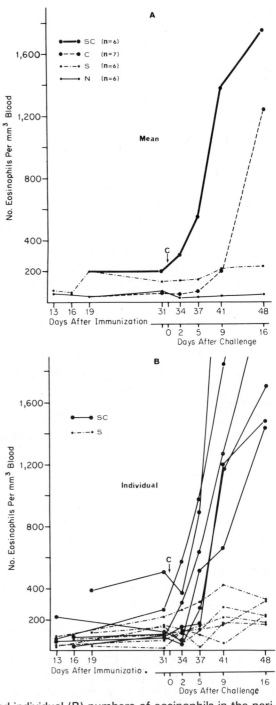

Figure 1 Mean (A) and individual (B) numbers of eosinophils in the peripheral blood of guinea pigs following an oral inoculation of 2500 infective larvae and 32 days later a challenge infection with 20,000 larvae. "C" with an arrow indicates the time when the challenge infection was given.

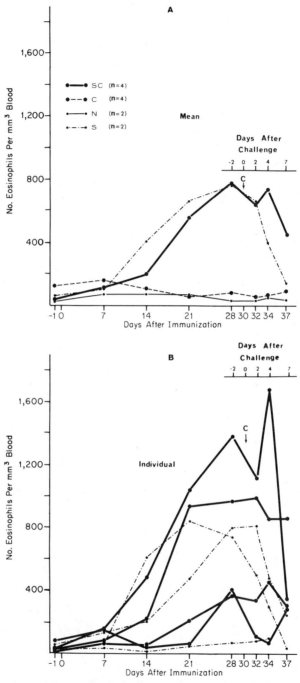

Figure 2   Mean (A) and individual (B) numbers of eosinophils in the peripheral blood of guinea pigs following an oral inoculation of 2500 infective larvae and 30 days later a challenge infection with 2000 larvae. One S animal was not included in the mean for this group because of its nonreactivity. "C" with an arrow denotes the challenge infection.

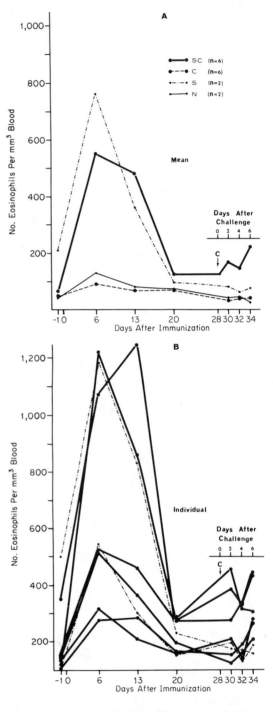

Figure 3 Mean (A) and individual (B) numbers of eosinophils in the peripheral blood of guinea pigs following a series of subcutaneous injections of larval sonicate and a challenge infection with 20,000 larvae on day 28. "C" with an arrow denotes the challenge infection.

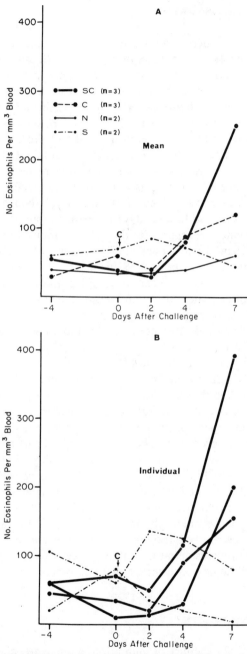

Figure 4 Mean (A) and individual (B) numbers of eosinophils in the peripheral blood of guinea pigs following an intraperitoneal injection of 4 ml anti-*Trichinella* serum and 24 hr later a challenge infection with 20,000 infective larvae. "C" with an arrow denotes the challenge infection.

Discussion

In these experiments, animals previously immunized by infection, by injection of antigen, or passively with antiserum responded to a challenge infection with a rise in eosinophilia detectable within 2–4 days after the challenge infection. By contrast, an eosinophilia was not noted for challenge controls until days 6 to 9 in these experiments. These data indicate that the intestinal stages of *T. spiralis* (preadult and adult) do contribute to the blood eosinophilia of this infection.

These data also support the concept that eosinophilia in helminthic infections is an immune mediated response of the host. Hence, our immunized guinea pigs were immunologically prepared to react promptly to *Trichinella* antigens at the time of challenge, whereas the controls needed several additional days to permit a similar reaction. The rapid development of *T. spiralis* in the gut, i.e., four molts and maturation in 2 days (Ali Khan, 1966; Kozek, 1971), seems to be associated with the release of a number of antigens as has been observed for other nematodes (Soulsby, 1963). Evidence that developing and molting *T. spiralis* are releasing significant amounts of antigens is the development of some immunity in mice to challenge after the immunizing infection was terminated after 20-hr (Campbell, 1965) or after 72- and 96-hr duration (Denham, 1966). Also, at least 7 antigens have been recognized in 18- to 20-hr cultures of infective larvae (Crandall and Zam, 1968).

Subsequent to completion of this study, Basten and Beeson (1970) reported that the thoracic duct lymphocytes from rats with a 3- to 5-day infection of *T. spiralis* could transfer the stimulus to eosinopoiesis. This finding supports the view in the present study that the intestinal stages of this parasite initiate the eosinophilia in trichinellosis. It was surprising, however, that the same cells from shorter ($\frac{1}{2}$- to $2\frac{1}{2}$-day) as well as longer (11- to 15-day, and 35-day) infections were inactive in this regard. It was also learned recently from Despommier (1972, personal communication) that premuscle larvae of *T. spiralis* (from the adult females) provoked no blood eosinophilia in rats in the first 10 days or so when injected intramuscularly although they migrate and eventually encyst in the skeletal muscle as in natural infection. In an earlier report by Despommier (1971), these newborn larvae were shown to lack immunogenicity.

Summary

The ability of immunized animals to accelerate their reactions to challenge was the basis of an attempt to demonstrate an eosinophil response to the intestinal phase of trichinellosis. Guinea pigs were immunized (4 weeks prior to challenge) by infection, injection of larval sonicate, or injection of homologous antiserum. In the first week after a challenge infection, all groups of immunized animals showed higher blood eosinophilia than nonchallenged controls, while cell counts for nonimmunized controls remained normal. Some animals immunized by infection or injection of sonicate responded to challenge with an eosinophilia within 2 or 4 days. These results indicate that the intestinal stages of *Trichinella spiralis* can induce an eosinophilia.

References

Ali Khan, Z. (1966). The postembryonic development of *Trichinella spiralis* with special reference to ecdysis. *J. Parasitol.* **52**, 248–259.

Archer, G. T., and Binet, J. L. (1971). Mast cell hyperplasia and eosinophilia induced by ascaris body fluid. *Brit. J. Exp. Pathol.* **52**, 696–702.

Archer, R. K. (1963). "The Eosinophil Leukocytes." Davis, Philadelphia, Pennsylvania.

Basten, A., and Beeson, P. B. (1970). Mechanism of eosinophilia. II. Role of the lymphocyte. *J. Exp. Med.* **131**, 1288–1305.

Basten, A., Boyer, M. H., and Beeson, P. B. (1970). Mechanism of eosinophilia. I. Factors affecting the eosinophil response of rats to *Trichinella spiralis*. *J. Exp. Med.* **131**, 1271–1287.

Boyer, M. H., Basten, A., and Beeson, P. B. (1970). Mechanism of eosinophilia. III. Suppression of eosinophilia by agents known to modify immune responses. *Blood* **36**, 458–470.

Brown, T. R. (1897). Studies on trichinosis. *Bull. Hopkins Hosp.* **8**, 79–81.

Campbell, D. H. (1942). Experimental eosinophilia with keratin from *Ascaris suum* and other sources. *J. Infec. Dis.* **71**, 270-276.

Campbell, W. C. (1965). Immunizing effect of enteral and enteral-parenteral infections of *Trichinella spiralis* in mice. *J. Parasitol.* **51**, 185–194.

Cambell, W. C., and Cuckler, A. C. (1966). Further studies on the effect of thiabendazole on trichinosis in swine, with notes on the biology of the infection. *J. Parasitol.* **52**, 260–279.

Castro, G. A., and Olson, L. J. (1967). Relationship between body weight and food and water intake in *Trichinella spiralis*-infected guinea pigs. *J. Parasitol.* **53**, 589–594.

Cohen, S. G., and Sapp, T. M. (1968). Tissue eosinophil response to complexes of antigen and antibody of varying character. *Ann. Allergy* **26**, 531–535.

Cohen, S., and Ward, P. A. (1971). *In vitro* and *in vivo* activity of a lymphocyte and immune complex-dependent chemotacic factor for eosinophils. *J. Exp. Med.* **133**, 133–146.

Crandall, R. B., and Zam, S. G. (1968). Analysis of excretory-secretory products of *Trichinella spiralis* larvae by disc-electrophoresis and immunodiffusion. *Amer. J. Trop. Med. Hyg.* **17**, 747–751.

Denham, D. A. (1966). Immunity to *Trichinella spiralis*. I. The immunity produced by mice to the first four days of the intestinal phase of the infection. *Parasitology* **56**, 323–327.

Despommier, D. D. (1971). Immunogenicity of the newborn larva of *Trichinella spiralis. J. Parasitol.* **57,** 531–534.

Gould, S. E. (1945). "Trichinosis." Thomas, Springfield, Illinois.

Harley, J. P., and Gallicchio, V. (1971). *Trichinella spiralis:* Migration of larvae in the rat. *Exp. Parasitol.* **30,** 11–21.

Ismail, M. M., and Tanner, C. E. (1972). *Trichinella spiralis:* Peripheral blood, intestinal, and bone-marrow eosinophilia in rats and its relationship to the inoculating dose of larvae, antibody response and parasitism. *Exp. Parasitol.* **31,** 262–272.

Kozek, W. J. (1971). The molting pattern in *Trichinella spiralis.* I. A light microscope study. *J. Parasitol.* **57,** 1015–1028.

Lin, T. M., and Olson, L. J. (1969). Prolonged toxic effect of *Trichinella spiralis* larval sonicate on the absorption of glucose by guinea pig intestine. *J. Parasitol.* **55,** 223–224.

Litt, M. (1961). Studies in experimental eosinophilia. III. The induction of peritoneal eosinophilia by the passive transfer of serum antibody. *J. Immunol.* **87,** 522–529.

Olson, L. J., and Schulz, C. W. (1963). Nematode induced hypersensitivity reactions in guinea pigs: Onset of eosinophilia and positive Schultz-Dale reactions following graded infections with *Toxocara canis. Ann. N.Y. Acad. Sci.* **113,** 440–455.

Opie, E. L. (1904a). An experimental study of the relation of cells with eosinophile granulation to infection with an animal parasite *(Trichinella spiralis). Amer. J. Med. Sci.* **127,** 477–493.

Opie, E. L. (1904b). The relation of cells with eosinophile granulation to bacterial infection. *Amer. J. Med. Sci.* **127,** 988–1010.

Pollay, W., Wein, B., and Hartmann, H. A. (1954). Effect of ACTH upon artificially induced trichinoisis in rats with special references to eosinophilia. *Proc. Soc. Exp. Biol. Med.* **86,** 577–580.

Soulsby, E. J. L. (1963). The relative value of differences in antigens from various stages of helminth parasites as used in diagnostic tests. *Amer. J. Hyg. Monogr. Seri.* **22,** 47–59.

Spry, C. J. F. (1971). Mechanism of eosinophilia. V. Kinetics of normal and accelerated eosinopoiesis. *Cell Tissue Kinet.* **4,** 351–364.

Villella, J. B. (1970). Life cycle and morphology. In S. E. Gould (ed.), "Trichinosis in Man and Animals." Thomas, Springfield, Illinois, pp. 19–60.

Zaiman, H., and Villaverde, H. (1964). Studies on the eosinophilic response of parabiotic rats infected with *Trichinella spiralis. Exp. Parasitol.* **15,** 14–31.

Zaiman, H., Scardino, V., Berson, P., and Stern, R. C. (1963). Further studies on the eosinophilic response of rats infected with irradiated *Trichinella. Exp. Parasitol.* **14,** 1–8.

Immunological Characterization of Antigenic Fractions of *Trichinella spiralis* Larvae

Fernando Beltrán-Hernández, Alberto Gómez-Priego, and Velia Estela Figueroa-Villalva

Immunoparasitology Laboratory
Department of Human Ecology
Faculty of Medicine
National University of Mexico
Mexico City

Introduction

Although human trichinellosis exists in the Mexican Republic, it is not considered to be an important public health problem. Taking into account the data reported by Perrín (1942), Mazzoti (1944), Beck (1953), and Biagi and Robledo (1962), the incidence of human infection is probably between 5 and 15%.

In our opinion, many cases of intestinal infection presented annually are erroneously diagnosed as originating from alimentary intoxication or infection by enterobacteria, which present symptoms similar to the intestinal phase of clinical trichinellosis. This situation cannot be clarified as yet because of the lack of sufficiently pure antigenic material specific for use in serologic diagnosis.

Sadun (1962) critically analyzed the antigenic characteristics of material obtained from *Trichinella spiralis* using different extraction methods. Of these methods, the most commonly utilized is that described by Melcher (1943). The antigenic material may be considered partially purified when the acid-soluble fraction is used. In recent years there have been important advances in the field of immunobiology of trichinellosis. Nevertheless, the necessity of adequate handling of immunodiagnostic techniques has not yet been completely achieved.

At present, there are no methods of extraction of antigenic material which could be used to give consistent results in any laboratory. Also, specific antigenic fractions have not yet been identified and characterized sufficiently to permit their large-scale use in serologic diagnosis.

There have also been important advances in basic research in trichinel-

175

losis in recent years, e.g., the observations of Cypess *et al.* (1971) on the participation of migration inhibitory factor (MIF), a soluble chemical mediator, in the phenomenon of cellular hypersensitivity in experimental trichinellosis. The *in vitro* work of Berntzen (1965) opens up great possibilities for immunobiological studies. Despommier (1971) and Despommier and Müller (1970) have demonstrated that the stichocytes, present only in muscle-stage larvae and in adults, contain secretory granules of various types, which probably represent deposits of functional antigens. Unfortunately, advances at the clinical level have been much slower.

We consider that at the present time, the principal necessities which must be satisfied are related to three major fields: (1) immunological surveillance at the veterinary level, (2) seroepidemiology in human populations, and (3) serodiagnosis of human trichinellosis.

To begin to solve any of the problems so far mentioned, it is first necessary to overcome the obstacles presented by the antigenic material now being used. For the last 29 years, the Melcher process for obtaining antigens from different helminths has been continuously utilized. Other methods, e.g., that of Chaffee *et al.* (1954), have been described. These have certain advantages, but give rise to a technical problem, as does the Melcher antigen.

In this chapter, we present some preliminary results obtained using crude soluble somatic antigen of *T. spiralis*–somatic antigen, sucrose-acetone (SASA), which is prepared using the method described by Clark and Casals (1958). With this antigenic material it is possible to study the humoral immune response of experimentally infected rats. Although rats are not good antibody producers, they are natural hosts for *T. spiralis* and were used for this study. We also present some preliminary results with fractions obtained from crude material.

Materials and Methods

Preparation of Crude Antigen

This was prepared from *T. spiralis* larvae encapsulated in the muscular tissue of white rats, 8 weeks after infection. The larvae were obtained by artificial digestion of the tissue at 37°C for 5 hr using a pepsin and hydrochloric acid mixture (Gursh, 1948). After several washes with saline solution and saline solution plus antibiotics, the larvae were homogenized in four volumes of 8.5% (0.24 M) sucrose in an ice bath for 2–3 min. The homogenate was then added to acetone at −20°C, using a 50 ml syringe. Twenty volumes of acetone were used for each volume of homogenate. The vessel was agitated vigorously for 15 sec, and then placed in an ice bath. The milky supernatant was decanted and the process was repeated until the acetone was clear. The sediment was then suspended in a small volume of acetone, homogenized again for 1 min, and then centrifuged at 0° C, at 300 g for 15 min to obtain a fine, pink-colored sediment. The supernatant was decanted, and the sediment was placed in a vacuum system at -60° C for approximately 12 hr to evaporate all the acetone remaining in the sediment. The powder produced was then suspended in phosphate buffered saline (PBS) at pH 7.2 in a proportion of 0.4 ml of PBS to one volume of original homogenate in sucrose. The suspension was then agitated continuously for 18 hr. The opalescent supernatant (SASA), was then stored in aliquots, at 0° C, or lyophilized.

Melcher Antigen

Antigen prepared at the Parasitology Section of the Microbiological Branch of the Center for Disease Control, Atlanta, Georgia was used. This was kindly supplied by Dr. Irving G. Kagan.

Chemical Analysis

The protein content was estimated following the method described by Lowry *et al.* (1951). The concentration of nucleic acids was determined using the orcinol method for RNA, and the *p*-nitrophenylhydrazine method for DNA. The Anthrone reaction was used to estimate the concentration of polysaccharides (Kabat and Mayer, 1961).

Fractionation

Gel filtration was carried out with glass columns 1×60 cm. The amount of antigen used in this procedure was 1.5 ml containing 2.0 mg protein/ml. The column of Sephadex G-100 was equilibrated with PBS, pH 7.2, and the flow rate used was 0.38 ml/min. The total effluent volume was 120 ml. The optical density of the effluent was measured at 280 nm. Each series of tubes representing a peak was concentrated to a final protein content of 1 mg/ml (Fig. 6).

Electrophoresis

Both the crude antigen (SASA) and each of the fractions obtained from this material were analyzed by electrophoresis using as support, RS-multi-separative Cellogel with Tris-veronal buffer, pH 9.0, at 300 V, 20 mA, with a running time of 90 min. The strips were stained with amido black.

Serum

Whole blood was obtained by cardiac puncture from rats infected with 1500 larvae. Samples were taken 13, 28, 45, and 65 days, and 17 and 36 weeks after infection and stored at -20° C. The serum was collected after centrifugation.

Serologic Tests

Double diffusion in agar gel, following the microtechnique procedure described by Wadsworth (1957) was used. Agar gel (1.2%) in PBS, pH 7.2, was prepared, and applied to 7.5 × 2.5 cm glass slides in 3.0 ml amounts. The diameter of the wells was 3 mm, and the distance between them 4 mm. The preparation was incubated at room temperature for 24–48 hr. The slides were dried with filter paper strips and then stained with 1% amido black. Immunoelectrophoretic analysis was done before electrophoresis of the antigen using 2% agar gel in veronal buffer, pH 8.6, with an ionic strength of 0.075, following the technique described by Scheidegger (1955). Agar was applied in 5-ml volumes to slides measuring 7.5 × 2.5 cm. The diameter of the wells was 3 mm; 150 V and 20 mA were applied for 60 min to the system containing veronal buffer, pH 8.6.

Results

Chemical Characteristics of the Crude Antigen

Table I summarizes the results obtained after chemical analysis of seven batches of antigen (SASA). It was observed that the protein content of SASA was high, but it is very interesting to note that the nucleic acid content was also high, an important characteristic of this antigenic material. Moreover, the relationship of nucleic acid to total protein content was much higher in SASA than in Melcher. The carbohydrate content of SASA was extremely high; this is probably related to the homogenization procedure in which sucrose is used.

Electrophoretic Analysis

Figure 1 schematically represents the distribution pattern of the protein component of SASA antigen compared with Melcher antigen. It was observed that the number of protein components present in the Melcher antigen was very low, whereas in SASA antigen, at least 17 components

Table I Comparative Chemical Characteristics of Two
Trichinella spiralis Soluble Somatic Larvae Antigen[a]

Method	Protein	Polysaccharides	RNA [b]	DNA
SASA antigen	4.940[c]	8.55[c]	2.54	1.56
Melcher	1.790	0.73	0.415	0.19

[a] The concentration is given in mg/ml.
[b] To avoid the problem of the presence of high polysaccharide content, the RNA determination was made with diluted material.
[c] Average of seven antigen sets

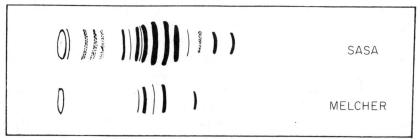

Figure 1 Electrophoretic analysis of SASA compared with Melcher antigen in RS-multiseparative Cellogel. Migration time 90 min; 300 V, 20 mA, Tris-veronal buffer, pH 9.0.

were present. Obviously, the Melcher antigen represented a more purified material than SASA.

Immunological Characterization of Crude Material SASA

1. *Immunodiffusion test.* Figure 2 represents the immunodiffusion patterns of both antigens, Melcher and SASA, against rat sera obtained from 10 days to 36 weeks after experimental infection with *T. spiralis*. It was possible to demonstrate specific immunoglobulins from day 10 after infection. After this time, the precipitation bands were more defined and increased in number on day 28 to reach a maximum on day 45. After day 45, the number of bands decreased, so that after 17 weeks of infection, only two bands were visible with SASA and one with Melcher. On the week 36 after infection it was possible to obtain a well-defined band with SASA antigen only. At this time, the Melcher antigen presented a barely perceptable line. Considering these results, the immune response of the rat appears to fall into two well-defined periods: the first from 10–45 days in which the most

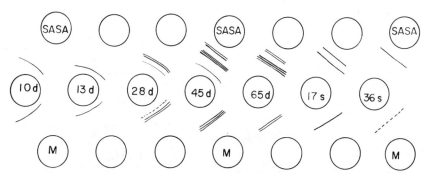

Figure 2 Identity and nonidentity reactions between Melcher (M) antigen, and soluble antigen extracted by the sucrose–acetone method (SASA) against rat sera obtained at different times after experimental infection.

important sensitization of the host occurs and represents the stage when the parasite is migrating through the host tissue; the second, from 45 days to 36 weeks, when the parasite has reached its definitive position in the host, where comparatively little antigenic stimulation occurs, and the circulating detectable antibody eventually disappears.

Figure 3 presents the immunological relationship between the two antigens with rat sera 10 days, 65 days, and 36 weeks after infection. This further illustrates the results described above. More importantly, it shows identity reactions between Melcher and SASA. Figure 4 shows the same relationship, and it also includes excretion and secretion products (ES) obtained after incubation of the muscle-stage larvae in sterile saline solution at 37° C against pooled rat sera taken 65 days after infection. There appears an identity band between ES and SASA. Considering the difficulty of preparing ES, it was decided in the future to use material purified from the identity band in SASA.

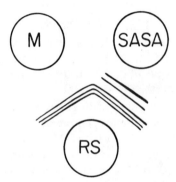

Figure 3 Immunological relationship between two different *T. spiralis* antigens (Melcher and SASA) in reaction against rat sera obtained at different times after infection.

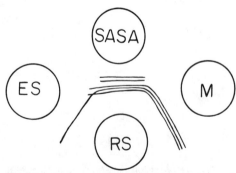

Figure 4 Immunological relationships between different *T. spiralis* antigens in double diffusion (Ouchterlony) against immune rat sera.

2. *Immunoelectrophoretic analysis.*   The results of the immunoelectrophoretic analysis demonstrated that of the 17 components present in
SASA antigen only six stimulate host antibody production (Fig. 5). On the
other hand, the Melcher antigen, a partially pure material, presents five

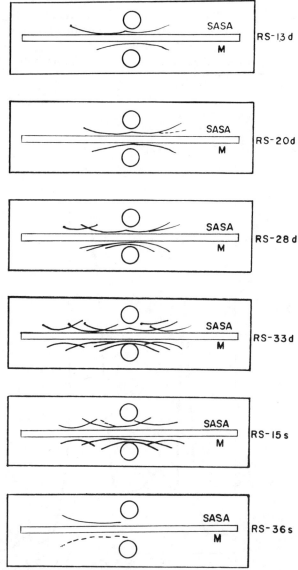

Figure 5   Immunoelectrophoretic analysis in agar of SASA and Melcher
(M) antigen with sera obtained from rats at different times after infection.
Migration time 90 min; 150 V, 20 mA, Veronal buffer, pH 8.6, ionic
strength 0.075.

active components. In both cases, the maximum response occurred 33 days after infection. After 36 weeks, only single precipitin arcs were present in each case, which, considering their different relative positions and intensities, probably represent two different proteins.

3. *Fractionation.* The optical density of material obtained from gel filtration through Sephadex G-100 is presented in Fig. 6. Three main peaks are present. Occasionally, in the ascending portion of peak 3, it was possible to observe a further peak, but this was not a constant feature under the experimental conditions used. It is important to mention that the exclu-

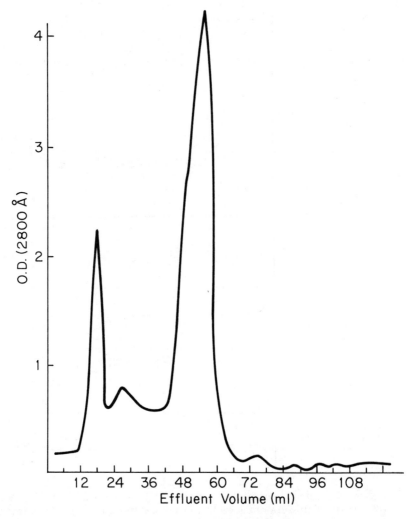

Figure 6 Elution pattern of SASA from Sephadex G-100 chromatography column.

sion volume is mainly represented by fraction I and II. The proteins present in fraction III probably have a molecular weight above 100,000.

4. *Electrophoretic analysis of antigenic fractions.* Figure 7 schematically represents the different components present in each SASA antigen chromatographic fraction. The major part of the protein content was found in fractions II and III. The center part of Fig. 7 shows the total number of protein components in the fractions. Under the experimental conditions used, almost all of the components present in the crude antigen were present in the fractions.

5. *Immunological characterization of antigenic fractions.* Figure 8 shows the results obtained in the gel diffusion analysis, using pooled rat sera from 38–50 days of infection, against SASA and Melcher antigen as well as against chromatographic fractions I, II, and III. In the left figure an identity band between F-II component and SASA is evident. However, the right figure this band, although still present, shows no identity with Melcher antigen. Fraction III contains an antigenic component present in both Melcher and SASA antigen. Since chromatographic fraction II contains a protein that gives a nonidentity reaction with a Melcher component, we are especially interested in isolating and purifying this substance, which is possibly related to the component found in gel diffusion 36 weeks after infection.

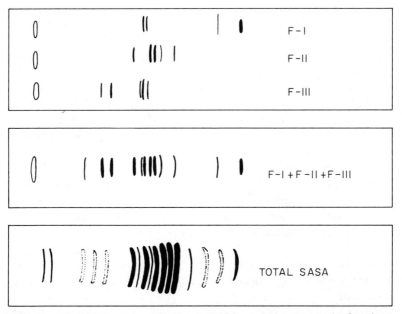

Figure 7 Electrophoretic analysis of SASA and the antigenic fractions showing the different protein components. A summation of the protein components of the fractions is also shown.

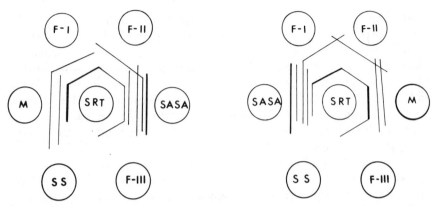

Figure 8 Immunodiffusion of the fractions, SASA and Melcher (M) antigen against pooled immune rat sera (SRT). Saline solution (SS) is used as control.

Discussion

From the results, we consider that the antigenic material SASA, which can be described as a crude soluble somatic antigen of *T. spiralis* larvae, is a very good material from which further isolation of the more specific proteins and polysaccharides that participate in the natural infection of the host can be attempted.

It is especially advantageous that the technique for obtaining SASA antigen can be accomplished in 48–72 hours. Moreover, this technique does not require skilled or experienced personnel, or sophisticated equipment. For this reason, it can be applied in any laboratory with facilities for routine work. The proceedure is completed at low temperatures and in conditions that prevent the denaturation of protein. We have maintained SASA antigen obtained from different species of parasites for over a year. The only effect encountered was a decrease in the protein content. However, the serologic characteristics were maintained.

The results expressed in Figs. 1, 2, and 5 demonstrates that almost all the proteins present in the acid-soluble fraction of Melcher antigen are also present in SASA, and that some of the SASA proteins are not found in the Melcher antigen. These data are especially interesting when obtained with sera from rats infected for more than 36 weeks. A definite band occurs against SASA, whereas that against Melcher antigen is barely perceptible. If these results are consistent, the use of this purified protein is indicated in seroepidemiological work to demonstrate antibodies remaining after infection.

Recently, it has been demonstrated by Despommier (1971) and Despommier and Müller (1970) that granules in the stichocyte cells of *T. spiralis* muscle larvae and adults contain antigenic material. Apparently these antigens are excreted and induce an immune response which protects against reinfection (Berntzen, 1972, personal communication). At present, we are initiating a series of experiments in which the principal objectives are to determine whether any of these functional stichocyte antigens are isolated and preserved in SASA. Results of initial experiments separating antigen by gel filtration in Sephadex G-100 expressed in Fig. 6, 7, and 8 indicate the necessity of further purification of fraction II using, e.g., DEAE-cellulose, or DEAE-cellulose plus Sephadex.

It is important to point out that some excretion and secretion products are present in SASA, as demonstrated in Fig. 4. Taking into account that excretion and secretion antigen is rather difficult to obtain, we believe that SASA may be used as a source for this antigen.

Summary

Clark and Casals (1958) described a procedure useful for obtaining antigen of arbovirus from cerebral tissue. A crude soluble somatic antigenic material (SASA) obtained from the larvae of *Trichinella spiralis* by the above method is described. The chemical characteristics of this material are compared with those of antigenic material from *T. spiralis* prepared by the Melcher procedure (1943). By electrophoresis on RS-multiseparative Cellogel, the antigen in the acid-soluble fraction of the Melcher preparation was demonstrated to have five protein components whereas SASA contained at least 17 components. The immunological characteristics of both antigens are determined, using serum of rats experimentally infected with 1500 larvae. Rats were used although they are considered to be poor antibody producers because they are a natural host of *T. spiralis*.

Using double diffusion in agar gel and electrophoretic analysis, the immunological relationships existing between the Melcher antigen, SASA, and an antigen of excretions and secretions (ES) were established. All the components present in Melcher antigen are present in SASA, but two components of the latter are not present in the Melcher antigen. SASA was fractionated on a column of Sephadex G-100; three peaks were obtained which were analyzed against immune rat sera. From electrophoretic studies, it was concluded that all the components present in the crude material were present in the fractions.

References

Beck, J. W. (1953). Xenodiagnostic technique as an aid in diagnosis of Trichinosis. *Amer. J. Trop. Med. Hyg.* **2,** 97–101.

Berntzen, A. K. (1965). Comparative growth and development of *Trichinella spiralis in vivo* and *in vitro* with a redescription of the life cycle. *Exp. Parasitol.* **16,** 74–106.

Biagi, F., and Robledo, E. (1962). Estado actual de conocimientos sobre triquinosis en México. *Wiad. Parazit.* **8**, 585–588.

Chaffee, E. F., Bauman, P. M., and Shapilo, J. J. (1954). Diagnosis of schistosomiasis by complement-fixation. *Amer. J. Trop. Med. Hyg.* **3**, 905–913.

Clarke, D. H., and Casals, J. (1958). Techniques for hemagglutination and hemagglutination-inhibition with arthropod-borne viruses. *Amer. J. Trop. Med. Hyg.* **7**, 561–573.

Cypess, R. H., Larsh, J. E., Jr., and Peagram, C. (1971). Macrophage inhibition produced by guinea pigs after sensitization with a larval antigen of *Trichinella spiralis. J. Parasitol.* **57**, 103–106.

Despommier, D. D. (1971). Immunogenicity of the newborn larvae of *Trichinella spiralis. J. Parasitol.* **57**, 531–534.

Despommier, D. D., and Müller, M. (1970). The stichocyte of *Trichinella spiralis:* its structure and function. *Proc. 2nd Int. Congr. Parasitol. J. Parasitol.* **56** (Sect. II), 76–77.

Gursh, O. F. (1948). Effect of digestion and refrigeration on the ability of *Trichinella spiralis* to infect rats. *J. Parasitol.* **34**, 394–395.

Kabat, E. A., and Mayer, M. M. (1961). "Experimental Immunochemistry," 2nd Ed. Thomas, Springfield, Illinois, p. 905.

Lowry, O. H., Rosebrough, N.J., Farr, A. L., and Randall, R. J. (1951). Protein measurement with the Folin phenol reagent. *J. Biol. Chem.* **193**, 265–275.

Mazzotti, L. (1944). Examen de 400 diafragmas humanos en la ciudad de Mexico para investigar Triquinosis. *Rev. Inst. Salubr. Enferm. Trop. Mex.* **5**, 157–161.

Melcher, L. R. 1943. An antigenic analysis of *Trichinella spiralis. J. Infec. Dis.* **73**, 31–40.

Perrín, T. (1942). Algunos estudios sobre Triquinosis ignoradas. *Ciencia* **3**, 108–114.

Sadun, E. H. (1962). Recent advances on the serological diagnosis of Trichinellosis. *In:* Z. Kozar (ed.), "Trichinellosis," *Proc. 1st Int. Conf. Trichinellosis,* pp. 266–274.

Scheidegger, J. J. (1955). Une micro-methode de l'immune-electrophorese. *Int. Arch. Allergy* **7**, 103–110.

Wadsworth, C. (1957). A slide microtechnique for the analysis of immune precipitates in gel. *Int. Arch. Allergy* **10**, 355–360.

Trichinella spiralis: Isolation and Purification of the Main Functional Antigen from Decapsulated Larvae

G. A. Ermolin and
E. E. Efremov

Laboratory of Biochemistry
The All-Union K. I. Skryabin
Institute of Helminthology,
Moscow

Introduction

Proceeding from the theory of "one gene—one enzyme," one may suggest that in monohybrid and dihybrid inheritance of infectivity (virulence) the main role in the pathogenic effect is played by only a few substances produced by parasites and that the passive and active immunity are produced just against these (Efroimson, 1971). All other antigens play in this case only a secondary role or even a ballast one.

The isolation of immunologically functional antigens, "decisive substances of infectivity," from one or more parasites will increase not only the sensitivity of serologic tests, but also the specificity of diagnostic preparations. The immunodiagnosis of trichinellosis with the use of "fractionated" antigens began with the basic work of Melcher (1943) who was the first to accomplish the chemical separation of protein extract from larvae.

Later studies on the antigenic structure of the extract and on the isolation of the "main precipitating antigen" were carried out with methods which reflected the development in biochemistry and immunochemistry (Kagan and Bargai, 1956; Van Peenen and Kent, 1960; Mills and Kent, 1965; Labzoffsky et al., 1959; Sleeman and Muschel, 1961; Tanner, 1962, 1970; Dymowska et al., 1965; Biquet et al., 1965; Ermolin, 1967, 1969, 1971; Dusanic, 1966; Crandall and Zam, 1968).

The aim of the present study was to isolate the main antigen from decapsulated larvae of reproductively isolated species of *Trichinella spiralis*

(Owen, 1835) (Britov *et al.,* 1971; Britov and Boev, 1972) and its purification under the control of immune sera from *Trichinella*-infected pigs.

Materials and Methods

The strain of *Trichinella* larvae used was maintained in the All-Union K. I. Skryabin Institute of Helminthology for 14 years (during the last 7 years it passed only through common white rats).

Decapsulated larvae were isolated by peptic digestion from carcasses of infected rats. From the digest the larvae were isolated by Baermann's method and were washed repeatedly in saline; 5 ml of larvae were suspended in 10 ml of Tris-glycine buffer solution (pH 8.3) and treated in the ultrasolic disintegrator MSE-100 for 30 min at 50–60 kHz and at 8 μm vibration amplitude of the piezoelement. The homogenate was centrifuged for 30 min in a refrigerated centrifuge (+4°C) at 15,000 rpm. The supernatant was removed, was dialyzed for 24 hr against the same buffer solution, and was stored at −35°C.

Immune sera were collected from pigs infected with the above-mentioned strain of *Trichinella spiralis* at the dose rate of two larvae per gram of body weight. Sera from one piglet, one cat, and four rats infected with *Trichinella nativa* larvae recovered from a bear and with *Trichinella spiralis* larvae recovered from a domestic pig were also used. Sera from rabbits hyperimmunized by excretory–secretory products of decapsulated larvae were used in some tests.

Preparative and analytic disc electrophoresis in polyacrylamide gels were carried out in chambers constructed by the present authors as described earlier (Ustinnikov and Ermolin, 1972). In preparative electrophoresis samples of the extract were introduced into the chamber in 5-ml aliquots (0.56% of protein content). After electrophoresis the gel was cut in the differential system (10 and 7.5%) in 1-cm long segments and in the monopore system (5%) in 0.5-cm long ones. The slices were then homogenized and eluted three times with Tris-HCl buffer solution (pH 6.7). The second and the third step in the purification of antigenic components included the preparative electrophoresis of eluates.

The immunodiffusion tests were carried out according to the method of Gusev and Tsvetkov (1961), the microvariant of immunodiffusion test according to Abelev and Tsevtkov (1960) and disc immunoelectrophoresis according to Maurer (1971).

For estimation of lactate dehydrogenase activity in the whole extract and the fractions, the gel slices were washed in cold 0.1 M Tris—HCl buffer solution (pH 8.3) and incubated for 1 hr at 37°C in a mixture of 0.036 M sodium $L(+)$-lactate, 0.3 mg/ml of NAD$^+$, 0.8 mg/ml of nitroblue tetrazolium and 0.14 mg/ml of phenazine methosulfate in the same buffer system. After developing, the stained gel slices were fixed in 7% acetic acid and were photographed.

Results

Larval extracts with protein contents of 0.52 and 1.57% were used in the present study. Nineteen protein bands were revealed in the extract by analytic differential disc electrophoresis; these bands differed from one another in electrophoretic mobility and relative protein content (Table 1). Up to 10 protein components were demonstrated in 10% gel (electrophoretic mobility of more than 0.5), the pore radium of which did not exceed 13 Å, and nine protein components were revealed in 7.5% gel with pore radius of about 15 Å.

In preparative electrophoresis each of the 10 gel fractions was heterogeneous in its protein composition (Fig. 1). Using the given method of elution, the recovery of protein from gel was 39.8%. In 10% gel the re-

Table I Protein Content (%) and the Electrophoretic Mobility of Components of the Extract from *Trichinella spiralis* Larvae after Analytic Disc Electrophoresis

Nos. of protein components (beginning from the anode end of gel)	Protein content (%) according to the absorption of the stained zones	Relative electrophoretic mobility
0	3.5	0.98
1	7.0	0.92
2	2.5	0.87
3	9.0	0.83
4	2.0	0.78
5	2.5	0.75
6	3.5	0.726
7	13.0	0.684–0.61
8	4.0	0.60
9	5.0	0.57–0.547
10	3.0	0.537
11	10.0	0.517–0.452
12	8.0	0.442–0.39
13	9.0	0.337
14	6.0	0.305
15	4.5	0.284–0.21
16	2.5	0.17
17	2.0	0.126
18	0.5	0.034
19	2.5	0.0105

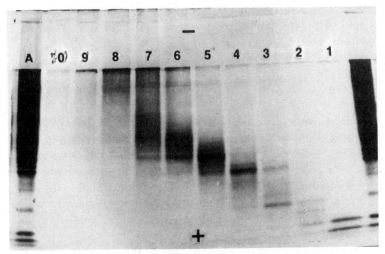

Figure 1 Analytic disc electrophoresis of the extract from *Trichinella spiralis* larvae and eluates of gel fractions obtained by preparative disc electrophoresis. Anion buffer system. Differential electrophoresis. A, Extract; numbers 1–10 are the eluates of the gel fractions.

covery of protein components was 29.31% (or 12.4% of the sample protein), and in 7.5% gel it was 54.34% (22.7% of the sample protein). Of the extracted protein, 10.7% (4.5% of the sample protein) had been retained in the mesh of the large-pored gel (3.5%), and 5.65% of it (2.3% of the sample protein) had been left at the origin.

With the sera of pigs infected with *Trichinella spiralis* (VIGIS strain), two antigenic components were demonstrated in the extract and five components in its fractions; these components differed from one another in serologic specificity.

The main antigenic component reacting with sera from pigs (15–63 days after infection) was located in the gel fractions 8 and 9 of the extract (Fig. 2). These fractions included protein components with electrophoretic mobility of 0.01–0.17. The main antigenic component was also demonstrated with sera from different animals infected with *Trichinella nativa, Trichinella spiralis* (VIGIS strain), or *Trichinella spiralis* isolated from a domestic pig (Fig. 3).

With an aim of further purification of the main antigenic component, electrophoresis of concentrated eluates of fractions 6, 7, 8, and 9 was made. With the resulting fractions the sera of infected pigs, in immune disc electrophoresis and immunodiffusion test, revealed only one antigenic component (Figs. 4 and 5). However, with sera from rabbits hyperimmunized by *Trichinella* excretory–secretory products this reactive fraction

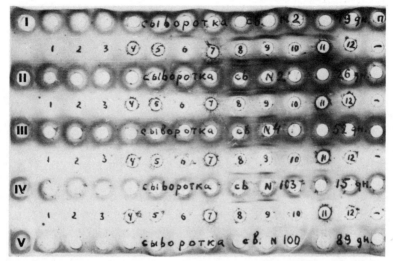

Figure 2 Immunodiffusion tests of eluates of gel fractions against sera from infected pigs. I–V, Undiluted sera taken 19, 26, 52, 75, and 89 days after infection. 1–12, Eluates corresponding to the gel fractions.

has been shown to contain not only the main antigenic component but also two other components of fully antigenic value (Fig. 5).

The eluates of antigenically active fractions were electrophoresed for a second time in 5% gel after which they were subjected to immunodiffusion test using sera of a pig (60 days after infection) and of rabbits hyperimmunized by *Trichinella* excretory–secretory products. It was demonstrated that the substance of the main antigen was immunochemically homogeneous (Figs 6 and 7). The mixtures of antigenically active fractions showed in the analytic disc electrophoresis (5% gel) after the first preparative electrophoresis 12 components, after the second electrophoresis 9 components, and after the third one only 5 components with a characteristic staining for protein. The relative electrophoretic mobility of these proteins was from 0.07 to 0.31 and their molecular weight was about 220,000.

After staining the disc gels for lactate dehydrogenase (LDH) at least two isozymes of LDH were revealed in the extract and antigenic fractions after their preparative electrophoresis and the second electrophoresis; these isozymes corresponded in their instability to the "slowest" isozymes of pig muscle. When the gels of the extract stained for either LDH or protein were compared, it was noticed that two components of the protein spectra of the extract (with a relative electrophoretic mobility of 0.056 and 0.21) corresponded to the two isozymes of LDH of the extract in their electrophoretic mobility.

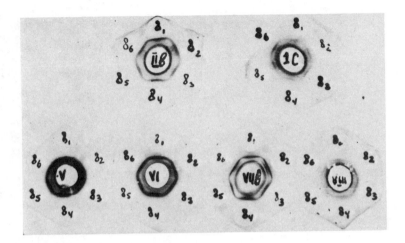

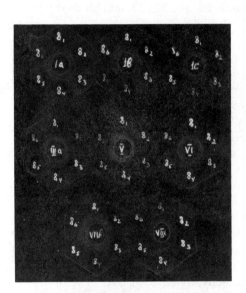
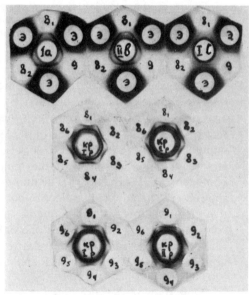

Figure 3 Immunodiffusion tests of fractions 8 and 9 against sera from animals infected with different *Trichinella* strains. A, Eluates of gel fractions 8 and 9 isolated in six tests and placed in peripheral wells. The surrounding figures (8_1, 8_2, etc.) are numbers of tests. B, Sera in the central wells: 1 a, 1 b, 1 c are sera of pig infected with *T. spiralis* (domestic pig strain) at different periods of infection. IIIa, Serum from a kitten 1 month after *T. spiralis* infection; V–VI, pooled sera of five rats 1 month after *T. nativa* infection; VIIb, serum from a rabbit repeatedly hyperimmunized with *T. spiralis* (strain VIGIS); VIII, pooled sera of five rats 1 month after *T. spiralis* infection. C, Kp Ip and Kp IIp are serum from a rabbit hyperimmunized with the extract.

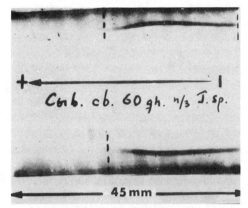

Figure 4 An immune disc electrophoregram after electrophoresis of gel fraction 8 against pig serum (obtained 60 days after infection).

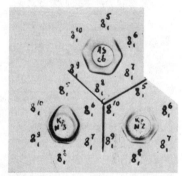

Figure 5 Immunodiffusion test reaction of gel fraction 8 after preparative electrophoresis. Eluates of gel fraction in the peripheral depressions. Sera in the central depressions: AS cb, serum of a pig obtained 60 days after *T. spiralis* (strain VIGIS) infection. Kp N2 and Kp N3, sera of rabbits 2 and 3 hyperimmunized with secretory–excretory products of decapsulated *T. spiralis* larvae.

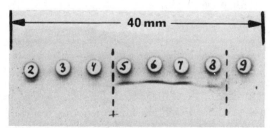

Figure 6 Immunodiffusion test reaction of eluates from fractions after second electrophoresis against serum of a pig obtained 60 days after *T. spiralis* (strain VIGIS) infection.

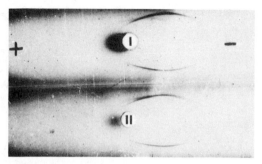

Figure 7 An immunoelectrophoregram of eluates from an antigenically active fraction after first and second electrophoresis against sera from rabbits hyperimmunized with excretory–secretory products.

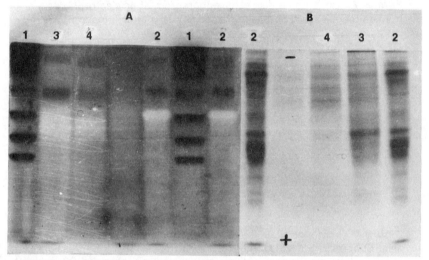

Figure 8 Analytic disc electrophoresis of (1) crystalline lactate dehydrogenase (LDH) from pig muscle (supplied by Reanal, Hungary), (2) extract from decapsulated *T. spiralis* larvae, (3) mixtures of antigenically active fractions after the second electrophoresis, (4) mixtures of antigen active fractions after the third electrophoresis; A, staining for LDH; B, staining for protein with Amido-Black 10B.

Discussion

The analysis of the electrophoregrams after their preparative electrophoresis in the differential gel system (7.5 and 10%) showed that it was not possible to obtain homogeneous fractions after a single disc electrophoresis process. This was due, probably, to the fact that during the preparative fractionation of large quantities of protein (50 and 100 mg in the present study), bands representing different fractions were quite large and overlapping resulting in a decreased resolution.

Using sera of different animal species infected with *Trichinella spiralis* the main antigenic component was found in fractions with relative electrophoretic mobility from 0.01 to 0.17, that is, in fractions which had either high molecular weight or low electrophoretic mobility which is apparent with the data of Crandall and Zam (1968). Therefore, a 5% gel was used in the second electrophoresis in order to increase the path length and to achieve better separation.

Three consecutive steps resulted in the isolation of an immunochemically homogeneous antigen (Figs. 6 and 7). The analytic disc electrophoresis of the substance of the main antigen after the third step showed five protein components. This fact, apparently, is connected with the phenomenon of molecular polymorphism (Tanner, 1970).

The results of the immunodiffusion test with sera of different animal species infected with *Trichinella spiralis* or *Trichinella nativa* demonstrated (Fig. 3) that the main precipitating antigen was serologically identical for the two *Trichinella* species: *T. spiralis* and *T. nativa.*

Our results with staining for LDH (Fig. 8) do not agree with Dusanic's opinion (1966) that the LDH activity is connected with the main precipitating antigen, as the main antigen has a molecular polymorphism and its location along the path in the disc electrophoresis process does not coincide with the location of the two LDH isozymes of the extract.

Summary

The extract of decapsulated *Trichinella spiralis* larvae was fractionated into nineteen protein fractions by analytic disc electrophoresis in polyacrylamide gels. The isolation of the main functional antigen was performed by preparative disc electrophoresis of the extract and by two successive electrophoreses of eluates of antigenic fractions in 5% polyacrylamide gels. Immunodiffusion, immunoelectrophoresis, and immune disc electrophoresis methods revealed the main antigen in protein fractions with relative electrophoretic mobility from 0.07 to 0.31. The main antigen was demonstrated by sera from pigs, rats, and cats infected with *Trichinella spiralis* and *Trichinella nativa,* and by sera from a rabbit hyperimmunized with excretory–secretory products of *Trichinella spiralis*. The main functional antigens from *Trichinella spiralis* and *Trichinella nativa* were serologically identical. Two isozymes of lactate dehydrogenase with relative electrophoretic mobility of 0.05 and 0.21 were revealed on disc electrophoregrams of the extract by characteristic coloration for lactate dehydrogenase (LDH).

References

Abelev, G. I., and Tsvetkov, V. S. (1960). The isolation of the specific antigen of the transplanted hepatoma in mice by method of immunofiltration. *Vop. Onkol.* **6,** 62.

Biguet, J., Tran Van Ky, P., Moschetto, Y., and Gnamey-Koffy, D. (1965). Contribution a l'etude de la structure antigenique des larves de *Trichinella spiralis* et des precipitines experimentalles du lapin. *Wiad. Parazitol.* **11,** 299–315.

Britov, V. A., and Boev, S. N. (1972). The taxonomic rank of various *Trichinella* strains and the character of their circulation. *Vestn. Akad. Nauk Kaz. S.S.R.* **4,** 27–32.

Britov, V. A., Ermolin, G. A., Tarakanov, V. I., and Nikitina, T. L. (1971). The genetic isolation of two *Trichinella* varieties. *Med. Parazitol. Parazit. Bol.* **5,** 515–521.

Crandall, R. B., and Zam, S. G. (1968). Analysis of excretory–secretory products of *Trichinella spiralis* larvae by disc electrophoresis and immunodiffusion. *Amer. J. Trop. Med. Hyg.* **11,** 201–215.

Dusanic, D. G. (1966). Serologic and enzymatic investigations of *Trichinella spiralis*. I. Precipitin reactions and lactic dehydrogenase. *Exp. Parasitol.* **19,** 310–319.

Dymowska, Z., Aleksandrowicz, J., and Zakrzewska, A. (1965). Antigens of *Trichinella spiralis*. I. Methods of preparation of antigenic fractions. *Acta Parazitol. Pol.* **13,** 183–190.

Efroimson, V. N. (1971). Immunogenetics. Izdatelstvo "Meditsina," Moskva.

Ermolin, G. A. (1967). Immunochemical studies of the antigenic structure of decapsulated *Trichinella spiralis* larvae. Dissertatsiya na soiskanie utchenoi stepeni kandidata biologitcheskikh nauk, Moskva, Biblioteka VIGIS.

Ermolin, G. A. (1969). Antigenic structure of decapsulated larvae of *Trichinella spiralis*. *Wiad. Parazitol.* **15,** 5–6.

Ermolin, G. A. (1971). Antigens excreted by *Trichinella spiralis* larvae during the process of their incubation in artificial nutrient media. *Tr. Vses. Inst. Gelmintol. imeni Skryabina* **17,** 271-277.

Gusev, A. I., and Tsvetkov, V. S. (1961). To the technique of conducting of microprecipitation test in agar. *Lab. Delo* **2,** 43.

Kagan, I. G., and Bargai, U. (1956). Studies on the serology of trichinosis with hemagglutination, agar diffusion tests and precipitin ring tests. *J. Parasitol.* **42,** 237-245.

Labzoffsky, N. A., Kuitunen, E., Morrissey, L. P., and Hamvas, I. I. (1959). Studies on the antigenic structure of *Trichinella spiralis* larvae. *Can. J. Microbiol.* **5,** 395–403.

Maurer, R. (1971). Disc. Electrophoresis. The theory and practice of electrophoresis in polyacrylamide gel. "Mir," Moskwa.

Melcher, L. R. (1943). An antigenic analysis of *Trichinella spiralis*. *J. Infec. Dis.* **73,** 31–39.

Mills, C. K., and Kent, N. H. (1965). Excretions and secretions of *Trichinella spiralis* and their role in immunity. *Exp. Parasitol.* **16,** 300–310.

Sleeman, H. K., and Muschel, L. H. (1961). Studies on complement fixing antigens isolated from *Trichinella spiralis* I. Isolation, purification and evaluation as diagnostic agents. *Amer. J. Trop. Med. Hyg.* **10**, 821–833.

Tanner, C. E. (1962). Immunochemistry of the functional precipitating antigens of *Trichinella spiralis* larvae. *J. Parasitol.* **48** (Sect. 2), 18.

Tanner, C. E. (1970). Immunochemical study of the antigens of *Trichinella spiralis* larvae. IV. Purification by continuous-flow paper electrophoresis and column chromatography. *Exp. Parasitol.* **27**, 116–135.

Ustinnikov, B. A., and Ermolin, G. A. (1972). The method of disc electrophoresis in polyacrylamide gel for fractionation and studies of protein. *Tsent. Nauch. Issled. Inst. Pishtshevoy Prom. Mosk.*

Van Peenen, P. F. D., and Kent, N. H. (1960). Extraction of immunologically active protein complexes from *Trichinella spiralis* larvae. *J. Parasitol.* **46** (Sect. 2), 23.

The Antigens of *Trichinella spiralis* Larvae Incubated and Cultivated under *in Vitro* Conditions

G. A. Ermolin and V. I. Tarakanov

*The All-Union K.I. Skryabin Institute of
Helminthology, Moscow
and The Helminthological Laboratory
of the Academy of Sciences of
U.S.S.R., Moscow*

Introduction

The isolation of specific antigens is a very important problem in the development of immunodiagnostic methods for helminthic infections. The main difficulty in this problem is the complexity of antigens.

Kent (1963) considers the low sensitivity and doubtful specificity of antigens to be due to the complex nature and uncertain biochemical characteristics of whole-body homogenates or extracts from helminths used in serologic tests. Chandler (1937), Shults and Davtyan (1951), Soulsby (1960) and Thorson (1963) think that the immunity to helminths is mediated by the inhibition of vitally important enzyme systems of the parasites. Taliaferro and Sarles (1939) confirmed the presence of antibodies to the excretory–secretory products of *Nippostrongylus braziliensis.* McCoy (1935) observed higher immunity in rats infected intraperitoneally with live *Trichinella* larvae than in rats immunized by larvae dried and heat-killed. Oliver-Gonzalez and Levine (1962) failed to inhibit the protective activity of immune serum by adsorption with dead *Trichinella* adults or larvae in spite of the fact that the serologic tests were negative with exhausted sera. Soulsby (1960) concluded that the antigenic components were excreted and secreted by helminths during molting. Campbell (1953, 1955) and Chute (1956) obtained a partial protection in mice after injection of a medium in which *Trichinella* larvae were incubated. Tanner and Gregory (1961), Briggs (1963), Crandall (1965), Mills and Kent (1965), Norman and Sadun (1959), and Kozar, *et al.* (1964) incubated *Trichinella* larvae in various media and studied their excretory-secretory products.

A comparison of spectra of antigens excreted and secreted by larvae of *Trichinella spiralis* Britov, 1971; (Britov *et al.,* 1971) during *in vitro* incubation and cultivation is given in the present paper.

199

Material and Methods

Trichinella larvae were isolated by digestion of the infected carcasses of white rats, washed with saline, and treated with antibiotics. Twenty thousand *Trichinella* larvae per 1 ml of Hanks' solution were incubated for 9 hr at $37°$ C in Erlenmeyer flasks agitated at 50–60 shakes/min. Then the *Trichinella* larvae were isolated by centrifugation and the supernatant liquid was dialyzed for 48 hr against double distilled water. The spectrum of proteins of excretory–secretory products (ESP) was analyzed by disc electrophoresis in polyacrylamide gel (Ermolin, 1971; Ermolin and Ustinnikov, 1972).

Five thousand *Trichinella* larvae per milliliter medium were cultivated in 300-ml chambers for 7 days at $37°$ C. Fifty ml of the medium was renewed every 6 hr. A gas phase consisting of 85% nitrogen, 10% oxygen, and 5% carbon dioxide (Berntzen, 1965) was maintained in this cultivation system.

Media 102B (Berntzen, 1965) and 115 (Berntzen and Mueller, 1964) were slightly modified. The modifications for 102B consisted of the following: sodium β-glycerophosphate instead of α-glycerophosphate, ζ-aminobutyric acid instead of hydroxybutyric acid and the ommission of aminto-n-butyric choline chloride. Chick embryo extract was prepared in Hanks' solution rather than in distilled water. The modifications for medium 115 were as follows: γ-aminobutyric acid instead of DL-β-hydroxybutyric acid, cattle serum without preservatives instead of A-γ calf serum and the ommission d-ribose, thymidylic acid, α- and β-globulin Cohn fraction IV and γ-amino-n-butyric choline chloride. The pH of the media was adjusted to 7.0–7.2 with $NaHCO_3$ and then sterilized by means of Zeitz filters. Excretory and secretory products (ESP) of larvae were collected in aliquots during the renewals of the main bulk of the culture medium every 6 hr and at the end following the separation of the worms from the medium. Fresh and lyophilized unused media served as control. The antigens were isolated by double diffusion in agar gel (Gusev and Tsvetkov, 1961) and immunoelectrophoresis (Grabar and Burten, 1963). The larvae were disintegrated at $0°$ C by using ultrasonic disintegrator MSE 100 for 10 min. Immune sera from singly infected or superinfected rabbits, sheep, or polar foxes were used in the tests.

Results

Trichinella larvae during 9 hr of incubation excreted and secreted ESP in which the protein content was 130–150 μg/ml. Dialysis decreased the protein content to 50–70 μg/ml. Seventeen protein fractions were demonstrated in the extracts and 14 protein fractions in the ESP. The main bulk of proteins from the extract was located in fractions C and D, and from ESP in the fractions of A and B. With hyperimmune sera, 17 antigenic components were demonstrated in the extracts, and 5 in ESP of which 2 were major components.

The larvae underwent one incomplete molting and were all motile during 72 hr of incubation. Later their motility diminished and they began to die. After 96 hrs of incubation in media 102B and 115, 11.7% and 10.2% of *Trichinella* larvae, respectively, became nonmotile; after 7 days of incubation 94% and 97%, respectively, were nonmotile.

The protein content (in relation to dry weight) increased in medium 102B by 1.7% and in medium 115 by 0.9% during 60 hr of incubation. During 60 hr of incubation antigenic components were demonstrated in both media using sheep sera (obtained 89 days after infection). The double diffusion test showed that precipitins to antigenic components of *Trichinella* extract appeared in the sera on the tenth to sixteenth day up to day 240 to 280 after infection of sheep. Antigens from *Trichinella* extract and from ESP demonstrated the test of identity. The sera of polar foxes up to day 70 after infection were weakly reactive with antigens from the extract of decapsulated *Trichinella* larvae. The protein content of *Trichinella* extract was 0.35% after 7 days of cultivation. Seven protein fractions were demonstrated in the extract of cultured *Trichinella* larvae during its electrophoresis in polyacrylamide gel and four protein fractions were demonstrated during disc electrophoresis (7.5 polyacrylamide gel). Three antigenic components were demonstrated by immunoelectrophoresis of the extract.

Discussion

Immunoelectrophoregrams of ESP showed that sera of infected animals had small quantities of antibodies to antigens of *Trichinella* larvae. However, even these small quantities of ESP antigens were effective in demonstrating antibodies in sera of infected animals.

An increase in protein content in modified media 102B and 115 was possibly due to *Trichinella* ESP. An analysis of ESP in media during the cultivation of *Trichinella* larvae showed that the excretion and secretion of antigen occurred from the first hours of cultivation and were present in subthreshold quantities up to the sixtieth hour of cultivation. Since the media were uniformly renewed every 6 hr we think that the maximal excretion and secretion of antigens by *Trichinella* larvae took place between hours 27 and 30 of cultivation. After 60 hr of cultivation these antigens disappeared from the media. Antibodies to *Trichinella* ESP were present in the sera of infected sheep from day 10–16 to 32–50 days after a single infection and were still present until days 79–150. In the sera of superinfected sheep the antibodies were detectable up to 226 days after the primary infection. However, the titer of antibodies varied widely in different animals infected and superinfected with equal doses.

Summary

Trichinella spiralis larvae during 9 hr of incubation at a concentration of 20,000 larvae/ml of Hanks' solution excreted and secreted five antigen components of which two induced synthesis of humoral antibodies in rabbits. *Trichinella* larvae during 60 hr of incubation at a concentration of 5000 larvae/ml of modified media 102B and 115 excreted and secreted at least three antigenic components of various serologic activity.

References

Berntzen, A. K. (1965). Comparative growth and development of *Trichinella spiralis in vitro* and *in vivo* with redescription of the life cycle. *Exp. Parasitol.* **16,** 74–106.

Berntzen, A. K., and Mueller, J. F. (1964). *In vitro* cultivation of *Spirometra mansonoides* (Cestoda) from procercoid to the early adult. *J. Parasitol.* **50,** 705–711.

Briggs, N. T. (1963). Immunological injury of mast cells in mice actively and passively sensitized to antigens from *Trichinella spiralis. J. Infec. Dis.* **113,** 22–32.

Britov, V. A., Ermolin, G. A., Tarakanov, V. I., and Nikitina, T. L. (1971). The genetic isolation of two *Trichinella* varieties. *Med. Parazitol. Parazit. Bolez* **5,** 515–521.

Campbell, C. H. (1953). The use of collodion particle agglutination test for detecting antibodies formed in response to *Trichinella spiralis* infection. *J. Parasitol.* **39** (Section 2), 34.

Campbell, C. H. (1955). The antigenic role of the excretion and secretion of *Trichinella spiralis* in the production of immunity in mice. *J. Parasitol.* **41,** 483–891.

Chandler, A. (1937). Studies on the nature of immunity to intestinal helminths. VI. General resume and discussion. *Amer. J. Hyg.* **26,** 309–321.

Chute, R. M. (1956). The dual antibody response to experimental trichinosis. *Proc. Helminthol. Soc. Wash.* **23,** 27–30.

Crandall, R. B. (1965). Chemotactic response of polymorphonuclear leukocytes to *Trichinella spiralis* and *Ascaris suum* extraxts. *J. Parasitol.* **51,** 397–404.

Ermolin, G. A. (1971). Immunochemical analysis of antigenic structure of decapsulated *Trichinella* larvae. *Sb. Rab. Gelmintol. Posvyashchennyi 90-Letiyu So Dnya Rozhdeniya K.I. Skryabina. Izdatel'stvo "Kolos" Mosk.* 134–141.

Ermolin, G. A., and Ustinnikov, B. A. (1972). The method of disc electrophoresis in polyacrylamide gel for fractionation and examination of proteins. *Tsent. Nauch. Issled. Inst. Pishtshevoy Prom. Mosk.*

Grabar, P., and Burten, P. (1963). Immunoelectrophoretic analysis. Moscow.

Gusev, A. I., and Tsvetkov, V. S. (1961). The technique of conduction the microprecipitation test in agar. *Lab. Delo.* **2,** 43.

Kent, N. H. (1963). Fractionation, isolation and definition of antigens from parasitic helminths. *Exp. Parasitol.* **13**, 45–56.

Kozar, Z., Karpiak, S., Krzyzanowski, M., and Kozar M. (1964). Metabolism of *Trichinella spiralis* larvae. *Wiad. Parazytol.* **10**, 280–281.

McCoy, O. R. (1931). Immunity of rats to reinfection with *Trichinella spiralis*. *Amer. J. Hyg.* 14, 484–494.

McCoy, O. R. (1935). Artificial immunization of rat against *Trichinella spiralis*. *Amer. J. Hyg.* **21**, 200–213.

Mills, C. K., and Kent, N. H. (1965). Excretion and secretion of *Trichinella spiralis* and their role in immunity. *Exp. Parasitol.* **16**, 300–311.

Norman, L., and Sadun, E. H. 1959. The use of metabolic antigens in the flocculation tests for the serologic diagnosis of trichinosis. *J. Parasitol.* **45**, 485–489.

Oliver-González, J., and Levine, M. (1962). Stage specific antibodies in experimental trichinosis. *Amer. J. Trop. Med. Hyg.* **11**, 241–244.

Shults, R. S., and Davtyan, E. A. (1951). To the question of helminth antigens. *Izv. Akad. Nauk Arm. SSR* **4**, 533–542.

Soulsby, E. J. L. (1960). Immunity to helminths—recent advances. *Vet. Rec.* **72**, 322–327.

Taliaferro, W. H., and Sarles, M. P. (1939). The cellular reactions in the skin, lungs and intestine of normal and immune rats after infection with *Nippostrongylus muris*. *J. Infec. Dis.* **64**, 157–192.

Tanner, C. E., and Gregory, J. (1961). Immunochemical study of the antigens of *Trichinella spiralis*. I. Identification and enumeration of antigens. *Can. J. Microbiol.* **7**, 473–481.

Thorson, R. E. (1963). The use of "metabolic" and "somatic" antigens in the diagnosis of helminthic infections. *Amer. J. Hyg. Monogr. Ser.* **22.**

Immunological Aspects of *Trichinella spiralis* Infection in the Rat

E. J. Ruitenberg

Laboratory of Pathology
National Institute of Public Health
Bilthoven

Introduction

In a *Trichinella spiralis* infection both humoral and cell-mediated immunity is provoked (Catty, 1969; Ruitenberg and Duyzings, 1972).

Ruitenberg and Duyzings describe the changes in various lymphatic tissues of the rat after *T. spiralis* infection. From these studies it might be concluded that in *T. spiralis* infection in the rat both types of immunity are induced. The humoral response is more marked, but this does not necessarily imply that this type of immunity is more important for host protection.

It might be assumed that at least a part of the immunological response is functional, i.e., directed toward one or more stages of the parasite. In this paper the results relevant to the effect of host immunity on the muscle phase and the intestinal phase will be described.

Results and Discussion

Immunity against the Muscle Phase

First, studies were performed to examine whether the induced immunity is directed toward the muscle phase. By means of (enzyme) histochemical studies the reaction pattern of encysted muscle larvae was studied at 1, 3, 12, and 24 months after infection in the rat. It was assumed that an alteration in the staining pattern of the larvae would indicate a diminished viability of the larva, possibly due to the immunological defense of the host (Ruitenberg and Loendersloot, 1971).

For histochemical studies cryostat sections (10 μm thick) of pieces of tongue and diaphragm from infected rats were cut and stained with hematoxylin and eosin (H&E) and periodic acid–Schiff (PAS) stain for the demonstration of neutral mucopolysaccharides and glycoproteins.

The following enzymatic reactions were studied: alkaline phosphatase (Burstone, 1958); acid phosphatase (Barka and Anderson, 1965); adenosine triphosphatase (Wachstein and Meisel, 1957); succinate dehydrogenase (Nachlas *et al.,* 1957); nicotinamide adenine dinucleotide (NADH) oxi-doreductase (Barka and Anderson, 1965); nicotinamide adenine dinucleo-tide phosphate (NADPH) oxidoreductase (Barka and Anderson, 1965); glucose-6-phosphate dehydrogenase (Nachlas *et al.,* 1958); leucine amino-peptidase (Pearse, 1961); phosphorylase (Takeuchi and Kuriaki, 1955). In Table I the results of this study are summarized. No alterations in the enzyme histochemical staining pattern at the various observation times could be established.

This finding could indicate that the immunity is not functional against the muscle larvae. On the other hand, it is possible that the technique used is not sensitive enough to detect a possible small change in the enzyme pattern of the larvae. Therefore, the experiment was repeated using poly-acrylamide gel electrophoresis. The isoenzyme pattern of acid phos-phatase and esterase (substrate: α-naphthylacetate) at 6 weeks postinfec-tion were studied (Edwards *et al.,* 1971; Ruitenberg, 1972).

In a homogenate of *T. spiralis* larvae, 6 weeks after infection, two vague-ly staining bands representing two isoenzymes of acid phosphatase were observed. The esterase pattern at 6 weeks after infection was compared with that at 3 and 6 months postinfection. However, no differences could be observed. Next, a quantification of these data was reached by measur-ing the intensity of the color of the bands by means of a Vitatron densi-tometer (Ruitenberg, in press).

Figure 1 represents a graph of a densitometer reading of electrophore-sis bands of esterase of a homogenate of *T. spiralis* larvae, 3 months after infection. Comparing the data at 6 weeks, 3 and 6 months after infection

Table I Enzyme histochemistry of *T. spiralis* larva (1, 3, 12 and 24 months after infection)

Enzymes	Reaction
PAS	+++
Alkaline phosphatase	−
Acid phosphatase	+++
Adenosine triphosphatase	++
Succinate dehydrogenase	+++
NADH oxidoreductase	+++
NADPH oxidoreductase	++
Glucose-6-phosphate dehydrogenase	−
Leucine aminopeptidase	±
Phosphorylase	+++

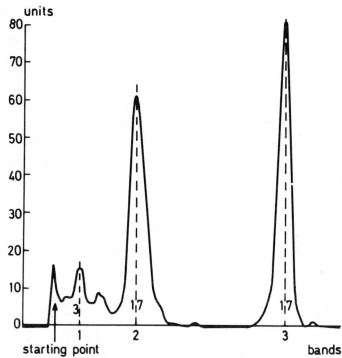

Figure 1 Densitometer plot of isoenzyme pattern of esterase activity (substrate: α-naphthylacetate) obtained from homogenate of *T. spiralis* larvae (3 months postinfection).

it was evident that no difference in the isoenzyme pattern of esterase could be established. From the results of the enzyme studies of the muscle larvae it might be concluded that no change in activity occurs in the course of a *T. spiralis* infection in the rat.

Next it was decided to determine whether immunoglobulins would be present around the larvae. With the aid of immunofluorescence, no immunoglobulins could be detected. Since the cuticle of muscle larvae possesses antigenic properties (Ruitenberg *et al.*, 1968), these results could indicate that indeed no immunoglobulins were present. On the other hand, it is conceivable that the immunofluorescence technique is not sensitive enough to detect very small amounts of immunoglobulins.

From these experiments the conclusion might be drawn that immunity does not influence the muscle phase. A possible explanation could be found in the presence of the capsule. The capsule is presumably virtually impermeable to the immunologically defensive tools of the host (immunoglobulins and sensitized lymphocytes).

In order to study the role of the capsule, *T. spiralis*—infected rats were treated with thiabendazole. A number of larvae were killed by this treatment (oral administration of 500 mg/kg for 5 days) (Ruitenberg and Steerenberg, 1972).

Within thin capsules remnants of muscle larvae were still present. Around these capsules a granuloma was observed. It might be speculated that it is mainly composed of lymphocytes specifically sensitized against *T. spiralis* and attracted by the presence of antigenic material from the larvae. Using the immunofluorescence technique it was possible to detect immunoglobulins on the cuticle of the larva. It is conceivable that the capsule is not maintained by the host after the death of the larva and that it becomes permeable.

In conclusion it is evident that muscle larvae are well protected against the immunity of the host. It is conceivable that the capsule plays an important role in this protection.

Immunity against the Intestinal Phase

Kozar and co-workers (1971) indicated that the functional immunity is primarily directed toward the intestinal phase. The adult worms leave the intestinal tract of the host because they are forced to do so for immunological reasons and not because they possess a limited viability. In order to study this, rats were treated with ALS (antiserum prepared against thymus cells) at 3-day intervals starting with day 3; the *T. spiralis* infection was performed at day 0.

From the results presented in Table II it is evident that normally the immunity exerts a marked influence on the expulsion of the adult *T. spiralis* worms from the intestinal tract. The presence of *T. spiralis* adult worms was studied by histological examination of the entire length of the small intestine with a swiss-roll technique (Reilly and Kirsner, 1965).

In a further series of experiments, it became evident that neonatal

Table II Effect of ALS on Expulsion of *T. spiralis* Adult Worms from the Intestinal Tract of Rats Infected with 250 Larvae Each (Swiss-Roll Technique)

Days post infection	Treatment results [a]	
	None [b]	ALS [b]
12	1	4
13	0	4
14	1	4
15	0	4
16	0	4
17	0	4

[a] Data given are number of rats harboring *T. spiralis* adult worms.
[b] Groups of four rats at each postinfection day.

thymectomy yielded the same results. The intestinal phase was distinctly prolonged if neonatally thymectomized rats were infected at 6 weeks of age.

Apparently the adult worms are subject to the immunological defense mechanism of their host; the expression of this immunological reaction is the expulsion of the adult worms from the intestinal tract. Another important conclusion seems to be that these results suggest that the functional (protective) antigens of *T. spiralis* are T cell dependent. After removing immunocompetent thymus-derived or thymus-dependent lymphoid cells, no protective immunity is observed.

Since it is known that killed suspensions of *Corynebacterium parvum* stimulate the lymphoreticular system (Halpern *et al.*, 1964) and may exert an adjuvant effect (Neveu *et al.*, 1964) resulting in protection against infections with *Plasmodium* (Nussenzweig, 1967) and *Brucella* (Adlam *et al.*, 1972), it seemed interesting to study the effect of *C. parvum* on the expulsion time of *T. spiralis* adult worms. For this purpose rats were injected intravenously with 1 ml of a formalin-killed *C. parvum* suspension.* Three days later 250 *T. spiralis* larvae were administered orally by means of a syringe.

In the first experiment the presence of *T. spiralis* adult worms was studied histologically. The intestinal phase was prolonged by several days in the *C. parvum*-treated animals (Table III). In the second experiment the number of *T. spiralis* adult worms was determined after isolation of the

Table III Effect of *C. parvum* on Expulsion of *T. spiralis* Adult Worms from the Intestinal Tract of Rats Infected with 250 Larvae Each (Swiss-Roll Technique)

Days post-infection	Treatment results[a]	
	None[b]	*C. parvum*[b]
7	4	4
8	4	4
9	3	4
10	0	4
11	1	3
12	0	1
13	0	0
14	0	0
15	0	0

[a] Number of rats harboring *T. spiralis* adult worms.
[b] Groups of four rats at each postinfection day.

* A generous gift of *C. parvum* from the Wellcome Foundation is gratefully acknowledged.

Table IV Effect of *C. parvum* on Expulsion of *T. spiralis* Adult Worms from the Intestinal Tract of Rats Infected with 250 Larvae Each (Isolation Technique)

Days post-infection	Treatment results[a]	
	None[b]	*C. parvum*[b]
8	241	320
9	279	207
10	120	173
11	9	270
12	7	349
13	0	120
14	6	76
15	0	0

[a] Number of *T. spiralis* adult worms isolated from the intestinal tract of all rats from one group.
[b] Groups of four rats at each postinfection day.

worms from the intestinal tract with the Baermann technique (Schmid and Hieronymi, 1955). In the *C. parvum*-treated animals the intestinal phase was distinctly prolonged by several days (Table IV).

The results indicate that in the experimental conditions chosen *C. parvum* exerts an immunosuppressive effect on a *T. spiralis* infection. The observations are in contrast with the adjuvant activity of *C. parvum* in other host–parasite relationships *(Plasmodium, Brucella)*. Recent studies by Scott (1972) indicate that *C. parvum* has no stimulatory effect on T cells. Consequently, our observations could be interpreted as partially suporting the suggestion that protective antigens of *T. spiralis* are T cell dependent.

Summary

The muscle phase of *T. spiralis* infection is protected against the immune response by the capsule. Host protective immunity is directed, particularly, against the intestinal phase of the infection. Functional antigens of *T. spiralis* are probably T cell dependent.

References

Adlam, C. J., Broughton, E. S., and Scott, M. T. (1972). Enhanced resistance of mice to infection with bacteria following pretreatment with *Corynebacterium parvum. Nature New Biol.* **235**, 219–220.

Barka, T., and Anderson, P. J. (1965). "Histochemistry: Theory, Practice and Bibliography." Harper and Row, New York.

Burstone, M. S. (1958). The relationship between fixation and techniques for the histochemical localization of hydrolytic enzymes. *J. Histochem. Cytochem.* **6**, 322–339.

Catty, D. (1969). The immunology of nematode infections. Trichinosis in guinea pigs as a model. *Monogr. Allergy* **5**, 134 pp.

Edwards, A. J., Burt, J. S., and Ogilvie, B. M. (1971). The effect of immunity upon some enzymes of the parasitic nematode *Nippostrongylus brasiliensis*. *Parasitology* **62**, 339–349.

Halpern, B. N., Prévot, A. R., Biozzi, G. Stiffel, C., Mouton, D., Morard, J. C., Bouthillier, Y., and Decreusefond, C. (1964). Stimulation de l'activité phagocytaire du système réticuloendothélial provoquée par *Corynebacterium parvum*. *J. Reticuloendothel. Soc.* **1**, 77–96.

Kozar, Z., Karmańska, K., Kotz, J., and Seniuta, R. (1971). The influence of anti-lymphocytic serum (ALS) on the course of trichinellosis in mice. *Wiad. Parazytol.* **17**, 541–548.

Nachlas, M. M., Tsou, K. C., Souza, E. de, Chang, S. S. and Seligman, A. M. (1957). Cytochemical demonstration of succinic dehydrogenase by the use of a new *p*-nitrophenyl substitute of ditetrazole. *J. Histochem. Cytochem.* **5**, 420–437.

Nachlas, M. M., Walker, D. G. and Seligman, A. M. (1958). The histochemical localization of triphosphopyridine nucleotide diaphorase. *J. Biophys. Biochem. Cytol.* **4**, 467–474.

Neveu, T., Branellec, A., and Biozzi, G. (1964). Propriétés adjuvantes de *Corynebacterium parvum* sur la production d'anticorps et sur l'induction de l'hypersensibilité retardée envers les proteines conjugées. *Ann. Inst. Pasteur* **106**, 771–777.

Nussenzweig, R. S. (1967). Increased nonspecific resistance to malaria produced by administration of killed *Corynebacterium parvum*. *Exp. Parasitol.* **21**, 224–231.

Pearse, A. G. E. (1961). "Histochemistry, Theoretical and Applied," 2nd Ed. Churchill, London .

Reilly, R. W., and Kirsner, J. B. (1965). Runt intestinal disease. *Lab. Inves.* **14**, 102–107.

Ruitenberg, E. J. Quantification of iso-enzyme patterns in polyacrylamide gels. *J. Histochem. Cytochem.* (in press).

Ruitenberg, E. J. (1972). Acid phosphatases in the intestinal cells of two nematode larvae: Anisakis sp. and *Trichinella spiralis*: In: "Comparative Biochemistry of Parasites," Academic Press. New York, pp. 283-295.

Ruitenberg, E. J., and Duyzings, M. J. M. (1972). An immuno-histological study of the immunological response of the rat to infection with *Trichinella spiralis*. *J. Comp. Pathol.* **82**, 401-407.

Ruitenberg, E. J., and Loendersloot, H. J. (1971). Enzymhistochemisch onderzoek van *Anisakis sp.* larven. *Tijdschr. Diergeneek.* **96**, 247–260.

Ruitenberg, E. J., and Steerenberg, P. A. (1972). De invloed van thiabendazol op een *Trichinella spiralis* infectie. *Versl. Meded. Volksgezondh.* **24**, 242–246.

Ruitenberg, E. J., Kampelmacher, E. H., and Berkvens, J. M. (1968). The indirect fluorescent antibody technique in the serodiagnosis of pigs infected with *Trichinella spiralis*. *Neth. J. Vet. Sci.* **1**, 143–153.

Schmid, F., and Hieronymi, E. (1955). "Die parasitaren Krankheiten der Haustiere," 6th Ed. Paul Parey, Berlin and Hamburg.

Scott, M. T. (1972). Biological effects of the adjuvant *Corynebacterium parvum.* I. Inhibition of PHA, mixed lymphocyte and GVH reactivity. *Cell. Immunol.* **5,** 459–468.

Takeuchi, T., and Kuriaki, H. (1955). Histochemical detection of phosphorylase in animal tissues. *J. Histochem. Cytochem.* **3,** 153–160.

Wachstein, M., and Meisel, E. (1957). Histochemistry of hepatic phosphatases at a physiologic pH. *Amer. J. Clin. Pathol.* **27,** 13–23.

Immunity in Mice against *Trichinella spiralis* after Administration of Benzimidazoles: Development of Immunity during the Intestinal and Early Migration Stages of Infection

J. Čorba and R. Špaldonová

Helminthological Institute
of the Slovak Academy of
Sciences,
Košice

Introduction

Benzimidazole derivatives are highly effective against experimental *Trichinella spiralis* infections in laboratory animals. Campbell and Cuckler (1964) were the first to prove the marked anthelminthic effect of thiabendazole on all developmental stages of this parasite. A similar effect of another derivative of benzimidazole, parbendazole, has been observed by Theodorides and Laderman (1969). Campbell and Hartman (1968) showed tetramisole to be effective on the intestinal stage of trichinellosis in mice, and its effect on the muscle stage has been described by Campbell and Cuckler (1967). Campbell and Yakstis (1970) and Duckett and Denham (1970) described the recently synthesized cambandazole as the most effective benzimidazole derivative against enteral and parenteral *Trichinella spiralis* infection.

This work is based on our own experimental results with parbendazole (Špaldonová and Hovorka, 1972) and tetramisole (Špaldonová *et al.,* 1970) used in experimental infection of *T. spiralis* in mice. The purpose of this work was to determine if during the intestinal and early migratory stages of *T. spiralis* resistance arises against reinfection in experimentally infected mice after the primary infection has been treated by the administration of several doses of parbendazole or the less effective tetramisole.

213

Materials and Methods

Assays were carried out in white male mice weighing 20–22 gm, which were infected with 300 *T. spiralis* larvae by a stomach tube. The *Trichinella* used was our strain HELU. The larvae were obtained by muscle digestion of infected mice in artificial gastric juice, containing 1% pepsin with an activity of 10,000 IU, according to the standard method. Each group consisted of 15 mice, which were given 100 mg/kg parbendazole (Smith, Kline and French, U.S.A.) and 40 mg/kg tetramisole (ICI, England). The anthelminthics were administered by a stomach tube according to the time scheme given in Table I. Seven days after the last dose all experimental and corresponding control groups were reinfected with 300 *T. spiralis* larvae each. In addition to these groups, there were also control groups which were given a single dose of 300 *T. spiralis* larvae each. On day 40 after challenge the animals were killed and their muscles were digested according to the previously described method (Špaldonová *et al.,* 1965). The amount of muscle larvae in each group was evaluated by the *t*-test. Simultaneously the reduction of the amount of muscle larvae in the experimental animals was calculated and compared to the corresponding control group.

Results

The results are presented in Table I. It is evident that marked immunity ($P < 0.001$) developed in group I of experimental animals which received parbendazole 24 and 48 hours after infection; the number of muscle larvae as compared to the reinfected control was markedly reduced (83.6%). The immunity was still more significant in groups II and III, which had been given doses of parbendazole at intervals of 72, 96, and 120 hr, and 144, 168 and 192 hr after infection, respectively. The reduction of the amount of muscle larvae as compared to the controls in this stage was about 96% ($P < 0.001$).

In the following stage of development of *Trichinella,* i.e., group IV, in which parbendazole had been administered on days 9–11 after infection, its immunizing effect was significantly lower (28.9% reduction). In group V where parbendazole had been given in 12- to 14-day intervals, the reduction rate was somewhat higher (59.3%).

In the group of animals in which tetramisole had been given, the reduction of the muscle larvae was insignificant as compared to the reinfected controls. It ranged from 21.4 to 49.3%. In the controls infected with a single dose, the average number of larvae was 26,780 ($\pm$ 2350).

Table I Development of Immunity Against Challenge in Mice Experimentally Infected with 300 *Trichinella spiralis* larvae after Administration of Parbendazole and Tetramisole at Different Developmental Stages of the Parasite

Experimental group	Time of administration of anthelminthics (days)	Challenge day/dose	Parbendazole (100 mg/kg)		Tetramisole (40 mg/kg)		Control (Average number of larvae/mouse)	
			Average number of larvae/mouse	% Reduction	Average number of larvae/mouse	% Reduction	Reinfected	Primary infection
I	1–2	9/300	6028 ± 1038 *a*	83.6	27,920 ± 5311	21.4	36,734 ± 3421	
II	3–5	12/300	1424 ± 621	96.1	20,833 ± 7368	49.3	40,689 ± 7426	
III	6–8	15/300	1465 ± 375	96.0	15,722 ± 375	38.8	25,666 ± 7694	26,780 ± 2900
IV	9–11	18/300	13388 ± 2518	28.9	21,430 ± 2101	21.8	13,820 ± 7,697	
V	12–14	21/300	11890 ± 1147	59.3	20,037 ± 7951	31.5	29,192 ± 2744	

a Standard deviation of the mean

This coincides with our standard numbers after an infection with 300 *T. spiralis* larvae.

Discussion

Together with the endeavor to synthesize new and highly effective anthelminthics the question arises whether the use of these substances could have an unfavorable effect on the mechanism of the host resistance. Anthelminthics deplete the host of the whole sensitive parasite population and thus the stimulus leading to the mobilization of its immune mechanism is also removed. Gibson *et al.* (1970) found that the development of resistance against *Trichostronglyus colubriformis* was entirely suppressed if infected sheep were given thiabendazole at weekly intervals throughout a period of 24 weeks. Administration of the less effective anthelminthic phenothiazine enabled a small number of parasites to survive in the host organism. These animals revealed a marked immunity against the challenge with *T. colubriformis*. In his experiments, Wakelin (1969) stimulated the development of immunity against *Trichuris muris* by eliminating the primary invasion by the administration of methyridine 7–14 days after infection. He found, however, that the challenge infection of *T. muris* in mice survived for a longer period than in untreated control animals. He suggested that this difference represents the time span which is absolutely necessary for the accumulation of an adequate antigenic stimulus in the host.

The method of chemical abbreviation of the infection has also been used by other authors. Dineen and Wagland (1966) working with *Haemonchus contortus* interrupted the sensitizing infection by thiabendazole. When after a short time the sheep were challenged, a significant immune response of these animals could be observed. On the basis of their results, the authors suggest that at the challenge a stage of immunological exhaustion of the organism occurred in the untreated animals, which, since their primary infection, had been exposed to a constant antigenic stimulus.

Our experiments with *T. spiralis,* which because of the different localizations of its developmental stages presents a good model, were carried out with the aim to elucidate some of the problems mentioned. The therapeutic doses were chosen on the basis of our previous work. Our results with tetramisole Špaldonová *et al.,* 1970) do not agree with those of Campbell and Hartman (1968) and Campbell and Cuckler (1967), since the effectiveness of tetramisole administered at a dose of 40 mg/kg at different stages of the life cycle was insignificant (5–31.2%). The high effectiveness of parbendazole administered at a dose of 100 mg/kg in our experiments (Špaldonová and Hovorka, 1972) is similar to that reported by Theodorides and Laderman (1969).

The immunizing effect of the different developmental stages of *T. spiralis* after administration of the anthelminthics thiabendazole and methyridine has been examined by Campbell (1965) and by Denham (1966), respectively.

The significance of the intestinal stage of trichinellosis on the development of immunity against the challenge has been proved by the results of our experiments with parbendazole. In group I, in which *Trichinella* persisted in the gastrointestinal tract for only 24 hr, a marked immunity was observed as evidenced by an 83.6% reduction in the muscle larvae. If the worms were left in the gastrointestinal tract for 72–144 hr (groups II and III), the immune response against the challenge was still higher (96%). Campbell (1965), also observed a high degree of immunity in the enteral stage of infection which lasted for only 20 hr. Our results are in agreement with the opinion of Soulsby *et al.* (1959) that the growing and molting stages of some nematodes are highly immunogenic.

Since it has been claimed that adult and juvenile stages of *Trichinella* have similar antigens (Oliver-González and Levine, 1962), it could be presumed that the mice of group V, which had been given parbendazole on days 12–14 when some larvae of the new generation could already be present in the muscle, were stimulated by larger amounts of adult and juvenile *Trichinella* antigens and thus could reveal a more marked immunity against the challenge. However, the degree of immunity as shown by the reduction of the number of muscle larvae, was much lower (59.3%) than in animals challenged after a primary infection for only 24 hr (group I). Our results, therefore, seem to support the view of Campbell (1965) who claimed that parenteral *Trichinella* infection in mice does not increase their resistance against reinfection already induced by the enteral stage. On the basis of our results we share the view of some authors (Ogilvie, 1965; Denham, 1966) that stimulation of the immune response of the host is more or less confined to a certain stage of the life cycle of the parasite.

Since in our experiments the effect of anthelminthics on *Trichinella* from the challenge dose has been excluded by reinfection of the animals 7 days after the treatment, the reduction rate of muscle larvae, particularly with parbendazole, in groups I–III can be explained by stimulation of the defense mechanism of the host. The latter may become evident by its effect on the reproductive ability of *Trichinella* (Rappaport and Wells, 1951) and by a decreased ability of the larvae to develop in the muscle tissues (Chute, 1956).

The comparison of the number of muscle larvae between the control group that received a single challenge and the reinfected control groups did not confirm the view of some authors on the possibility of inducing immunity with a single dose of *T. spiralis* larvae. The resistance induced by a single dose is too weak and persists only for a short time. Therefore, Larsh and co-workers (1952) did not find any marked immune response as early as 7 days after such an immunization. In our case the interval between the primary infection and the challenge was 9–21 days.

Summary

The development of immunity against reinfection has been investigated in mice experimentally infected with *Trichinella spiralis* and given benzimidazole derivatives parbendazole in a dose of 100 mg/kg and tetramisole in a dose of 40 mg/kg during the intestinal and the early migratory stages of infection. It was found that the development of immunity is mostly affected by the intestinal stage of infection since, as early as 24 hr after infection, marked immunity could be observed in animals which received parbendazole. After 3–6 days of infection, i.e., up to the time when anthelminthics were applied, the muscle trichinellae originating from the challenge had been reduced by 96%. With regard to the development of immunity, the administration of parbendazole was much more effective than tetramisole.

References

Campbell, W. C. (1965). Immunizing effect on enteral and enteral-parenteral infections of *Trichinella spiralis* in mice. *J. Parasitol.* **51,** 185–194.

Campbell, W. C., and Cuckler, A. C. (1964). Effect of thiabendazole upon the enteral and parenteral phase of trichinosis in mice. *J. Parasitol.* **50,** 481–488.

Campbell, W. C., and Cuckler, A. C. (1967). Comparative studies on the chemotherapy of experimental trichinosis in mice. *Z. Tropenmed. Parasitol.* **18,** 408–417.

Campbell, W. C., and Hartman, R. K. (1968). Changes in the efficacy of three anthelminthics during the maturation of a nematode *(Trichinella spiralis). J. Parasitol.* **54,** 112–116.

Campbell, W. C. and Yakstis, J. J. (1970). Efficacy of cambendazole against *Trichinella spiralis* in mice. *J. Parasitol.* **56,** 186–188.

Chute, R. M. (1956). The dual antibody response to experimental trichinosis. *Proc. Helminth. Soc. Wash.* **23,** 49–58.

Denham, D. A. (1966). Immunity to *Trichinella spiralis* I. The immunity produced by mice to the first four days of the intestinal phase of the infection. *Parasitology* **56,** 323–327.

Dineen, J. K., and Wagland, B. M. (1966). The dynamics of the host-parasite relationship V. Evidence for immunological exhaustion in sheep experimentally infected with *Haemonchus contortus. Parasitology* **56,** 665–667.

Duckett, M. G., and Denham, D. A. (1970). The effect of cambendazole on *Trichinella spiralis* infections in mice. *J. Helminthol.* **44,** 211–218.

Gibson, T. E., Parfitt, J. W., and Everett, G. (1970). The effect of Anthelminthics treatment on the development of resistance of *Trichostrongylus colubriformis* in sheep. *Res. Vet. Sci.* **2,** 138–145.

Larsh, J. E., Jr. Gilchrist, H. B., and Greenberg, B. G. (1952). A study of the distribution and longevity of adult *Trichinella spiralis* in immunized and non-immunized mice. *J. Elisha Mitchell Scient. Soc.* **68**, 1–11.

Ogilvie, B. M. (1965). Role of adult worms in immunity of rates to *Nippostrongylus brasiliensis. Parasitology* **55**, 325–335.

Oliver-Gonzalez, J., and Levine, D. M. (1962). Stage specific antibodies in experimental trichinosis. *Amer. J. Trop. Med. Hyg.* **11**, 241–244.

Rappaport, I., and Wells, H. S. (1951). Studies in trichinosis. I. Immunity to reinfection in mice following a single light infection. *J. Infec. Dis.* **88**, 248–253.

Soulsby, E. J. L., Sommerville, R. J., and Stewart, D. F. (1959). Antigentic stimulus of exsheathing fluid in self-cure of sheep infected with *Haemonchus contortus. Nature, London* **183**, 533–554.

Špaldonová, R., and Hovorka, J. (1972). Wirkung des Parbendazols bei experimenteller Trichinellose. *Angew, Parasitol.* **13**, 207–213.

Špaldonová, R., Podhájecký, K., and Tomašovičová, O. (1970). Research on the helminth specificity from the point of view of anthelminthic efficacy in different phases of onthogenesis. *Final Rep., Helmintol. Inst. Kosice Czech.* pp. 40–47.

Špaldonová, R., Corba, J., and Podhájecký, K. (1965). Chemotherapy of experimental trichinosis in mice. *Final Rep, Helminthol. Inst. Kosice, Czech.* pp. 23–27.

Theodorides, V. J., and Laderman, M. (1969). Activity of parbendazole upon *Trichinella spiralis* in mice. *J. Parasitol.* **55**, 678.

Wakelin, D. (1969). Studies on the immunity of albino mice to *Trichuris muris.* The stimulation of immunity by chemically abbreviated infections. *Parasitology* **59**, 549–555.

Immunological Studies of Rat Skeletal Muscles in the Course of *Trichinella spiralis* Infection Treated with Thiabendazole

Krystyna Jarczewska, Miroslaw Gorny, and
Jan Zeromski

Department of Pathological Anatomy
Institute of Biostructure
Medical Academy
Poznań

Introduction

Treatment of trichinellosis both in intestinal and muscular stages of disease has been symptomatic up to recent time. There was no drug that would specifically destroy the larvae. The introduction of thiabendazole (Thb-Minthezol) has dramically changed the therapeutic approach to this disease (Campbell and Cuckler, 1962; Stone *et al.*, 1964). The drug acts primarily on the intestinal phase of trichinellosis by destroying both the adult and larval forms of the parasite, thereby reducing muscle invasion (Kociecka, 1971). Administration of thiabendazole (Thb) to the muscular phase, especially the later stages of the disease was of little value and, moreover, was dangerous for the patient, causing fever, allergic skin rashes, and even shock (Kozar *et al.*, 1966). Morphological studies of the skeletal muscles of both humans and animals have shown that the drug causes disintegration of the larvae in the muscles. Disintegrated larvae are surrounded by massive inflammatory aggregates consisting of lymphocytes and macrophages, the latter with marked activity of hydrolytic enzymes (Gabryel *et al.*, 1971). On the other hand, the specific immune response, both humoral and cellular, is expressed early, starting from 10–14 days after infection (Larsh, 1967). This antigenic stimulation makes early immunological diagnosis of trichinellosis possible (Baratawidjaja *et al.*, 1963; Wegesa *et al.*, 1971).

Marked disintegration of the larvae in the course of Thb therapy suggests that during treatment large amounts of antigenic substances of the parasite are released into the bloodstream with subsequent antigen–antibody reaction resulting in sensitization of the host. Such immunological reactivity is probably of significance to the general status of the patient.

The purpose of this study was to detect possible local immune reactions in the muscles of infected animals in the course of Thb therapy.

Materials And Methods

Tissue Source

Sixty Wistar rats were infected orally with 3000 *T. spiralis* larvae. Thiabendazole (Merck) suspension was administered directly into the stomach by means of a plastic tube in doses of 150 mg/animal for 5 days. The drug was given 24 hr, 5, 10, 15, 20 days, 3 months, and 1 and 2 years after infection. Tissue specimens were collected on 2, 4, and 8 days after completion of Thb treatment. For immunofluorescent studies the tongue and the diaphragm were used. The tissue specimens were quickly frozen in Dry Ice–acetone mixture. A portion of the material was fixed in 0.4% ethanol solution of acridine hydrochloride and embedded in paraffin.

Conjugated Reagents

The following conjugates were used: (1) Rabbit immune globulin against *T. spiralis* (T.S.) larvae homogenate labeled with fluorescein isothiocyanate (FITC-isomer I, Sigma), (R.a.T.S. FITC). The antigen and antiserum were prepared as previously described (Zeromski and Jazbor, 1969a). (2) Rabbit immune globulin against guinea pig globulin labeled with FITC (R.a.G.P. glob.FITC). (3) Rabbit immune globulin against rat γ-globulin labeled with FITC (R.a.Rat glob.FITC).

Serum globulins were prepared by precipitation of whole serum by half-saturated ammonium sulfate solution. Proteins were conjugated and purified in essentially the same way as described previously (Zeromski and Jazbor, 1969 a, b). Fluorescein: protein (F:P) ratio of obtained reagents ranged from 2 to 5.

Immunofluorescent Studies

Heterologous complement-fixing indirect and direct reactions with other labeled reagents were carried out as described in preceding papers (Zeromski and Jazbor, 1969a,b). Appropriate control reactions were always performed in parallel.

Histochemical Reactions and Histological Staining

Metachromasia with toluidine blue was carried out on frozen sections for examining the mast cells. Paraffin sections were stained with hematoxylin–eosin and also by Dominici method for examining the eosinophils.

Fluorescent Microscopy and Photomicrography

Tissue specimens were viewed in a Reichert Zetopan research microscope and photographed as described previously.

Results

The data concerning immunofluorescent fixation of heterologous complement are summarized in Table I. The larvae and surrounding muscle were fixing complement in the group of animals which were given Thb soon after infection (from the tenth day) and sacrificed 3–5 days later. Immunofluorescent reaction was evident in the larval body and adjacent portions of the muscle fiber in which the larva had settled (Figs. 1 and 2). *Trichinella spiralis* antigens and rat γ-globulins could be detected at the same sites by means of appropriate reagents (Fig. 3). The larvae were often surrounded by a rim of cells with green-yellow cytoplasmic fluorescence (Fig. 4). Control reactions have, however, revealed that the latter was nonspecific. Dominici staining identified these cells as eosinophils.

In animals which received Thb later (20 days or later after infection) specific fluorescence became more and more limited to the larval body or its fragments (Table I). In sites of heterologous complement fixation, antigens of the parasite were still evident. At late periods after infection (1–2 years), fixation of heterologous complement in larvae and in muscles could not be detected in either Thb treated or untreated rats.

In cellular aggregates surrounding larvae and also among sarcolemmal sheaths of neighboring muscles, large cells showing apparent but weak cytoplasmic fluorescence with various conjugates were noticeable, thus

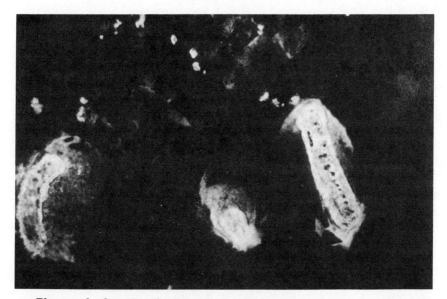

Figure 1 Specific fluorescence of transverse section of *Trichinella* larva and its vicinity. Fluorescent fixation of heterologous complement. Thb-treated rat, 17 days after infection. × 200.

Table I Immunofluorescent Fixation of Heterologous Complement (IFHC) in Thiabendazole Treated Rats

Time interval between infection and Thb administration	Time interval between infection and sacrifice (days)	IFHC	Presence of *T. spiralis* antigen	Presence of larvae
24 hr	7		No S.F.	Lacking
	9	No S.F.[a]	Marginal S.F. of larvae	Very few if any
	13			
5 days	12	No S.F.	S.F. of larval body	Present
	14	S.F. of larval body		
	18			
10 days	17	S.F. of larvae and surrounding muscular fiber	S.F. of larvae and vicinity	Present
	19	As above, but weaker F. of surroundings		
	23			
15 days	22	Distinct S.F. limited to larval body	S.F. of larval body	Numerous encapsulated larvae
	24			
	28			
20 days	27	Weak S.F. limited to fragments of larval body	S.F. of larvae	As above
	29			
	33			
3 months	100	No S.F.	S.F. of larvae	Encapsulated larvae Capsule with features of hyalinization calcification
1 year	375	No S.F.	As above	As above
2 years	740	No S.F.	As above	As above

[a] S.F., specific fluorescence.

224

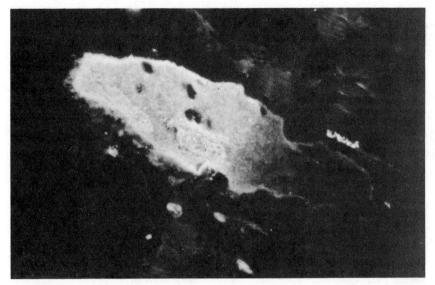

Figure 2 Specific fluorescence of the larva and its vicinity. Reaction as above in the Thb-treated rat, 19 days after infection. × 360.

being devoid of specificity. These cells were identified as mast cells by means of toluidine blue reaction. They were also visible but not conspicious in muscles of healthy control rats.

The evaluation of eosinophilis in inflammatory aggregates has shown that they were much more numerous (up to 40%) in rats treated with Thb, especially at early periods after infection, in comparison to untreated animals. Metachromatic reaction with toluidine blue and also the Dominici stain demonstrated numerous mast cells in muscles of infected rats. There were more mast cells in Thb treated animals; the phenomenon was not, however, assessed quantitatively. The frequency of degranulation of these cells was similar in both groups of treated and untreated rats.

Discussion

Results of our study indicate that the destruction of *T. spiralis* larvae in the course of Thb therapy is a complex process involving defense mechanisms of the host. This is evident from the fact that antigen–antibody complexes are present in muscles of infected rats. Deposits of the components of the complexes, such as parasite antigens and rat γ-globulin, and also fixation of heterologous complement could be detected not only within the larva but also in the host muscle. The latter could indicate the range of reaction within individual muscle fibers. It seems probable that the toxic effect of Thb against *Trichinella* becomes synergistically

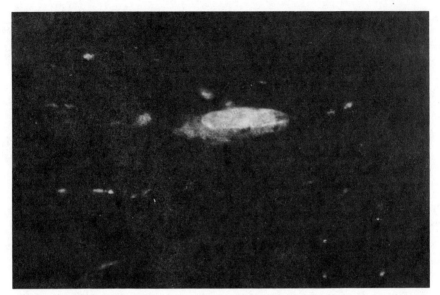

Figure 3 Specific fluorescence of a portion of the larva and its surroundings. Reaction with immunofluorescent reagent against *Trichinella* antigens. R.a.T.S. FITC, Thb-treated rat, 17 days after infection. × 200.

reinforced by immunological mechanisms at some stage of parasitic growth. This immunological reactivity is apparently strictly dependent on emergence of a specific anti-*Trichinella* immunity in the host. In our experiments it was most marked in animals in which Thb was administered from the tenth day following infection. Perhaps the drug itself mediates the intensity and the type of emerging immunity. The direct effect of Thb on larvae probably facilitates access of immune humoral factors to antigenic elements of the parasite body, which is manifested by the immune complex formation. Occurrence of the latter in trichinellosis, without the influence of Thb, has been demonstrated by isotope techniques (Dusanic and Lewert, 1963), immunofluorescence (Nowoslawski *et al.*, 1969), and from our previous work (Zeromski and Jazbor, 1969b). The immunological reactivity of the muscular fibers in the vicinity of the larvae may be partly autoimmune in nature. Gross antigenic similarities between *T. spiralis* larvae and striated muscles have been noticed (Kozar, 1971).

Additional indirect evidence for immunological response of the host against *Trichinella* is the presence of eosinophil aggregates. The latter are common in trichinellosis but their number and intensity in animals treated with Thb was far greater than in control infected animals. Their significance in trichinellosis is not fully explained; it is known, however,

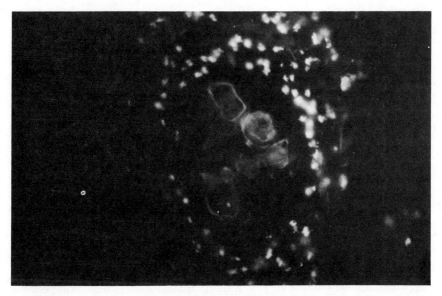

Figure 4 A rim of nonspecific fluorescent cells (eosinophils) around transverse sections of larva. R.a.T.S. FITC, Thb-treated rat, 24 days after infection. × 200.

that eosinophil-attracting histamine diminishes muscle invasion by the parasite (Ismail and Tanner, 1969). It is also known that eosinophils have a high affinity for antigen–antibody complexes (Hirsch, 1965).

As far as mast cells are concerned, the evaluation of their role is very difficult on the basis of our experiments. Frequency of degranulation of mast cells was visually similar in both experimental and control animals. Presence of mast cells and their degranulation in trichinellosis is a distinct phenomenon, especially noticeable in muscles (Briggs, 1963; Karmanska *et al.,* 1971). The lack of increased degranulation in the course of Thb therapy with concomitant features of immunological reactivity may indicate another type of host immunity. Mast cell degranulation is a significant sign of anaphylactic type hypersensitivity (type I according to Roitt, 1971). Formation of immunological complexes with concomitant massive inflammatory reaction corresponds to type III of Roitt (1971), i.e., hypersensitivity mediated by antigen-antibody complexes. The features of the latter, such as deposition of immune complexes and inflammatory cell exudate with hydrolytic enzymes activity, could be found in the local inflammatory reaction around larva in the course of Thb treatment. Thus, it seems likely that coexisting host hypersensitivity toward larval antigens is one of the factors mediating the course of Thb therapy. The role of specific immune complexes may be relevant here. The pathogenic role of the latter in disease in general, in a well-known and established phenomenon (Dixon, 1962; Cochrane, 1971) but it still needs clarification in relation to trichinellosis.

Summary

Trichinella spiralis-infected rats were treated at various intervals with thiabendazole (Thb). Frozen sections of muscles were examined by means of immunofluorescence for the fixation of heterologous complement, the presence of *Trichinella* antigens, and host γ-globulin. Paraffin sections were examined for the presence of eosinophils and mast cells by means of Dominici and toluidine blue methods, respectively. It has been found that larvae settled in muscles were coated and surrounded by specific *Trichinella* antigen-antibody complexes. This phenomenon was evident in the rats which received Thb therapy soon after infection (from the tenth day). It became less distinct in the groups of animals treated at later periods and it eventually waned. Eosinophils, which composed a large portion of the cellular aggregate around the larvae (up to 40%) were much more numerous in Thb-treated than in untreated animals. There was no distinct difference in degranulation of mast cells in both groups of animals. It is postulated that Thb therapy may be partly mediated by specific immune status of the host.

Acknowledgment

This study was supported by a research grant CDC-E-P-2, Center for Disease Control. U.S. Public Health Service.

References

Baratawidjaja, R. K., Hewson, A., and Labzoffsky, N. A. (1963). Fluorescent antibody staining in the serodiagnosis of trichinosis. *Can. J. Microbiol.* **9,** 625–628.

Briggs, N. T. (1963). Immunological injury of mast cells in mice actively and passively sensitized to antigens from *Trichinella spiralis. J. Infec. Dis.* **113,** 22–32.

Campbell, W. C., and Cuckler, A. C. (1962). Thiabendazole treatment of the invasive phase of experimental trichinosis in swine. *Ann. Trop. Med. Parasitol.* **56,** 500–505.

Cochrane, C. G. (1971). Initiating events in immune complex injury. *In*: B. Amos (ed.). "Progress in Immunology." Academic Press, New York, pp. 143–153.

Dixon, F. J. (1962). Tissue injury produced by antigen–antibody complexes. *In*: P. Grabar and P. Miescher (eds.), "Mechanism of Cell and Tissue Damage Produced by Immune Reactions." Schwabe, Basel, pp. 71–87.

Dusanic, D. G., and Lewert, R. M. (1963). Detection of soluble and insoluble antigen–antibody complexes of isotopically labelled *Trichinella spiralis* and *Schistosoma mansoni* extracts following electrophoretic separation. *J. Parasitol.* **49.** 34–35.

Gabryel, P., Gustowska, L., Blotna, M., and Kociecka, W. (1971). Odczyny tkankowe przy stosowaniu Thiabendazolu w poznej fazie miesniowej zakazenia wlosniem kretym. *Proc. 5th Meet. Pol. Soc. Pathol. Katowice*, pp. 208–209.

Hirsch, J. G. (1965). Neutrophil and eosinophil leucocytes. *In*: B. W. Zweifach L. Grant, and R. T. McCluckey (eds.), "Inflammatory Process." Academic Press, New York, pp. 245–280.

Ismail, M. M., and Tanner, C. E. (1969). The relation between eosinophilia, serotonin and histamine in experimental trichinellosis *Wiad. Parazytol.* **15**, 700–701.

Karmánska, K., Kozar, Z., Seniuta, R., and Czajkowska, J. (1971). Behavior of mast cells in experimental trichinellosis in mice. *Wiad. Parazytol.* **17**, 593–607.

Kocięcka, W. (1971). Behaviour of *Trichinella spiralis* larvae in animals treated by thiabendazole and hydrocortisone. *Wiad. Parazytol.* **17**, 625–640.

Kozar, Z. (1971). Some current immunologic aspects of trichinellosis. *Wiad. Parazytol.* **17**, 503–540.

Kozar, Z., Jackowska-Klimowicz, J., and Sladki, E. (1966). Thiabendazole therapy in human trichinellosis. *Wiad. Parazytol.* **12**, 605–617.

Larsh, J. E., Jr. (1967). The present understanding of the mechanism of immunity to *Trichinella spiralis*. *Amer. J. Trop. Med. Hyg.* **16**, 123–132.

Nowoslawski, A., Brzosko, W. J., and Gancarz Z. (1969). Immunopathological aspects of experimental trichinellosis. *Wiad. Parazytol.* **15**, 642–643.

Roitt, I. M. (1971). "Essential Immunology." Blackwell, Oxford, pp. 105–132.

Stone, O. J., Stone, C. T., and Mullins, J. F. (1964). Thiabendazole-probable cure for trichinosis. *J. Amer. Med. Ass.* **187**, 536–537.

Wegesa, P., Sulzer, A. J., and Van Orden, A. (1971). A slide antigen in the indirect fluorescent antibody test for *Trichinella spiralis*. *Immunology* **21**, 805–808.

Zeromski, J., and Jazbor, A. (1969). Diagnosis of systemic lupus erythematosus. Semiquantitative immunofluorescent method of LE factor determination in frozen and paraffin sections. *Pol. Med. J.* **8**, 1282–1287.

Zeromski, J., and Jazbor, A. (1969a). Localization of antigens of developing *Trichinella spiralis* larvae in the tissue of infected rats. I. Comparative studies on direct and indirect immunofluorescence. *Acta Parasitol. Pol.* **17**, 119–125.

Zeromski, J., and Jazbor, A. (1969b). Localization of antigens of developing *Trichinella spiralis* larvae in the tissue of infected rats. II. Immunofluorescent fixation of heterologous complement by larval antigens. *Acta Parasitol. Pol.* **17**, 127–130.

Immunogenicity of the Stichosome of *Trichinella spiralis* in Mice

W. J. Kozek* and Catherine A. Crandall

*Department of Immunology and Medical Microbiology and
Department of Pathology, College of Medicine, University
of Florida, Gainesville, Florida*

Introduction

Recent reports have indicated that the stichosome of *Trichinella spiralis* contains functional antigens which may be of significance in the acquired resistance to this helminth (Despommier and Müller, 1969, 1970a, b; Despommier, 1971). Because little is known about the antigenic development of the stichosome, and the chronology of host response to stichosome antigens, this study was undertaken to determine (1) when, during the intramuscular development of the larva, the stichosome becomes antigenic, (2) how soon, after infection of muscle by the larvae, antibodies against the stichosome can be detected in the circulation, and (3) whether circulating antibodies could have access to the intramuscular larva.

Materials and Methods

Unless otherwise noted, 8- to 10-week-old CD female mice (Charles River, Wilmington, Massachusetts) were used in these investigations. The mice were maintained in facilities fully accredited by the American Association for Accreditation of Laboratory Animal Care. Frozen sections 4 μm thick of *T. spiralis* larvae in tongue and/or diaphragms of rats harboring a 6-to 8-month-old infection were used as antigen for direct and indirect fluorescent antibody (FA) tests. *Trichinella spiralis* hyperimmune rabbit serum was obtained from a rabbit inoculated six times with 10,000–14,000 *T. spiralis* larvae at monthly intervals. The preparation of anti-immunoglobulin sera, conjugation of antisera with fluorescein isothio-

*Present address: California Primate Research Center, University of California, Davis, California.

cyanate, and staining procedures have been described in detail elsewhere (Crandall, *et al.,* 1967; Crandall and Crandall, 1971, 1972).

Experimental Procedures and Results

Detection of Antigenic Components in the Stichosome of the Developing Larvae

Eight mice were inoculated by stomach intubation with approximately 400 *T. spiralis* larvae and divided into four groups containing two mice per group. One or both mice of each group were killed on day 9, 11, 14, and 16 after inoculation. The diaphragms were excised, quick frozen, and kept at $-20°C$ until sectioned with a cryostat. To detect antigen in the stichosome of the developing larvae the frozen sections were stained with fluorescein-conjugated γ-globulin prepared from a *T. spiralis* hyperimmune rabbit. Fluorescein-labeled normal rabbit globulin was used for the control.

Some internal organ(s) which could not be identified in the larvae of 9- and 11- day-old infections fluoresced; at 14 and 16 days, the stichosome, intestine, and outermost cuticle were well stained. No fluorescence was observed in any sections stained with fluorescein-labeled normal rabbit globulin.

Detection of Circulating Antibodies against Stichosome Products during Larval Infection

Muscle-infecting larvae (MIL-newborns) were obtained from gravid females according to a modified procedure of Dennis *et al.* (1970). Our culture media consisted of 70 ml of Hanks' balanced salt solution, 30 ml of decomplemented ($56°C$, 30 min) normal rabbit serum, 10,000 IU of penicillin and 10 mg of streptomycin (Grand Island Biological Co., Grand Island, New York). The pH was adjusted to approximately 7.8 with 2% $NaHCO_3$. MILs were separated from the adults by straining the culture medium through a #500 stainless steel or copper bolt cloth with a pore dimension of approximately 20×20 μm (W. S. Tyler, Inc., Mentor, Ohio). The adults were transferred to fresh medium every 10–12 hr for 2–3 days. MILs were collected each time the medium was changed.

Three experiments were carried out to determine how soon circulating antibodies to the stichosome products (SP) could be detected following inoculation with MILs. In the first experiment five mice were inoculated with approximately 6000 MILs through a tail vein in 0.2 ml of the incubation medium. One mouse was exsanguinated on day 6, 10, 15, 23, and 37 after inoculation. Sera obtained from uninfected mice were used as controls. All sera were diluted 1:40 with phosphate-buffered saline, pH 7.5, and the indirect FA test was done with fluorescein-labeled antimouse globulins specific for the different immunoglobulin classes.

Antibodies in IgG_1 were first detected to the stichosome at 37 days following the injection of the MIL; no stichosome antibodies in IgM or IgA were detected in any of the sera. IgA antibodies to the muscle and hypodermis were detected at 23 days and to the muscle and hypodermis as well as the cuticle at 37 days. IgM antibodies were not detected in any sera.

In the second experiment 10 mice were inoculated with approximately 7300 MILs through a tail vein in 0.2 ml of incubation medium. Five of these mice (nos. 1–5) were bled from the suborbital sinus for approximately 0.2 ml of blood at 2, 4, and 6 weeks after inoculation; the remaining five (nos. 6–10) were bled at 3 and 5 weeks after inoculation. At the end of the experiment all mice in this group were killed and the muscle larvae collected by a modified method used by Larsh and Kent (1949) for rats. The mice were skinned and eviscerated. Each mouse carcass was ground separately in a Waring blender containing between 100 to 150 ml of digest fluid (1% pepsin containing 1% HCl). The ground carcass and the wash from several rinses of the blender with the digested fluid were pooled in a glass container so that the final volume was 200–250 ml. Digestion was carried out overnight at $37°$ C. The next day approximately one-half of the fluid at the top was carefully removed, the remaining digest was made up to a constant volume and the total number of larvae in each carcass was determined by counting larvae in measured aliquots of the digest mixture.

The numbers of intestine-infecting larvae (IILs) recovered 6 weeks after inoculation from mice 1–5 were 4800, 2530, 2700, 3740, and 3530 and from mice 6–10, the numbers were 4060, 2370, 4700, 4700, and 5930, respectively. Antibodies to the stichosome were first detected in sera of three of five mice at 4 weeks, in four of five mice at 5 weeks, and in all five sera at 6 weeks, postinoculation. Antibodies to some stromal components of the larvae were detected in mice 6–10 at 3 weeks, postinoculation, and to the muscle of larvae at 2 weeks, postinoculation in the serum of mouse 5.

All serum samples of mouse 1 and 6 were tested for antibodies belonging to the IgA and IgM classes. IgA antibodies were not detected in any of the sera tested. IgM antibodies to the larval membranes were detected at 5 (mouse 6) and 6 (mouse 1) weeks, postinoculation. There was no correlation between the number of IILs recovered and the time when antibodies to the stichosome were detected, nor between the number of larvae presumably destroyed and the time of detection of antistromal antibodies.

In the third experiment, mice (nos. 1–3) were inoculated with approximately 33,000, 36,000, and 16,000 MILs, respectively, through a mesenteric vein in approximately 1 ml of incubation medium. Two additional mice (nos. 4 and 5) received approximately 50,000 MILs each through a tail vein in 0.25 ml of the medium. Mice were bled from the suborbital sinus at weekly intervals for 6 weeks, beginning 2 weeks after inoculation. Indirect FA tests on the sera and larval counts were performed as described above.

Mice 1, 2, and 3 had detectable antibodies to the stichosome at 5 weeks after inoculation; the number of the IIL recoved from these mice was 19,800, 10,900, and 2000, respectively. Mouse 4 had demonstrable antibodies at 4 weeks, mouse 5 at 6 weeks; from each of these mice approximately 2000 IILs were recovered. In most of these mice IgG antibodies to somatic structures (cuticle, hypodermis, muscle) could be detected 2 weeks earlier than the antibodies to the stichosome.

Uptake of Globulins by Infected Muscle Fibers

To determine whether the infected muscle fibers and/or the cysts are permeable to antibodies during any part of the intramuscular developmental phase of the larvae, 20 female, 6- to 8-week-old ICR mice (Flow Labs., Dublin, Virginia) were inoculated with approximately 380 *T. spiralis* larvae. The mice were divided into five groups, four mice per group. Permeability studies were carried out at 9, 12, 16, 19, and 27 days after inoculation. In a group, two mice received 2 ml of normal rabbit serum injected intraperitoneally, the other two received 2 ml of *T. spiralis* rabbit hyperimmune serum which had an antistichosome titer of 1:640 previously determined by the indirect FA test. Fifteen to 24 hr after injection, to allow for equilibration of serum, one or two mice from each subgroup were necropsied. The tongues and the diaphragms were quick-frozen and cryostat sections were stained with fluorescein-labeled goat antirabbit-IgG. The IgG of the normal and hyperimmune sera was readily detected in the intercellular spaces of the tongue and the diaphragm. There was no indication that the γ-globulins penetrated into or were taken up by the normal (uninfected) muscle fibers. At 10 days after inoculation, infected fibers apparently did not take up any globulins, but at 13 and 17 days infected fibers were slightly more fluorescent than the background stain of normal cells. In addition to a uniform fluorescence, discrete areas of more intense fluorescence were observed within the infected fiber whether the mice received hyperimmune or normal serum. The cuticle and cell membranes of the larvae stained faintly in the infected muscle fibers of mice which received hyperimmune serum, and comparable but weaker staining was observed in the larvae of mice which received normal serum.

At 20 and 28 days after inoculation no evidence was found that IgG from either the normal or the hyperimmune serum was taken up by the infected fibers.

Discussion

The results of this study demonstrate that stichosome antigens are present in larvae by the third week of infection and antibodies to the stichosome products are induced during the muscle phase of infection. In addition, γ-globulins from the circulation are detectable within infected muscle fibers during a limited period of larval development.

The morphological studies of Wu (1955) and Ali Khan (1966) showed that stichocytes can be recognized as early as 6 days postinoculation and by 16 days postinoculation the stichosome has all the morphological characteristics of fully developed intestine-infecting larvae (IIL). The demonstration of stichosome staining at 14 days postinoculation indicated the presence of antigens at least by the time these cells reach maturity by morphological criteria. If the fluorescent staining areas observed in larvae of 9- and 11-day infections prove, on further study, to be stichocytes, it would indicate that some antigens appear extremely early in development.

Antibodies to stichosome were not detected until 4–6 weeks after inoculation of MILs; in contrast, antibodies to other organs of the larvae were detected much earlier. These findings are consistent with the observation that stichosome antigens are present only after maturation of the larvae; the earlier appearing antibodies were undoubtedly induced by antigens released from dead newborn larvae soon after injection. The usual way in which the host is exposed to the stichosome antigens during larval infection is unknown. Antigens may be available on death of the larvae or, as suggested by Despommier (1971), there may be some release of antigens during intramuscular development.

IgG was not detected within the infected muscle at any time after the third week of infection, which confirms the report by Jackson (1959) that mature, living cysts are impermeable to γ-globulin. In contrast, permeability of the cysts to certain small molecules has been well established (Hanks and Stoner, 1958; Kozar *et al.,* 1969; McCoy *et al.,* 1941; Stoner and Hanks, 1955; Zarzycki *et al.,* 1968). In addition, it has been reported that albumin may penetrate the cyst (Zarzycki *et al.,* 1966). The detection of fluorescent staining within infected fibers during the third week, and the more intense staining of intracellular larvae following injection of immune sera than following normal sera suggests that intact antibody may enter the fiber during this period. However, it cannot be stated with certainty whether the staining was due to the presence of the intact immunoglobulin or due to peptide fragments from IgG which could still bind with the FA reagent. During the third week of infection the greatest growth and organ development of larvae as well as marked organizational changes within the muscle fibers occur (Read, 1970), which, it may be conjectured, is associated with an increase in membrane permeability and permits entry of immunoglobulins. In addition, the localized areas of more intense fluorescence within the infected fibers suggest that the uptake is not just a result of increased permeability, but that there is a localized reaction, probably pinocytosis.

The detection of antigens to the stichosome during intramuscular development and the detection of antibody to stichosome induced by the muscle larvae support the report of Despommier (1971) that stichosome antigens of larvae are released during intramuscular development. The early detection of antibody to structures other than the stichosome indicates that the newborn larvae are potentially antigenic.

Summary

Fluorescent antibody studies were done to determine (1) when the stichosome becomes antigenic during intramuscular development of *T. spiralis* larvae, (2) when antibodies to the stichosome are detected in the sera of mice after an intravenous inoculation of newborn larvae, and (3) whether intramuscular larvae are accessible to circulating antibodies.

Some internal organ(s) which could not be identified in the larvae of 9- and 11-day-old infections fluoresced when frozen sections of mouse diaphragm were stained with labeled γ-globulin from a rabbit hyperinfected with *T. spiralis*. At 14 and 16 days, the stichosome, intestine, and outermost cuticular layer were well stained.

The serum of mice which received intravenous inoculations varying from 5,000 to 50,000 newborn *T. spiralis* larvae was tested for the presence of antibodies in the different Ig classes by the indirect fluorescent antibody technique from 6 days to 6 weeks postinoculation. Antibody in the IgG_1 class to the stichosome or its products was usually detected during and after the fourth week, but those to the stromal elements were detectable as early as 2 weeks after inoculation. Antibodies to the stichosome were not detected in the IgA and IgM classes.

Following intraperitoneal injection, rabbit γ-globulin was observed within the infected muscle fibers of mice only during the third week of infection.

Acknowledgment

Supported in part by Public Health Service Grants AI-03212 and AI-05345 from the NIAID and NIH Training Grant 5TI AI 0128.

References

Ali Khan, Z. (1966). The postembryonic development of *Trichinella spiralis* with special reference to ecdysis. *J. Parasitol.* **52**, 248–259.

Crandall, C. A., and Crandall, R. B. (1971). *Ascaris suum:* Immunoglobulin response in mice. *Exp. Parasitol.* **30**, 426–437.

Crandall, R. B., and Crandall, C. A. (1972). *Trichinella spiralis*: Immunologic response to infection in mice. *Exp. Parasitol.* **31**, 378–398.

Crandall, R. B., Cebra, J. J., and Crandall, C. A. (1967). The relative proportions of IgG-, IgA- and IgM-containing cells in rabbit tissues during experimental trichinosis. *Immunology* **12**, 147–158.

Dennis, D. T., Despommier, D. D., and Davis, N. (1970). Infectivity of the newborn larva of *Trichinella spiralis* in the rat. *J. Parasitol.* **56**, 974–977.

Despommier, D., and Müller, M. (1969). Particle associated, functional antigens of *Trichinella spiralis* larvae and immunity in mice. *Wiad. Parazytol.* **15**, 612.

Despommier, D., and Müller, M. (1970a). Functional antigens of *Trichinella spiralis*. *J. Parasitol.* **54** (Sect. II, Part 1), 76.

Despommier, D., and Müller, M. (1970b). The stichosome of *Trichinella spiralis*: Its structure and function. *J. Parasitol.* **54** (Sect. II, Part 1), 76.

Despommier, D. D. (1971). Immunogenicity of the newborn larva of *Trichinella spiralis*. *J. Parasitol.* **57**, 531–534.

Hanks, L. V., and Stoner, R. D. (1958). Incorporation of DL-Tyrosine-2-C-$_{14}$ and DL-Tryptophan-2-C-$_{14}$ by encysted *Trichinella spiralis* larvae. *Exp. Parasitol.* **7**, 92–98.

Jackson, G. J. (1959). Fluorescent antibody studies of *Trichinella spiralis* infections. *J. Infec. Dis.* **105**, 97–117.

Kozar, Z., Zarzycki, J., Czechowicz, K., and Teppa-Szumowska, E. (1969). Autoradiographic studies on incorporation of amino acids in the muscular phase of trichinellosis. *Wiad. Parazytol.* **15**, 662–666.

Larsh, J. E., Jr., and Kent, D. E. (1949). The effect of alcohol on natural and acquired immunity of mice to infection with *Trichinella spiralis*. *J. Parasitol.* **35**, 45–53.

McCoy, O. R., Downing, V. F., and Van Voorhis, S. N. (1941). The penetration of radioactive phosphorus into encysted *Trichinella* larvae. *J. Parasitol.* **27**, 53–58.

Read, C. P. (1970). Some physiological and biochemical aspects of host–parasite relations, *J. Parasitol.* **56**, 643–652.

Stoner, R. D., and Hankes, L. V. (1955). Incorporation of C^{14}-labeled amino acids by *Trichinella spiralis* larvae. *Exp. Parasitol.* **4**, 435–444.

Wu, L. Y. (1955). The development of the stichosome and associated structure in *Trichinella spiralis*. *Can. J. Zool.* **33**, 404–446.

Zarzycki, J., Kozar, Z., and Czechowicz, K. (1966). An attempt to use the autoradiographic method for studying host–parasite relationships in trichinellosis. *Wiad. Parazytol.* **12**, 553–560.

Zarzycki, J., Kozar, Z., Czechowicz, K., and Teppa-Szumowska, E. (1968). Autoradiographic studies with P^{32} of the muscular tissue in *T. spiralis* infected mice. *Wiad. Parazytol.* **14**, 145-154.

The Stichocyte of *Trichinella spiralis* during Morphogenesis in the Small Intestine of the Rat

Dickson D. Despommier

Division of Tropical Medicine
School of Public Health
College of Physicians and Surgeons
Columbia University
New York

Introduction

Acquired resistance against trichinellosis can be induced by infection of the host with the intestinal phase only (Campbell *et al.,* 1963; Denham, 1966), with the first 7–8 hr of exposure being sufficient to elicit protection (Denham, 1966).

Further, it is now well established that the stichocyte of the mature muscle larva contains antigens (Jackson, 1959; Brzosko *et al.,* 1965; Despommier and Müller, 1970) and that these are associated with two morphologically and antigenically distinct populations of secretory granules (α and β) which, in turn, stimulate the infected host to produce precipitating antibodies against them at some time during the course of the infection (Despommier and Müller, 1970).

This chapter describes our study undertaken to ascertain the temporal nature of the secretion of stichocyte granules by muscle and intestinal stages of *Trichinella spiralis,* and to correlate this pattern of secretion with earlier studies on the induction of protective resistance. It will be shown that all intestinal stages actively secrete granule product and that nearly all larval-derived secretory granules (α and β) are exhausted by 30–40 hr after oral infection, with over half the granules secreted by the 8th hr. It will further be demonstrated that the stichocyte undergoes extensive morphological changes during the worms' first 48 hr in the intestine, culminating in the synthesis of new granules which are then secreted by the mature adult.

239

Materials and Methods

Infection of Rats with *Trichinella spiralis*

Muscle larvae were obtained from stock-infected mice by digestion in a solution of 1% pepsin (Sigma Chem., St. Louis, Missouri) and 1% HCl (Fisher Scientific, New York) for 1 hr at 37° C. Known numbers of larvae were then administered orally to anesthetized 200 gm male Wistar rats via an 18° gauge blunted needle and a 1-ml tuberculin syringe.

Collection of Intestinal Stages of *Trichinella spiralis*

All intestinal stages of *T. spiralis* were collected using a circular thermal migration device (Despommier, 1973) based upon concepts developed by McCue and Thorson (1964).

At varying times after oral infection, rats were killed with ether; then the first half of the small intestine was removed and split open. The gut was then placed in the apparatus and all worms migrated to the center within 25 min. Worms were then carefully pipetted into a test tube, gently washed three times in 0.85% NaCl, and fixed for electron microscopy.

Electron Microscopy

All worms were fixed for 1–2 hr in a mixture of 4% gluteraldehyde–2.5% paraformaldehyde in 0.1 M collidine buffer (pH 7.2). All procedures were carried out at room temperature. Worms were then washed for the same length of time in 0.25 M collidine buffer before being postfixed for 1 hr in potassium dichromate-buffered (pH 7.2) 1% osmium tetroxide.

Following postfixation, worms were dehydrated for 10 min each in a graded series of increasing concentrations of ethanol. Final dehydration in propylene oxide was followed by leaving the worms in a 3:1 mixture of propylene oxide and Durcopan (Fluka AG Chemische Fabrik, Buchs, Switzerland) or Epon-812 (Fisher Scientific, New York) for 1 hr, a 1:1 mixture for 1 hr, and then overnight in a 1:3 mixture. The propylene oxide was allowed to vaporize from the samples for 24 hr beginning on the following day.

The worms were then placed in freshly mixed Durcopan or Epon-812 for 3 hr and embedded. Embedding was carried out as follows. Worms in fresh embedding medium were placed into a 50-ml screw cap centrifuge tube and sedimented at 15,000 rpm for 15 minutes at 20° C. The excess embedding medium was discarded and the pellet of worms was removed with a glass stirring rod and placed in a beam capsule. More embedding mixture was poured on top of the pellet of worms and the top of the beam capsule was then closed. The beam capsule was placed into a specially constructed wooden adaptor fitted to a 50-ml plastic centrifuge tube and sedimented again at 15,000 rpm for 15 min at 20° C. This procedure resulted in a tightly packed pellet of worms in the bottom of the beam capsule.

After teasing the pellet to the center of the capsule with a small dissection needle, the capsule was placed in the curing oven for 3 days at 60° C.

Silver-gray sections were obtained on the embedded samples using a diamond knife (I. E. DuPont de Nemours and Co., Inc., Wilmington, Delaware).

After the sections of worm were stained with lead citrate (Reynolds, 1963) and uranyl acetate (Watson, 1958), they were observed with the aid of a Philips-300 electron microscope operating at 80 kV. Observations were made on many individual worms in each group on both thick- and thin-sectioned material. The figures presented in the text represent the situation most commonly observed in any given group of worms.

Single, mature female worms were also flat embedded, sectioned, and studied, but observations on many worms of a given time point showed that there were no morphological differences of the stichocytes between these and male worms.

Results

Forty-five rats were each orally infected with 8000 muscle larvae. Worms were collected from each of five rats at each of the following time points after infection: 0, 8, 20, and 34 hr, and 2–6, 8, and 10 days.

Muscle larvae, 17 and 35 days old, respectively, were fixed and sectioned *in situ,* and the later served as the zero time point. It is to this time point that all changes occurring in the stichocyte are compared after oral infection has begun.

A 17-day-old muscle larve, *in situ,* is shown in Fig. 1. The stichocyte fills the entire center portion of the larva and contains secretory granules of the α variety. In addition, large amounts of glycogen are present (Beckett and Boothroyd, 1961).

The prominent nucleus is centrally located and possesses a distinct large nucleolus. Secretion product fills the lumen of the esophagus. The cell is engaged in granulogenesis at this time.

A characteristic feature of the stichocyte is the canaliculi, located adjacent to the esophagus (Fig. 3). A duct (Figs. 2, inset, and 4) connects these vesicular structures to the esophageal lumen. Each cell apparently has only one duct (Richels, 1955). It is through this system of canaliculi that the secretory granule contents exits from the cell, through the duct, and into the esophagus, eventually leaving the worm via the oral route. A stichocyte from a 35-day-old muscle larva, *in situ,* containing β granules is shown in Fig. 2.

The cytoplasm is now completely filled with secretory granules and the esophageal lumen is empty. The stichocyte at this stage has well-defined rough endoplasmic reticulum (RER) and many mitochondria, suggestive of

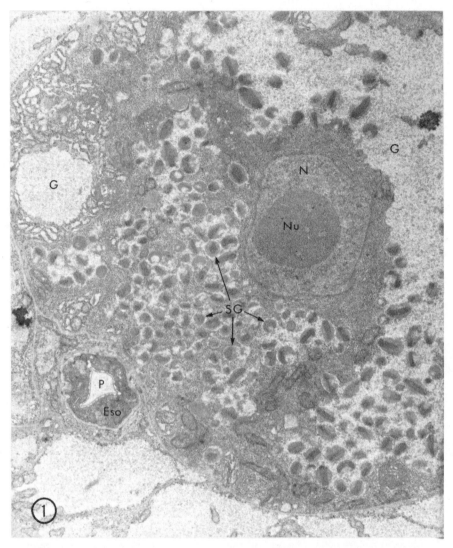

Figure 1 Cross section of a stichocyte of a 17-day-old muscle larva *in situ.*
The cytoplasm of the stichocyte is filled with glycogen (G) and α secretory
granules (SG). The nucleus (N) contains a prominent nucleolus (Nu). Canaliculi are not seen in this view. The esophageal lumen is filled with secretory
granule contents (P). The cell at this stage is still in an active state of granulogenesis. Eso, Esophagus. × 2800.

a high degree of protein synthetic capability, although no further granule
synthesis activity was observed.

The stichocyte of a worm which has been in the small intestine for 8 hr
is seen in Fig. 4. Several major morphological differences are evident between the stichocyte of the 35-day-old muscle larva, *in situ,* and the stich-

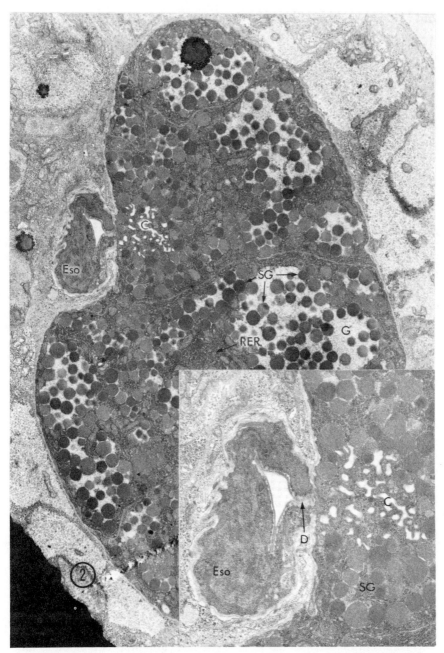

Figure 2 A stichocyte containing only β secretory granules (SG) is seen in this oblique section of a 35-day-old mature muscle larva *in situ.* Canaliculi (C) are seen adjacent to the esophagus (Eso). The esophageal region (enlarged in the inset) shows a part of the duct (D) which connects the canaliculi with the lumen of the esophagus. Masses of glycogen (G) are also present. Rough endoplasmic reticulum (RER) is despersed throughout the cell. × 2900.

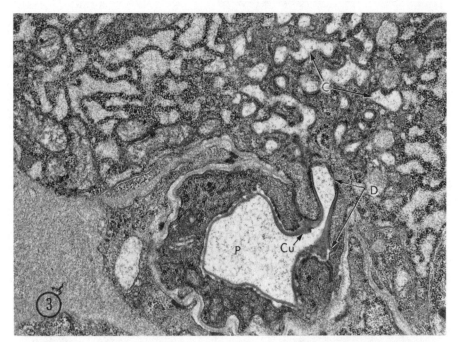

Figure 3 The duct (D) of a stichocyte of a 17-day-old muscle larva *in situ* is seen in cross section. The canaliculi (C) and the esophageal lumen are filled with secretory granule contents (P.). A dense cuticle (Cu) lines the esophagus and duct, terminating at a canalicular vesicle. × 6300.

ocyte of the 8-hr-old larva. A large portion of the secretory granules have, by 8 hr, been utilized by the developing worm. This is evidenced, in general, by the collapsed appearance of the cell, fewer granules in the cytoplasm, and the presence of much granule contents in the canaliculi and gut lumen.

Further, the granules appear to be grouped around the periphery of the cell and particularly high concentrations are observed around the canaliculi, again giving the overall impression that a high degree of secretory activity is occurring at this time. Although only the β granules are shown in Fig. 4, both varieties of granules are being simultaneously secreted (Fig. 5a and b).

There is little glycogen left in the cytoplasm at 8 hr as compared to the mature muscle larva. The cytoplasm appears to be filling in the space vacated by the glycogen and secretory granules with RER and mitochondria. Secretory granules are seen in the lower half of the cell at 20 hr (Fig. 6). The majority of granules have now been secreted by the developing worm. The glycogen reserves of the *in situ* larva have apparently been completely utilized. The cytoplasm has expanded and filled in the cell periphery with RER and mitrochondria. The cisternae of the RER are highly distended and filled with product.

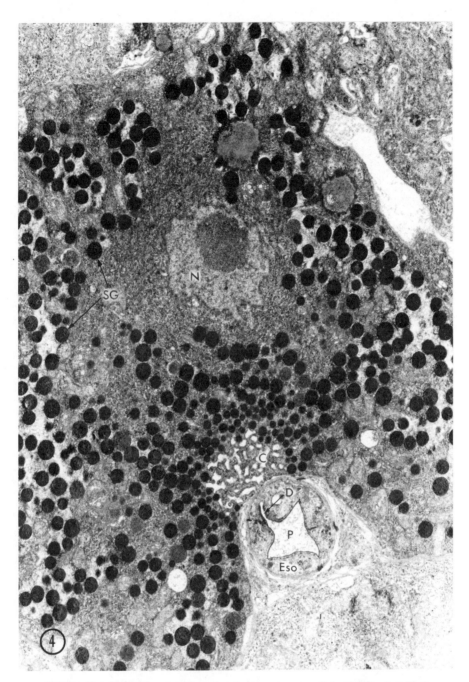

Figure 4 A stichocyte of a developing worm after 8 hr of infection in the small intestine. Note the overall collapsed appearance of the cell and nucleus (N). The β secretory granules (SG) are mostly in the cell periphery and give the impression of "streaming" toward the canaliculi (C). The cytoplasm surrounding the nucleus consists mostly of rough endoplasmic reticulum. Two large inclusions are seen in the upper portion of the cell. D, duct; P, granule contents; Eso, esophagus. × 2900.

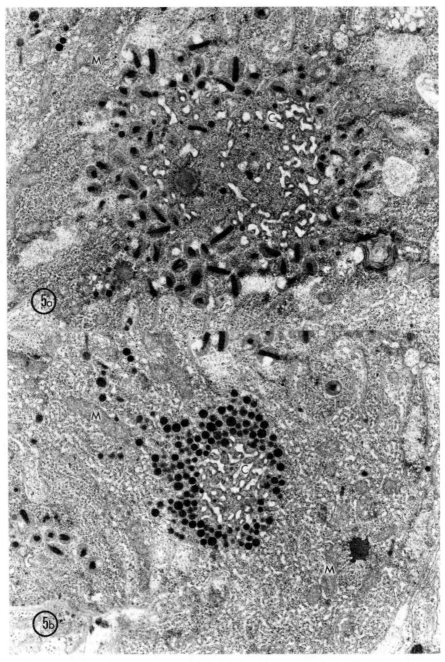

Figure 5 Evidence for simultaneous secretion of α (5a) and β (5b) granules is seen in this longitudinal section of two adjacent stichocytes in a single larva at 8 hr after infection. C, Canaliculi; M, mitochondria. $\times$ 9800.

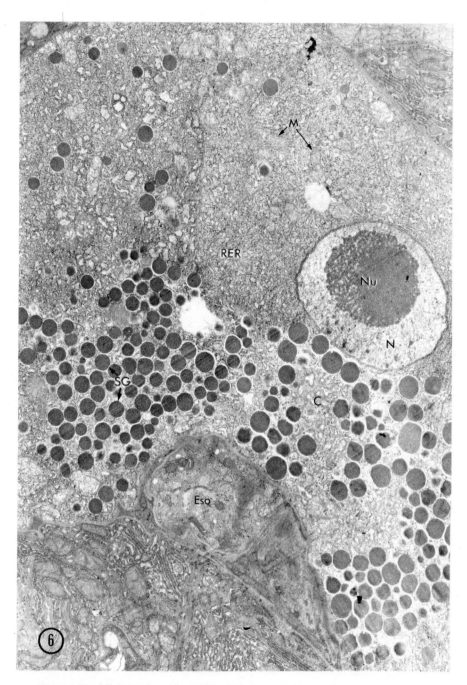

Figure 6 The stichocyte at 20 hr after oral infection contains some β secretory granules (SG) which are mostly localized in the lower half of the cell. The nucleus (N) is still prominent and centrally located. Rough endoplasmic reticulum (RER) with distended cisternae and numerous mitochondria (M) are now the predominant features of the cytoplasm. No visible glycogen deposits are present. Eso, Esophagus; C, canaliculi; Nu, nucleolus. × 3500.

A stichocyte from a 34-hr-old worm is shown in Fig. 7. A large cluster of granules is present in the lower half of the cell. However, more granules are now located in the peripheral region of the cell than at 20 hr. The cytoplasm gives the typical appearance of a functioning secretory cell, with one notable exception. No typical Golgi membranes were observed in any portion of the cytoplasm.

These morphological features indicate that all the granules seen at 34 hr in the cell periphery may not be larval-derived, but may actually represent *de novo* synthesis of secretory granules. More evidence for this view is seen in the fully mature adult stichocyte.

From the second until the ninth day after infection, all adult stichocytes closely resemble the one from a 3-day-old adult female worm shown in Fig. 8. By 3 days the transformation from larval to adult stichocyte is complete. The cytoplasm contains secretory granules and their contents can be observed in the canaliculi, duct, and esophageal lumen (Fig. 9).

Occasionally, the adult-derived granules appear irregular in shape, as seen in the canalicular region. However, most stichocytes of the adult contained spherically shaped granules as seen in the upper right portion of Fig. 10.

Discussion

The outward effects of host resistance against challenge infections of *Trichinella spiralis* are by now well characterized and include (1) reduced numbers of muscle larvae (McCoy, 1931) (2) reduced numbers of adults (McCoy, 1931), and (3) stunting of adult females (Larsh *et al.,* 1956; Despommier and Wostmann, 1969).

It was demonstrated in the present studies that both the muscle and intestinal stages of *Trichinella spiralis* secrete products derived from granules in the stichocyte. These observations were similar to those of Bruce (1972 personal communication). In the case of the muscle larva, these granules are of two major kinds, α and β, the products of which are antigenic during the natural course of infection (Despommier and Müller, 1970). The adult cell possesses no recognizable α granules, but does synthesize a granule morphologically similar to the larval β granule.

Since protective resistance can be induced by both short and long term exposure of the host to the intestinal stages, it was necessary, in the present work, to collect and study intestinal stages which correlated in age to the exposure times used by earlier investigators in studying this resistance.

In studies employing short-term host infections, Denham (1966) showed that as little as 8 hr of exposure was necessary to induce protection. Because only larval-derived secretory granule products are being exported during the early gut phase it is probable that antigens derived from the α and/or β granules are responsible for the observed protection.

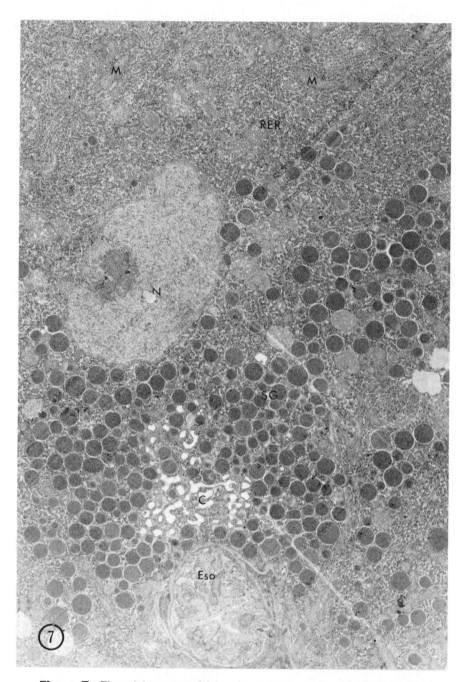

Figure 7 The stichocyte at 34 hr after infection has changed little from 20 hr. Again, most of the secretory granules (SG) are localized to the lower half of the cell cytoplasm. The cisternae of the rough endoplasmic reticulum (RER) are somewhat less distended than at 20 hr, but product is still evident in them. C, Canaliculi; N, nucleus; Eso, esophagus; M, mitochondria. ✕ 3500.

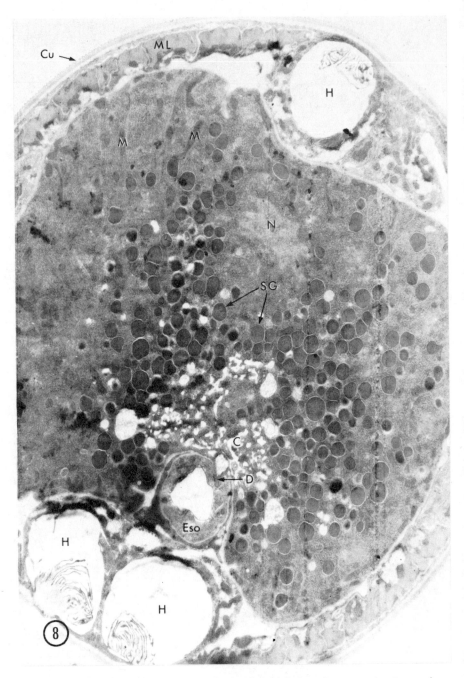

Figure 8 The stichocyte of a 3-day-old adult female worm is shown in cross section. The peripheral cytoplasm is characterized by inward-directed columns of rough endoplasmic reticulum with elongated mitochondria (M) interspersed between these regions. The secretory granules (SG) appear to originate somewhere near the cell periphery and migrate toward the canaliculi (C) in the lower half of the cell. N, Nucleus; D, duct; Eso, esophagus; ML, muscle layer; Cu, cuticle; H, hypodermal gland cell. × 3500.

250

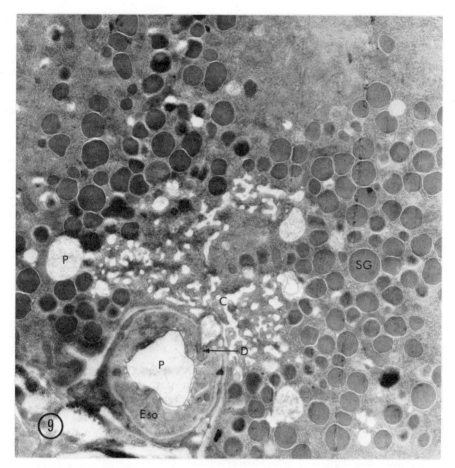

Figure 9 An enlarged view of the 3-day-old adult stichocyte shown in Fig. 8 is seen here at higher magnification. Granule contents (P) is seen in the canalicular vesicles (C), duct (D), and esophageal lumen. Eso, Esophagus, SG, Secretory granules. × 4300.

This hypothesis is supported by *in vitro* studies which showed that the secretions of the muscle larva induce a strong protection in mice (Campbell, 1955: Mills and Kent, 1965). Further, preliminary studies indicate that the β granule, isolated via cell fractionation techniques, is capable of eliciting a strong acquired resistance in mice. (Despommier and Müller, 1970).

Since one of the major effects of host immunity is to directly limit adult worm fecundity (Despommier and Wostmann, 1969; Denham and Martinez, 1970), host immune responses therefore would act to hinder larval development which later on would reflect in a decreased reproductive potential.

Immunity induced by long-term exposures (4 days or more) to the in-

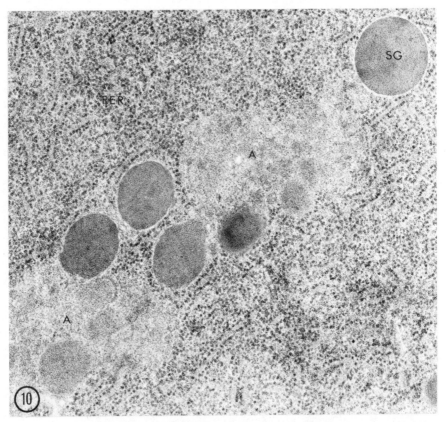

Figure 10 A typical area of peripheral cytoplasm is shown here at high magnification. Rough endoplasmic reticulum (RER), secretory granules (SG), and regions of amorphous material (A) predominate.

testinal stages of *T. spiralis* (Campbell 1965; Campbell *et al.,* 1963) must also be induced, at least, by larval-derived granule antigens if the above hypothesis is correct. However, because a new adult-derived secretory granule is present in the stichocyte after day 2 of infection, it is possible that products from these new granules may contribute substantially to the stimulation of protective resistance. Again, *in vitro* studies seem to support this conjecture, as it is known that injections of secretions collected from 3-day-old adults will result in acquired resistance (Chipman, 1957). From the two studies cited, however, the relative efficacy of immunization with larval and adult secretions cannot be compared, since no mention was made of the quantity of secreted protein necessary to induce the protection obtained in either case. However, in another study, Denham (1972, personal communication) has shown that equal amounts of adult and larval secretions protect equally well. The underlying biochemical and physiological changes induced by host immunity in the worm which must ultimately result in reduced fecundity, stunting, and early worm egression are still unknown. However, now that the temporal relationship between granulogenesis and secretion by the stichocyte is established, it will be possible to begin investigations into the nature of these secreted products and to discover the functions that the granule contents are serving for the developing worm and the adult. This approach should result in a detailed understanding of the effects of host immunity on the life cycle of *T. spiralis.*

Summary

Evidence for secretory granule utilization and synthesis was examined for at the ultrastructural level in mature muscle larvae, *in situ;* and in various stages of the intestinal infection.

Granulogenesis was occurring in the stichocyte of the larva at 17 days after infection. By 35 days of the infection, the stichocyte of the muscle larva had completely filled with secretory granules.

After 8 hr in the small intestine, over one-half of the α and β granules had been secreted by the developing worm. In addition, there was a marked reduction of glycogen in all tissues. The developing worm had secreted nearly all granules by 20–34 hr of infection.

The stichocyte of the mature adult worm (i.e. 2–9 days after infection) contained adult-derived secretory granules. Secretory granule content was observed in the canalicular vesicles, duct, and esophageal lumen at all stages of infection, except in the 35-day-old muscle larva.

The role of granule secretion and biogenesis in the induction of protective resistance is discussed.

Acknowledgments

I wish to express my appreciation to Miss Lorna Aron for her excellent technical assistance, and to Dr. James Jamieson and to Dr. Miklos Müller of the Rockefeller University for their helpful comments in the interpretation of observations made on granulogenesis.

This work was supported in part by grants 5-R01-AI-10627 and RR-05449, U.S. Public Health Service.

The author was a recipient of Career Development Award 1 K04-AI-70255-01 from the U.S. National Institutes of Health.

References

Beckett, E. B., and Boothroyd, B. (1961). Some observations on the mature larva of the nematode *Trichinella spiralis. Ann. Trop. Med. Parasitol.* **55,** 116–124.

Brzosko, W., Gancarz, Z., and Nowoslawski, A. (1965). Immunofluorescence in the serological diagnosis of *Trichinella spiralis* infection. *Med. Doswi. Mikrobiol.* **17,** 325–332.

Campbell, C. H. (1955). The antigenic role of the excretions and secretions of *trichinella spiralis* in the production of immunity in mice. *J. Parasitol,* **41,** 483–491.

Campbell, W. C. (1965). Immunizing effects of enteral and enteral-parenteral infections of *Trichinella spiralis* in mice. *J. Parasitol.* **51,** 185–194.

Campbell, W. C., Hartman, R. K., and Cuckler, A. C. (1963). Induction of immunity to trichinosis in mice by means of chemically abbreviated infections. *Exp. Parasitol.* **14,** 29–36.

Chipman, P. B. (1957). The antigenic role of the excretions and secretions of adult *Trichinella spiralis* in the production of immunity in mice. *J. Parasitol.* **43,** 593–598.

Denham, D. A. (1966). Immunity to *Trichinella spiralis.* I. The immunity produced by mice to the first four days of the intestinal phase of the infection. *J. Parasitol.* **56,** 323–327.

Denham, D. A., and Martinez, A. R. (1970). Studies with Methyridine and *Trichinella spiralis.* II. The use of the drug to study rate of larval production in mice. *J. Helminthol.* **44,** 357–363.

Despommier, D. D. (1973). A circular thermal migration device for the rapid collection of large numbers of intestinal helminths. *J. Parasitol.* **59,** 933–935.

Despommier, D. D., and Müller, M. (1970). The stichosome of *Trichinella spiralis:* its structure and function. *J. Parasitol.* **56,** (Sect. II, Part I. *2nd Int. Cong. Parasitol.),* 76–77.

Despommier, D. D., and Wostmann, B. S. (1969). *Trichinella spiralis:* Immune elimination in mice. *Exp. Parasitol.* **24,** 243–250.

Jackson, G. J. (1959). Fluorescent antibody studies of *Trichinella spiralis* infections. *J. Infec. Dis.* **105,** 97–117.

Larsh, J. E., Jr., Race, G. J., and Jefferies, W. B. (1956). The association in young mice of intestinal inflammation and the loss of adult worms following an initial infection with *Trichinella spiralis. J. Infec. Dis.* **99,** 63–71.

McCoy, O. R. (1931). Immunity of rats to reinfection with *Trichinella spiralis. Amer. J. Hyg.* **14,** 484–494.

McCue, J. F., and Thorson, R. E. (1964). Behavior of parasitic stages of helminths in a thermal gradient. *J. Parasitol.* **50,** 67–71.

Mills, C. K., and Kent, N. H. (1965). Excretions and secretions of *Trichinella spiralis* and their role in immunity. *Exp. Parasitol.* **16,** 300–310.

Reynolds, E. S. (1963). The use of lead citrate at high pH as an electronopaque stain in electron microscopy. *J. Cell Biol.* **17,** 208–212.

Richels, I. (1955). Histologische Studien zu den Problemen der Zellkonstanz: Untersuchungen zut mikroskopische Anatomie im Lebenszklus von *Trichinella spiralis. Zentralbl. Bakteriol. Parasitenk. Krankh. Hyg.* **163,** 46–84.

Watson, M. L. (1958). Staining of tissue sections for electron microscopy with heavy metals. *J. Biophys. Biochem. Cytol.* **4,** 475–478.

Immunocytoadherence Test for the Detection of Cellular Immune Response Against *Trichinella spiralis* Antigens

Wojciech S. Plonka

Department of Medical Parasitology
National Institute of Hygiene,
Warsaw

Introduction

An indirect immunocytoadherence (IICA) test described by Duffus and Allen (1969) and by Howard *et al.* (1969) for detection of lipopolysaccharide antigens of *Salmonella galinarum* and polysaccharide antigens of *Diplococcus pneumoniae,* respectively, was adopted to use in the study of soluble antigens of *Trichinella spiralis* larvae.

Materials and Methods

Animals and Immunization

Fifty female white mice 10–12 weeks of age were immunized intraperitoneally with 500 living *T. spiralis* larvae in 0.1 ml saline. Ten animals were used as nonimmunized controls.

Preparation of Antigen for Coating of SRBC

A 1% suspension of dried, powdered *T. spiralis* larvae in distilled water was frozen and thawed 10 times, and centrifuged. After dialysis for 24 hrs against distilled water, it was lyophilized and used as the antigen. Protein was determined by the Biuret method (Kabat and Meyer, 1961) with colorimetric readings at 540 nm. The protein content per milligram of the lyophilized material was 0.58 mg.

Sheep red blood cells (SRBC) were coated with 5 mg of lyophilized antigen per milliliter of washed and packed erythrocytes, according to the procedure of tanning and coating cells for the passive hemagglutination test of Stavitsky (1954). Freshly prepared tannic acid-treated and antigen-coated SRBC were suspended in Hanks' balanced salt solution to prepare the 1% suspension of erythrocytes.

Preparation of Spleen Cell Suspension

Spleen cells were obtained from mice at daily intervals for 10 days after immunization. Erythrocytes in the suspension were lysed by osmotic shock; the remaining cells were washed and suspended in Hanks' balanced salt solution to obtain a final concentration of 2×10^7 cells/ml.

Rosette Formation

A suspension of spleen cells (0.05 ml) was mixed with 1 ml of Hanks' balanced salt solution and 0.1 ml of the 1% suspension of coated SRBC and incubated in small test tubes which were shaken every 10 min. After 1 hr incubation at 37° C the cells were counted in a Burker chamber and the number of rosettes was calculated per 1000 nucleated spleen cells.

All the experiments were controlled by examining mixtures of spleen cells from immunized mice with uncoated erythrocytes and mixtures of spleen cells from nonimmunized mice both with coated and uncoated sheep erythrocytes. The values for all these control tests were the same as for unimmunized mice.

Rosette Inhibition

To demonstrate inhibition of rosette formation, 0.05 ml of spleen cell suspension, plus 1 ml of Hanks' balanced salt solution was preincubated for 60 min at 37° C with 5 mg/ml of lyophilized antigen. Following this, 0.1 ml of the 1% suspension of coated SRBC was added and the mixture was incubated for an additional 60 min at 37° C. Rosette formation was calculated as above.

Results

Rosette formation by spleen cells and the inhibition of rosette formation at various intervals after intraperitoneal injection of 500 *T. spiralis* larvae is presented in Table I.

The average rosette counts for 10 control mice was 0.38 rosette-forming cells (RFC)/1000 spleen cells. The mean number of rosettes rose above control level to 0.8 RFC/1000 spleen cells at 24 and 48 hr and to 1.6 RFC/1000 spleen cells 3 days following immunization. Rosette formation increased rapidly to reach a peak of 7.5 RFC/100 spleen cells on the fifth day after immunization. Thereafter, the number of rosettes decreased slowly to 2 RFC/1000 spleen cells on the tenth day. As can be seen from Table I, preincubation of the spleen cells with *T. spiralis* antigen inhibited the formation of rosettes.

Discussion

From the results presented here, it is apparent that RFC response of mouse spleen increased during the first 5 days after intraperitoneal injection of larvae and decreased during the next 5 days. Preincubation of spleen cells with the antigen inhibited formation of rosettes throughout the period of observation.

Simultaneously, studies of the antibody levels using the hemagglutination test (Plonka *et al.*, 1972) of the serum samples taken at the same time as the harvest of spleen cells showed no change in the titers as compared with control animals for the 10 days of observation. Consequently, it is concluded that RFC response in mice is a useful and valid cytoimmunological test for the study of the early period of *T. spiralis* infection when other immunological tests, e.g., hemagglutination, fail to detect an immune response. Such studies may provide a more detailed insight into the kinetics of antibody formation by lymphoid cells in this infection.

Summary

Sheep red blood cells (SRBC) sensitized with soluble *Trichinella spiralis* antigen were used as indicators for rosette-forming cells in mouse spleen after inoculation of living *Trichinella spiralis* larvae into the peritoneal cavity. After inoculation the number of rosette-forming cells rapidly rose to a peak on the fifth day. On incubation at $37°$ C a proportion of rosette-forming cells acquired several layers of adherent sensitized SRBC.

Table I Rosette-Forming Cells (RFC) Response in Mouse Spleen after Intraperitoneal Inoculation of 500 Living *T. spiralis* Larvae

Days after inoculation	Number of RFC/1000 spleen cells		Number of RFC/1000 spleen cells after pre-incubation with antigen	
	Mean	SD	Mean	SD
0	0.38	±0.09	0.43	±0.09
1	0.80	±0.19	0.31	±0.08
2	0.80	±0.27	0.28	±0.06
3	1.60	±0.38	0.47	±0.10
4	5.30	±1.13	0.32	±0.08
5	7.50	±1.79	0.38	±0.08
6	7.00	±1.31	0.44	±0.09
7	6.40	±1.22	0.30	±0.05
8	3.50	±0.83	0.31	±0.06
9	2.50	±0.54	0.40	±0.07
10	2.00	±0.39	0.33	±0.06

This suggested that such cells were actively producing antibodies against *Trichinella* antigen.

Acknowledgment

This work was supported in part by grant CDC-E-P2 from the Communicable Diseases Center, U.S. Public Health Service.

References

Duffus, W. P. H., and Allen, D. (1969). A study of the ontogeny of specific immune responsiveness amongst circulating leucocytes in the chicken. *Immunology* **16,** 337–347.

Howard, J. G., Elson, J., Christie, G. H., and Kinsky, R. G. (1969). Studies on immunological paralysis. II. The detection and significance of antibody-forming cells in the spleen during immunological paralysis with type III pneumococcal polysaccharide. *Clin. Exp. Immunol.* **4,** 41–53.

Kabat, E. A., and Meyer, M. (1961) "Experimental Immunochemistry," (2nd ed.). Thomas, Springfield, Illinois.

Plonka, W. S., Gancarz, Z., and Zawadzka-Jedrzejewska, B. (1972). A rapid screening hemagglutination test in the diagnosis of human trichinosis. *J. Immunol. Methods* **1,** 309–312.

Stavitsky, A. B. (1954). Micromethods for the study of proteins and antibodies. I. Procedure and general application of hemagglutination and hemagglutination-inhibition reactions with tannic acid and protein-treated red blood cells. *J. Immunol.* **72,** 360–367.

Leukocytes and *Trichinella spiralis*. I. *In Vivo* Adhesion of Peritoneal Exudate to Newborn Larvae, Infective Larvae, and Adults

Miroslaw Stankiewicz*

Veterinary Medical Research Institute
Iowa State University
Ames, Iowa

Introduction

Larsh *et al.* (1964a,b, 1966, 1969, 1970a,b) indicated that leukocytes are very important for expulsion of adult *Trichinella spiralis* from the mouse intestine. Others (Keller and Keist, 1972; Kelly and Dineen, 1972; Larsh, 1967) also considered white cells to be important factors in the host defense against parasitic nematodes. The direct effect of the host cells on the parasite is preceeded by the migration of the cells and in many cases by the adherence of the cells to the parasite. Despite numerous publications concerning adhesion of the cells to different parasites, little is known about the mechanisms of adherence. Several authors emphasize the role of previous contact of the host with the parasites and especially antibodies. Moreover, eosinophils were most often reported to be the adherent cell type. Although some reports indicated that cells will adhere to parasites in nonimmune animals, almost nothing is known about their ability to affect the parasites. *Trichinella spiralis* is a parasite which maintains intimate contact with the tissues and cells of the host during a major part of its life cycle. This would provide ample opportunity for various cells to adhere. In this report, results are presented which indicate that cell adherence can occur with various manifestations in the different stages of the life cycle of *T. spiralis*. In further publications of this series evidence for the direct effect of cells on the parasite and the mechanism of cell adherence will be discussed.

*Present address: Department of Parasitology, Zoological Institute, University of Warsaw.

Materials and Methods

Host Animals

Mice used in all experiments were ARS ICR albino males with a weight of 20–30 gm. Rats used were female, Sprague Dawley, 110–140 gm. Both mice and rats were parasite-free. Mainly noninfected animals were used for these experiments, and only several were immunized. Mice were given successive oral infections with 250, 400, and 600 *T. spiralis* infective larvae at 30-day intervals and 2 months later were tested for cell adherence. Rats received two infections (5000 and 7000) and were tested 1 month later.

Infective Larvae

The parasites were maintained in a colony of Sprague Dawley female rats which had been orally infected. Infective larvae were obtained after overnight digestion of infected tissue with constant agitation according to Zimmermann *et al.* (1961). After digestion, larvae were filtered through two layers of cheesecloth and washed several times in water. Then larvae were filtered through four layers of cheesecloth and washed three times in phosphate buffered saline (pH 7.2). Larvae were counted by dilution techniques and six samples of 1 cm^3 each were counted. The final volume of the larval suspension was adjusted so that 1000 larvae were in 1 cm^3 of solution.

Mice and rats were injected intraperitoneally with 1 and 5 cm^3 of larval suspension, respectively. At varying intervals following the injections, animals were killed with carbon dioxide, and 3 cm^3 of phosphate buffered saline (PBS) with 1% sodium citrate was injected into the peritoneal cavity of the mice and 10 cm^3 into the peritoneal cavity of the rats. The abdomens were palpated for 1 min and the peritoneal cavity was then opened by an incision along the linea alba. Fluid present therein was removed by Pasteur pipette into the tubes containing 10–15 cm^3 of cold PBS (ice bath). Care was taken not to disturb the interface between fluid from the peritoneal cavity and the PBS in the tubes. In that way larvae settled down very rapidly and were separated from nonadherent cells.

Adult *Trichinella spiralis*

Rats were orally inoculated with approximately 5000, 6000, or 7000 infective larvae. Rats were fasted on the fifth day postinfection and then were killed on the sixth day. The entire small intestine was removed, slit longitudinally, cut into 3-cm sections and placed in a modified Baermann apparatus containing 0.15 M saline solution at 37° C. After 1 hr of incubation at 37° C, adult *T. spiralis* were collected, washed in saline plus merthiolate, and PBS in a technique similar to that used for the infective larvae. Mice were inoculated intraperitoneally with 500–1000 parasites and rats with 3000–5000 worms. Parasites were recovered following the procedure used with infective larvae.

Differentiation of Cells Adhering to the Parasite

One-tenth percent or 0.01% of neutral red and 0.01% of crystal violet was used for that purpose. Usually one or two drops of stain were mixed with one drop of solution containing larvae and cells and this mixture was examined under the microscope at different intervals. Moreover, smears of larvae covered by cells were prepared and stained with methyl-green-pyronin and Wright's stains (Pearse, 1960). Cells were also examined with a phase contrast microscope.

Cell Adhesion with Newborn Larvae

Mice orally infected with 400 larvae and rats infected with 7000 larvae were killed at various intervals following infection. The peritoneal cavities of the mice were washed out with 3-5 cm³ and the rats with 15-20 cm³ of PBS with 1% sodium citrate. Fluids containing newborn larvae were centrifuged and the sediment was resuspended in a small amount of the supernatant. The supernatant was placed on slides and examined microscopically. Only small numbers of larvae were available from orally infected mice. Therefore, to be able to observe sufficient numbers of larvae, adult forms obtained from oral infection (6 days postinfection) were inoculated intraperitoneally into the mice and rats. Adults produced numerous larvae in these conditions.

Results

Cell Adherence to *T. spiralis* Infective Larvae

Noninfected Mice. After ½ hr the first cells attached to the larvae were observed. However, only a few parasites with single cells were seen at that time. Usually they were not flattened on the surface of the larvae. After 1 hr the number of larvae with attached cells increased considerably (Table I). The number of cells adhering to the larvae also increased (Fig.

Table I   Cell Adherence in Peritoneal Cavities of Mice to *T. spiralis* Infective Larvae

No. of cells per covered parasite	Percent of parasites covered[a]			
	1	2	3	4
More than 10	50	57	70	88
	(8–81)	(36–72)	(62–74)	(75–96)
Less than 10	25	17	14	8
	(5–61)	(3–34)	(9–22)	(0–20)
None	25	26	16	6
	(2–50)	(20–30)	(16–17)	(2–8)
Number of mice	10	10	10	10

[a] Data given at 1, 2, 3, and 4 hr after injection, are the average, with the range given in parentheses.

1). Some of the parasites became completely covered by cells. After 1 hr postinjection, additional layers of cells (attached to adherent cells) were created. However, many of the larvae remained uncovered. After 2, 3, and particularly 4 hr, the cell adherence reaction became increasingly intense. After 4 hr postinjection most of the larvae were covered by many layers involving hundreds of cells (Fig. 2). Some of the larvae were also trapped in large cell clusters at that time. All the larvae were apparently alive. However, larvae trapped in the cell clusters were prevented from normal motility. Increasing numbers of adherent cells resulted in increasingly sluggish movements of the parasites. Adhesion was very firm and convulsive movements of the larvae failed to dislodge the adherent cells. Cells were usually equally distributed on the surface of the *T. spiralis*. No specific places for adherence were observed.

Noninfected Rats. A similar but weaker cellular reaction was observed in rats (Table II). It was still visible 4 hr after inoculation. Usually later than in mice, cells adhering to the parasite became flattened. Smaller clusters with the trapped larvae were noticed. It was more clear than in the mice that some of the dead larvae or injured parasites were not covered by cells or were covered by significantly smaller numbers of cells.

Noninfected Rats and Dead Larvae. In order to determine whether living worms reacted more readily than did dead worms with cells, the larvae were killed by exposure to 50% ethyl alcohol or alternate freezing and thawing at $-70°C$ and room temperature. The treated larvae were compared with unaltered larvae (Table II). The experiment confirmed previous observations. The number of leukocytes attached to the larvae was smaller and considerably fewer larvae were covered by cells. In addition with the alcohol-treated larvae, more of the cells were found on the concave surface of the slightly covered larvae than on the convex side.

Infected Rats. Rats infected for 1 or 3 months with 7000 larvae were used in these experiments. A comparison of the results obtained from infected and noninfected animals showed that the reaction in infected animals was stronger and faster (Table II). Adhesion of cells to the natural openings was seen more often than in nonimmune animals.

Cell Adherence to *T. spiralis* Adult Worms

Noninfected Mice. After 1 hr in the peritoneal cavity of mice, no cell adherence to the adult *T. spiralis* was observed. After 2 hr, only solitary cells on individual parasites were noticed. Even after 3 hr, less than 0.5% of the parasites had shown cells on their surface. Moreover, those cells apparently did not adhere very firmly because motile parasites were able to free themselves from the cells. Only 3–15% of the parasites were covered

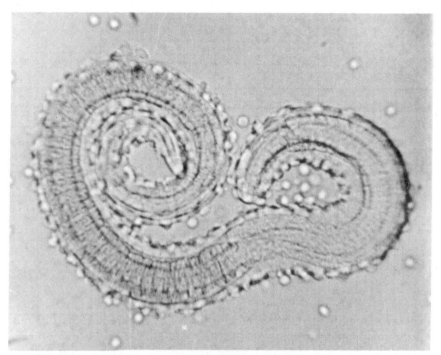

Figure 1 Cell adherence to *Trichinella spiralis* infective larva 1 hr after injection into the peritoneal cavity of nonimmunized mouse.

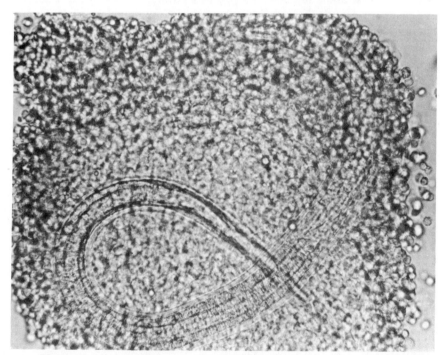

Figure 2 Cell adherence to *Trichinella spiralis* infective larva 4 hr after injection into the peritoneal cavity of nonimmunized mouse.

263

Table II Cell Adherence in the Peritoneal Cavities of Rats to *T. spiralis* Infective Larvae

No. of cells per covered parasite	Percent of parasites covered at different hours after injection[a]					
	1	1 [b]	2	3	4	4 [c]
More than 10	4	64	.8	47	63	30
	(0–14)	(25–92)	(2–18)	(26–61)	(51–86)	(9–47)
Less than 10	12	21	14	12	11	11
	(2–22)	(7–37)	(9–13)	(3–25)	(6–18)	(7–14)
None	84	15	78	41	26	58
	(73–97)	(0–43)	(66–88)	(30–56)	(8–38)	(43–65)
Number of rats	10	14	12	8	12	12

[a] Data are given as average with range given in parentheses.
[b] Rats infected for 1 or 3 months with 7000 *T. spiralis*.
[c] Dead larvae.

by more than 10 cells 4 hr after injection. The adherence was still not great after 6 hr of incubation (12–33%). Only a few adults were entirely covered at that time. It is interesting to note that in many cases certain areas of the adult *T. spiralis* were more readily attacked by cells than others (Fig. 3). These areas included the regions around the mouth, the anus, and just proximal to the ovary. Cells were also found relatively often in different regions of the stichosome. Results described in this experiment were based upon investigation of 40 mice.

Immunized Mice. In contrast to noninfected animals, about 9% of the recovered adults from six investigated animals had shown cell adherence 2 hr after inoculation but only 0.5% were entirely covered.

Association of Cell Adhesion with Time of Development of the Parasite. The aim of this experiment was to determine when in the development of infective larvae in the rat intestine did the changes take place which resulted in different cell adherence reactions after inoculation into the peritoneal cavities of mice. Rats were orally infected with 6000 infective larvae. Twelve hr, 1, 2, 3, 4, and 6 days after infection parasites were removed from the intestine and injected into the peritoneal cavity of noninfected mice. Parasites were removed from the peritoneal cavity of the mouse 3 hr after injection. Results are presented in Table III. Slight decreases in intensity of adherence occurred with parasites obtained 12 hr after infection but the cells could still adhere to the whole surface of the parasites. A tremendous decrease in intensity of adherence was seen 48 hr later (after infection). Primarily the mouth area of the parasite was covered by cells at that time (Fig. 4).

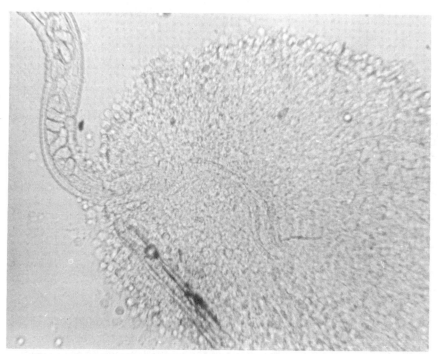

Figure 3 Cell adherence to anterior part of *Trichinella spiralis* 6-day-old female, 4 hr after injection into the peritoneal cavity of nonimmunized mouse.

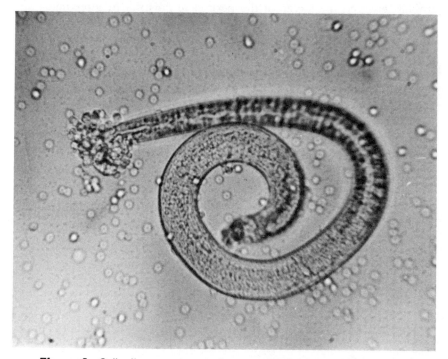

Figure 4 Cell adherence to anterior part of *Trichinella spiralis* 48-hour-old male, 3 hr after injection into the peritoneal cavity of nonimmunized mouse.

Table III   Mouse Peritoneal Cell Adherences to *T. spiralis* after Various Intervals of Development in the Rat Intestine

No. of cells per covered parasite	Percent of parasites covered at different times (in hours) of development[a]						
	Infective stage	12	24	48	72	96	144
More than 10	59	48	18	6	1	0.2	0
	(47–65)	(25–74)	(6–32)	(1–14)	(0–3)	(0–1)	0
Less than 10	18	19	8	6	1.5	0.4	0.2
	(12–21)	(6–28)	(3–12)	(2–10)	(0–7)	(0–2)	(0–1)
None	23	33	74	88	97.5	99.4	99.8
	(20–27)	(20–47)	(66–88)	(86–97)	(98–100)	(97–100)	(99–100)
Number of rats	6	6	6	6	6	6	6

[a] Data given as average with range given in parentheses.

Cell Types Adhering to *T. spiralis* Infective Larvae

Rats.   In noninfected rats 4 hr after injection, almost exclusively neutrophils were attached to the larvae. Only a few eosinophils, basophils, and mononuclear cells were seen. None of the monoclear cells were pyroninophilic. Two hr after injection, neutrophils were predominant but not to the same extent as 4 hr after. Also in immunized rats, primarily neutrophils covered the larvae in the peritoneal cavity 4 hr after injection. However, more eosinophils and mononuclear cells were observed at this time. It is interesting that more mast cells were attached to the larvae 2 hr after injection than 4 hr after injection. Many of them were flattened on the larvae and some were degranulated or degranulating. In some cases mast cells were not seen on the larvae but granules with the shape and staining characteristics of mast cells were seen. It is difficult to decide if mast cells degranulated as a result of contact with the parasite because some of the mast cells were also degranulating spontaneously. Only a few mononuclears were visible with the very vague pyroninophilic cytoplasm in adhering to the parasite in immune animals.

Mice.   Both 2 and 4 hr after injection, larvae were covered by mononuclears and neutrophils. Few eosinophils and basophils were noticed. In noninfected animals, no pyroninophilic cells were visibly sticking to the parasites. In immunized animals however, many of the pyroninophils surrounded the parasite. More basophils and eosinophils were seen in immunized animals than in nonimmune animals.

Cell Adherence to *T. spiralis* Newborn Larvae

Cell adherence also occurred on the surface of the newborn larvae (Fig. 5), whether these were introduced into the peritoneal cavity by nor-

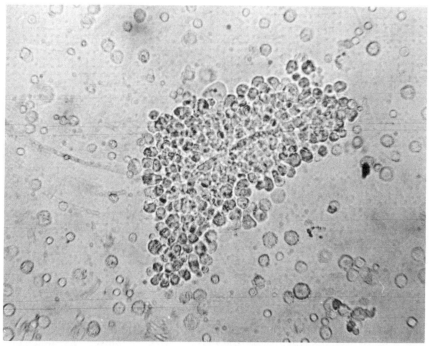

Figure 5   Cell adherence to *Trichinella spiralis* newborn larva in the peritoneal cavity of nonimmunized mouse.

mal infection (Tables IV and V) or by injection of adult forms (Table VI). However, in contrast to the very intense reaction that was seen with infected larvae, only a few newborn larvae were seen with the cells on their surfaces shortly after infection or injection. As it was shown in Table VI (where more larvae than from normal infection were investigated) much more extensive cell adherence occurred 6 and 8 days after injection. The

Table IV   Cell Adherence to Larvae Migrating through Peritoneal Cavities of Normal Mice after Oral Infection with 400 *T. spiralis* Infective Larvae

Days after infection	No. of larvae counted	No. of larvae with adherence	No. of clusters which may contain larvae	No. of mice
7	48	6	5	3
9	253	6	12	6
10	163	6	8	3
11	521	17	38	6
12	119	8	25	2
13	78	0	37	6
14	74	2	65	2

Table V Cell Adherence to Larvae Migrating through the Peritoneal Cavities of Normal Rats after Oral Infection with 6000 or 7000 *T. spiralis* Infective Larvae

Days after infection	No. of larvae counted	No. of larvae with adherence	No. of clusters which may contain larvae	No. of rats
7	112	3	–	5
9	761	10	–	5
11	929	43	21	8
13	226	23	40	7
14	140	4	20	1

same phenomenon was observed with 26 rats injected with *T. spiralis* adults, although the larvae produced by these adults were not counted. Cells adhered to the whole surface of the larvae and natural openings or they attacked the larvae from a certain distance by pseudopodia. It was observed that even a few cells could considerably decrease the mobility of a newborn larva. It seems that partially immobilized larvae are more readily attacked by increasing numbers of cells so that eventually a large cluster is created. Very often clusters of cells were so large that the larvae were completely covered. Movement was the sole indication that a larva was present inside. Larvae covered by many cells died and only the shape of the cluster indicated that adherence had taken place. After many observations, it was possible to recognize them from other clusters of cells that did not contain larvae. There is however, the possibility of making errors in evaluation. Therefore, this type of adherence was separated in an additional column (Tables IV–VI). Newborn larvae seem to be completely and rapidly destroyed by cells. Fragments or ghosts of larvae were often all that could be observed.

In order to check how many larvae from experimentally injected adults could reach muscle tissue, five mice were injected with 1000 and four rats with 5000 *T. spiralis* adults. Each was killed 40 days later and the

Table VI Cell Adherence to Newborn Larvae after injection of 500 Adult *T. spiralis* into Peritoneal Cavity of Normal Mice

Days after injection	No. of larvae counted	No. of larvae with adherence	No. of clusters which may contain larvae	No. of mice
2	1562	12	20	5
3	752	4	44	2
4	2676	8	32	5
5	1520	7	110	2
6	4248	44	650	6
8	828[a]	190	1349	7[a]

[a] All larvae counted.

whole carcass was digested. Only 283 larvae per mouse and 6930 larvae per rat were found.

Discussion

The results presented here strongly suggest that in nonimmunized rats and mice, cell adherence to various stages of *T. spiralis* may take place. Both pyroninophilic and nonpyroninophilic mononuclear cells were seen to adhere to the infective larvae. Eosinophils in immune and nonimmune animals also were adherent, but these did not appear to be selectively attracted to the parasites. The population of cells covering the parasite is a function of the host. In the rat, the majority of the cells consisted of neutrophils. In mice however, both neutrophils and mononuclear cells were found. In this respect, present results are different from those obtained by Lancastre and Bazin (1967), indicating that *Trichinella spiralis* larvae were covered only by polymorphonuclear cells in the peritoneal cavity of mice. These data support observations of Jackson and Bradbury (1970) who found mononuclear and polymorphonuclear leukocytes on the third stage of *Neoaplectana glaseri* in the peritoneal cavity of rats. According to Jeska (1969), only mononuclears adhere to the larvae of *Haemonchus contortus, Ascaris suum,* and *Turbatrix aceti.* From the available literature, only Jeska (1969), Jackson and Bradbury (1970), and Lancastre and Bazin (1967) used nonimmune animals in their experiments and found adherent leukocytes on the parasites. Jackson and Bradbury reported cells on *Neoaplectana glaseri* in rats 1 day after injection, Lancastre and Bazin, 12 hrs after injection of *T. spiralis,* and Jeska in mice after 4 hr. Reaction of cells as it can be concluded from present data can be even faster. After 1 hr cells were observed on the infective stage larvae. *In vitro* investigations (unpublished data) reveal that peritoneal exudate cells from noninfected animals can adhere to *T. spiralis* in 5–10 min.

Of the granulocytes, mainly eosinophils had been reported *in vitro* or *in vivo* adhering to different parasites (Soulsby, 1961, 1962, 1963; Fros and Liqui Lung, 1953; Bang *et al.,* 1962; Reddy *et al.,* 1969; Higashi and Chowdhury, 1970). Adhesion of polymorphonuclear cells to antibody-sensitized third or second stage larvae of *Ascaris suum* has been reported by Morseth and Soulsby (1969). It seems that mast cells are also able to adhere to the parasite. However, relatively few of these cells were observed on the larvae injected into the peritoneal cavities of animals. This was observed more frequently however, in rats which were previously infected. More cells were seen 2 hr after infection than 4 hr. Cellular fragility and inclination to degranulation, which were also observed, were probably the reasons that mast cells were not observed on the surfaces of the parasite. Our knowledge concerning the mechanism of adhesion of cells is very limited. Results obtained from infected animals could suggest that perhaps antibodies are associated with cell adherence. However, cell adherence reaction in noninfected mice and rats indicate other mechanisms which may also influence adherence of cells. Because the investigation of the mechanisms of cell adherence was not the major purpose of this study, the full discussion and data from *in vitro* tests on the roll of cells alone, with heat-labile and heat-stable substances in cell adherence, will be published separately.

Besides the above-mentioned factors, a very important role in cell adherence reactions is played by the parasite. As indicated by Crandall (1965), antigen obtained from *T. spiralis* is chemotactic for polymorphonuclear cells in the presence of serum. In the present study, considerable variations in cell adherence were observed with different stages in the life cycle of *T. spiralis*. The developmental stage most readily covered by cells is the infective stage and the equal distribution of cells indicates that the whole surface of this stage is very active.

Much weaker adhesion was observed with adult forms than with infective larvae when studied by experiments lasting equal lengths of time. In addition, certain areas of the adult were covered earlier and with more cells than others. It is intriguing that those areas correspond to the regions of adult *T. spiralis* which reacted positively with the fluorescent antibody technique observed by Catty (1969). Many factors may be responsible for the weakened adherence with the adult forms. First, the surface of the adult forms may not be as biologically active as that of the larvae. Second, adults may excrete some substances acting as suppressive or cytotoxic agents. The existence of host antigens in adult *Trichinella* is less probable because adult forms were transferred from rats to mice, unless these antigens are common to both. From Denham's work (1966), it is known that the adult *Trichinella* is immunogenic. An explanation of why the adult is not attacked by cells as readily as is the infective stage may also help to explain parasite survival in a host with a well-developed immune system. The two phenomena (first, the apparently less reactivity of adults with cells and, second, the slower and lesser cellular reaction of rats as compared to mice when exposed to *T. spiralis* rat strain) are considered to be significant and more detailed investigations of both are underway.

The least cell adherence was observed with the newborn larvae immediately after infection or injection. The exceptionally weak reaction of this stage could be explained by the apparently very poor immunogenicity of newborn larvae. Despommier (1971) did not obtain any resistance when mice were immunized with killed newborn larvae. Lancastre and Bazin (1967) and Lancastre *et al.* (1970) did not observe cells adhering to the young larvae and suggested that the larvae are not antigenic as long as they don't have reproductive systems. The development of reproductive organs does not seem to be a necessary structure for immunogenicity and/or reactivity with cells. Adult forms have a mature reproductive system but they are not as well covered by cells when compared to larvae. Adhesion to the newborn larvae is apparently connected with certain developments of this stage. In fact, adherence became more pronounced when larvae were placed in the peritoneal cavity for 6 to 8 days. Many of them could probably be destroyed by cells and therefore only a few of these larvae will reach the muscles. The results of our studies support a previous report (Dennis *et al.*, 1970) of low infectivity (2–9%) of newborn larvae when injected into the peritoneal cavity of rats. No morphological changes of infective larvae or adults were observed in present studies. The possibility of complete destruction of parasites by cells from normal nonimmune mice are presented in the next chapter.

Summary

It was found that in normal nonimmune mice and rats, cell adherence reactions took place with infective larvae, adult forms and newborn larvae. The most rapid and extensive cell adherence occurred with the infective larvae, and cells were usually equally distributed on the surface. Weaker adherence was observed with adult forms and certain areas were covered faster and with more cells than others. The weakest reaction occurred with the newborn larvae. It was also observed that newborn larvae could be killed by the adherent cells. No visible morphological changes were seen in the adult or infective stage larvae after 4–6 hr exposure to cells, although parasites trapped in big clusters of cells were immobilized. Cell adherence occurred faster in previously infected or immunized rats and mice. Dead infective larvae were covered by smaller numbers of cells than were living larvae.

Acknowledgments

I would like to thank Dr. E. L. Jeska for his suggestions, advice, and for providing research facilities. To W. J. Hubbard and M. E. Alls for aid in preparation of this manuscript, and to K. Smith for his technical assistance, and Dr. W. J. Zimmermann for providing *Trichinella*.
This investigation received financial support from the World Health Organization.

References

Bang, F. B., Saha, T. K., and Bandyopadhaya, A. K. (1962). Reactions of eosinophils with helminthic larvae in tropical eosinophilia. *Bull. Calcutta Sch. Trop. Med.* **10**, 152–153.

Catty, D. (1969). The immunology of nematode infectious trichinosis in guinea pigs as a model. *Monogr. Allergy* **5**, 101.

Crandall, R. B. (1965) Chemotactic response of polymorphonuclear leukocytes to *Trichinella spiralis* and *Ascaris suum* extracts. *J. Parasitol.* **51**, 397–404.

Denham, D. A. (1966). Immunity to *Trichinella spiralis*. II. Immunity produced by the adult worm in mice. *Parasitology* **56**, 745–751.

Dennis, D. T., Despommier, D. D., and Davis, N. (1970). Infectivity of the newborn larva of *Trichinella spiralis* in the rat. *J. Parasitol.* **56**, 974–977.

Despommier, D. D. (1971). Immunogenicity of the newborn larva of *Trichinella spiralis. J. Parasitol.* **57**, 531–534.

Fros, J., and Liqui Lung, M. A. V. (1953). Sheathless *Microfilaria bancrofti* and eosinophilic granulocytes. *Doc. Med. Geogr. Trop.* **5**, 116–118.

Higashi, G. I., and Chowdhury, A. B. (1970). *In vitro* adhesion of eosinophils to infective larvae of *Wuchereria bancrofti. Immunology* **19**, 65-83.

Jackson, G. J., and Bradbury, P. C. (1970). Cuticular fine structure and molting of *Neoaplectana glaseri* (Nematoda) after prolonged contact with rat peritoneal exudate. *J. Parasitol.* **56**, 108–115.

Jeska, E. L. (1969). Mouse peritoneal exudate cell reactions to parasitic worms. I. Cell adhesion reactions. *Immunology* **16**, 761–771.

Keller, R. and Keist, R. (1972). Protective immunity to *Nippostrongylus brasiliensis* in the rat. Central role of lymphocytes in worm expulsion. *Immunology* **22**, 767–773.

Kelly, J. D. and Dineen, J. K. (1972). The cellular transfer of immunity to *Nippostrongylus brasiliensis* in inbred rats (Lewis strain). *Immunology* **22**, 199–210.

Lancastre, F. A., and Bazin, J. (1967). Trichinose experimentale. Survive et reproduction des différents stades de *Trichinella spiralis* dans la cavité péritoneale de la souris. *Ann. Parasitol. Paris* **42**, 525–532.

Lancastre, F., Bazin, J., and Mougeot, G. (1970). Comportement de *Trichinella spiralis* la cavité péritoneale de la souris. *J. Parasitol.* **56**, 438.

Larsh, J. E. (1967). Delayed (cellular) hypersensitivity in parasitic infections. *Amer. J. Trop. Med. Hyg.* **16**, 735–745.

Larsh, J. E., Jr., Goulson, H. T., and Weatherly, N. F. (1964a). Studies on delayed (cellular) hypersensitivity in mice infected with *Trichinella spiralis*. I. Transfer of lymph node cells. *J. Elisha Mitchell Sci. Soc.* **80**, 133–135.

Larsh, J. E., Jr., Goulson, H. T., and Weatherly, N. F. (1964b). Studies on delayed (cellular) hypersensitivity in mice infected with *Trichinella spiralis*. II. Transfer of peritoneal exudate cells. *J. Parasitol.* **50**, 496–498.

Larsh, J. E., Jr., Race, G. J., Goulson, H. T., and Weatherly, N. F. (1966). Studies on delayed (cellular) hypersensitivity in mice infected with *Trichinella spiralis*. III. Serologic and histopathologic findings in recipients given peritoneal exudate cells. *J. Parasitol.* **52**, 146–150.

Larsh, J. E., Jr., Goulson, H. T., Weatherly, N. F., and Chaffee, E. F. (1969). Studies on delayed (cellular) hypersensitivity in mice infected with *Trichinella spiralis*. IV. Artificial sensitization of donors. *J. Parasitol.* **55**, 726–729.

Larsh, J. E., Jr., Goulson, H. T., Weatherly, N. F., and Chaffee, E. F. (1970a). Studies on delayed (cellular) hypersensitivity in mice infected with *Trichinella spiralis*. V. Tests in recipients injected with donor spleen cells 1, 3, 7, 14, or 21 days before infection. *J. Parasitol.* **56**, 978–981.

Larsh, J. E., Jr., Goulson, H. T., Weatherly, N. F., and Chaffee, E. F. (1970b). Studies on delayed (cellular) hypersensitivity in mice infected with *Trichinella spiralis*. VI. Results in recipients injected with antiserum of "freeze-thaw" spleen cells. *J. Parasitol.* **56,** 1206–1209.

Morseth, D. J., and Soulsby, E. J. L. (1969). Fine structure of leukocytes adhering to the cuticle of *Ascaris suum* larvae. II. Polymorphonuclear leukocytes. *J. Parasitol.* **55,** 1025–1034.

Pearse, A. G. E. (1960). "Histochemistry—Theoretical and Applied," (2nd Ed.). Little, Brown and Co., Boston, Massachusetts.

Reddy, C. R. R. M., Parvathi, G., and Sivaramappa, M. (1969). Adhesion of white blood cells to guinea-worm larvae. *Amer. J. Trop. Med. Hyg.* **18,** 379–381.

Soulsby, E. J. L. (1961). Immunity to helminths and its effect on helminth infection. *Colston Pap.* **13,** 165–188.

Soulsby, E. J. L. (1962). Antigen-antibody reactions in helminth infections. *Advan. Immunol.* **2,** 265–303.

Soulsby, E. J. L. (1963). The nature and origin of the functional antigens in helminth infections. *Ann. N.Y. Acad. Sci.* **113,** 492–509.

Zimmermann, W. J., Schwarte, L. H., Biester, H. E. (1961). On the occurrence of *Trichinella spiralis* in pork sausage available in Iowa (1953–1960). *J. Parasitol.* **47,** 429–432.

Leukocytes and *Trichinella spiralis.* II. Effect of Peritoneal Exudate Cell Adherence on Larvae and Adults

Miroslaw Stankiewicz*

Veterinary Medical Research Institute
Iowa State University
Ames, Iowa

Introduction

Much has been written concerning immunity in trichinellosis (see review articles: Larsh, 1967, 1968, 1970; Kozar, 1971). However, direct effects of leukocytes of immunized and nonimmunized animals on *Trichinella spiralis* were not intensively investigated. There is only the short communication of Lancastre *et al.* (1970) and the publication of Lancastre and Bazin (1967) which reported that larvae and adult forms of *T. spiralis* injected into the peritoneal cavity of mice were covered by leukocytes and destroyed (infective larvae in 48 hr and adults in 3–5 days). Newborn larvae, according to Lancastre and Bazin (1967) and Lancastre *et al.* (1970). were not attacked by cells. Stankiewicz (Part III, this volume) was able to demonstrate adhesion of cells to newborn and infective larvae and adult forms. The possibility of destruction of newborn larvae by adherent cells was also discussed by Stankiewicz (Part III, this volume).

It is difficult to conclude from the experiments conducted by Lancastre and Bazin (1967) that the parasites injected into the peritoneal cavity died because of the action of cells or because of other unfavorable conditions, since that environment is not natural for infective or adult stages. This chapter describes an investigation of the viability of infective stage and adult *T. spiralis* in the peritoneal cavities of mice which were treated by methods known to suppress leukocyte activity as well as in the peritoneal cavities of untreated mice. In addition, two strains of *T. spiralis,* rat and mouse, were used to study the effect of cells on *T. spiralis.* To provide a broader applicability, rats and guinea pigs were also used as experimental animals. Results strongly suggested that in nonimmunized rats and mice, leukocytes were able to destroy both adult and infective stages of *T.*

*Present Address: Department of Parasitology, Zoological Institute, University of Warsaw.

275

spiralis, while in mice with suppressed leukocyte activity, larvae can develop to adult forms in the peritoneal cavity.

Materials and Methods

Unless specifically indicated, materials and methods in these experiments were used as previously described (Stankiewicz in Part III, this volume.

Cortisone Treatment and X-irradiation of Mice

One group of animals received daily doses (2.5 mg, subcutaneously) of cortisone (cortisone acetate) beginning 4 days prior to injection of larvae. A second group of animals received one injection (10 mg, subcutaneously) 1 day prior to inoculation of larvae. The third group received an intraperitoneal injection (10 mg) 1 day prior to inoculation. After injection of larvae, all animals received daily doses (2.5 mg) of cortisone subcutaneously and intraperitoneally, respectively. Effective dosage levels of cortisone were determined after Coker (1956). The cortisone treatments were recorded as a single group of animals when analyzing the data. The mice used to determine the effect of X-irradiation on the cell adherence were irradiated with 500 R and tested according to Yarinksy (1962) and Larsh *et al.* (1962) 4 days later.

In experiments to determine the influence of cortisone on cell adherence, 8-week-old white Swiss mice (from the colony of the Parasitology Department, School of Public Health, University of North Carolina), were used. In this and another experiment as indicated in the results, mice were injected with the mouse strain of *T. spiralis* obtained from the abovementioned laboratory. In the rest of the experiments, *T. spiralis* maintained in rats were used.

Mice were injected intraperitoneally with 1000 infective larvae in 1 cm^3 of phosphate buffered saline (PBS); rats with 5000 larvae in 5 cm^3 of PBS. Adult *T. spiralis* were administered 500–1000 per mouse and 3000–5000 per rat. On the average, six to nine animals were used each time for observation unless otherwise indicated.

Results

Adult *T. spiralis* in the Peritoneal Cavity of Nonimmune Mice

First Day. Almost all parasites were covered by a very heavy coat of cells and were trapped in a big cluster and immobilized. No visible pathological changes could be seen in the parasites.

Second Day. An intense cellular reaction was still evident (Fig. 1). The anterior part of some parasites appeared to be digested. Observation of the parasite, however, was very difficult because of the tremendous number of adherent cells. Only about 5–10% of the observed parasites were motile and some of these were not covered by cells.

Third Day. The parasites were still covered by thousands of cells. In addition to existing adherent small cells, giant cells appeared on the parasites. In many cases considerable amounts of the internal parts of the parasite were missing (Fig. 2). Both females and males were being degraded. Some parasites with only one-fourth of their body intact were still able to move. Generally, most of them did not show any motility.

Fourth Day. Many fragments of parasites and numerous giant cells were present. Highly degraded parasites and cuticles alone were not heavily covered with cells and free cuticles were seen (Fig. 3). The cuticles were fragile and pressure on the cover glass caused disruption. Whole worms were seldom seen.

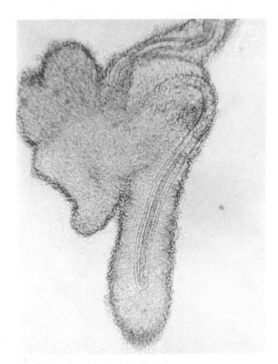

Figure 1 Cell adherence to adult *Trichinella spiralis* removed from the peritoneal cavity of a normal mouse (not previously infected) 2 days after inoculation.

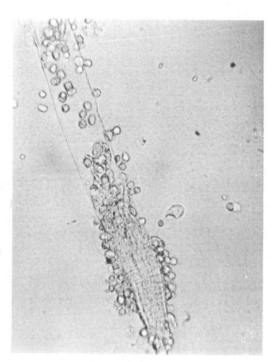

Figure 2 Fragment of adult *Trichinella spiralis* removed from the peritoneal cavity of normal mouse 3 days after inoculation.

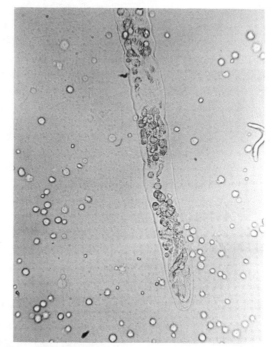

Figure 3 Fragment of *Trichinella spiralis* adult removed from the peritoneal cavity of normal mouse 4 days after inoculation.

Fifth Day. Only a few intact parasites were visible. Primarily only fragments were present and often mainly the ends of the fragments were covered by cells. Sporadic movements of single parasites or fragments were visible.

Sixth, Seventh, and Eighth Days. A decreasing number of fragments were present. Generally cell adherence to both fragments and partially degraded parasites was weak. Despite the effects of cell adherence on the adult worms, numerous newborn larvae were present in the peritoneal cavity of investigated animals. Some of the newborn larvae were covered by leukocytes as described by Stankiewicz (Part III, this volume).

Adult *T. spiralis* in the Peritoneal Cavity of Immunized Mice

Second Day. Parasites were covered by a thicker layer of cells as compared to nonimmunized animals. Cells adhering directly to the parasite created a uniform band and the shape of single cells could not be recognized. Observation was extremely difficult because of the compactness of the band and cells. Only a few parasites were seen through the coats of the cells and pathological changes were observed. None of the parasites was able to move.

Fourth Day. Most of the parasites were in large clusters of cells and no internal organs were distinguishable. Only a uniform mass was visible inside the parasites. In contrast to nonimmunized animals, no free cuticles were found.

Sixth and Eighth Days. More parasites were observed in this group of mice, at this period in time than in the nonimmunized group. Many of the parasites were still in clusters and very heavily coated by cells. Only fragments or completely destroyed adults were not covered. Visible cuticles were not covered by cells or were covered by very few cells. No newborn larvae were found in the peritoneal cavities on days 2–8 of this investigation.

Adult *T. spiralis* in the Peritoneal Cavity of Nonimmune Rats

Cell adhesion to the adult stage in the rats is very weak. Many parasites were not covered by cells and usually only a few were entirely covered (Table I).

First through Third Days. Cells were adherent primarily to the anterior and to the posterior part of the parasite. Most of the parasites were alive, although changes in the inner structure of the worm's body occurred. Frequently however, more damage was seen in the anterior than in the posterior part of the parasite.

Table I Cell adherence to Adult *Trichinella spiralis* Injected into the Peritoneal Cavity of Nonimmune Rats

	Average percent of parasites at different days after injection					
	1	2	3	4	5	6
Coverage of parasites by cells						
Complete	6	6	9	13	6	4
Partial	46	48	34	46	30	25
Not covered or covered by only a few cells	48	46	57	41	64	71
Approximate percent alive	90–99	85–95	70–84	60–80	10–60	5–50
Number of rats	4	5	4	5	4	4

Fourth Day. Numbers of recoverable whole parasites were lower than on the previous days and the number of fragments increased.

Fifth and Sixth Days. The number of degenerating and dead parasites increased considerably but many of them were still motile.

As it was shown, adult forms are not as readily attacked by cells in the peritoneal cavity of rats as in mice and they survive longer in rats than in mice. Moreover, in rats, giant cells were not observed on the surface of the parasite.

Infective Larvae in the Peritoneal Cavity of Nonimmune Mice

First Day. Very few larvae were found without adherent cells. Generally, larvae were surrounded by a very compact coat of cells. Some larvae were in the process of molting and a few parasites with two sheaths were seen. Larvae were motile and no cuticular or internal changes were visible. Cells did not appear to dissolve or cause lesions in the cuticle and the molting larvae were separated from the cells by cuticles.

Second Day. Larvae were still heavily covered (Fig. 4) and both mouth and anus could be seen plugged by cells. It seems that some of the larvae however, could free themselves from the cells by shedding the cuticle. The beginning of pathological changes inside the larvae were seen at this time. Some of the larvae appeared to be digested, especially in the region of the stichosome.

Third Day. Many larvae were still in large cell clusters. Only free cuticles were usually covered by smaller numbers of cells than cuticles containing larvae (Fig. 5). Giant cells were also seen on the parasites. Most of the larvae did not move and pathological changes were more pro-

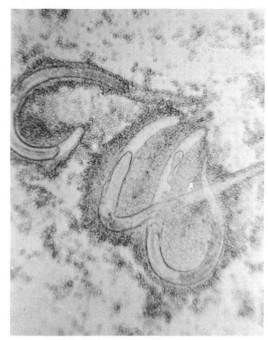

Figure 4 Cell adherence to infective *Trichinella spiralis* larvae in the peritoneal cavity of normal mouse, 2 days after inoculation.

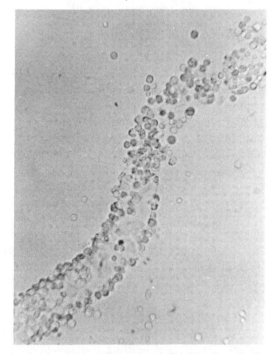

Figure 5 Cell adherence to the fragment of cuticle of *Trichinella spiralis* larva in the peritoneal cavity of normal mouse 3 days after inoculation.

nounced than on the second day. There appeared to be a disruption, fragmentation, and breakdown of internal structures.

Fourth Day. Larvae were primarily in the clusters surrounded by numerous cells. Many fragments of larvae or only cuticles with small fragments of larvae remaining were seen. Only sporadic movements of larvae were observed. Giant cells were more numerous than on the third day (Fig. 6).

Fifth Day. Smaller numbers of larvae were recovered from the peritoneal cavities of mice than on previous days. It was almost impossible to distinguish the internal organs in the worms, and only a few fragments were able to move.

Sixth Day. The general picture is similar to that found on the fifth day. However, some of the cells adhering to the larvae have lost their morphology and a very thick band was seen in this place.

Seventh, Eighth, and Twelfth Days. Further decreases in number of larvae or fragments recoverable from the peritoneal cavities was observed. In fact, only a few small fragments of parasites were obtained in exudates of some of the animals on day 12.

Infective Larvae in the Peritoneal Cavities of Nonimmunized Rats

First Day. Larvae were covered by cells but usually fewer cells were involved than in mice. Simultaneously, in the same animal, larvae were seen which were heavily covered by a single layer of cells or not covered at all. Cells covered not only the surface of the parasite, but also the natural orifices. More larvae were observed molting than in the mouse. Movement of larvae was sluggish and some larvae were immobile.

Second Day. More cells covered the parasites than during the first day and nearly all larvae found were covered by cells. Larvae were trapped, several at a time, in large cell clusters. Many larvae were seen undergoing interior fragmentation. Cuticle sheaths which were pulled away from the surface were usually covered by fewer cells than parts of the cuticle that were in contact with the worm body. Giant cells adhering to the larvae were also present. More larvae appeared to be dead than during the first day.

Third Day. Internal organs of many larvae were indistinct and disrupted (Fig. 7) and motility was gone. Most of the larvae were in large cell clusters formed by many layers of cells. Pseudopodia of cells could be seen in the mouth and anus of the larvae (Fig. 8).

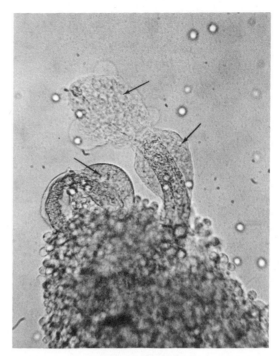

Figure 6 Giant cells adhering to the *Trichinella spiralis* larvae in the peritoneal cavity of normal mouse 4 days after inoculation.

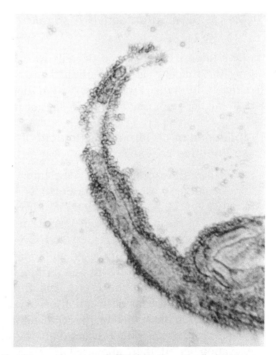

Figure 7 Disruption of the inner tissues of *Trichinella spiralis* larva removed from the peritoneal cavity of normal rat 3 days after inoculation.

Fourth Day. The number of whole, undamaged worms decreased while the number of fragments of various sizes increased considerably. Very solid plugs of cells were seen at the ends of some of the larval fragments (Fig. 9). Some of the highly destroyed larvae were not covered by cells. Many free cuticles were not covered or were covered by a few cells. Usually parts of cuticles that still contained pieces of larvae were covered by more cells than those parts that did not.

Fifth, Sixth, Seventh, and Twelfth Days. Further decreases in the numbers of parasites present in the peritoneal cavity occurred. The numerous fragments were usually reduced in size and only sporadic, highly damaged larvae and fragments were seen to move on the fifth day. Some of the larvae were covered by a various size cyst created by cells and only very small fragments of parasites were found inside the cysts in sampled animals on the twelfth day.

Infective Larvae in the Peritoneal Cavity of Nonimmunized Guinea Pigs

Observations conducted on the fourth, sixth, and eighth days had shown that larvae could also be destroyed in guinea pigs. General reactions were similar to those previously described in mice and rats.

Mouse Strain of Infective *T. spiralis* Larvae in the Nonimmune Mouse

Less intensive adherence of cells was observed to the mouse strain during the first day after injection than to the rat strain. Otherwise no significant differences were observed in the adherence of cells and in the fate of the larvae during the next 6 days of investigation.

Influence of Different Treatments of Mice on Cell Adherence to Infective Larvae

Influence of X-irradiation. The clearest difference between irradiated and normal mice was seen on the first day. Numerous larvae were molting and only a few cells adhered to them. Movement of larvae was more vigorous than in the nonirradiated. During the next 2 days, differences between the two groups decreased and larvae became covered by cells, although fewer cells were involved and more larvae were in the process of molting (Fig. 10) and motile in the X-irradiated mice. Motile larvae were also more frequent on the fourth and fifth days in X-irradiated mice, nevertheless, significant destruction of larvae already appeared from the third day on. On the sixth day, detectable differences were not observed in cell adherence or parasite destruction in the two groups. During the entire observation period, there appeared to be more macrophages in comparison to other cells adhering to worms in irradiated animals.

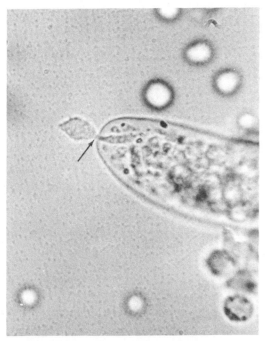

Figure 8 Cell pseudopod plugging the anus of *Trichinella spiralis* larvae recovered from the peritoneal cavity of normal rat 3 days after inoculation.

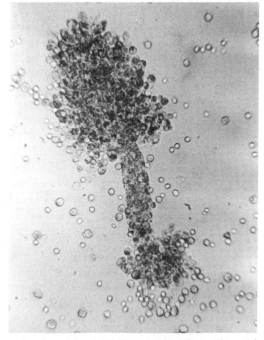

Figure 9 Cell adherence to the fragment of larva removed from the peritoneal cavity of a normal rat 4 days after inoculation.

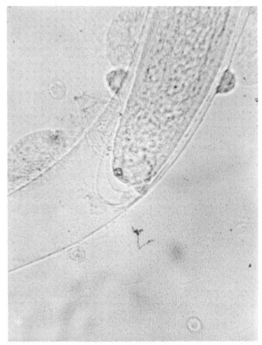

Figure 10 *Trichinella spiralis* larva with several sheaths removed from the peritoneal cavity of irradiated mouse 3 days after inoculation.

Influence of Cortisone.   Very strong inhibition of cell adherence was observed from 1–7 days after injection of larvae into cortisone-treated mice (Table II). Numerous larvae seemed to undergo normal development when cell adherence was inhibited by cortisone and only a few were destroyed. During the first day after injection, molting of larvae occurred frequently and usually larvae with one sheath were visible. Larvae with two and three sheaths plus some young males and females were seen on the second day. Numerous parasites with sheaths and fully developed adults were observed on the third day. On the sixth and seventh days, parasites were still motile and a few newborn larvae in the peritoneal cavities of examined mice were noticed. However, in none of the several throughly examined females were larvae found inside the parasite, although, some of the females appeared to contain developing embryos.

Discussion

In normal nonimmunized mice, rats, and guinea pigs, parasites are surrounded by huge numbers of cells, immobilized, and destroyed. Immobilization can occur in the large clusters of cells containing several parasites or single parasites can be coated by hundreds of cells. The quality and quantity of cell adherence is a function of animals used and the stage of the parasite as discussed by Stankiewicz (Part III, this volume). The infective stage of *T. spiralis* is the most attractive stage to the host cells and only very small differences were observed between the rat and the mouse strains in a particular species. There was a difference in the reaction of the cells of mice and rats to the adult form of the rat strain of *T. spiralis*. Cell adherence in the rats was much weaker as compared to the mouse; moreover, adult *T. spiralis* survived longer in rats than in mice. This suggested that unless the parasite is intensely attacked by cells, it may survive longer, and deliberate suppression of cell adherence with X-irradiation or cortisone supports the premise. When cell adherence was decreased by administration of cortisone, the larvae not only survived but also underwent almost normal development and reached maturity.

Cell adherence is more intense in immunized animals than in nonimmunized. Usually when adult forms were injected into the nonimmunized animals, numerous live, newborn larvae were present in the peritoneal cavity. They were either larvaposited or released by disruption of the adult forms. In immunized animals however, newborn larvae were not seen because the reaction was so destructive that larvae were probably killed inside the adults since none of them were seen in the body fluid.

Many factors can be involved in the destruction of the parasites by cells. These factors can be summarized as: (1) Certain substances can be excreted by cells that interact directly with the parasites. (2) Normal metabolic functions of the parasite (gas exchange, transport of nutritional materials and excretion of metabolic products) can be arrested due to tremendous numbers of cells covering not only the surface but the natural openings. Very slow diffusion of the neutral red stain inside the clusters of cells containing larvae seems to support this suggestion (unpublished data). (3) Changes in pH also cannot be excluded. (4) Unfavorable conditions created by cells could trigger autolytic and other changes destructive to the parasite. The rapid destruction of the parasites covered by cells in the nonimmune animals may exclude antibodies as an initiating factor of these effects. Further experiments must be performed to elaborate the destructive mechanisms.

The possibility of enzymatic activity of the cells and their interference with the cuticular transport are discussed by Jackson and Bradbury (1970). In their system utilizing *Neoaplectana glaseri*, which is not a natural parasite of mammals, distinct cuticular changes of the third stage were observed 4 or 5 days after injection into the peritoneal cavity of rats. If such larvae were placed in a favorable culture, the nematodes survived but did not develop to mature stages. The possibility of destruction of microfilariae by leukocytes is also discussed by Bagai and Subrahmanyam (1970). Alterations of the cuticle by polymorphonuclear cells were reported by Morseth and Soulsby (1969). In the present study, light microscope observations suggested that changes in the soft tissues beneath the cuticle occurred faster than in the cuticle.

A certain protective role may be ascribed to the cuticle, especially since the larvae appear to release themselves from cells during molting by rejecting the cuticle together with the adherent cells. From the following observations, it is tempting to speculate that the cuticle by itself may not be as attractive to peritoneal exudate cells as are the substances which may diffuse through the cuticle. The facts which substantiate this argument are: (1) Free cuticles were usually covered by smaller numbers of leukocytes or not covered at all. (2) Those parts of the cuticles that contained the parasites were usually heavily covered by cells. (3) In many cases, when the parasites were broken, the ends of the fragments had more cells than the surface.

Pathological changes can occur inside the whole parasite. However, it seems that the anterior part is more rapidly destroyed than the posterior. In the case of larvae, some parasite would be completely deprived of this part of the body whereas the posterior end was untouched and motile. The movement was one of the most unexpected things observed during these experiments. Some of the almost completely destroyed parasites or fragments were also able to move. This seemed to indicate that movement is probably one of the last vital signs to be lost. In experiments conducted by Lancastre and Bazin (1967), larvae in the peritoneal cavity of mice did not survive longer than 48 hr unless injections of protein were administered while adults survived 3–5 days in mice. In our experiments with normal mice, most of the larvae and adults lost their motility within 2–3 days. These differences may be due to the different strains of animals and due to the use of PBS for injection of parasites instead of serum.

Summary

Trichinella spiralis infective larvae were injected into the peritoneal cavities of normal mice, guinea pigs, rats and X-irradiated or cortisone-treated mice. In peritoneal cavities of normal animals, the larvae were heavily coated by leukocytes and rapidly destroyed. Infective larvae injected into X-irradiated mice survived longer than in nonirradiated mice but they were eventually destroyed also. Larvae placed in the peritoneal cavities of mice treated with cortisone, not only survived longer but also many of them reached maturity and both males and females were seen.

Trichinella spiralis adults were injected into the peritoneal cavities of normal mice, immune mice, and normal rats. The adults were heavily covered by peritoneal exudate cells and were destroyed in normal and im-

Table II Cell Adherence in the Peritoneal Cavities of Mice Treated with Cortisone

	Average percent of parasites at different days after injection						
	1	2	3	4	5	6	7
Coverage of parasites by cells							
Complete	9	6	8	10	0	1	0
Partial	56	34	20	54	32	17	19
Not covered or covered by only a few cells	35	60	72	36	68	82	81
Number of mice	9	9	9	4[a]	9	9	8

[a] Only one group of mice injected subcutaneously was investigated.

munized mice. In rats however, these stages were not as heavily covered and they survived longer.

Acknowledgments

The author wishes to express his gratitude to Drs. E. L. Jeska, J. E. Larsh, Jr., and N. F. Weatherly for their interest and encouragement and for providing research facilities. Appreciation is also extended to Mr. W. J. Hubbard, Mr. K. Smith, and Ms. M. E. Alls for aid in preparation of this manuscript. I also want to thank Dr. M. A. Emmerson for irradiating the animals.

This investigation received financial support from the World Health Organization.

References

Bagai, R. C., and Subrahmanyam, D. (1970). Nature of acquired resistance to filarial infection in albino rats. *Nature London* **228**, 682–683.

Coker, C. M. (1956). Some effect of cortisone in mice with acquired immunity to *Trichinella spiralis*. *J. Infec. Dis.* **98**, 39–44.

Jackson, G. J., and Bradbury, P. C. (1970). Cuticular fine structure and molting of *Neoaplectana glaseri* (Nematoda) after prolonged contact with rat peritoneal exudate. *J. Parasitol.* **56**, 108–115.

Kozar, Z. (1971). Some current immunologic aspects of trichinellosis. *Wiad. Parazytol.* **12**, 503–540.

Lancastre, F. A. and Bazin, J. (1967). Trichinose expérimentale. Survie et reproduction des différents stades de *Trichinella spiralis* dans la cavite peritonéale de la souris. *Ann. Parasitol. Paris* **42**, 525–532.

Lancastre, F., Bazin, J., and Mougeot, G. (1970). Comportement de *Trichinella spiralis* la cavité péritonéale de la souris. *J. Parasitol.* **56**, 438.

Larsh, J. E., Jr. (1967). The present understanding of the mechanism of immunity to *Trichinella spiralis*. *Amer. J. Trop. Med. Hyg.* **16**, 123–132.

Larsh, J. E., Jr. (1968). Experimental trichiniasis. *In:* B. Dawes (ed.), "Advances in Parasitology," vol. 6. Academic Press, New York, pp. 351–372.

Larsh, J. E., Jr. (1970). Immunology. *In:* S. E. Gould (ed.), "Trichinosis in Man and Animals." Thomas, Springfield, Illinois, pp. 129–146.

Larsh, J. E., Jr., Race, G. J., and Yarinsky, A. (1962). A histopathologic study in mice immunized against *Trichinella spiralis* and exposed to total-body X-irradiation. *Amer. J. Trop. Med. Hyg.* **11,** 633–640.

Morseth, D. J., and Soulsby, E. J. L. (1969). Fine structure of leukocytes adhering to the cuticle of *Ascaris suum* larvae. II. Polymorphonuclear leukocytes. *J. Parasitol.* **55,** 1025–1034.

Yarinsky, A. (1962). The influence of X-irradiation on the immunity of mice to infection with *Trichinella spiralis. J. Elisha Mitchell Sci. Soc.* **78,** 29–43.

Mechanism of the Transfer of Delayed Hypersensitivity to *Trichinella spiralis:* The Effect of Immune Serum

Charles W. Kim, Mahendra P. Jamuar,* and L. D. Hamilton

Department of Microbiology, Health Sciences Center, State University of New York, Stony Brook, and Division of Microbiology, Medical Research Center, Brookhaven National Laboratory, Upton, New York

Introduction

That a typical delayed type of hypersensitivity to crude saline extract or acid-soluble protein fraction of *Trichinella spiralis* larvae has been induced in the guinea pig is evidenced by: (1) delayed skin reaction, (2) perivascular infiltration of predominantly mononuclear cells at the skin test site, (3) absence of precipitating antibody, and (4) transfer of the delayed hypersensitive state from sensitized donors to normal recipients by means of splenic cells (Kim, 1966a,b) and lymph node cells (Kim *et al.,* 1967a, b, 1970). Transfer of delayed hypersensitivity to *T. spiralis* antigen by means of splenic cells has also been reported in mice (Larsh *et al.,* 1969, 1970a, b).

Transfer of delayed hypersensitivity has been attributed to cellular factors rather than to humoral factors. However, some reports implicate humoral serum factors or cell extracts in the passive transfer of delayed hypersensitivity. A plasma fraction identified as an α-globulin albumin passively transferred to normal guinea pigs a delayed type skin sensitivity to tuberculin PPD (Cole and Favour, 1955). More recently, plasma from sensitized, irradiated donors passively transferred PPD sensitivity (Dupuy *et al.,* 1969, 1970). Also interesting are reports of a synergic effect of immune serum on the passive transfer of delayed hypersensitivity to bovine γ-globulin, bovine serum albumin, ovalbumin, and hemocyanin, but not to PPD (Asherson and Loewi, 1966; Asherson, 1967a, b).

In view of the finding that immune serum may be synergic in transfer of delayed hypersensitivity—at least to certain antigens—it seemed desirable

---

*Present address: Department of Zoology, Patna University, Patna, Bihar

to determine the effect of immune serum in the passive transfer of delayed hypersensitivity to *T. spiralis.*

Materials and Methods

Sensitization and Skin-Testing in Donors (Kim *et al.,* 1970)

Albino, pen-inbred guinea pigs of both sexes weighing on the average 514 gm were sensitized once with *T. spiralis* antigen (76 μg total protein of crude saline extract of larvae) plus complete adjuvant (Difco's H37 Ra) and were skin-tested 7 days later with the homologous antigen (76 μg total protein). The second group of animals was sensitized with 380 μg of total protein plus complete adjuvant and skin-tested with 76 μg of total protein. The third group of animals was sensitized four times at 2-week intervals with 1.5 mg total protein plus complete adjuvant and skin-tested 2 weeks after the last sensitiztion (56 days after initial sensitization) with 76 μg total protein.

Detection of Antibody in Donors (Kim *et al.,* 1970)

Donor animals were bled (intracardiac) approximately 24 hr after the skin test, just before removal of lymph nodes for transfer. Passive cutaneous anaphylaxis (PCA) and precipitin ring tests served to detect antibody.

Preparation of Antiserum

To prepare 7-day serum, guinea pigs were sensitized once with 76 μg total protein, skin-tested 7 days later, and bled (intracardiac) at the height of the skin test reaction.

To prepare immune serum, guinea pigs were hypersensitized with *T. spiralis* antigen (1.5 mg total protein) plus complete adjuvant four times at 2-week intervals. They were bled (intracardiac) 2 weeks after the last immunization and the serum was obtained and stored at −20° C until needed.

X-irradiation of Recipients (Kim, 1966b)

Normal guinea pigs of both sexes weighing on the average 496 gm were exposed to sublethal doses (150 R, and 200 R) of total body X-irradiation at 250 kV, 30 mA, at 60 cm distance with 0.5 mm Cu–1 mm Al added filter, and with HVL 1.25 mm Cu approximately 18 hr before transfer of cells. For 150 R, the dose rate measured from 119.3 R/min to 125 R/min, and for 200 R from 118 R/min to 122.5 R/min.

Passive Transfer of Lymph Node Cells (Kim *et al.,* 1970)

Approximately 24 hr after the skin test in the donors, the lymph nodes (cervical, axillary, popliteal, and inguinal) were removed, trimmed, teased, strained, and standardized. The cells ($> 1 \times 10^8$) were inoculated intraperitoneally to X-irradiated (150 R, 200 R) and nonirradiated recipients. To one group 1 ml of immune serum was injected intravenously (marginal ear vein) immediately after cell transfer. The other group received only cells. A third group received only the immune serum (1 ml intravenously). In one experiment, 7-day serum was used rather than the immune serum. The sex as well as the approximate weights of recipients were matched with those of donors.

Skin-Testing of Recipients

The recipient animals were skin-tested with 76 μg total protein 3 days after transfer of cells and/or serum.

Histopathology in Recipients

Stretch preparations were made of some of the animals of the loose connective tissue between the dermal and musculofascial layer at the site of the skin test approximately 25 hr after the skin test and were stained with hematoxylin–eosin–azure II.

Antibody Detection in Recipients

Irradiated and nonirradiated animals that received only cells were bled (intracardiac) from day 4 after transfer through day 13 and at days 17, 24, 31, and 38. PCA and precipitin ring tests were used to detect antibody in the serum. Serum samples were used undiluted for both tests.

Results

Skin-Test Reactions in Donors

Delayed skin reactions were observed in animals skin-tested 7 days after one sensitization with 76 μg total protein (Table I). The reaction began to appear at 3 hr after the skin test, peaked (17 × 21 mm) between 22 and 24 hr, and was typically erythematous and indurated with a blanched or necrotic center in some animals. When the sensitizing dose was increased fivefold to 380 μg, the reaction was almost identical, beginning at 3 hr and peaking (17 × 22 mm) between 21 and 24 hr.

When the donor animals were hypersensitized (four times at 2-week intervals), the skin-test reaction was accelerated, beginning at 1 hr as small, strawberry-red spots, and reaching its peak before 12 hr (Table II). At its peak, the reaction was slightly hemorrhagic, circumscribed by a diffuse pale edema, and significantly smaller in size (7 × 9 mm) than the typical delayed reaction. Skin tests of control animals not sensitized previously were always negative.

Detection of Antibody in Donors

Antibody was detected by PCA in 50% of the donors sensitized once with 76 μg when serum was diluted 1:5, 25% when serum was diluted 1:20, and 9% when serum was diluted 1:80 (Table III). However, in donors sensitized once with a higher dosage (380 μg), antibody was detected by PCA in 100% of the animals when serum was diluted 1:5, 50% when serum was diluted 1:20, and 22% when serum was diluted 1:80. In each of the dilutions the percentage of positives was greater than in the 76 μg group. In both groups, the average size of the reactions decreased correspondingly with higher dilutions of serum.

When the donor animals were hypersensitized, antibody was detected by PCA in all (100%) of the serum samples in each of the dilutions: 1:20, 1:40, 1:80, and 1:320 (Table IV).

Precipitating antibody was not detected by the ring test in the sera of animals sensitized once with 76 μg and skin-tested (Table V). However, in the sera of animals sensitized once with a higher dosage (380 μg), antibody was detected by the ring test in all (100%) of the samples with 1:100 dilution of antigen and in 93% with 1:200 dilution of antigen. Higher dilutions of antigen, however, gave negative results. In the sera of hypersensitized animals, antibody was detected in all (100%) of the samples with antigen dilutions of 1:100 to 1:1600, and in 85% of the samples with 1:3200 dilution of antigen.

Skin-Test Reactions in Recipients

The skin-test reactions in recipients 3 days after transfer of lymph node cells from donors sensitized once with 76 μg are shown in Table VI. The reaction began at 3 hr after the skin test in X-irradiated (150 R, 200 R) and nonirradiated animals that received cells plus immune serum and cells alone. The reactions at 22–24 hr were smaller in animals receiving cells plus immune serum than in those receiving cells alone, irrespective of X-irradiation. Similarly, the skin test reactions in X-irradiated and non irradiated animals that received cells from donors sensitized once with 380 μg were generally smaller in those that received cells plus immune serum as opposed to those that received cells alone (Table VII). However, the skin-test reactions in X-irradiated and nonirradiated animals that received cells from hypersensitized donors, were slightly larger in size in those that received cells plus immune serum than in those that received cells alone (Table VIII). The difference in size of the reactions was less apparent in the animals X-irradiated with 200 R.

Interestingly, when 7-day serum was used (Table IX), the skin-test reactions in the recipients were similar to those in which immune serum was used (Table VI), i.e., in X-irradiated (150 R) and nonirradiated animals, the reactions were either the same or smaller in those that received

Table I Skin-Test Reaction to *T. spiralis* Antigen in Sensitized Donors[a]

Sensitizing antigen (μg total protein)	Days between sensitization and skin test	Average reaction in mm, at different hours after skin test							
		½–2	3	4	5	6	21	22	24
76	7	–	4 × 5	5 × 6	6 × 7	6 × 7	16 × 21	17 × 21	17 × 21
380	7	–	4 × 4	5 × 5	6 × 7	8 × 8	17 × 22	17 × 22	17 × 22

[a] Skin-test dose, 76 μg (total protein).

Table II Skin-Test[a] Reaction to *T. spiralis* Antigen in Hypersensitized[b] Donors

Sensitizing antigen (mg total protein)	Days between initial sensitization and skin test	Average reaction in mm, at different hours after skin test					
		1–2	3–7	12	21	22	24
1.5	56	6 × 7	7 × 9	7 × 8	6 × 7	6 × 6	5 × 5

[a] Skin-test dose, 76 μg (total protein).
[b] Four times at 2-week intervals.

Table III Detection of Antibody by Passive Cutaneous Anaphylaxis (PCA) in Donors Sensitized with *T. spiralis* Antigen

Sensitizing antigen (μg total protein)	Days between sensitization and skin test[a]	serum dilutions	No. positive/ No. samples[b]	Average reaction (mm)
76	7	1:5	22/44 (50%)	14 × 37
		1:20	11/44 (25%)	10 × 26
		1:80	4/44 (9%)	9 × 18
380	7	1:5	18/18 (100%)	16 × 41
		1:20	9/18 (50%)	15 × 37
		1:80	4/18 (22%)	10 × 20

[a] Skin-test dose, 76 μg (total protein).
[b] Percent is given in parenthesis.

Table IV Detection of Antibody by Passive Cutaneous Anaphylaxis (PCA) in Donors Hypersensitized[a] with *T. Spiralis* Antigen

Sensitizing antigen (mg total protein)	Days between initial sensitization and skin test[b]	Serum dilutions	No. positive/ No. samples	Average reaction (mm)
1.5	56	1:20	34/34	26 × 80
		1:40	34/34	24 × 71
		1:80	33/33	27 × 71
		1:320	33/33	23 × 60

[a] Four times at 2-week intervals.
[b] Skin-test dose, 76 μg (total protein).

cells plus 7-day serum than in those that received only cells. As expected, the skin test was essentially negative in control animals that received only immune serum.

Histopathology in Recipients

The skin-test sites of X-irradiated (200 R) and non-irradiated animals receiving cells plus immune serum and cells alone from donors sensitized once (76 µg) showed a predominance of mononuclear cells (lymphocytes, monocytes, and macrophages) as in a typical delayed response even though the skin-test reactions (Table VI) were not the same in all of the groups.

Detection of Antibody in Recipients

Antibody was detected earlier by both PCA and precipitin ring tests in animals receiving cells from hypersensitized donors than in those receiving cells from donors sensitized only once, as expected. Furthermore, antibody was detected earlier by both tests in nonirradiated than in X-irradiated recipients. In one instance in which antibody was detected on the same day (day 4 after transfer by PCA in the sera of X-irradiated (150 R) and non-irradiated animals that received cells from hypersensitized donors, a greater percentage of positives was obtained with serum samples from non-irradiated animals than with those from irradiated animals. Recipient animals X-irradiated with 200 R did not live beyond 10 days after transfer, whereas those X-irradiated with 150 R lived as long as the nonirradiated controls (38 days following transfer), at least in one of the experiments. Hence, X-irradiation not only delayed the appearance of antibody following transfer but it also decreased the longevity of the animals.

Discussion

As the guinea pigs became hypersensitized by repeated sensitizing doses of antigen and also produced antibody, particularly precipitating antibody, the skin-test reaction appeared earlier and waned sooner, somewhat like the Arthus type reaction although it was not typical of that type of reaction. It would be more accurate to describe it as an accelerated delayed hypersensitivity response, confirming earlier work (Kim *et al.*, 1970) in which the presence of precipitating antibody interfered with manifestation of a typical delayed response. The skin test appears to be less sensitive than the PCA test in distinguishing the reactions caused by different dosages of a single sensitization, i.e., there was no difference in the time of initiation and the peak of the delayed skin reaction in donors sensitized with 76 µg and with 380 µg, whereas in the PCA test the percentage of positives was doubled with sera from animals sensitized with 380 µg as compared to those from animals sensitized with 76 µg. However, the

Table V Detection of Antibody by Precipitin Ring Test in Donors Sensitized with *T. spiralis* Antigen

Sensitizing antigen (total protein)	Days between initial sensitization and skin test[a]	No. positive/No. samples					
		Antigen dilutions					
		1:100	1:200	1:400	1:800	1:1600	1:3200
1 × 76 µg	7	0/44	0/44	0/44	0/44	0/44	0/44
1 × 380 µg	7	18/18	15/18	0/18	0/18	0/18	0/18
4 ×[b] 1.5 mg	56	34/34	34/34	34/34	34/34	34/34	29/34

[a] Skin-test dose, 76 µg (total protein).
[b] At 2-week intervals.

skin test is sufficiently sensitive in distinguishing the reaction in animals sensitized only once (irrespective of dosage) from that in hypersensitized animals, although here too the serologic findings by PCA and precipitin ring tests are much more sensitive in distinguishing the two groups.

For transfer studies, the recipients were X-irradiated with sublethal dosages (150 R, and 200 R) to suppress immune activity. Previous study (Kim, 1966b) had shown that a total body X-irradiation of 200 R of donors partly inhibited the appearance of PCA antibody, inhibited the appearance of precipitating antibody altogether, and somewhat suppressed the skin-test reaction. In the present study, X-irradiation indeed suppressed the immune activity in the recipients as evidenced by a delay in the appearance

Table VI Skin-Test[a] Reaction in X-irradiated and Nonirradiated Recipients After Transfer of Lymph Node Cells (1 × 10⁸) and Immune Serum

Donors Sensitization	X-irradiation (R)		Average reaction in mm, at different hours after skin test						
			½–2	3	4	5	6	22	24
1×	150	Cells + immune serum[b]	–	3 × 3	3 × 4	3 × 4	3 × 4	3 × 4	3 × 4
		Cells	–	3 × 4	3 × 4	3 × 4	4 × 4	4 × 4	4 × 4
76 µg	200	Cells + immune serum[b]	–	3 × 4	3 × 4	4 × 4	4 × 4	2 × 2	2 × 2
		Cells	–	3 × 5	3 × 5	4 × 5	4 × 5	4 × 5	4 × 5
(total protein)	Nonirrad.	Cells + immune serum[b]	–	3 × 4	4 × 4	4 × 4	4 × 4	4 × 4	4 × 4
		Cells	–	4 × 4	4 × 4	4 × 4	4 × 5	6 × 7	6 × 7

[a] Skin-test dose, 76 µg (total protein).
[b] One ml of immune serum (intravenous).

Table VII Skin-Test[a] Reaction in X-irradiated and Nonirradiated Recipients After Transfer of Lymph Node Cells (1 × 10^8) and Immune Serum

Donors Sensitization	X-irradiation (R)		Average reaction in mm, at different hours after skin test							
			½-1½	2	3	4	5	6	22	24
1X	150	Cells + immune serum[b]	–	4 × 4	4 × 4	4 × 5	4 × 5	4 × 5	4 × 5	3 × 4
		Cells	–	4 × 4	4 × 5	4 × 5	4 × 5	4 × 5	6 × 7	5 × 6
380 μg (total protein)	Nonirrad.	Cells + immune serum[b]	–	4 × 4	4 × 4	4 × 4	4 × 5	4 × 4	3 × 4	3 × 4
		Cells	–	3 × 3	3 × 3	4 × 5	5 × 6	5 × 6	6 × 7	6 × 7

[a] Skin-test dose, 76 μg (total protein).
[b] One ml of immune serum (intravenous).

Table VIII Skin-Test[a] Reaction in X-irradiated and Nonirradiated Recipients After Transfer of Lymph Node Cells (1 × 10⁸) and Immune Serum

Donors Sensitization	X-irradiation (R)		Average reaction in mm, at different hours after skin test								
			1½	2	3	4	5	6	12	22	24
4×	150	Cells + immune serum[b]	4 × 5	4 × 5	4 × 5	6 × 7	6 × 7	6 × 6	5 × 6	4 × 5	4 × 5
		Cells	–	–	3 × 4	4 × 5	4 × 5	4 × 5		3 × 4	2 × 3
1.5 mg	200	Cells + immune serum[b]	3 × 4	3 × 4	4 × 5	4 × 5	4 × 5	4 × 5	4 × 6	4 × 5	3 × 4
		Cells	–	–	3 × 4	3 × 4	4 × 5	4 × 4		3 × 3	2 × 2
(total protein)	Nonirrad.	Cells + immune serum	–	–	4 × 5	4 × 7	4 × 7	4 × 8	6 × 8	5 × 5	5 × 5
		Cells	–	–	3 × 4	4 × 5	4 × 5	4 × 5	3 × 5	3 × 4	3 × 4

[a] Skin-test dose, 76 µg (total protein).
[b] One ml of immune serum (intravenous).

299

of PCA and precipitating antibodies in X-irradiated animals as compared to nonirradiated animals. The suppressive effect of X-irradiation on the skin-test reactions in the recipients was also evident; the difference being more significant between those X-irradiated with the higher dosage (200 R) and those not irradiated.

Whether the donor animals had been sensitized with 76 or 380 μg, the addition of immune serum to the cells at the time of passive transfer of cells did not have a synergic effect on the skin-test reactions in the recipients; in fact, the reactions were usually smaller in these groups. Hence, our findings accord with the PPD findings of Asherson and Loewi (1966) and Asherson (1967a, b) in which they were unable to show a synergic effect of immune serum on passive transfer of delayed hypersensitivity to that antigen. Asherson (1967a) attributed the failure of serum to increase the passive transfer of delayed hypersensitivity to tuberculin to be related to the poor antibody response to that antigen at the time of transfer (3 weeks after immunization). If indeed failure of synergic effect of serum on transfer of delayed hypersensitivity is attributable to poor antibody response, the results with 7-day serum are tenable. However, the failure of the immune serum to exhibit a synergic effect on the passive transfer cannot be attributed to this since the antibody response at this stage is not poor. Our present findings contrast with the findings of Asherson and Loewi (1966) and Asherson (1967a, b) with other antigens, such as bovine serum albumin, bovine γ-globulin, ovalbumin and hemocyanin, in which the synergic effect of the immune serum on passive transfer of delayed hypersensitivity to these antigens was attributed to the action of the antibody in the serum which caused local inflammation and retention of the antigen. Since antibody was know to be present in our immune serum, the failure of the immune serum to exhibit a synergic effect on the passive transfer may be due not only to the difference in the antigen but

Table IX Skin-Test[a] Reaction in X-irradiated and Nonirradiated Recipients After Transfer of Lymph Node Cells (1 × 10^8) and 7-Day Serum

Donors Sensitization	X-irradiation (R)		Average reaction in mm, at different hours after skin test				
			½–2	3–4	5–6	21–22	24
1X	150	Cells + 7-day serum[b]	–	3 × 3	4 × 4	5 × 6	5 × 6
76 μg		Cells	–	3 × 4	4 × 5	5 × 6	5 × 6
(total protein)	Nonirrad.	Cells + 7-day serum[b]	–	3 × 3	4 × 4	3 × 5	3 × 5
		Cells	–	3 × 4	4 × 5	6 × 7	6 × 9

[a] Skin-test dose, 76 μg (total protein).
[b] One ml of 7-day serum (intravenous).

may be partly due to differences in the procedure, e.g., (1) only 1 ml was injected as opposed to 3 ml, and (2) serum was injected after, rather than before, transfer of cells. Interestingly enough, the skin-test results in animals that received cells from hypersensitized donors suggested that the addition of immune serum may have a slight synergic effect on the transfer of accelerated delayed hypersensitivity since those receiving cells plus immune serum manifested slightly larger skin reactions than those receiving cells alone. However, hypersensitized animals have been shown to be the least effective donors for transfer of delayed hypersensitivity since the delayed skin reactions in the donors are at best accelerated delayed responses due to the very presence of antibody (Kim *et al.*, 1970).

The mechanism involved in the transfer of delayed hypersensitivity remains obscure, but it is evident from the present findings that passive transfer of delayed hypersensitivity to *T. spiralis* is not enhanced by the presence of antibody, i.e., the addition of immune serum to the cells does not synergize passive transfer.

Summary

To test the possible synergic effect of immune serum on the transfer of delayed hypersensitivity by lymphocytes, guinea pigs were sensitized once (76 μg or 380 μg total protein) or hypersensitized (1.5 mg total protein) with crude saline extract of *T. spiralis* larvae plus complete adjuvant. Lymph node cells (1×10^8) from sensitized and hypersensitized donors were injected, either alone or with immune serum (1 ml), into X-irradiated (150 R, 200 R) and nonirradiated recipients, and skin tested 3 days later. The skin-test reactions in animals that received cells from sensitized donors were smaller when immune serum was added to the cells, irrespective of X-irradiation. The skin-test reactions in X-irradiated and nonirradiated animals that received cells from hypersensitized donors were slightly larger in size in those that received cells plus immune serum than in those that received cells alone; however, the reactions in donors and recipients were not typically delayed. The skin test sites of X-irradiated (200 R) and nonirradiated animals receiving cells plus immune serum and cells alone from sensitized donors (76 μg) both showed a predominance of mononuclear cells as in a typical delayed response even though the skin-test reactions were not typical. As expected, antibody was detected earlier by both passive cutaneous anaphylaxis and precipitin ring tests in animals receiving cells from hypersensitized donors than in those receiving cells from donors sensitized only once. Also, antibody was detected earlier by both tests in nonirradiated than in X-irradiated recipients. These findings suggest that the transfer of delayed hypersensitivity to *T. spiralis* is not enhanced by the presence of antibody, i.e., the addition of immune serum to the cells does not have a synergic effect on the passive transfer.

Acknowledgments

The authors thank J. P. Shanley and D. van der Kolk for technical assistance. This work was supported by the U.S. Atomic Energy Commission.

References

Asherson, G. L. (1967a). The passive transfer of delayed hypersensitivity in the guinea pig. II. The ability of passively transferred antibody to cause local inflammation and retention of antigen and the role of these phenomena in the passive transfer of delayed hypersensitivity. *Immunology* **13**, 441–451.

Asherson, G. L. (1967b). The role of serum factors in the passive transfer of delayed hypersensitivity. *Immunopathology Vth Int. Symp.,* pp 290–294.

Asherson, G. L., and Loewi, G. (1966). The effect of irradiation on the passive transfer of delayed hypersensitivity. *Immunology* **13**, 509–512.

Cole, L. R., and Favour, C. B. (1955). Correlations between plasma protein fractions, antibody titers, and the passive transfer of delayed and immediate cutaneous reactivity to tuberculin PPD and tuberculopolysaccharides. *J. Exp. Med.* **101**, 391–420.

Dupuy, J. M., Good, R. A., Kalpaktsoglou, P., and Perey, D. Y. (1969). Passive transfer of cell-mediated immunity with cell-free plasma. *Fed. Proc.* **28**, 563.

Dupuy, J. M., Stutman, O., and Good, R. A. (1970). Effector mechanisms of plasma transfer of cell mediated immunity. *Fed. Proc.* **29**, 702.

Kim, C. W. (1966a). Delayed hypersensitivity to larval antigens of *Trichinella spiralis. J. Infec. Dis.* **116**, 208–214.

Kim, C. W. (1966b). Delayed hypersensitivity to *Trichinella spiralis* antigens in irradiated guinea pigs. *J. Parasitol.* **52**, 722–726.

Kim, C. W., Savel, H., and Hamilton, L. D. (1967a). Delayed hypersensitivity to *Trichinella spiralis.* I. Transfer of delayed hypersensitivity by lymph node cells. *J. Immunol.* **99**, 1150–1155.

Kim, C. W., Jamuar, M. P., and Hamilton, L. D. (1967b). Delayed hypersensitivity to *Trichinella spiralis.* II. The antibody response in recipients after transfer of delayed hypersensitivity. *J. Immunol.* **99**, 1156–1161.

Kim, C. W., Jamuar, M. P., and Hamilton, L. D. (1970). Delayed hypersensitivity to *Trichinella spiralis.* III. Effect of repeated sensitization in donors and recipients. *J. Immunol.* **105**, 175–186.

Larsh, J. E., Jr., Goulson, H. T., Weatherly, N. F., and Chaffee, E. F. (1969). Studies on delayed (cellular) hypersensitivity in mice infected with *Trichinella spiralis.* IV. Artificial sensitization of donors. *J. Parasitol.* **55**, 726–729.

Larsh, J. E., Jr., Goulson, H. T., Weatherly, N. F., and Chaffee, E. F. (1970a). Studies on delayed (cellular) hypersensitivity in mice infected with *Trichinella spiralis.* V. Tests in recipients injected with donor spleen cells 1, 3, 7, 15, or 21 days before infection. *J. Parasitol.* **56**, 978–981.

Larsh, J. E., Jr., Goulson, H. T., Weatherly, N. F., and Chaffee, E. F. (1970b). Studies on delayed (cellular) hypersensitivity in mice infected with *Trichinella spiralis.* VI. Results in recipients injected with antiserum or "freeze-thaw" spleen cells. *J. Parasitol.* **56**, 1206–1209.

Fine Structure of Lymphocytes from Animals Hypersensitized to *Trichinella spiralis* Antigen

Mahendra P. Jamuar,* Charles W. Kim,† and L. D. Hamilton

Division of Microbiology, Medical Research Center, Brookhaven National Laboratory, Upton, New York

Introduction

Our earlier fine structure studies showed that lymphocytes from guinea pigs sensitized to *Trichinella spiralis* antigen combined with complete adjuvant and skin-tested 7 days later showed certain changes: they were usually large and had a greater nucleocytoplasmic ratio with an eccentric nucleus and patches of compact chromatin around the periphery; the cytoplasm had many ribosomes with a few scattered channels of endoplasmic reticulum, mitochondria, Golgi bodies and some dark granules (Jamuar *et al.,* 1968).

When animals were hypersensitized at 1-, 2-, or 3-week intervals with antigen plus Freund's complete adjuvant, then skin-tested 28, 56, or 84 days after initial sensitization, preliminary fine structure studies suggested that antigen not only mobilized lymphocytes to produce antibody but a correlation was noted between the degree of antigenic stimulus and proliferation of cellular organelles associated with protein synthesis in lymphocytes (Kim *et al.,* 1970). Indeed, with the largest dose and optimal interval of antigenic stimulation, fine structure studies indicated the production of lymphocytes very much like plasma cells. Therefore, this finding was studied further.

Materials and Methods

Sensitization and Skin–Testing

Albino, pen-inbred guinea pigs of both sexes weighing on the average 460 gm were injected into the digital spaces in the footpads intradermally

*Present address: Department to Zoology, Patna University, Patna, Bihar.
†Present address: Department of Microbiology, Health Sciences Center, State University of New York, Stony Brook, New York

with 0.1 ml of crude saline extract of *T. spiralis* larvae emulsified in 0.1 ml of Freund's complete adjuvant (Difco's H37 Ra). Three groups of animals were sensitized four times at 1-, 2-, or 3-week intervals (1.5 mg protein) and skin-tested 28, 56, or 84 days after initial sensitization, respectively. The skin-test dose was 76 μg total protein.

Electron Microscope Preparation

Approximately 24 hr after the skin test, lymph nodes (cervical, axillary, and inguinal) were removed and placed in MEM (Hyland). They were trimmed, teased, strained, and centrifuged. The cells, washed with Tyrode solution and centrifuged at 1500 rpm for 10 min, were fixed in 6% glutaraldehyde and 1% osmium tetroxide in Sorenson's buffer (pH 7.2), dehydrated in ethanol and propylene oxide, and embedded in Epon 812. Thin sections, cut with Porter-Blum ultramicrotome and stained with uranyl acetate and lead citrate, were examined under the RCA-EMU 3G microscope.

Results

Skin-Test Reactions

As reported (Kim *et al.,* 1970) skin-test reactions in hypersensitized animals were accelerated, i.e., the reaction began at 1 hr as a small, strawberry-red spot, peaking before 12 hr. At its peak, the reaction was slightly hemorrhagic circumscribed by a diffuse pale edema, and significantly smaller in size than the typical delayed reaction.

Electron Microscopy of Cells

Most lymph node cells from animals sensitized at 1-week intervals were unstimulated, small lymphocytes (Fig. 1) characterized by a large nucleus and a thin rim of cytoplasm. However, several stimulated lymphocytes (Fig. 2) larger than the normal lymphocytes were observed. The nucleus of these lymphocytes had compact peripheral chromatin in addition to the patches scattered in the nucleoplasm, and a distinct nucleolus. The rest of the nucleoplasm was occupied by lighter chromatin or euchromatin, extending up to the nuclear pores. The cytoplasm contained endoplasmic reticulum, a few mitochondria, and ribosomes.

Other large cells (Fig. 3) resembling plasma cells had an eccentric nucleus, and a cytoplasm filled with channels of endoplasmic reticulum in continuity with the perinuclear space indicative of protein-secreting cells. There were also a large area of Golgi apparatus, several vesicles, and mitochondria. In the nucleus the euchromatin occupied a larger area and the nucleolus had increased in size such that very often several sections of nucleolus were seen in one nucleus. These transitional cells were identical to the lymphoplasmacytes of Avrameas and Leduc (1970).

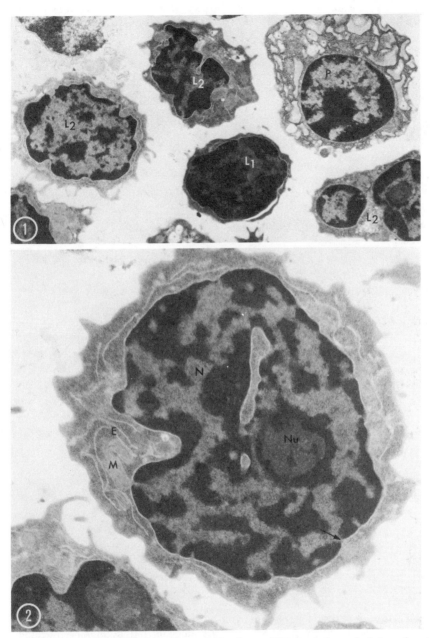

Figure 1 Lymphocytes from animal sensitized at 1-week intervals at various stages of development—a non-stimulated small lymphocyte (L_1), a few large, stimulated lymphocytes (L_2), and a plasma cell (P). $\times$ 4080.

Figure 2 This is a large, stimulated lymphocyte of L_2 type from animal sensitized at 1-week intervals as shown in Fig. 1. Note the patches of compact chromatin, a distinct nucleolus (Nu) and a nuclear pore (arrow) in the nucleus (N). The cytoplasm contains endoplasmic reticulum (E), a few mitochondria (M), and ribosomes. $\times$ 17,280.

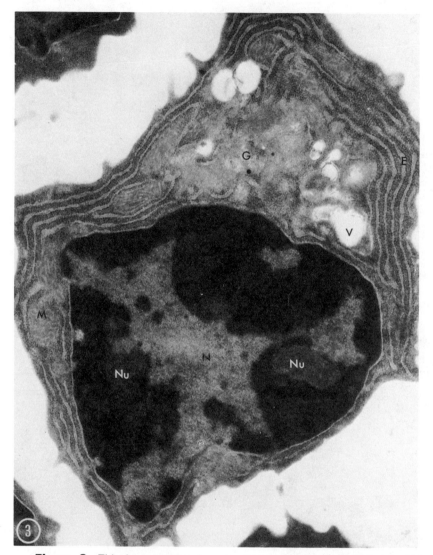

Figure 3 This is a mature lymphoplasmacyte from animal sensitized at 1-week intervals with an eccentric nucleus (N) containing nucleolus (Nu). The cytoplasm is filled with well-developed endoplasmic recticulum (E) in addition to several mitochondria (M), Golgi bodies (G), and vesicles (V). × 24,840.

There were also typical mature plasma cells (Fig. 4) seen in this group. These cells had a prominent nucleus and cytoplasm filled with distended cisternae of endoplasmic reticulum containing electron dense material.

Lymphocytes from animals sensitized at 2-week intervals were more advanced than those from animals sensitized at 1-week intervals. They

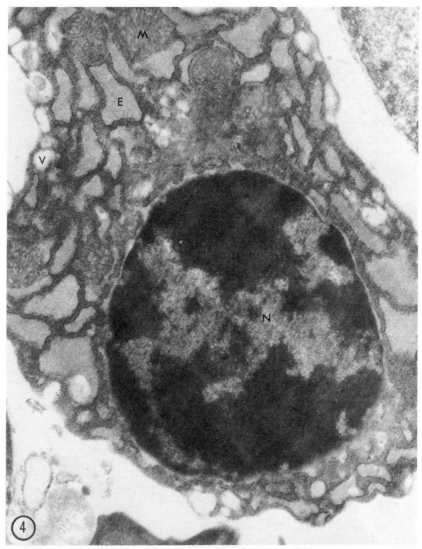

Figure 4 This is a mature plasma cell from animal sensitized at 1-week intervals with a nucleus (N) and a large cytoplasm filled with distended cisternae of endoplasmic reticulum (E), several mitochondria (M) and vesicles (V). × 24,840.

contained more of the structures generally associated with synthetic function (Figs. 5 and 6); they had a more differentiated appearance: the ribosomes were in aggregates as polyribosomes and individual ribosomes lined the channels of endoplasmic reticulum. The cytoplasm also contained several mitochondria and vesicles. The nucleus contained clumped dense chromatin, a large area of euchromatin, and a large nucleolus (Figs. 5–7).

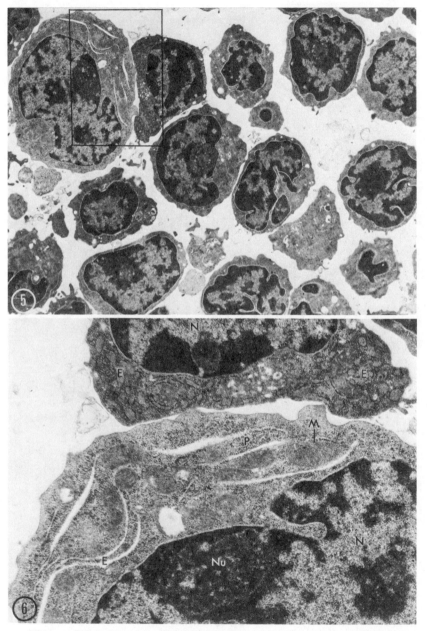

Figure 5 A large, stimulated lymphocyte and other lymphocytes at various stages of development from animal sensitized at 2-week intervals. × 6040.

Figure 6 A part of the inset of Fig. 5 at a higher magnification showing the cytoplasm of the large lymphocyte containing channels of endoplasmic reticulum (E), polyribosomes (P), mitochondria (M), as well as part of the nucleus (N) with a prominent nucleolus (Nu). × 17,280.

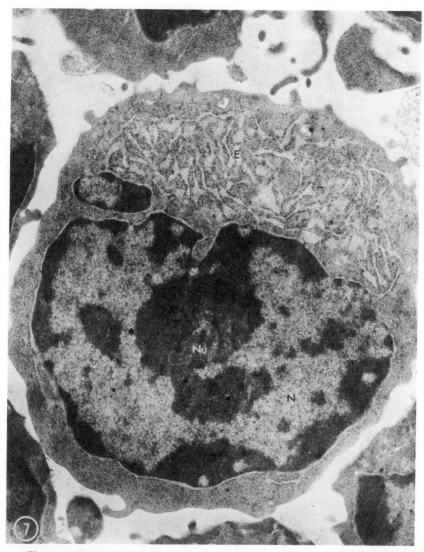

Figure 7 A stimulated lymphocyte from animal sensitized at 2-week intervals with a more differentiated appearance: an eccentric nucleus (N) with a prominent nucleolus (Nu), and ergastoplasm (E) arranged in short pieces of reticulum localized in one part of the cell. × 18,720.

In some cells the ergastoplasm was arranged as short pieces of reticulum localized in one part of the cell (Fig. 7). Lymphocytes at different stages of development were seen (Fig. 8): small lymphocytes (L_1), and advanced cells (L_2), characterized by the presence of polyribosomes, as well as channels of endoplasmic reticulum. Other cells more like plasma cells, the so-called lymphoplasmacytes (LP) were found more frequently in

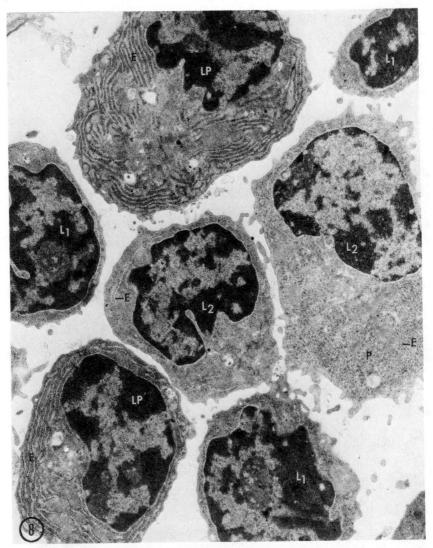

Figure 8 Several lymphocytes from animal sensitized at 2-week intervals at various stages of development (L_1, L_2). The stimulated lymphocytes (L_2) show prominent polyribosomes (P) as well as channels of endoplasmic reticulum (E). The two cells with more of the well-developed endoplasmic reticulum are lymphoplasmacytes (LP). $\times$ 11,120.

animals sensitized at 2-week intervals than in the other two groups. They had an eccentric nucleus and concentric lamellae of endoplasmic reticulum around the nucleus that filled the rest of the cytoplasm (Figs. 8 and 9). The nucleus had a prominent nucleolus and clumped chromatin showing nuclear pores. The cisternae of the endoplasmic reticulum were distended and contained electron dense material—protein, probably antibody (Fig.

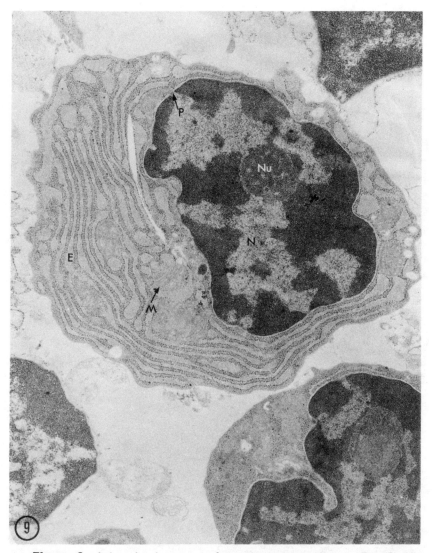

Figure 9 A lymphoplasmacyte from the same group as Fig. 8. Note the well-developed endoplasmic reticulum (E), several mitochondria (M), a nucleus (N) with a prominent nucleolus (Nu), and a nuclear pore (P). × 18,750.

9). These cells appeared to be ready to release their antibody. The cytoplasm also contained several mitochondria and vesicles.

Lymphocytes from animals sensitized at 3-week intervals showed less development of synthetic structural units compared with the previous two groups. However, nuclear and cytoplasmic changes were still quite prominent in these lymphocytes (Figs. 10 and 11). Stimulated lymphocytes

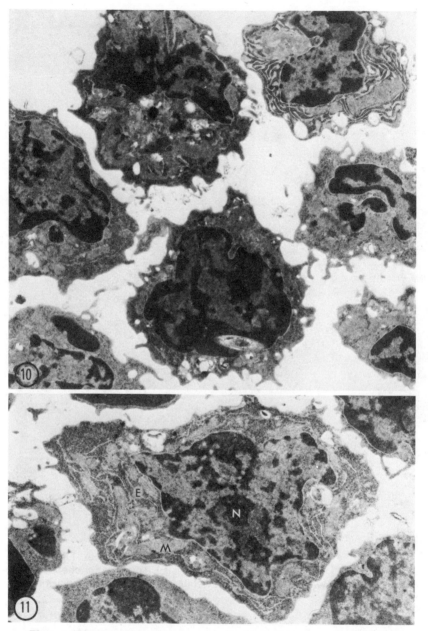

Figure 10 Lymphocytes from animal sensitized at 3-week intervals with less development of the synthetic structural units compared with those in the previous two groups. However, nuclear and cytoplasmic changes are still quite prominent. × 11,120.

Figure 11 A stimulated lymphocyte from the same group as in Fig. 10 showing a large nucleus (N), channels of endoplasmic reticulum (E) and mitochondria (M). × 13,000.

showed channels of endoplasmic reticulum, several mitochondria, and a characteristic nucleus (Fig. 11). The so-called lymphoplasmacytes were also present in this group but were fewer in number than in the other two groups (Fig. 12). The most distinguishing feature of this cell, as in the other groups, was its eccentric nucleus encircled by concentric lamellae of endoplasmic reticulum that filled the rest of the cytoplasm.

Discussion

These morphological changes confirm our earlier findings (Kim *et al.,* 1970) that with optimal interval of antigenic stimulation, namely 2 weeks, the sites of synthesis in individual lymphocytes develop to where they resemble plasma cells with their development of an elaborate endoplasmic reticulum. Also, with optimal antigenic stimulation, the total plasma cell population increased—a well-recognized reaction, especially if the antigen is given in combination with Freund's adjuvant (Balfour *et al.,* 1965). The increase in transitional cells under optimal antigenic stimulation correlated well with the percentage of cells that fluoresced in an earlier study (Kim *et al.,* 1971) suggesting that these cells synthesize γ-globulin (Zucker-Franklin, 1969). These transitional cells were called "lymphoplasmacytes" by Avrameas and Leduc (1970) which is an accurate description since in size and densities of their nuclei and cytoplasm they resemble more closely small and medium lymphocytes; yet they contain structural units, especially endoplasmic reticulum indicative of active protein synthesis, very like plasma cells. With progressive development of the endoplasmic reticulum there was concomitant loss of condensation of chromatin in the nucleus, along with an increase in the size of the cell, change in the original spherical shape, and eccentricity of the nucleus as reported by Hummeler *et al.* (1966b). Furthermore, the eccentric nucleus had a large nucleolus. Since the increase in the size of the nucleolus goes along with increased ribosomal RNA in the cytoplasm (Brachet and Mirsky, 1961), we can conclude that the large transitional cells (lymphoplasmacytes) exhibiting these changes are probably antibody-synthesizing cells. Other investigators (Feldman and Nordquist, 1967; Harris and Harris, 1949; Harris *et al.,* 1945, 1966; Hummeler *et al.,* 1966a, b; Schooley, 1961) have reported small lymphocytes with unusually well-developed endoplasmic reticulum capable of synthesizing and releasing antibody.

Avrameas and Leduc (1970) proposed that since lymphoplasmacytes were derived from small lymphocytes, they are the memory cells and that memory and antibody synthesis are two different activities of the same cell. Although we did not specifically label cells to determine sites of antibody synthesis, the well-developed, distended endoplasmic reticulum with channels in continuity with the perinuclear space indicated that these were indeed protein-secreting cells and were very likely antibody-secreting cells.

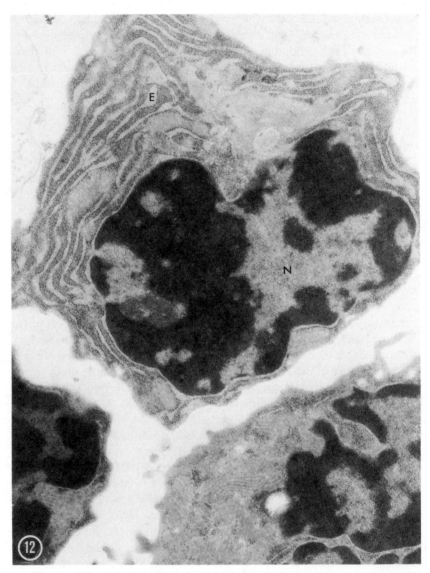

Figure 12 A lymphoplasmycyte from animal sensitized at 3-week intervals with an eccentric nucleus (N) and well-developed endoplasmic reticulum (E). × 25,920.

Many investigators (Balfour *et al.*, 1965; Vazquez, 1964; Wissler *et al.*, 1957) have reported the presence in stimulated lymphoid organs of cells with morphological characteristics of small lymphocytes which contained antibodies and were able to divide. The development of lymphocytes into cells so like plasma cells suggests that lymphocytes may indeed transform into plasma cells — at least into one type of plasma cell. Whether they divide with eventual formation of small lymphocytes again (Uhr, 1966) remains an open question; we did not study cell kinetics or whether they were from the medullary or subcortical region of lymph nodes. However, our observations show that when animals are sensitized to *T. spiralis* antigen, lymphocytes very like plasma cells are found in a suspended cell population from lymph nodes; these cells are probably derived from small lymphocytes as a result of antigenic stimulation.

Summary

Preliminary fine structure studies suggested that antigen not only mobilized lymphocytes to produce antibody but that with increasing antigenic dose synthetic structures of individual lymphocytes increased; indeed with the largest dose and optimal time interval, lymphocytes similar to plasma cells were produced. To study this finding further, three groups of guinea pigs were sensitized four times at 1-, 2- or 3-week intervals with crude saline extract to *T. spiralis* larvae (1.5 mg total protein) and complete adjuvant, and skin-tested 28, 56, or 84 days after initial sensitization, respectively. Approximately 24 hr after the skin test, lymph nodes (cervical, axillary, and inguinal) were removed and processed for electron microscopy: the cells were fixed in 6% glutaraldehyde and 1% osmium tetroxide in Sorenson's buffer (pH 7.2), dehydrated in ethanol and propylene oxide, embedded in Epon 812, and stained with uranyl acetate and lead citrate. Lymphocytes from animals sensitized at 1-week intervals were larger than normal lymphocytes. The nucleus showed patches of compact peripheral chromatin with a distinct nucleolus, and the cytoplasm contained many ribosomes together with a small amount of ergastoplasm showing no apparent organization, mitochondria, vesicles and Golgi bodies. Several classical plasma cells were also observed in this group. Lymphocytes from animals sensitized at 2-week intervals were more advanced than those from animals sensitized at 1-week intervals, and contained more of the structures generally associated with synthetic function. These cells had a more diffentiated appearance, i.e., in some the ribosomes occurred in aggregates, and the ergastoplasm was arranged in some cases as short pieces of reticulum localized in one part of the cell, while in others it appeared more generally distributed throughout the cytoplasm. The nucleus contained one or two nucleoli and clumped chromatin. Many more classical, mature antibody-forming plasma cells, in which the cytoplasm was filled with dilated ergastoplasmic sacs arranged in concentric lamellae around the nucleus, were observed in this group than in the first group. Lymphocytes from animals sensitized at 3-week intervals showed less development of the synthetic structural units in comparison to the previous two groups. These changes confirm that with optimal interval of antigenic stimulation, the sites of synthesis in individual lymphocytes develop to where they resemble plasma cells. Development of lymphocytes to cells so like plasma cells suggests that lymphocytes may indeed transform into plasma cells—at least into one type of plasma cell.

Acknowledgments

The authors thank John P. Shanley for technical assistance.
This work was supported by the U.S. Atomic Energy Commission.

References

Avrameas, S., and Leduc, E. (1970). Detection of simultaneous antibody synthesis in plasma cells and specialized lymphocytes in rabbit lymph nodes. *J. Exp. Med.* **131,** 1137–1168.

Balfour, B. M., Cooper, E. H., and Alpen, E. L. (1965). Morphological and kinetic studies on antibody-producing cells in rat lymph nodes. *Immunology* **8,** 230–244.

Brachet, J., and Mirsky, A. E. (1961). "The Cell," Vol. 11. Academic Press, New York.

Feldman, J. D., and Nordquist, R. E. (1967). Immunologic competence of thoracic duct cells, II. Ultrastructure. *Lab. Invest.* **16,** 564–579.

Harris, S., and Harris, T. N. (1949). Influenzal antibodies in lymphocytes of rabbits following the local injection of virus. *J. Immunol.* **61,** 193–207.

Harris, T. N., Grimm, E., Mertens, E., and Ehrich, W. E. (1945). The role of the lymphocyte in antibody formation. *J. Exp. Med.* **81,** 73–85.

Harris, T. N., Hummeler, K., and Harris, S. (1966). Electron microscopic observations on antibody-producing lymph node cells. *J. Exp. Med.* **123,** 161–172.

Hummeler, K., Harris, S., and Harris, T. N. (1966a). Fine structure of some antibody-producing cells. *Fed. Proc.* **25,** 1734–1738.

Hummeler, K., Harris, T. N., Tomassini, N., Hechtel, M., and Farber, M. B. (1966b). Electron microscopic observations on antibody-producing cells in lymph and blood. *J. Exp. Med.* **124,** 255–262.

Jamuar, M. P., Kim, C. W., and Hamilton, L. D. (1968). Fine structure of lymphocytes sensitized to *Trichinella spiralis* antigen. *J. Immunol.* **100,** 329–337.

Kim, C. W., Jamuar, M. P., and Hamilton, L. D. (1970). Delayed hypersensitivity to *Trichinella spiralis.* III. Effect of repeated sensitizations in donors and recipients. *J. Immunol.* **105,** 175–186.

Kim, C. W., Jamuar, M. P., and Hamilton, L. D. (1971). Transformation of lymphocytes from animals sensitized to *Trichinella spiralis. J. Immunol.* **107,** 1382–1389.

Schooley, J. C. (1961). Autoradiographic observations of plasma cell formation. *J. Immunol.* **86,** 331–337.

Uhr, J. W. (1966). Delayed hypersensitivity. *Physiol. Rev.* **46,** 359–419.

Vazquez, J. J. (1964). Kinetics of proliferation of antibody-forming cells. *In:* R. A. Good and A. E. Gabrielson (eds.), "The Thymus in Immunobiology." Hoeber Medical Division, Harper & Row, New York, pp. 298–316.

Wissler, R. W., Fitch, F. W., Lavia, M. F., and Gunderson, G. H. (1957). The cellular basis for antibody formation. *J. Cell. Comp. Physiol.* **50** (Suppl. 1), 265–301.

Zucker-Franklin, D. (1969). The ultrastructure of lymphocytes. *Semin. Hematol.* **6,** 4–27.

Protection against *Listeria monocytogenes* in Mice Following Infection with *Trichinella spiralis*

Raymond H. Cypess, Rolando Zapata, and David Gitlin

Department of Epidemiology and Microbiology
Graduate School of Public Health
University of Pittsburgh
Pittsburgh, Pennsylvania

Introduction

Chronic infection with intracellular parasites has been shown to provide nonspecific protection against phylogenetically unrelated intracellular organisms (Ruskin and Remington, 1968a; Kagan *et al.,* 1968; Ruskin *et al.,* 1969). This protection has been shown to be mediated through cellular as opposed to humoral factors (Ruskin and Remington, 1968b). According to Mackaness (1968), living agents that can induce this protection have been shown to have the following characteristics: (1) they are intracellular parasites; (2) they persist in the host's tissues; and (3) they provoke a state of cell-mediated hypersensitivity. Since *Trichinella spiralis,* an obligate multicellular parasite, produces a chronic intracellular infection of host muscle cells and has been shown by *in vivo* and *in vitro* reactions to induce cell-mediated hypersensitivity (Kim, 1966; Cypess *et al.,* 1971), experiments were undertaken to determine if *T. spiralis* could produce this type of protection.

Materials and Methods

Host

Eight-week-old female mice of the strain $B_6D_2F_1$ obtained from the Jackson Laboratory, Bar Harbor, Maine were used throughout this study.

319

Organisms

Listeria monocytogenes strain #984, was obtained from the American Type Culture Collection, Rockville, Maryland, and maintained in brain-heart infusion broth and agar. To obtain solubilized antigens from *L. monocytogenes,* the bacteria were killed in 5% formalin, washed, suspended in distilled water, and then sonicated in the presence of 100 glass beads; the suspension was cleared by centrifugation; and the supernatant antigens in solution were sterilized by filtration through a Millipore filter (Millipore Filter Corporation, Bedford, Massachusetts) with a pore size of 0.22 μm. Mice were immunized by an intraperitoneal injection of live LM every 2 weeks starting with 0.05 LD_{50}; the dose was gradually increased to 10 LD_{50} over a 10-week period (Hasanclever and Karakawa, 1957). The survivors were used as donors for serum 2 weeks after their last injection. Antibodies specific for *L. monocytogenes* were estimated by a radial immunodiffusion method (Mancini *et al.,* 1965).

The strain of *Trichinella spiralis* and the methods of isolating larvae for infection and recovering adult worms and larvae were those used by Larsh and Kent (1949).

Serologic Tests

Two types of *T. spiralis* antigens were utilized for detection of precipitating antibodies. The first was a Melcher's antigen and the second was a crude larval saline extract prepared according to the method of Larsh *et al.* (1969). Sera containing precipitating antibodies to *T. spiralis* were obtained from mice given three infections of 200 *T. spiralis* larvae at 21-day intervals (Hendricks, 1950). The bentonite flocculation test (BFT) was performed according to the method of Norman and Kagan (1963).*

Reticuloendothelial Activity

The rate of uptake of colloidal carbon by the reticuloendothelial system was measured by the method of Biozzi *et al.* (1953). Briefly, individual mice were injected with 0.2 ml of colloidal carbon (1:8 dilution in physiological saline of Pelikan ink, C11/1431A, Gunther Wagner, Hanover, Germany) and were bled with a Pasteur pipette washed in heparin from the venous orbital plexus at 30 seconds and 2, 5, 10, and 15 min after injection of the carbon suspension. Fifty μliters of each blood sample was diluted in 2.0 ml of 0.1% Na_2CO_3 and mixed well. The optical densities of each sample were read at 650 nm in a Coleman Jr. 6B Spectrophotometer using 10 $\times$ 75 mm microcuvettes. A blank of 0.1% Na_2CO_3 containing 50 μliters of normal mouse blood was used to obtain the extinction value.

---

*The *Trichinella* antigen and positive sera used for this test were kindly supplied by Dr. I. Kagan and Miss Lois Norman of the Center for Disease Control.

Experimental Design

Experiment I Mice were randomly divided into six groups of 10 mice. Five groups (experimentals) were orally infected with 200 *T. spiralis,* while five groups (controls) received sham inoculations. At 14, 21, 28, 35, and 56 days following infection, both experimentals and controls were injected intraperitoneally with an LD_{50} of *L. monocytogenes* (the various time periods tested represent replicate experiments with the same design).

Experiment II Twenty-eight days after infection with 200 *T. spiralis,* one group of experimental mice were given a second (challenging) infection of 200 *T. spiralis* to determine if the mice developed acquired immunity to the parasite. The controls received only the challenging infection.

Experiment III Mice immune to *L. monocytogenes* were challenged with 200 *T. spiralis* to determine if mice immune to *L. monocytogenes* were protected against infection by *T. spiralis*

Experiment IV Serologic cross reactivity between *T. spiralis* and *L. monocytogenes* antigens was determined using Ouchterlony and BFT methods.

Results

Experiment I

Mice infected orally with 200 *T. spiralis* larvae were protected against challenge with the intracellular bacteria, *Listeria monocytogenes* at days 21, 28, 35, and 56 days following infection (Table I).

Experiment II

The average number of adult worms recovered from both the experimental and control mice that received two infections of 200 *T. spiralis* were significantly different [experimentals 71.5 (56–82); controls 155 (172–141), $P < 0.01$]. Therefore, mice that were orally infected with 200 *T. spiralis* developed a demonstrable resistance to reinfection with the same agent.

Experiment III

The average number of larvae recovered from both mice immune to *L. monocytogenes* and control mice that received sham injections were not significantly different (Table II). Therefore, mice immune to *L. monocytogenes* did not show any evidence of protection against infection by *T. spiralis.*

Table I Challenge of Mice with *Listeria monocytogenes*

No. of cells of *Listeria*	Interval between infection and challenge (days)[a]	No. of mice that died/no. inoculated
6×10^7	14[b]	0/7
6×10^7	Control	1/7
2×10^8	14	4/7
2×10^8	Control	7/7
3×10^8	14	7/7
3×10^8	Control	7/7
6×10^7	21	0/10
6×10^7	Control	0/10
4×10^8	21	3/10
4×10^8	Control	10/10
6×10^8	21	4/10
6×10^8	Control	10/10
6×10^7	28	0/10
6×10^7	Control	0/10
2×10^8	28	1/10
2×10^8	Control	7/10
2×10^8	28	2/10
2×10^8	Control	8/10
6×10^7	35	0/10
6×10^7	Control	0/10
1.8×10^8	35	0/10
1.8×10^8	Control	10/10
3×10^8	35	8/10
3×10^8	Control	8/10
6×10^7	56	0/10
6×10^7	Control	0/10
1.8×10^8	56	2/10
1.8×10^8	Control	10/10
3×10^8	56	10/10
3×10^8	Control	10/10

[a] Animals had been infected orally with 200 *T. spiralis* the listed number of days before they were challenged intraperitoneally. Controls had not received *T. spiralis*.
[b] Day 14 not significantly different.
Days 21, 28, 35, 56 significantly different at $P < .01$.

Experiment IV

Serologic cross reactions between *Trichinella* and *Listeria* were absent as determined by bentonite flocculation and immunoprecipitation reactions. Therefore, cross protection to *L. monocytogenes* in mice following infection with *T. spiralis* does not appear to be mediated by humoral antibody.

Experiment V

The results of the carbon clearance stuides are presented in Table III. The rate of clearance *(K)* in control animals is fairly constant over

Table II Number of *T. spiralis* Larvae in Mice 28 Days after Oral Challenge with 200 *T. spiralis*

Mouse		Total count
Experimental[a]	1	4,680
	2	7,950
	3	9,750
	4	5,000
	5	13,100 .
	6	5,390
	7	8,060
	8	17,000
	9	2,250
	Av.	8,131
Control[b]	1	6,700
	2	9,200
	3	8,000
	4	8,780
	5	5,850
	6	12,200
	7	9,500
	8	7,800
	9	4,950
	Av.	8,109

[a] Animals had been injected intraperitoneally three times with *Listeria monocytogenes*.
[b] Controls had received sham injections

Table III Carbon Clearance in *T. spiralis*-Infected Mice

Time after infection[a]	K[b]	
	Control[c]	*T. spiralis*
0	0.060[d]	ND[e]
7	0.055	0.052
14	0.047	0.076
21	0.050	0.075
28	0.056	0.074
49	0.065	0.063

[a] Time in days after oral infection with 200 *T. spiralis* larvae

[b] $K = \dfrac{\log C_1 - \log C_2}{T_2 - T}$ (clearance constant), where C_1 = concentration (OD) of colloidal carbon in the blood at time, T_1, and C_2 = concentration of colloidal carbon (OD) in the blood at time T_2.
[c] Noninfected animals.
[d] Average K value for six mice.
[e] ND, not determined.

the 56-day test period. In *T. spiralis*-infected animals the rate of clearance is similar to controls at 7 days after infection but becomes accelerated at 14 days after infection and remains accelerated at 28 days after infection. By 49 days after infection the clearance rate of *T. spiralis*-infected animals has returned to control values.

Discussion

It is generally accepted that immunity to *L. monocytogenes* in mice is dependent entirely upon cellular mechanisms (Mackaness and Blanden, 1967). Although our failure to detect serologic cross reactions between *T. spiralis* and *L. monocytogenes* by the Ouchterlony or bentonite flocculation test does not entirely rule out the possibility that these two organisms share common functional antigens, our findings suggest that infection with *T. spiralis* confers nonspecific protection to a phylogenetically unrelated intracellular organism. This nonspecific protection was still present at 35 and 56 days following infection with *T. spiralis*. It is possible that this protection following *T. spiralis* infection could function as long as *Trichinella* antigen persisted in the host since following infection of mice with *Toxoplasma* and *Besnoita* nonspecific protection remained functional as long as parasitic infection remained patent in the host (Ruskin and Remington, 1968a).

Mice immune to *L. monocytogenes* did not show any nonspecific resistance to challenge with *T. spiralis*. This is in accordance with previous reports that vaccination of mice with Freund's complete adjuvant did not confer protection against this nematode (Larsh *et al.*, 1969), nor that *Listeria* infection conferred protection against challenge with *Toxoplasma* (Ruskin and Remington, 1968a).

The experiments on carbon clearance indicate that the nonspecific resistance to *Listeria* following *Trichinella* infection was not a function of increased phagocytic properties in the fixed cells of the reticuloendothelial system. This failure to correlate nonspecific protection with fixed RES activity has also been noted by Ruskin *et al.* (1969) and Lucia and Nussenzweig (1969).

In the case of nonspecific resistance to intracellular bacteria following protozoan infections, the peritoneal macrophage appears to be the effector arm of this resistance (Ruskin *et al.*, 1969). This same effector mechanism may be operating following *Trichinella* infections. Further work along these aspects appears to be warranted.

Summary

Trichinella spiralis, an obligate multicellular parasite, produces a chronic intracellular infection of host muscle cells. Mice given *Trichinella* were protected against challenge with the intracellular bacteria, *Listeria monocytogenes,* at days 21, 28, 35, and 56 following infection.

Conversely, mice immune to *Listeria* did not show any evidence of protection against infection by *Trichinella.* Serologic cross reactions between *Trichinella* and *Listeria* were absent as determined by bentonite flocculation and immunoprecipitation reactions. Carbon clearance determination failed to reveal any significant difference between *Trichinella*-infected animals and normal controls. These findings suggest that multicellular parasitic infection may confer nonspecific protection to unrelated intracellular organisms.

Acknowledgment

The work described in this chapter was supported by grant HD-01031 from the U.S. Public Health Service, and NIH grant AI-10490-02.

References

Biozzi, G., Benacerraf, B., and Halpern, B. (1953). Quantitative study of the granulopectic activity of the reticuloendothelial system II. *Brit. J. Exp. Pathol.* **34,** 441–457.

Cypess, R. H., Larsh, J. E., Jr., and Pegram, C. (1971). Macrophage inhibition produced by guinea pigs after sensitization with a larval antigen of *Trichinella spiralis. J. Parasitol.* **57,** 103–106.

Hasanclever, H. F., and Karakawa, W. W. (1957). Immunization of mice against *Listeria monocytogenes. J. Bacteriol.* **74,** 584–586.

Hendricks, J. R. (1950). The relationship between precipitin titer and number of *Trichinella spiralis* in the intestinal tract of mice following test infections. *J. Immunol.* **64,** 173–177.

Kagan, I. G., Norman, L., and Hall, E. C. (1968). The effect of infection with *Trypanosoma cruzi* on the development of spontaneous mammary cancer in mice. *In:* A. Anselmi (Ed.), p. 326–340. "Medicina Tropical" Mexico.

Kim, C. W. (1966). Delayed hypersensitivity to larval antigens of *Trichinella spiralis. J. Infec. Dis.* **116,** 208–214.

Larsh, J. E., Jr., and Kent, D. E. (1949). The effect of alcohol on acquired immunity to infection with *Trichinella spiralis. J. Parasitol.* **35,** 45–53.

Larsh, J. E., Jr., Goulson, H. T., Weatherly, N. F., and Chaffee, E. F. (1969). Studies on delayed (cellular) hypersensitivity in mice infected with *Trichinella spiralis* IV. Artificial sensitization of donors. *J. Parasitol.* **55,** 726–729.

Lucia, H. L., and Nussenzweig, R. S. (1969). *Plasmodium chabavdi* and *Plasmodium vinçkei:* Phagocytic activity of mouse reticuloendothelial system. *Exp. Parasitol.* **25,** 319–323.

Mackaness, G. B. (1968). The immunology of antituberculous immunity. *Amer. Rev. Resp. Dis.* **97,** 337–344.

Mackaness, G. B., and Blanden, R. V. (1967). Cellular immunity. *Progr. Allergy* **11,** 89–140.

Mancini, G., Carbonara, A. O., and Heremans, J. F. (1965). Immunochemical quantitation of antigens by single radial immunodiffusion. *Immunochemistry* **2,** 235–254.

Norman, L., and Kagan, I. G. (1963). Bentonite, latex and cholesterol flocculation tests for the diagnosis of trichinosis. *Publ. Health Rep.* **78,** 227–232.

Ruskin, J., and Remington, J. S. (1968a). Immunity and intracellular infection: Resistance to bacteria in mice infected with a protozoan. *Science* **160,** 72.

Ruskin, J., and Remington, J. S. (1968b). Role for the macrophage in acquired immunity to phylogenetically unrelated intracellular organisms. *Antimicrob. Ag. Chemother.* pp. 474–477.

Ruskin, J., McIntosh, J. and Remington, J. S. (1969). Studies on the mechanisms of resistance to phylogenetically diverse intracellular organisms. *J. Immunol.* **103,** 252–259.

Purification of a Leukoagglutinating Factor from *Trichinella spiralis* Larvae

Charles E. Tanner and Gaétan Faubert

Institute of Parasitology,
Macdonald College,
McGill University,
Province of Quebec

Introduction

Nonspecific inflammatory and specific immunological mechanisms reject incompatible skin grafts and neutralize toxinogenic bacteria. However, parasites seem to be able to escape the action of these mechanisms since they survive for considerable periods of time in the body of their hosts. There are a number of theories which attempt to explain this fascinating biological paradox. Sprent (1963) proposed that some parasites may escape rejection by containing or acquiring host antigens and, thus, impair the recognition of "not-self." This proposition has received support in the work of Damian (1964), Biguet *et al.* (1965), and Smithers *et al.* (1969). Recently, however, there have been reports that trypanosomes (Goodwin *et al.,* 1972), plasmodia (Greenwood *et al.,* 1972), and leishmania (Serebryakov *et al.,* 1972) suppress the immunological response of the infected host to foreign immunogens. The only nematode which induces this same phenomenon is *Trichinella spiralis.* Svet-Moldavsky *et al.* (1970) have found that trichinellosis in mice can prolong the acceptance time of skin homografts. We (Faubert and Tanner, 1971) have reported that *Trichinella* infections can suppress the capacity of mice to form antibodies to sheep erythrocytes; this capacity is possessed by the serum of infected mice, since normal animals treated with the serum of mice with trichinellosis are unable to respond fully to sheep erythrocytes.

In an attempt to relate this suppressive phenomenon to cellular immunological events, we discovered that the serum of mice infected with

327

Trichinella spiralis is capable of agglutinating and killing homologous lymph node cells.* We also discovered that these intriguing properties are possessed by crude saline extracts of *Trichinella* larvae. We immediately seized upon the possibility that this agglutinating property was due to the same substance which, during trichinellosis, inhibits the capacity of infected animals to respond to the normally immunogenic stimulus of foreign erythrocytes. This substance is of considerable interest because it also may be one of the substances by which the parasite is protected from the immunological response of the host.

We report here an attempt to purify this agglutinating principle from crude extracts of *Trichinella* larvae. The functional activity of chromatographic fractions rich in this factor, assayed in rabbits and in mice, indicates that it can enhance muscle trichinellosis.

Materials and Methods

The parasite used in this study was isolated 20 years ago from an infected pig. It has been kept since then by exclusive rat–rat passage in the Institute of Parasitology at McGill University.

Extraction of the Larvae

The preparation of the crude saline extract of muscle larvae was done as previously described (Tanner, 1970). Lyophilized larvae in the proportion of 1 gm/100 ml were suspended in phosphate-buffered saline, pH 7.2, and the antigens were extracted by ultrasounds from a 20 kHz 200 W Fisher BP-2 ultrasonic probe. The supernatant of the centrifuged extract was the crude antigen preparation.

Leukoagglutination Test

This test was done essentially as described by Greaves *et al.* (1969). Serial dilutions of chromatographic fractions of the extract were made in Medium 199 (Difco) in a volume of 0.2 ml. Pooled normal or infected mouse lymph node cells (2×10^5) in 0.2 ml of Medium 199 were added to each tube and the reaction was incubated for 60 min at 37° C. After incubation the agglutination titer was read as the highest dilution showing the agglutination of more than 10% of the cells added in the reaction. An illustration of the leukoagglutination obtained is shown in Fig. 1.

Chromatography

The crude buffered saline extract of *Trichinella* larvae was purified by passage through a 100×2.5 cm Sephadex G-200 column. Elution was

*A manuscript describing the biological properties of this factor is presently in preparation.

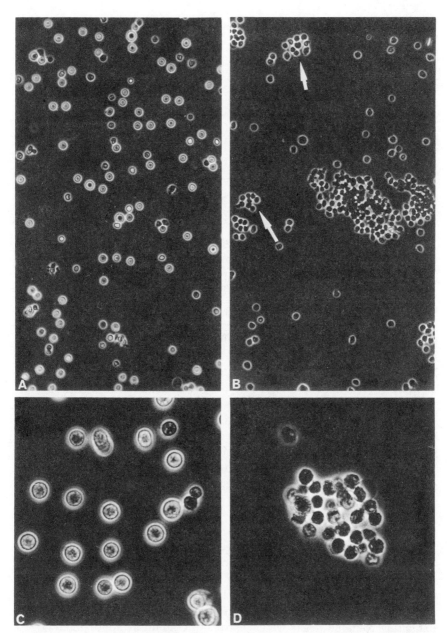

Figure 1 The agglutination of mouse lymph node cells by extracts of *Trinchinella* larvae. Lymph node cells suspended in medium 199 (A) × 360; (C) × 720. Lymph node cells suspended in medium 199 containing a crude extract of *Trichinella* larvae (B) × 360; (D) × 720. Phase-contrast.

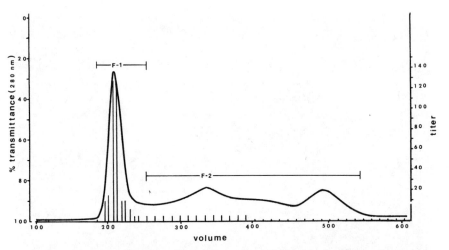

Figure 2 Elution profile of a crude extract of *Trichinella* larvae chromatographed through a 100 × 2.5 cm G-200 column, showing those fractions containing leukoagglutinating activity. Elution with phosphate–buffered saline, pH 7.2, at 5 ml/hr.

achieved at 5° C with the same buffer used to extract the larvae. The rate of elution was 5 ml/hr; the 10-ml fractions taken were collected by an LKB Ultro-Rac and the column effluents were monitored at 280 nm by an LKB Uvicord adsorptiometer. In one experiment two pooled fractions from the G-200 column were further fractionated through 100 × 2.3 cm DEAE-cellulose columns. The absorbant was prepared for chromatography as recommended by Peterson and Sober (1962) and the column was packed under 10 pounds pressure (Fahey *et al.*, 1958). Two fractions were taken from each of the G-200 fractions: one was eluted with 0.1 *M* and the other with 1.0 *M* NaCl the salt was dissolved in phosphate buffer pH 8.0.

Results

The G-200 elution profile of the components of the crude *Trichinella* extract (Fig. 2) is characterized by a prominent peak of macromolecules with a molecular weight of approximately 340,000 daltons. The rest of the components of the extract are dispersed along a series of elution volumes exhibiting rounded peaks which leave the column at approximately 350 and 500 ml. It is a curious fact that the large majority of the antigens against which antibodies are formed during infections are associated with the second peak; very few antigens can be discerned in pooled fractions of the first peak—even when the analysis is done with a serum of rabbits hyperimmunized with the parasite extract. The third peak is composed largely of polypeptides.

When individual fractions of the column are incubated with lymph node cells, only those eluting under the macromolecular first peak agglutinate the leukocytes. There is virtually no activity in any of the other fractions. The lethal activity of the parasite extract is also in the same macromolecular fraction.

The fractions collected under the first peak were pooled as G-200 Fraction 1 and the fractions under the second peak were pooled as G-200 Fraction 2. The two pooled G-200 fractions were further refined by refractionation through DEAE-cellulose columns. The biological activity of all of these components of the crude extract of *Trichinella* larvae was tested in mice. One hundred Swiss mice of the Charles River strain were divided into 10 groups of 10 animals each and were either not treated or injected with physiological saline, 5% sheep red blood cells, the whole crude extract of the larvae (TSE), the G-200 Fractions 1 or 2, or DEAE-cellulose fractions of these two. All the parasite antigen preparations were adjusted to contain 0.5 mg protein/ml; each animal was injected eight times with 0.1 ml intramuscularly: six injections were made in the 2 weeks preceeding inoculation with larvae, one other was made 24 hr before and another 24 hr after inoculation with larvae. Each animal received a total of 0.4 mg protein in the treatments. Freund's adjuvant was not used. The animals were each inoculated with 100 larvae; the mice were killed 30 days after inoculation and the number of larvae in each carcass was determined after peptic digestion. The results of this experiment are presented in Table I.

The results of this experiment clearly confirm that the crude extract of larvae protects the animals treated with it; fewer parasites were recovered from the mice treated with this substance than from the controls. On the other hand, the mice treated with G-200 Fraction 1 (the one which contained the agglutinating factor) bore considerably more larvae than the

Table I   The Mean Recovery of Muscle Larvae from Mice Treated with Purified Fractions of a Buffered Saline Extract (TSE) of *Trichinella spiralis* Larvae

Treatment	Recovery
—	3107
Saline	3117
TSE	2530
G-200F1	5030
G-200F2	1710
G-200F1 (DEAE 0.1M)	3445
G-200F1 (DEAE 1.0M)	2950
G-200F2 (DEAE 0.1M)	2195
G-200F2 (DEAE 1.0M)	3210
5% Sheep RBC	4319

controls. Those animals which had been treated with the second G-200 fraction were also protected from the parasite, since fewer larvae developed in these animals than in the controls.

The results obtained with the DEAE fractions were not as clear-cut, but one can discern a tendency to an enhancement of parasitism in animals treated with G-200 Fl eluted from DEAE with 0.1 M NaCl; G-200 F2 eluted from DEAE with the same 0.1 M buffer tended to protect the animals treated with it. It is significant to mention that the level of muscle infection was also enhanced in those control animals treated with sheep erythrocytes.

A similar experiment was done in a group of 14 rabbits. These animals were inoculated intramuscularly nine times with saline or the crude extract of the larvae (TSE) or the first or the second G-200 fractions. No adjuvant was used in the injections. Each animal received a total of 0.6 mg protein over a period of 3 weeks; 7 days after the last injection each animal was inoculated with 20 larvae per gram muscle (6000 larvae in a 1000-gm animal). The animals were killed 30 days after inoculation and the number of larvae in each carcass was determined after peptic digestion. The results of this experiment are presented in Table II.

These results indicate even more dramatically the protective action of both the crude extract of the larvae and the second G-200 fraction. The enhancing activity of the first G-200 fraction on the level of muscle infection is also clearly evident in this illustration.

Discussion

The factors which govern the establishment of *Trichinella spiralis* in the muscles of its host are still a tantalizing mystery. Because this highly organized animal lives within the very sophisticated environment of the host, the factors which control parasite numbers must be complex. Probably no one mechanism is primary in any one host–parasite association; each association may present quantive and qualitative differences in the

Table II The Mean Recovery of Muscle Larvae from Rabbits Treated with Purified Fractions of a Buffered Saline Extract (TSE) of *Trichinella spiralis* Larvae

Number of Animals	Treatment	Recovery[a]
3	Saline	194
4	TSE	1.7
4	G-200F1	467
3	G-200F2	5

[a] Larvae per gram muscle.

roles played by nonspecific inflammatory or by specific immunological phenomena.

The results of these experiments suggest that *Trichinella* larvae contain substances which are able to enhance or suppress muscle invasion. The interaction of these parasite substances with the protective mechanisms of the host may be one of the factors which can determine the intensity of infection. It is of considerable interest that the purified fraction from the *Trichinella* larvae which enhanced infection also contained a substance which agglutinates and kills lymph node cells. These results also suggest that the establishment and maintenance of *T. spiralis* in the tissues of an animal may be due, at least in part, to the action of this factor on lymphoid tissues.

The enhancing effect on muscle parasitism of injections with sheep erythrocytes clearly indicates that a phenomenon of antigenic competition may also operate to facilitate establishment of the worm. The deflection of the protective mechanisms by an immunogolical response to "nonessential" antigens derived from the parasite or from damaged host tissue would enhance the probability of a successful infection. Studies are currently underway to further characterize some of these substances.

Summary

Partial purification of a substance from *Trichinella* larvae which agglutinates mouse lymph node cells was achieved by G-200 chromatography. An assay of the biological activity of the gel fractions in mice and in rabbits revealed that the larvae contain substances which either enhance or suppress muscle parasitism. The enhancing fractions contained the leukocyte-agglutinating substance. It is probable that these substances play a role in the establishment and maintenance of *Trichinella* infections in experimental animals.

Acknowledgment

Supported by the Ministère des Affaires Sociales de la Province de Québec and the National Research Council of Canada.

References

Biguet, J., Rosé, F., Capron, A., and Tran Van Ky, P. (1965). Contribution de l'analyse immunoélectrophorétique á la connaissance des antigènes vermineux. Incidences pratiques sur leur standardisation, leur purification et le diagnostique des helminthioses par immunoélectrophorèse. *Rev. Immunol.* **29**, 5–30.

Damian, R. T. (1964). Molecular mimicry: antigen sharing by parasite and host and its consequences. *Amer. Natur.* **98,** 129–149.

Faubert, G., and Tanner, C. E. (1971). *Trichinella spiralis:* inhibition of sheep hemagglutinins in mice. *Exp. Parasitol.* **30,** 120–123.

Fahey, J. L., McCoy, P. F., and Goolian, M. (1958). Chromatography of serum proteins in normal and pathologic sera: The distribution of protein-bound carbohydrate and cholestrol, siderophilin, thyroxin-binding protein, B_{12}-binding protein, alkaline and acid phosphatases, radio-iodinated albumin and myeloma protein. *J. Clin. Invest.* **37,** 272–284.

Goodwin, L. G., Green, D. G., Guy, M. W., and Voller, A. (1972). Immunosuppression during trypanosomiasis. *Brit. J. Exp. Pathol.* **53,** 40–43.

Greaves, M. F., Tursi, A., Playfair, J. H. L., Torrigiani, G., Zamir, R., and Roitt, I. M. (1969). Immunosuppressive potency and *in vitro* activity of ALS globulin. *Lancet,* 11 Jan., pp. 6–72.

Greenwood, B. M., Bradley-Moore, A. M., Palit, A., and Bryceson, A. D. M. (1972). Immunosuppression in children with Malaria. *Lancet,* 22 Jan. pp. 169–172.

Peterson, E. A., and Sober, H. A. (1962). Column chromatography of proteins: substituted celluloses. *In:* "Methods in Enzymology," Vol. 5. Academic Press, New York, pp. 3–27.

Serebryakov, V. A., Karakhodzhaeva, S., and Dzhumaev, M. D. (1972). On the effect of leishmanial vaccinations on the dynamics of immunity to diptheria under conditions of second vaccination with ADPT vaccine. *Med. Parasitol. Parasit. Dis.* **41,** 303–307. (In Russ. w. Engl. summ.)

Smithers, S. R., Terry, R. J., and Hockley, D. J. (1969). Host antigens in schistosomiasis. *Proc. Roy. Soc.* **171,** 483–494.

Sprent, J. F. A. (1963). "Parasitism." Baillière, Tindal and Cox, Co., London.

Svet-Moldavsky, G. J., Shaghijan, G. S., Chernyakhovskaya, I. Y., Mkheidze, D. M., Litovchenko, T. A., Ozeretskovskaya, N. N., and Kadaghidze, Z. G. (1970). Inhibition of skin allograft rejection in *Trichinella* infected mice. *Transplantation* **9,** 69–70.

Tanner, C. E. (1970). Immunochemical study of the antigens of *Trichinella spiralis* larvae. IV. Purification by continuous-flow paper electrophoresis and column chromatography. *Exp. Parasitol.* **27,** 116–135.

The Immunosuppressive Effect of Freund's Adjuvant on Resistance of Chinese Hamsters to the Tissue Phase of *Trichinella spiralis*

Albert L. Ritterson

Department of Microbiology
University of Rochester School of Medicine
Rochester, New York

Introduction

Both golden *(Mesocricetus auratus)* and Chinese *(Cricetulus griseus)* hamsters are susceptible to primary infection with *Trichinella.* The response of the latter host differs from that of the golden hamster, and most other experimental hosts, in that it rejects all or most of the muscle phase of the parasite. This occurs after junveniles have effected penetration of the host cells and have begun to grow. The process of rejection is accompanied by an intense, focalized round cell infiltration at the site occupied by the worm. The granuloma, which is clearly evident by the ninth day of the infection, reaches maximum intensity by about the fourteenth day; thereafter, it gradually subsides. Tissue-dwelling worms can be recovered, in dimishing numbers, through the nineteenth day, but these juveniles rarely exceed 200 μm in length. At least 10% of the infecting dose persists as adults in the gut after 18 days of infection (Concannon and Ritterson, 1965.)

Functional and histological similarities between events which occur in tissues of Chinese hamsters with primary infections and those of other host species responding to reinfection (Larsh, 1963) suggests that resistance is dependent upon early activation of the immune response in this "abnormal" host. Alternatively, resistance of Chinese hamsters has been characterized as innate (Ritterson, 1959). In an attempt to evaluate these dissimilar though not inconsistent bases for resistance, it was decided to study some of the parameters of antibody response in *Trichinella*-infected Chinese hamsters.

Owing to the small size of Chinese hamsters, serum yields are low and are somewhat difficult to obtain. Therefore, the method described by Munoz (1957) for producing large volumes of ascitic fluid in mice by the intraperitoneal injection of Freund's adjuvant was employed. While failing

335

to produce significant amounts of ascitic fluid in the Chinese hamster, the adjuvant brought about an unexpected suppression of host resistance which initiated the present study.

Materials and Methods

Chinese hamsters used in this study were adult males approximately 3 months of age. Animals were maintained on Purina Laboratory Chow supplemented twice weekly with lettuce.

Infection and Carcass Larva Recovery

Trichinella spiralis is maintained in this laboratory by serial passage through golden hamsters. The techniques employed for transfer of infection and subsequent quantification of carcass larvae have been previously described (Ritterson, 1959). In all experiments, the infectious dose was administered *(per os)* at the level of approximately 200 larvae per animal. Carcass larva recoveries were carried out at 28–33 days of infection.

Adjuvants

A single injection (0.3 ml, intraperitoneally) of Freund's complete adjuvant (Difco) was given to each hamster in a series of experiments. Studies were carried out using animals which were treated 18 days prior to infection, on the day of infection, and 6, 14, and 21 days after infection. Two experiments were performed in which complete adjuvant was administered by the subcutaneous route (0.3 ml; groin) on the day of infection and on 0 and 1 of infection. One experiment was carried out using a single injection (0.3 ml, intraperitoneally) of Freund's incomplete adjuvant (Difco) which was administered on the day of infection.

Endotoxin (lipopolysaccharide B; *Escherichia coli* 055:B5; Difco) was prepared in sterile saline and given as a single injection (0.2 ml; 50 μg; intraperitoneally). In separate experiments, groups of hamsters were treated (once each) on days 1, 3, 6, 14, and 21 after infection. Each experiment was conducted with a group of infected, untreated controls.

Evaluation of Granulomas

In several experiments, granulomatous reactions to tissue-invading juveniles were appraised in the following way. Freund's treated (0.3 ml, intraperitoneally, day 0) Chinese hamsters were killed at weekly intervals beginning on the seventh day after infection. A similar series of untreated, infected controls was sacrificed for comparison. Cheek pouch retractor muscles were removed, fixed, stained, and mounted as previously described (Ritterson, 1957). By this method, the full expanse of each lesion and associated cellular responses can be observed. All lesions were drawn in outline using the camera lucida. Subsequently, drawings were classed according to the assessed age of lesions represented; a chronological sequence was compiled for purposes of illustration (Fig. 2). Photomicrographic representations of identical lesions have been published (Ritterson, 1959).

Results

Intraperitoneal administration of Freund's complete adjuvant induces the formation of an intense, rapidly developing abdominal granuloma in Chinese hamsters. Granulomas developed in over 70% of the treated animals; among these there was a 30% mortality within 20–30 days of treatment. Characteristically, the lesion localizes to form a tough mass which encases, compresses, and generally obscures the spleen. The reaction mass gradually extends to include the liver, spleen, and diaphragm in a thick encapsulated unit. The body wall becomes somewhat thickened and varying degrees of diffuse infiltration of other abdominal viscera develop. Ascites is minimal. There was no evidence of adjuvant-induced arthritis.

Of 20 hamsters receiving Freund's complete adjuvant intraperitoneally) on the day of infection, 17 developed abdominal granulomas and 15 survived the term of the experiment. Three animals showed no evidence of adjuvant-induced lesions; their carcasses yielded a mean of 151 worms recovered by digestion with pepsin (Fig. 1). Eleven hamsters showed the lesions described above and yielded a mean of 6300 carcass larvae (Fig. 1). In one animal, a portion of the spleen protruded from the granuloma as a large hypertrophied mass. In this case, full resistance was expressed; larvae were not recovered in the carcass digest.

Adjuvant administered 18 days prior to infection or as late as 6 days after infection resulted in corresponding suppression of host resistance. Of five animals receiving Freund's 18 days prior to infection, three survived yielding a mean recovery of 4300 carcass larvae (Fig. 1). Three animals which had been treated with adjuvant 6 days after infection yielded a mean of 3800 worms (Fig. 1); a fourth animal in this group died. Each of two groups of five animals treated at 14 and 21 days, respectively, survived the term of the experiment. Neither of the latter two groups revealed any evidence of suppression of resistance as measured by recovery of carcass larvae (Fig. 1); all had moderately developed abdominal granulomas at necropsy.

Each of a group of five animals was given Freund's complete adjuvant by subcutaneous injection (0.3 ml) on the day of infection. Of these, three developed large granulomas at the site of the injection; they yielded a mean of 720 carcass larvae (Fig. 1). The two remaining animals exhibited no lesions and yielded no carcass larvae. Of 10 animals receiving two

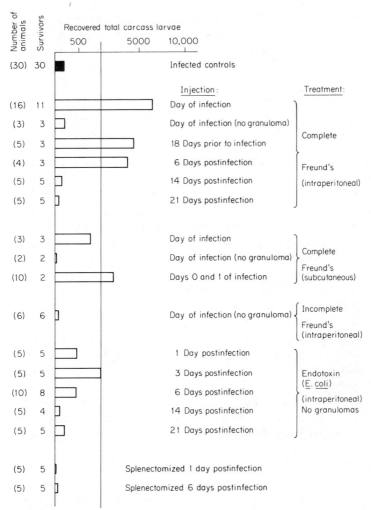

Figure 1 Effects of Freund's adjuvant, bacterial endotoxin, and splenectomy on recoveries of total carcass larvae from Chinese hamsters infected with *Trichinella spiralis*.

separate injections (0.5 ml, subcutaneously) on days 0 and 1 of infection, eight died within 24 hours of the second injection; presumably of a Shwartzman-like reaction. The two survivors had large, localized granulomas at necropsy; their carcasses yielded a mean of 2040 larvae (Fig. 1).

Six animals treated with Freund's incomplete adjuvant (0.3 ml, intraperitoneally) on the day of infection developed no abdominal lesions; their carcasses yielded a mean of 40 worms (Fig. 1).

Animals treated with bacterial endotoxin (*Escherichia coli*; 50 μg, intraperitoneally) exhibited a moderate suppression of resistance when the

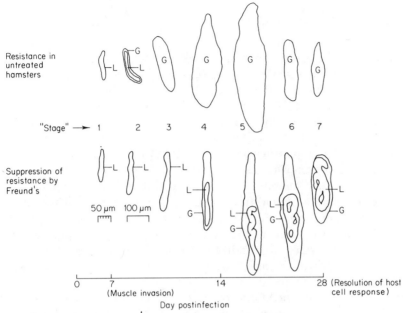

Resistance in untreated hamsters

"Stage" ⟶ 1   2   3   4   5   6   7

Suppression of resistance by Freund's

50 μm   100 μm

0   7   14   28 (Resolution of host cell response)
(Muscle invasion)
Day postinfection

Figure 2 Tissue response in cheek pouch muscle of Chinese hamster infected with *Trichinella spiralis* and suppression of innate resistance by Freund's adjuvant. L, larvae; G, granuloma. (Camera lucida outline drawings.)

injections were given at 1, 3, or 6 days after infection (Fig. 1). Recoveries of carcass larvae from animals treated at 14 or 21 days postinfection corresponded with those of the infected, untreated controls (Fig. 1)

Each of the preceding experiments was controlled with untreated, infected animals. Recoveries of their carcass larvae were averaged and expressed as a single value for convenience (Fig. 1; mean; 165; range, 0–260).

Splenectomies were performed on five animals the day after infection and five others on the sixth day. Neither of these groups showed impairment of resistance as measured by recovery of carcass larvae (Fig. 1).

Eighteen *Trichinella*-infected Chinese hamsters were sacrificed in groups of six at 10, 14, and 28 days postinfection. Camera lucida outline drawings were made of all lesions observed in stained whole mount preparations of cheek pouch retractor muscles. By comparing the range of intensity of lesions seen at each necropsy interval, an estimated chronological sequence of these foci was chosen and arranged for illustration (Fig. 2). Despite the arbitrary nature of this choice, it was clearly evident that juvenile trichinellae invaded host cells and appeared normal early in the infection. This was followed by some growth of the contained parasite; closely followed by an influx of host round cells. Although the host cell reaction could not be quantitatively differentiated as to cell type, it was evident that they were predominantly lymphoid-macrophage in character. Neutrophils were scant in the granulomatous foci. Subsequently, the focal lesions enlarged, reaching a peak size at about the second week of infection. Thereafter, the lesions subsided leaving no traces of the parasite. It was estimated that larvae did not persist beyond a few days after the development of the focal granuloma. At least, no larva was observed within well-developed lesions (Fig. 2).

Another group of 18 hamsters was injected with Freund's complete adjuvant (0.3 ml, intraperitoneally) on the day of infection. These animals were sacrificed in groups of six at 10, 14, and 28 days postinfection. Retractor muscle whole mounts were prepared and evaluated as before. In this series, larvae were found throughout the time sequence of the study (Fig. 2). The round cell infiltration was significantly delayed and never reached the intensity seen in the untreated group (Fig. 2). Indeed, the worm-containing lesions were indistinguishable from those seen in cortisone treated animals of an earlier study (Ritterson, 1959). Growth of tissue larvae appeared to be normal; as if, in a natural host.

In a parallel study, the effects of treatment with Freund's adjuvant on the growth of tissue juveniles was compared with that from infected, untreated Chinese hamsters. Each of eight animals was infected with 200 larvae; half were treated with adjuvant (intraperitioneally) on the day of infection. Animals were sacrificed, in pairs, at 8, 15, and 21 days after infection. At necropsy, 1 gm of muscle was taken from each animal and digested in trypsin. Slides were prepared from sediments of these digests by spreading the "mush" over uniform areas of several slides. The wet digest was fixed with hot Schaudin's fluid and stained with hematoxylin. For each animal, 100 larvae were drawn by camera lucida and subsequently measured with a calibrated caliper. An estimate was made of the area of the slides which had to be scanned in order to draw the worms. From the latter, the numbers of larvae recovered from each animal relative to those recovered from the 8-day untreated control could be estimated.

At 8 days of infection, there was no apparent difference between the sizes of larvae recovered from either animal (Table I). Larvae recovered from the Freund's treated animal were roughly equal in numbers to those from the untreated control. At 15 days of infection, worms derived from two untreated controls showed that growth of the intracellular parasite had occurred in the resistant host. Recovered larvae were about as numerous as those recovered from the control at 8 days of infection. However, the maximum lengths of worms recovered from adjuvant-suppressed animals, at the same time interval were considerably greater (Table I). This is taken to support the view, suggested above, that, in the Chinese hamster, the cut-off time for survival of tissue trichinellae occurs at about 2 weeks after infection. Worms recovered from Freund's-treated

Table I Size Ranges of Larvae Recovered from Freund's Treated and Untreated Chinese Hamsters by Tryptic Digestion

Day post infection	Treatment	No. larvae counted/measured	Size range of larvae (μm)		Median length (μm)
			Minimum	Maximum	
8	None	100	63	105	81
8	Freund's	100	60	102	82
15	None	100	57	117	78
15	None	100	61	126	82
15[a]	Freund's	100	58	150	80
15[a]	Freund's	100	81	205	107
21	None	(None found)	–	–	–
21[b]	Freund's	100	70	474	112

[a] Estimated to be five times more numerous than 8-day untreated control.
[b] Estimated to be 8 to 10 times more numerous than 8-day untreated control.

animals at 15 days of infection were estimated to be five times more abundant than the recovery from the control of the 8-day infection. After 21 days of infection, worms were not found in the trypsin digest of the untreated control (Table I). The corresponding adjuvant-treated hamster yielded larvae in numbers estimated to be 8 to 10 times the recovery from the untreated 8-day control. The maximum length of recovered worms reached 474 μm (Table I). The latter value is low owing to the fact that larger worms failed to adhere to the slides and were not measured. Moreover, the minimum size of recovered larvae and the relatively low value for median length of worms indicates persistence of productive females in the gut beyond expectation. This suggests that the immunosuppressive effect of adjuvant-induced granuloma was effective against both the tissue and gut phases of the parasite.

A final study was carried out in which five Chinese hamsters were immunized by infection with 200 larvae. After 35 days of infection, these animals were reinfected with 300 worms and simultaneously treated with Freund's as previously. At 28 days after the second infection, retractor muscle preparations were made from these animals. The lesions were found to contain developed larvae which were identical with those of corresponding Freund's treated animals (above) with primary infections. The mean recovery of carcass larvae from this group of animals was 2000. A group of five correspondingly reinfected controls yielded no larvae from total carcass digests.

Discussion

In his studies on the development of *Nippostrongylus muris* in abnormal hosts, Lindquist (1950) found that tissue invading larvae elicited a prompt granulomatous response which resulted in the loss of most parasites. Moreover, he indicate the similarity of this response to that seen after reinfection of the natural host.

In the same sense, the Chinese hamster is an abnormal host for *Trichinella,* at least, during its somatic phase. This animal readily accepts primary infection which it supports in an unremarkable way in the gut phase (Concannon and Ritterson, 1965); juveniles are abundantly produced and penetrate host muscle cells. Subsequently, there is a short period of growth of the intracellular parasite (Table I) followed by an intense focal granulomatous response (Fig. 2), chiefly lymphoid-macrophage, by the host. Host reaction reahces maximum intensity at about the second week of infection after which it subsides (Fig. 2), rarely leaving a trace of either the infectious agent or host response (i.e., scarring). It is noteworthy that this corresponds with the time of development of the supposedly immunogenic stichosome (Ali Khan, 1966; Despommier, 1971).

It has already been shown that the immunosuppressives, cortisone (Ritterson 1959) and methotrexate (Ritterson, 1968) impair resistance to the tissue phase of *Trichinella* in the Chinese hamster. The mechanisms of action of these agents offer a number of explanations; one of which, specific immune suppression, they have in common. Enhanced development of tissue juveniles in hamsters with separate granulomatous response to Freund's adjuvant can be interpreted in the same way. It has also been shown that cortisone, methotrexate, and adjuvant-induced granuloma impair resistance of Chinese hamsters to the luminal parasite *Hymenolepis microstoma* (Ritterson, 1971). Seemingly, the mechanism responsible for impairment of resistance by Freund's is that of preoccupying (drawing off) the host's cellular immune mechanism with the classically cellular response to mycobacterial antigens. Although adjuvant granulomas "draw off" large numbers of lymphoid-macrophage cells, the fact that several observed instances of splenic hypertrophy among these animals preserved resistance suggests a compensatory cellular response. In these few animals, extrasplenic pathological changes due to the granuloma were identical to those observed in hamsters not showing splenic hypertrophy. In one instance, loss of immunosuppressive effect of Freund's granuloma by splenic hypertrophy was observed in the *Hymenolepsis*-Chinese hamster system (Ritterson, 1971). Impairment of resistance of *Trichinella* by bacterial endotoxin (Fig. 1) supports the view that the host's immune mechanisms are being affected in a complex way by the agents employed in this study. Even though the means by which adjuvant-induced granulomas impair resistance are not clear, it would seem that, to some degree, it is dependent upon suppression of specific cellular immunity. It has recently been found (Lipton and Ritterson, unpublished) that there is a prompt, specific humoral response in Chinese hamsters infected with *Trichinella* and that the host responds anamnestically to reinfection. The present study shows that adjuvant-induced granuloma can override resistance to reinfection. Impairment of resistance in animals with preformed antibody by a procedure which "diverts" large numbers of cells of the lymphoid-macrophage series admits to the interpretation that cellular immunity is involved in rejection of the parasite (xenograft). It has also recently found (Ritterson, unpublished) that resistance to the tissue phase of *Trichinella* occurs in Chinese hamsters which have been infected only by direct inoculation of juveniles intracardially or into muscle. This finding clearly separates tissue resistance from immunologically complicating events which occur in the naturally infected host. It also emphasizes the generally neglected role of tissue resistance to the parenteral phase of *Trichinella*.

Summary

The Chinese hamster *(Cricetulus griseus)* is peculiarly refractory to establishment of the parenteral phase of infection with *Trichinella spiralis*. This host characteristically yields 0–200 carcass larvae after 30 days of infection by 200 or more worms. In this animal, it has been shown that injection of Freund's complete adjuvant (0.3 ml, intraperitoneally) usually induces an intense abdominal granuloma which encases and obscures the spleen. The granuloma itself becomes heavily infiltrated with cells of the lymphoid-macrophage series. Infected animals which develop granulomas lose resistance to the maturation of tissue larvae (mean of recoveries of carcass larvae: 6700). Rarely, the spleen escapes entrapment, in which case it undergoes marked hypertrophy. These animals maintain their normal resistance. Splenectomy of untreated, infected hamsters does not affect their resistance to tissue trichinellae. Adjuvant-treated animals which fail to develop granulomas also maintain their normal resistance. Granulomatous reactions which are induced later than 6 days postinfection are not effective as immunosuppressives.

Administration of complete adjuvant by the subcutaneous route often evokes a local response which is less intense than the abdominal lesions. The latter route of administration is correspondingly less effective as an immunosuppressive. Incomplete Freund's adjuvant does not induce granuloma and is not immunosuppressive. Bacterial endotoxin *(E. coli)*, which does not elicit a tissue response by the host, is moderately immunosuppressive when administered no later than the sixth day of infection.

Acknowledgment

This investigation was supported in part by grant AI-01042 from the U.S. Public Health Service.

References

Ali Khan, Z. (1966). The postembryonic development of *Trichinella spiralis* with special reference to ecdysis. *J. Parasitol.* **52**, 248–259.

Concannon, J., and Ritterson, A. L. (1965). Comparative recoveries of adult worms from Chinese and golden hamsters fed known doses of *Trichinella spiralis. J. Parasitol.* **51**, 938-941.

Despommier, D. D. (1971). Immunogenicity of the newborn larva of *Trichinella spiralis. J. Parasitol.* **57**, 531–534.

Larsh, J. E., Jr., (1963). Experimental trichinosis. *Advan. Parasitol.* **1**, 213–286.

Lindquist, W. D. (1950). Some abnormal host relationships of a rat nematode, *Nippostronglylus muris. Amer. J. Hyg.* **52**, 22–41.

Munoz, J. (1957). Production in mice of large volumes of ascites fluid containing antibodies. *Proc. Soc. Exp. Biol. Med.* **95**, 757–759.

Ritterson, A. L. (1957). The Chinese hamster *(Cricetulus griseus)* as an experimental host for *Trichinella spiralis. J. Parasit.* **43**, 542–547.

Ritterson, A. L. (1959). Innate resistance of species of hamsters to *Trichinella spiralis* and its reversal by cortisone. *J. Infec. Dis.* **105**, 253–266.

Ritterson, A. L. (1968). Effect of immunosuppressive drugs (6-mercaptopurine and methotrexate) on resistance of Chinese hamsters to the tissue phase of *Trichinella spiralis. J. Infec. Dis.* **118**, 365–369.

Ritterson, A. L. (1971). Resistance of Chinese hamsters to *Hymenolepsis microstoma* and its reversal by immunosuppression. *J. Parasitol.* **57**, 1247–1250.

The Stage Specificity of the Immune Response to *Trichinella spiralis*

E. R. James and D. A. Denham

Department of Helminthology,
London School of Hygiene and Tropical Medicine
London

Introduction

Oliver-González (1941) suggested that both intestinal adults and muscle larvae are immunogenic and that antibody production in *Trichinella spiralis* infections is, to a certain degree, stage specific. The intestinal phase of *T. spiralis* has been shown to be immunogenic by Kim (1957), Campbell (1965), and Denham (1966a,b). Immunogenicity of the muscle larvae has been demonstrated by Campbell (1955), Despommier and Wostman (1968), and by Despommier (1971).

Since Dennis *et al.* (1970) developed the technique for producing large numbers of newborn larvae it has been possible to work with the migrating stage larvae toward establishing the immunogenicity of this stage. Despommier (1971) showed that rats inoculated intravenously (iv) with newborn larvae had a significantly reduced muscle burden after a normal challenge infection. Rats immunized by muscle stage larvae contained in diffusion chambers and challenged by injection of newborn larvae iv harbored similar numbers of muscle larvae as did controls.

Using drug abbreviated intestinal infections and injections of newborn larvae the present studies were aimed at a further analysis of the stage specificity of immunity to *T. spiralis* infections in mice.

Materials and Methods

The London strain of *Trichinella spiralis* was used, and the experimental host animals were female albino mice of the T.O. strain, approximately 6 weeks old and weighing 25 gm at the beginning of each experiment.

The methods for obtaining viable muscle larvae by the standard digestion procedure, oral infection of mice with these larvae, and the enumeration of encysted muscle larvae were described previously by Denham (1965, 1968).

The method of obtaining viable newborn larvae differed from that described by Dennis *et al.* (1970) in some details. Rats or mice were killed on day 6 after oral inoculation with infective larvae, the entire small intestine was removed, cut lengthwise, and washed briefly in warm tap water to remove the digesta. The intestines were put into 0.85% saline at 37° C and incubated for 1 hr, then washed and discarded. The saline, and washings, were passed through 2 sieves; a 300-μm sieve removed any large unwanted particles, and adult worms were recovered from a 74-μm sieve and put into a Baermann apparatus containing culture medium for 1½ hr at 37° C. Adult worms were then run off into a 20-ml centifuge tube and allowed to settle. The supernatant was discarded and the worms were resuspended in culture medium supplemented with merthiolate at a concentration of 1:20,000; this washing was repeated twice more and all further operations were conducted in a sterile environment.

Each 100 ml of culture medium contained 88 ml of medium 199 (BDH), 2 ml sodium bicarbonate solution (BDH 4.4% v/w), and 10 ml heated horse serum no. 1 (Wellcome). Fifty mg of Penbritin ampicillin, Beecham Research Labs.) and 12,500 units of Mycostatin (Nystatin, Squibb) were added.

Approximately 2000 adult worms were added to the 100 ml of culture medium in a 200-ml roller bottle which was sealed and kept rotating at approximately 15 rph at 37° C.

After 24 hr, during which time newborn larvae were shed, the culture medium was passed through a 53-μm sieve to remove the adult worms and centrifuged at 1500 rpm for 5 min in 20-ml conical tubes. The supernatant was removed and the sedimented larvae were pooled and resuspended in medium 199. Samples of the suspension were counted for larvae using a bright line haemocytometer.

Suspensions of newborn larvae were injected into the lateral tail vein of the mice through a 26-gauge needle, generally in 0.2-ml volumes.

Statistical analysis of the data was conducted on an Olivetti Programma 101.

Results

Immunization with Parenteral Stages Only

Experiment 1 The aim of this experiment was to "immunize" mice by injecting newborn larvae iv and to challenge in the same way.

Sixteen mice were given an iv injection of approximately 2000 newborn larvae, a second injection of 2000 7 days later, and a third injection of approximately 2800 larvae 14 days later. Eight of these mice, together with 11 previously uninfected controls were challenged with 7200 newborn larvae on the twenty-eighth day after the first immunizing infection.

Fifty-six days after the initial immunizing injection the mice were killed and the muscle larvae were counted. The results are shown in Table I. No significant difference in larval counts was found between the immunized-unchallenged and the immunized-challenged groups. This suggests that the immunity gene:ated by the three previous inoculations completely prevented the establishment of the 5150 larvae resulting from the challenge infection.

Experiment 2   This experiment was designed to immunize mice with newborn larvae and then challenge with a normal infection.

Eighteen mice received the same immunizing injections of newborn larvae as given in experiment 1, and 10 of these together with 10 uninfected controls were challenged orally on the twenty-eighth day with 101 ± 23 viable excysted muscle larvae. The numbers of muscle larvae recovered from individual digestion are shown in Table II.

The difference between the immunized-challenged group and immunized control means that 8090 of the muscle larvae in the former group are due to the challenge infection. Previous immunization with parenteral stages has reduced the muscle larvae developing from the challenge infection by 63%.

Immunization with Intestinal Phase Only

Experiment 3   The object of this experiment was to immunize mice with the intestinal phase of *T. spiralis* only and to challenge with a normal infection.

Five mice each received 480 ± 30 viable excysted muscle larvae via the oral route. At 100, 104, and 108 hr after infection each mouse was given a subcutaneous injection of a 5% solution of methyridine in normal saline at a dose rate of 25 mg/kg. Denham (1965) has shown that this drug removes all adult worms from the intestine; and a control group of mice contained no adult intestinal worms at autopsy. The infection and treatment procedure was repeated 7 and 14 days after the first infection.

Twenty-one days after the start of the immunization procedure these mice, with five treated only with methyridine, and five uninfected, untreated mice were each given 57 ± 2 viable excysted muscle larvae via the oral route as a challenge infection.

At 56 days these 15 mice were killed and digested for recovery of muscle larvae. The results of the counts are given in Table III. The 1347 larvae recovered from the infected/treated/challenged group represents a development of only 13% of the challenge infection compared with the two unimmunized control groups; this means that the immunization was 87% effective against a normal challenge.

Table I Number of Muscle Larvae Recovered after Immunization and Challenge with Parenteral Stages of *T. spiralis*[a]

Immunized	Immunized/challenged	Challenge controls
1186	927	3619
1792	998	4017
2378	2112	4212
3136	3424	4223
3219	3563	4609
4479	3706	4815
5023	4531	5031
5340	6471	5346
		6249
		6970
		7557
3319 ± 537 [b]	3217 ± 656	5150 ± 383

[a] Immunizing infections given days 0, 7, and 14; challenge given day 28.
[b] Mean ±S.E.

Experiment 4 The aim of this experiment was to immunize mice with the intestinal phase of *T. spiralis* only and to challenge with an injection of newborn larvae.

Thirteen mice in three groups were prepared in the same way as for experiment 3. At 21 days a challenge infection of approximately 3000 newborn larvae was given iv to each mouse, and at 56 days the mice were killed for muscle larva recovery. The results are shown in Table IV. Although the infected/treated/challenged group is 15% lower than the two control groups this is not statistically significant.

Table II Number of Muscle Larvae Recovered after Immunization with Parenteral Stages and Challenge with a Normal Infection of *T. spiralis*[a]

Immunized	Immunized/challenged	Challenge controls
1186	4,125	7,020
1792	5,238	9,245
2378	6,507	10,076
3136	7,471	18,236
3,219	8,818	19,808
4479	9,325	19,887
5023	14,483	24,366
5340	14,867	25,475
	18,527	29,096
	24,724	50,065
3319 ± 537 [b]	11,409 ± 2085	21,327 ± 3949

[a] Immunizing infections given days 0, 7, and 14; challenge given day 28.
[b] Mean ±S.E.

Table III Number of Muscle Larvae Recovered after Immunization with Intestinal Stages and Challenge with a Normal Infection of *T. spiralis*[a]

Infected/ treated/challenged	Treated/ challenged control	Challenge control
(1 died)	3,746	6,327
707	6,920	7,967
780	11,117	8,092
1863	13,419	10,116
2038	16,672	14,420
1347 ±351 [b]	10,373 ±2295	9,384 ± 1395

[a] Immunizing infections given days 0, 7, and 14; methyridine treatment given days 5, 12, and 19; challenge given day 21.
[b] Mean ±S.E.

Discussion

Oliver-Gonzalez (1941) and Oliver-Gonzalez and Levine (1962) suggested that infections of *T. spiralis* produced antibodies specifically to either the intestinal or muscle stages.

These experiments were designed to determine whether stage specificity exists at a level where resistance generated by one stage will act against that stage and not on the other stages. In experiment 1 parenteral infections of newborn larvae stimulated an acquired immune response which did not allow a subsequent challenge of newborn larvae to develop to the muscle stage. From this it would appear that the migrating and encysting muscle larvae are effective in stimulating a response against a challenge of these same stages.

In experiment 3, mice exposed only to the intestinal phase of *T. spiralis* have acquired an immunity which produces an 87% reduction of

Table IV Number of Muscle Larvae Recovery after Immunization with Intestinal Stages and Challenge with Parenteral Stages of *T. spiralis*[a]

Infected/ treated/challenged	Treated/ challenged control	Challenge control
175	(1 died)	(1 died)
984	1504	1665
2016	2034	1801
2402	2362	2176
2412		
1598 ±441 [b]	1967 ±250	1881 ±152

[a] Immunizing infections given days 0, 7, and 14; methyridine treatment given days 5, 12, and 19; challenge given day 21.
[b] Mean ±S.E.

developed muscle larvae in a normal oral challenge infection. However, experiment 4 which tests the stage specificity of the immunity developed to the intestinal phase, shows that the number of muscle larvae which develop from a parenteral-only challenge is reduced by a statistically insignificant 15%. Thus it seems that immunity generated by adult worms is largely specific to this stage.

Fluorescent antibody studies by Jackson (1959) demonstrated the action of immune sera to adults and muscle larvae, but there was no reaction to newborn larvae. Despommier (1971) concluded that the newborn larva is not immunogenic and relates this to the absence of β_1 granules in this stage, while they do occur in the stichosome of the adult and muscle larva stages (Despommier and Müller, 1970 a,b.

An experiment similar to experiment 2 in which mice will be infected with newborn larvae, challenged orally with infective larvae, but autopsied during the intestinal phase has yet to be performed. However, experiment 2 suggests that the adult worms are capable of remaining for a sufficient time in the intestine to produce a reasonable muscle infection. In experiment 2 it is also observed that the resistance induced by the parenteral infections is not as strong as that produced in experiment 1. Unpublished experiments suggest that adult worms may facilitate the invasion of the muscles by the migratory stage and this may partly explain the results of experiment 2.

Summary

Mice infected with *Trichinella spiralis* were treated with methyridine before the adult worms had shed any newborn larvae, so that immunity to the intestinal phase only was stimulated. Newborn larvae obtained from *in vitro* culture of adult worms were injected iv into mice to produce acquired immunity only to the parenteral stages. Infected and control mice were challenged with normal infections orally or with newborn larvae given iv. The degree of immunity was gauged by the number of muscle larvae developing. An infection of intestinal stages only was 87% effective against a normal challenge but 15% effective against a parenteral-only challenge. An infection of parenteral stages was 100% effective when challenged parenterally but 63% effective against a normal challenge.

Acknowledgments

We wish to thank Professor G. S. Nelson, in whose department this work was carried out, for his advice and encouragement, and the Medical Research Council for their financial assistance.

References

Campbell, C. H. (1955). The antigenic role of the excretions and secretions of *Trichinella spiralis* in the production of immunity in mice. *J. Parasitol.* **41,** 483–491.

Campbell, W. C. (1965). Immunizing effect of enteral and enteral-parenteral infections of *Trichinella spiralis* in mice. *J. Parasitol.* **51,** 185–194.

Denham, D. A. (1965). Studies with methyridine and *Trichinella spiralis* I. Effect upon the intestinal phase in mice. *Exp. Parasitol.* **17,** 10–14.

Denham, D. A. (1966a). Immunity to *Trichinella spiralis* I. The Immunity produced by mice to the first four days of the intestinal phase of the infection. *J. Parasitol.* **56,** 323–327.

Denham, D. A. (1966b). Immunity to *Trichinella spiralis* II. Immunity produced by the adult worm in mice. *Parasitology* **56,** 745–751.

Denham, D. A. (1968). Immunity to *Trichinella spiralis* III. The longevity of the intestinal phase of the infection in mice. *J. Helminthol.* **42,** 257–268.

Dennis, D. T., Despommier, D. D., and Davis, N. (1970). Infectivity of the newborn larva of *Trichinella spiralis* in the rat. *J. Parasitol.* **56,** 974–977.

Despommier, D. D. (1971). Immunogenicity of the newborn larva of *Trichinella spiralis*. *J. Parasitol.* **57,** 531–535.

Despommier, D. D., and Müller, M. (1970a). Functional antigens of *Trichinella spiralis, J. Parasitol.* **56,** (Suppl), 76.

Despommier, D. D., and Müller, M. (1970b). The stichosome of *Trichinella spiralis:* its structure and function. *J. Parasitol.* **56,** (Suppl), 76–77.

Despommier, D. D., and Wostmann, B. S. (1968). Diffusion chambers for inducing immunity to *Trichinella spiralis* in mice. *Exp. Parasitol.* **23,** 228–233.

Jackson, G. J. (1959). Fluorescent antibody studies of *Trichinella spiralis* infections. *J. Infec. Dis.* **105,** 97–117.

Kim, C. W. (1957). Immunity to *Trichinella spiralis* in mice infected with irradiated larvae. *J. Elisha Mitchell Sci. Soc.* **73,** 308–317.

Oliver-González, J. (1941). The dual antibody basis of acquired immunity in trichinosis. *J. Infec. Dis.* **69,** 254–270.

Oliver-González, J., and Levine, D. M. (1962). Stage specific antibodies in experimental trichinosis. *Amer. J. Trop. Med. Hyg.* **11,** 241–244.

Enlargement of Lymph Nodes during Infection with *Trichinella spiralis:* A Preliminary Histological Study

Gaétan Faubert and Charles E. Tanner

Institute of Parasitology,
Macdonald College,
McGill University,
Province of Québec

Introduction

The consequences of antigenic stimulation are an increase in the size of the lymph nodes draining the site injected and a frequent drastic change in the numbers and cell types in the draining nodes (Gatti *et al.,* 1970). Such a change is due to the migration of cells from the central to the peripheral lymphoid organs. Neonatal thymectomy of mice has been used by many investigators to prevent the colonization of secondary lymphoid organs with thymocytes. Thymectomy can also be done in young adult (6-week-old) mice. At this age, however, thymus cells are well established in the secondary organs and must be killed with irradiation. This latter treatment also affects the stem cell compartment of the bone marrow and its final products, the mature peripheral blood cells, which are essential for life of the animal (Congdon, 1971) and, thus, irradiated animals must receive a transplant of bone marrow cells in order to survive. The immunogenicity of *Trichinella spiralis* infections is a very well-known phenomenon (Gould, 1970). Since this immunogenicity must be reflected in the lymph nodes of infected animals, one of the purposes of this communication is to report the effect of *T. spiralis* on the size of the lymph nodes of mice during infection. The effect of adult thymectomy on both the muscular phase of trichinellosis and on the size of the lymph nodes is also reported, since this primary lymphoid organ affects the development of secondary organs and the immunological system in general. The histology of the lymph nodes of infected animals was studied in a preliminary attempt to determine a cytological basis for the function of the lymphoid system in trichinellosis.

353

Materials and Methods

Animals and Infections

Young adult A/Jax and Charles River Swiss mice of both sexes (weighing 20–25 gm) were used in this study. They were usually maintained in groups of six and fed mouse chow and water *ad libitum*. The mice were orally inoculated with either 100 or 500 *Trichinella* larvae derived from rats, as has been previously described (Faubert and Tanner, 1971).

Digestion of the Muscle

The mice were decapitated immediately after cervical dislocation and the skin and the viscera were removed. Each carcass was homogenized in a 50 ml stainless steel chamber with a Serval "Omni-Mixer" in 25 ml of digesting fluid which contained 0.3% pepsin (w/v) and 0.4% concentrated HCl (v/v) in tap water. The muscle was digested in 300 ml digesting fluid for 150 min at 37° C while under continuous agitation with a magnetic stirrer. The muscle larvae were allowed to sediment from the digestion mixture for 90 min at room temperature; they were then collected by aspiration and washed three times in buffered saline, pH 7.2.

Isolation of Lymph Nodes

The two brachial, the two iliac (lumbar), and mesenteric lymph nodes were removed at autopsy and carefully cleaned of adhering fat and tissues. They were then weighed on a torsion balance and placed in individual Petri dishes containing ice cold TC Medium 199 (Difco).

Histology

The brachial, iliac, and mesenteric lymph nodes were cut in half and kept in 10% formol-saline for 48 hr. The tissue was then dehydrated in alcohol and passed through benzene and embedded in 58° C paraffin. Eight-μm sections were cut with a Cambridge rocking microtome and then stained with hematoxylin and eosin (Humason, 1967).

Histochemistry

The Feulgen reaction was done on some of the lymph node tissue sections. The Feulgen technique involves two chemical reactions: (1) the oxidation of 1,2-glycols and/or amino alcohol groups to aldehydes, and (2) the reaction of resulting aldehydes with Schiff reagent to form a purple-red color. Acid hydrolysis is required for the oxidation of the DNA. When nucleic acid is treated with warm HCl, aldehyde groups are exposed from the deoxypentose sugars of DNA but not from the pentose sugars of RNA. Thus, when treated with Schiff reagent, DNA reacts positively, but RNA does not react. The procedure followed was essentially that described by Humason (1967). Fast green dye (British Drug House) 1:2 (w/v) in 95% ethyl alcohol was used as counterstain.

The Schiff reagent was stored at 4° C in a brown bottle with a minimum of air space. The bleaching solution consisted of 1% hydrochloric acid (w/v) and 4% sodium bisulfite (w/v) (Shawinigan, The McArthur Chemical Co., Ltd., Montreal). Fresh bleaching solution was made every day.

Thymectomy

The mouse to be thymectomized was anesthetized with ether and then placed on its back on a wooden operating board and the fore- and hindlegs restrained with masking tape; the head of the animal was held back by a rubber band. A longitudinal incision was made in the midventral region along the upper part of the neck. The skin, muscles, and salivary glands were kept away from the trachea with retractors and a small incision was made into the sternum. The thymic lobes were clearly visible; they were easily detached with a soft round-end glass tube attached to a motor-driven aspirator. The wound was closed with small surgical wound clips (Auto-clips 9 mm, Clay-Adams Inc., New York). Bleeding and mortality were negligible and, with some practice, this operation could be performed in less than 5 min.

γ-Irradiation

Irradiation was carried out with a ^{60}Co source in an Atomic Energy of Canada Ltd. "Gamma-cell 220," at a dose rate of approximately 131,650 true rads/hr. The dose of 850 rads used in the present study was obtained by shielding the source with a 50% lead attenuator.

Bone Marrow Transplants

A/Jax mice were killed, their femurs removed and the ends of the bone cut. About 1 ml of cold sterile Medium 199 was forced through the bone by means of a tuberculin syringe fitted with a #26 intradermal needle. The cells obtained by this method were washed three times in cold (5° C) Medium 199 and counted with a Neubauer hemacytometer. About 3×10^5 bone marrow cells were injected intravenously into mice which had been irradiated 12 hr before.

Results

Relationship of Total Body Weight to the Weight of Lymph Nodes after Inoculation with *T. spiralis* Larvae

It is well known that mice (Yarinsky, 1962; Kozar and Kozar, 1963) and guinea pigs (Castro and Olson, 1967) lose weight following inoculation with *Trichinella* larvae. A relationship between the total body weight and the weight of lymph nodes was determined because the latter could reflect the immunological state of the host. For this purpose, 60 mice were each inoculated with 500 larvae and 15 of these were killed either 7, 15, 30, or

90 days later. These specific times were chosen deliberately in order to observe the effects of the parasite when the infection was primarily in the intestinal, migratory, or sedentary muscle stages.

The mesenteric, iliac, and brachial lymph nodes were carefully cleaned of adhering tissue and weighed. Twenty-five mice of the same age were used as controls; they were inoculated with saline and five animals from this group were killed at the same time post-inoculation as the experimental mice. Since there was a considerable variation in the size of the lymph nodes among the different animals, the weights of each node were divided by the total body weight of the animal; this value was then multiplied by 1000. This relationship is illustrated in Figs. 1 and 2.

The expected progressive decline in body weight (TBW) to a minimum, on day 15, and the return to nearly normal values by day 30, can be contrasted with the relative enlargement of the different lymph nodes. The mesenteric node increases earliest; the ratio of node weight to TBW rises from a value of 7 before inoculation with the parasite to a maximum of 40 by day 15 of the infection; it then declines to normal values by day 30. The two iliac and two brachial nodes enlarge later during the course of infection. The ratios of node weight to TBW rise to maximum values of 50 and 70, respectively, from normal values of 15 and 20 at day 0, by the thirtieth day of infection. There is a slight drop in weight after this time, but they are still heavier than normal on the ninetieth day.

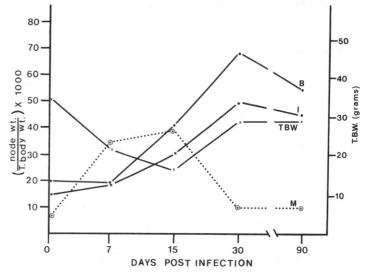

Figure 1 Relationship between the weight of the mesenteric (M), iliac (I), and brachial (B) lymph nodes and the total body weight (TBW) of mice infected with 500 *T. spiralis* larvae. Each dot on the graph represents the mean weight of 15 different animals.

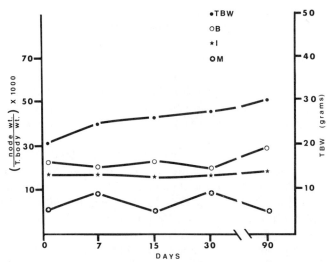

Figure 2 Relationship between the weight of the mesenteric (M), iliac (I), and brachial (B) lymph nodes and the total body weight (TBW) of control mice inoculated with saline. Each value on the graph represents the mean of five different animals.

This progressive enlargement of the different lymph nodes corresponds to the different phases in the development of *Trichinella* in the host. Thus, the draining mesenteric nodes enlarge in the first 7 days when the infection is primarily intestinal. Between day 7 and 15, when the infection is shifting from a primarily intestinal to a primarily somatic location, the iliac and brachial nodes begin to increase in size. These latter two nodes continue their increase and the mesenteric node decreases when the infection becomes primarily somatic after day 15. As expected, the total body weight of the control group increased in the 90 days of the experiment. There was, however, little change in the ratio of node to total body weight throughout this period in these animals.

The Effect of Adult Thymectomy and γ-Irradiation on the Size of Lymph Nodes and on the Number of Muscle Larvae

The influence of neonatal thymectomy on the course of trichinellosis in mice has been studied by Kozar *et al.* (1969). In their experiments BN mice were neonatally thymectomized 24 hr after birth and, 6 weeks later, the animals were each inoculated with 100 larvae. Their results indicated that neonatal thymectomy has no influence on the level of infection with *T. spiralis.*

In this present study, thymectomy was done on 31, 8-week-old A/Jax mice; 1 week after the operation, they were irradiated with 850 rads from a ^{60}Co source. Bone marrow cells (1.3×10^5) from normal syngeneic mice were transplanted to the treated animals 2 hr after irradiation; 25 of these mice were inoculated with a dose of 100 *Trichinella* larvae 3 weeks later (group A). The remaining six thymectomized and irradiated mice were not inoculated (group B). Fifteen normal mice, inoculated with 100 *Trichinella* larvae, served as controls (group C).

Five of the thymectomized and infected mice were each killed on day 7 or 15 or 30 after inoculation; the total body weight and the weight of the lymph nodes were taken as described above. The results are illustrated in Figs. 3 and 4.

The lymph nodes of thymectomized infected mice do not increase in size as they do in nonthymectomized animals. The ratio of lymph node to total body weight in these animals (Fig. 3) is virtually identical to that in normal uninfected mice (Fig. 2). The lymph nodes of the 15 nonthymectomized inoculated controls (group C) underwent the same cycle, and the same magnitude of enlargement of the nodes of the animals inoculated with 500 larvae (see above); the enlargement phenomenon is, therefore, not dose-dependent. The size of the lymph nodes of thymectomized, irradiated, but noninfected mice (group B) did not vary during the 30 days of the experiment. The mean total body weight of the mice in the three groups (Fig. 4) decreased at the same rate and reached similar low levels irrespective of whether the animals were only thymectomized, thymectomized and inoculated, or only inoculated. The mean number of muscle larvae obtained per gram of total body weight from the infected groups A and C is shown in Table I. The different mean numbers of larvae obtained

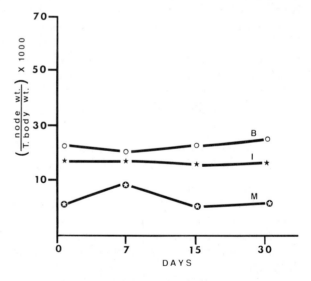

Figure 3 Relationship between the weight of the mesenteric (M), iliac (I), and brachial lymph nodes (B) and the total body weight (TBW) of thymectomized and infected A/Jax mice. Each value on the graph represents the mean of five different animals.

Table I Mean Number of Muscle Larvae Harvested per Gram Body Weight in Normal A/Jax Mice (Group C) and in Thymectomized A/Jax Mice (Group A) Infected with 100 *Trichinella* Larvae

	Group A (15 mice)	Group C (15 mice)
Mean number of muscle larvae $\pm$S.E.[a]	1680 $\pm$600	1762 $\pm$550

[a] Standard error.

in the two groups are not significantly different. This result confirms the report of Kozar *et al.* (1969), who showed that thymectomy does not affect the level of muscle invasion by *T. spiralis*.

Histology and Histochemistry

In all cases, the histological appearance of the tissue was correlated to the stage of the disease. The lesions observed in all the enlarged nodes are located in the paracortical zone and in the germinal center. These lesions are characterized by the presence of necrotic areas and by an increase in the depth of the paracortical zone due to an increase in the number of

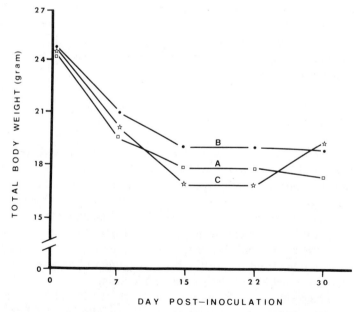

Figure 4 Mean total body weight, in grams, of A/Jax mice treated as follows: Group A, thymectomized and irradiated and infected with 100 *Trichinella* larvae (15 mice); group B, thymectomized and irradiated only (6 mice); group C, inoculated with 100 *Trichinella* larvae (15 mice).

blastoid cells. Cells in various stages of disintegration can be readily seen in both the germinal centers and in the paracortical zone.

When the infection is primarily in the intestinal phase 7 days after inoculation, the structure of the enlarged mesenteric lymph node is abnormal (Fig. 5A) in comparison to the normal lymph node (Fig. 5B). The partial disappearance of the germinal center and the presence of disintegrating cells (arrows) in small necrotic zones is evident in Fig. 5A. The normal mesenteric lymph node (Fig. 5B) shows many small dark lymphocytes in contrast with the pale and blast aspect of the cells in the infected node (Fig. 5A).

Adenopathy of the brachial node (Fig. 6A) is evident 15 days after inoculation, while in the iliac nodes, adenopathy does not become apparent until 30 days. The paracortical area of the brachial node is shown in Fig. 6A and B; many blast cells and many dark cells can be seen in these two micrographs. Remission of the pathology coincides with the return of the lymph nodes to normal weights. Thus, 30 days after inoculation, the structure of the mesenteric node is normal (Fig. 7A) as are the brachial and iliac nodes on the ninetieth day.

The small necrotic zones in the paracortical zone of iliac lymph nodes removed from animals inoculated 30 days before are shown in Fig. 7B (arrows). Numerous plasma cells are found in the cortical layer of iliac lymph nodes removed from mice infected for 30 days, many of them showing the diverse shapes of disintegrating cells (Fig. 8A). Paraffin sections stained for DNA by the Feulgen reaction showed the presence of clumps of Feulgen-positive material (Fig. 8B, arrows). These clumps presumably represent disintegrating nuclei. Similar material was not observed in normal brachial lymph nodes (Fig. 8C).

Discussion

The increase in the size of lymph nodes during infection with *Trichinella* could be due to the stimulation by the parasite of proliferating, functionally uncommitted lymphoid cells. Although Crandall *et al.* (1967) and Kozar *et al.* (1971) have observed the presence of globulin-containing cells in infected animals, there is no evidence that this globulin is specifically antiparasite. The increase in size could also be due to the migration of cells from other lymphoid sites. Alternatively, the hyperplasia could be induced by a "signal" from one of the primary lymphoid organs as a consequence of the stimulation of the parasitic infection.

The results reported here show clearly the influence of the thymus on the enlargement of the lymph nodes. These latter do not increase in size in A/Jax mice thymectomized prior to inoculation with *Trichinella* larvae. Furthermore, it has been observed that the thymus of mice infected with

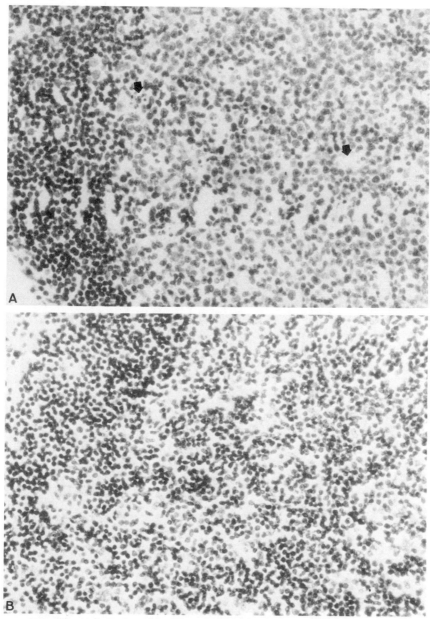

Figure 5 A, Subcortical area of the mesenteric lymph node in a 7-day-old infection. Notice the partial disappearance of the germinal center. Small necrotic zones with disintegrating cells in them are indicated (see arrow). (Feulgen reaction, × 450.) B, Subcortical area of a normal mesenteric lymph node. Note the absence of necrotic zones or of disintegrating or blast cells. Feulgen reaction, × 450.

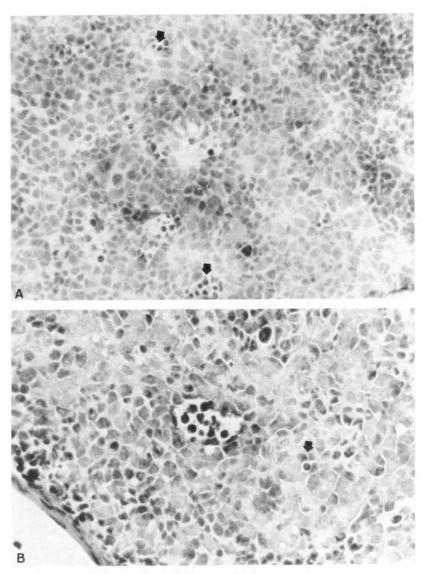

Figure 6 A, Adenopathy of the brachial lymph node from mice inoculated 15 days before. The arrows show the presence of dark cells. H & E, × 450. B, Higher magnification of (A). Notice the presence of dark cells in a necrotic zone (see arrow). H & E, × 800.

Trichinella for 40 days is very much smaller than in uninfected mice (I. Ljungström, personal communication). The fact that the production of sheep hemagglutinin is inhibited in mice infected with *Trichinella* (Faubert and Tanner, 1971) may very well be due to the involution of the thymus during infection; this involution may be due to a rapid emigration of cells

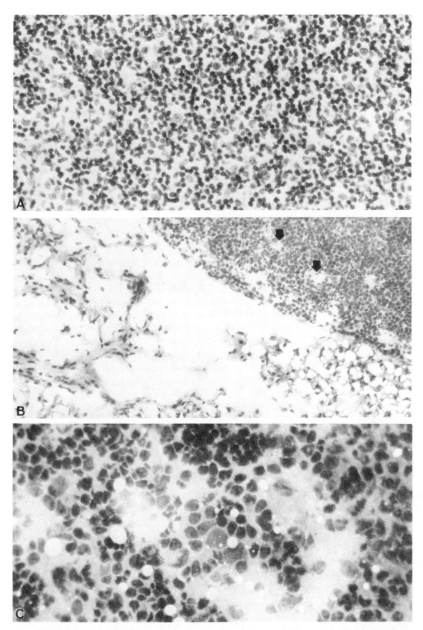

Figure 7 A, Histological aspect of the mesenteric lymph node removed from mice 30 days after inoculation. The germinal center of this node does now show any blast cells or necrotic zones. Feulgen reaction, × 450. B, Presence of small necrotic zones (see arrows) in the paracortical zone of iliac lymph nodes removed from animals inoculated 30 days before. H & E, × 450. C, Higher magnification of (B) (× 640). Notice the presence of plasma cells around the necrotic zones.

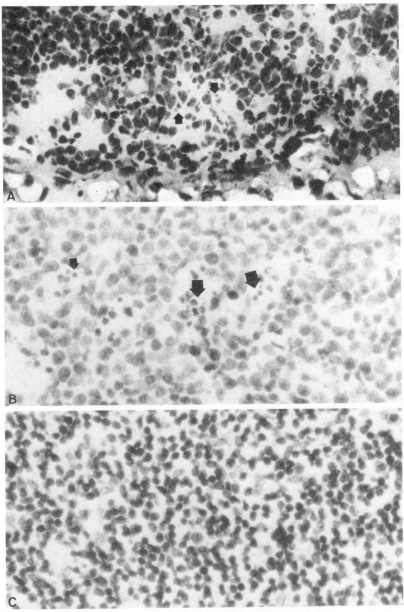

Figure 8   A, H & E stain of the brachial lymph node section of mice inoculated 30 days before. Many disintegrating cells can be seen in the pale area (see arrows). × 560. B, Brachial lymph node removed from mice inoculated with *Trichinella* 30 days before. Feulgen reaction showing the presence of extracellular chromatin (see arrows). × 640. C, Brachial lymph node removed from normal mice of the same age as the infected mice. The Feulgen reaction did not show any extracellular chromatin. × 640.

from this organ to the lymph node. However, the thymus is not the only central lymphoid organ affected in mice infected with *Trichinella*. We have found that bone marrow cells from infected A/Jax mice fail to reconstitute thymectomized and lethally irradiated syngenic mice (manuscript in preparation).

The lymph nodes of mice infected with *Trichinella* show lesions in the germinal center and in the paracortical zone of the node. These lesions are evident when the lymph node enlarges during the course of infection and, they disappear when the node returns to its normal size. Pambuccian *et al.* (1966) have previously reported similar lesions in the mesenteric lymph node of rats infected with *Trichinella*. Kozar *et al.* (1971) have reported that the mesenteric lymph nodes of mice treated with ALS and infected with *T. spiralis* show diverse stages of cellular disintegration and a proliferation of the reticulum cells. These changes increase in intensity until the thirtieth day after infection, but were diminished after 40 and 50 days.

It is impossible to evaluate at this time the influence of these lesions on the operation of the immunological system of the host. However, it is amazing that these lesions of lymph node levels are transitory, suggesting that the lesions in the peripheral lymphoid organs are due to the young migrating larvae en route to the muscles. There is no doubt that the lymph nodes are important organs of the immunological defense mechanisms of the host. In stimulating this system, the migrating larvae overcome powerful cells whose functions are to destroy any invaders. The result of this battle is probably the death of some migrating larvae and of some of the lymphoid cells involved in the antiparasite reaction.

Summary

The effect of *T. spiralis* on the size of the mesenteric, brachial, and iliac lymph nodes has been studied in 60 normal Swiss mice inoculated with 500 larvae and in 31 thymectomized A/Jax inoculated with 100 larvae. The results of this experiment show that lymph nodes increase in size during the course of the infection. The mesenteric nodes increase earliest (on day 7), reach a maximum by day 15 of the infection, and then decline to normal values by day 30. The two iliac and the two brachial nodes begin enlarging later during the course of infection and are still larger than normal on day 90. This phenomenon is not dose-dependent. The lymph nodes of thymectomized infected mice do not increase in size during the course of infection, suggesting that the enlargement of these organs is thymus dependent.

The lymph nodes of infected mice show lesions in the germinal centers and in the paracortical zone. These lesions become evident when the lymph node enlarges during the course of infection, and they disappear when the node returns to its normal size. The results reported here are discussed on the basis that migrating larvae overcome lymphoid cells whose function is to destroy the invading parasites.

Acknowledgment

This investigation has been supported by financial assistance from the Ministére des Affaires Sociales de la Province de Québec and the National Research Council of Canada.

References

Castro, G. A., and Olson, L. J. (1967). Relationship between body weight and food and water intake in *T. spiralis* infected guinea pigs. *J. Parasitol.* **53**, 589–594.

Congdon, C. C. (1971). Bone-marrow transplantation. *Science* **171**, 1116-1124.

Crandall, R. B., Cebra, J. J., and Crandall, C. A. (1967). The relative proportions of IgG, IgA and IgM containing cells in rabbit tissues during experimental trichinosis. *Immunology* **12**, 147–158.

Faubert, G., and Tanner, C. E. (1971). *Trichinella spiralis:* Inhibition of sheep hemagglutinins in mice. *Exp. Parasitol.* **30**, 120–123.

Gatti, R. A., Stutman, O., and Good, R. A. (1970). The lymphoid system. *Ann. Rev. Physiol.* **32**, 529–546.

Gould, S. E., Ed. (1970). "Trichinosis in Man and Animals." Thomas, Springfield, Illinois.

Humason, G. L. (1967). "Animal Tissue Techniques." Freeman and Co., San Francisco.

Kozar, Z., and Kozar, M. (1963). The course of experimental trichinellosis in mice. Methods of infection and the influence of various invasive doses on the mortality and weight of the animals. *Wiad. Parazytol.* **9**, 403–418.

Kozar, M., Karmánska, K., Kotz, J., Marciniec, D., and Sieniuta, R. (1969). Trichinellosis in thymectomized mice. *Wiad. Parazytol.* **15**, 634–637.

Kozar, Z., Karmánska, K., Kotz, K., and Sieniuta, R. (1971). The influence of anti-lymphocytic serum (ALS) on the course of Trichinellosis in mice. *Wiad. Parazytol.* **17**, 541–572.

Pambuccian, G., Cironeanu, I., and Motoc, F. (1966). The lesions of the lymph nodes in experimental trichinosis of white rats. *Wiad. Parazytol.* **12**, 561–568.

Yarinsky, A. (1962). The influence of X-irradiation on the immunity of mice to infection with *T. spiralis. J. Elisha Mitchell Sci. Soc.* **78**, 29–43.

Humoral and Cellular Factors in the Resistance of Rats to *Trichinella spiralis*

Rufus W. Gore, Hans-Jürgen Bürger,* and Elvio H. Sadun

Department of Medical Zoology
Walter Reed Army Institute of Research
Washington, D. C.

Introduction

Rats manifest a resistance to *Trichinella spiralis* by expelling adult worms from the intestinal tract after the seventh day of infection and by a reduction in the number of larvae which invade the muscles. Although a considerable number of investigations have been conducted in many host species infected with this parasite, descriptions of the mechanisms involved in the expulsion of adult worms from the intestine are still based largely on circumstantial evidence.

Delayed skin reactions have been reported in rabbits and guinea pigs after intradermal inoculation of *T. spiralis* larval extracts (Bachman, 1928; Augustine and Theiler, 1932; Melcher, 1943). Larsh and his co-workers were able to transfer resistance from previously infected mice to susceptible animals by transferring sensitized lymph node and peritoneal exudate cells. These studies were corroborated by histological investigations which revealed inflammation of the intestine compatible with delayed hypersensitivity (Larsh *et al.,* 1966). Kim (1966) showed that antigenic extracts of *T. spiralis* larvae with Freund's complete adjuvant can induce delayed hypersensitivity responses in guinea pigs. He observed a delayed skin reaction, perivascular infiltration of mononuclear cells at the skin test site, and the transfer of delayed hypersensitivity from sensitized donors to normal recipients by means of splenic and lymph node cells (Kim, 1966; Kim *et al.,* 1967, 1970).

On the basis of this and related evidence, it has been suggested that the expulsion of *T. spiralis* from the small intestine may be the result of a delayed hypersensitivity reaction (Larsh *et al,* 1964, 1966, 1972). On the other hand Catty (1969) working with infected guinea pigs suggested that resistance in trichinellosis "may have a strong anaphylactic involvement"

*Present address: Institut fur Parasitologie, Bünteway

resulting from the development of a "long-term sensitizing antibody with biological and physicochemical properties analogous to the reagin of humans and the reagin-like antibody of rats." Allergic sensitization has been demonstrated in experimentally infected guinea pigs (Sharp and Olson, 1962) and mice (Briggs, 1963; Briggs and DeGiusti, 1966). *Trichinella spiralis* has been shown to elicit the formation of reaginic antibodies in man (Zvaifler *et al.*, 1966), mice (Sadun *et al.*, 1968; Mota and Wong, 1968; Mota *et al.*, 1969a, b), rabbits (Sadun *et al.*, 1968), and guinea pigs (Catty, 1969).

In order to test these hypotheses, investigations were conducted to determine if the highly specific resistance which develops during trichinal infections is significantly reduced by procedures such as neonatal thymectomy and the use of antilymphocytic globulin which is known to reduce the number of circulating lymphocytes and the intensity of delayed hypersensitivity reactions. Conversely, attempts were made to determine whether or not the resistance is significantly increased by passive transfer of washed sensitized lymphocytes. The humoral response in terms of fluorescent and homocytotropic antibodies was determined in the various experimental groups and the role of passive transfer of serum from resistant animals was also assessed. Preliminary results of these experiments were published in abstract form (Gore *et al.*, 1970).

Materials and Methods

Thymectomy

Inbred Fischer rats* were used in these experiments. The pregnant females were given oxytetracycline and a multivitamin mixture in the drinking water beginning a few days before delivery and for up to 2 weeks after delivery in order to minimize the possibility of infection at the time of thymectomy. Thymectomy was performed on the newborn rats according to the principles of Jankovic *et al.* (1962) within 24 hr after birth. Successful removal of the thymus was determined by estimating the number of circulating small lymphocytes at 3–6 weeks of age and further verified at necropsy by searching for the remnants of thymus tissue. Animals with stitch abscesses or those that appeared cachetic were excluded from the study. Arnason and his co-workers (1962) have shown that thymectomized animals have a decreased number of lymphocytes. Therefore, rats were grouped according to their number of circulating small lymphocytes (Stechschulte, 1969). Thymectomized rats with a relatively low number of

---

*In conducting the research described in this report, the investigators adhered to the "Guide for Laboratory Animal Facilities and Care," as promulgated by the Committee on the Guide for Laboratory Animal Facilities and Care of the Institute of Laboratory Animal Resources, National Academy of Sciences–National Research Council.

small lymphocytes were assigned to the thymectomized group. Thymic remnants were found in less than 10% of these animals. Unsuccessfully thymectomized or sham operated rats with numbers of circulating small lymphocytes similar to those of untreated controls were assigned to the sham-operated group.

Antilymphocyte globulin (ALG)

Antilymphocyte serum was prepared as follows. Each of six New Zealand rabbits was injected in the foot pads with 10^8 rat lymphoid cells in Freund's complete adjuvant. They were reinjected intradermally with the same number of cells in Hanks' balanced salt solution 9 and 16 days afterward. The rabbits were bled 14, 21, and 28 days after the last injection and exsanguinated 1 week later. Sera collected from each bleeding were pooled and stored at $-72°$ C. Before the pooled sera were used in the experiment they were heated at $56°$ C for 45 min and absorbed twice with rat erythrocytes ($\frac{1}{3}$ packed volume) for 30 minutes at $37°$ C. The antilymphocyte globulin was precipitated with 40% saturated ammonium sulfate and washed twice in 50% saturated ammonium sulfate. The globulin was then dialyzed against phosphate buffered saline at a pH 7.4 for 48 hr with six changes of prechilled buffer. Normal rabbit globulin (NRG) was obtained by bleeding seven normal New Zealand rabbits. The globulin was precipitated, washed, and dialyzed as described above.

Lymphocytes The thymus and the anterior and posterior cervical, mediastinal, inguinal, and mesenteric lymph nodes were excised from rats immediately after they were bled under light ether anesthesia. The excised material was placed in a chilled nutrient solution consisting of Eagle Basal Medium with Hanks' balanced salt solution, minced, and teased into small pieces. The mixture was then passed through 50 and 100 mesh wire screens which retained the fibrous strands on the screen and allowed the cells to pass through. Spleen cell suspensions from the rats were prepared in the same manner. The cells collected were washed twice and resuspended in Hanks' balanced salt solution with 3–5 units of heparin per milliliter. Aliquots of each pool were counted in a hemocytometer, stained with Giemsa's stain for differential cell counting and also stained with 0.1% trypan blue to test the viability of the cells. Between 95 and 98% of the cells excluded the dye and were considered viable. A total of 10^9 viable lymphoid cells was given to each recipient rat 8–11 days before infection.

Rat globulins Immune rat globulin was obtained by collecting the blood of rats infected 6 weeks earlier with *T. spiralis*. The sera were collected, pooled, and stored, and the globulin was precipitated, washed, and dialyzed as described for the ALG preparation. The rat globulins were tested for antibodies by the SAFA and PCA tests and found to be positive.

Experimental Infections

Challenge infections were done using 10 *T. spiralis* larvae/gm of body weight in all experiments except one thymectomy experiment in which 20 larvae/gm of body weight were used. *Trichinella spiralis* larvae for infecting the animals and for preparing antigens were obtained from young adult rats 6–8 weeks after each was fed 3000–4000 washed larvae. The rats were killed and the larvae were separated from the muscles by artificial digestion in a pepsin-hydrochloric acid mixture. The entire carcass was digested except for the head, paws, and tail. Infection was determined by counting adult *T. spiralis* worms in the intestine and larvae in the muscles at appropriate intervals. Adult worms were recovered with strict adherence to the described technique. Immediately after killing each rat, the small intestine was removed, slit open, cut into small pieces, and placed in a Baermann funnel filled with warm saline. The funnel was kept in an incubator at 38° C for 5 hr. The worms that settled to the bottom of tube attached to the Baermann funnel during incubation were counted. Larvae in the muscles were collected after the individual rat carcasses were digested in pepsin-hydrochloric acid. Replicate samples representing one-thousandths of the total digest were taken and all larvae present were counted after they were immobilized in 1% agar.

Serologic Tests

Antibody levels to *T. spiralis* in various groups were determined by the soluble antigen fluorescent antibody (SAFA) technique and by the homologous passive cutaneous anaphylactic (PCA) test. These tests were conducted as described (Gore and Sadun, 1968; Sadun *et al.,* 1968). In both tests a lipid-free somatic extract of *Trichinella* larvae was prepared in Tris-buffered saline and stored in 1 ml aliquots at $-72°$ C, as described previously.

Results

Neonatal Thymectomy

A first series of experiments was conducted to determine the effect of neonatal thymectomy on the recovery of *T. spiralis* adults and larvae following infection. The results of three experiments involving a total of 96 rats are summarized in Table I. Although there was no significant difference in the number of adults harbored by animals in the two groups 7 days after infection, 5 days later (12 days after infection) considerably more adults were recovered from the intestines of the thymectomized animals than from the controls. The difference is significant at this time. Forty days after infection the average number of larvae in the thymectomized animals was greater than in the controls, although this difference is not statistically significant. Fluorescent antibodies were detected in a few rats as early as 7 days after infection (Table II). All of the rats became positive by the twelfth day and the titers increased reaching their maximum at the end of the experiment 40 days after the infection. Homocytotropic antibodies were occasionally detected 7 days after infection (Table II) in animals of either group. Beginning with the twelfth day after infection most sera were reacting in the PCA and among the controls all of the animals were positive 40 days after infection. No quantitative determinations of PCA antibodies were done.

Although neonatal thymectomy did not interfere with the production of fluorescent or homocytotropic antibodies in a consistent or significant manner, there was a slight indication of higher titers and greater numbers of reacting animals among the controls (Table II).

Antilymphocytic Globulin

In a subsequent experiment, the effect of thymectomy and of antilymphocytic globulin (ALG) was studied in relation to the *Trichinella spiralis* adult and larval burdens. A total of 162 rats was divided into four groups. Group I included 35 rats which were successfully thymectomized; Group II consisted of 36 rats which were successfully thymectomized and received antilymphocytic globulin; the 31 rats of Group III received only antilymphocytic globulin, and the 60 rats of Group IV received normal rabbit globulin and served as controls. As indicated in Fig. 1, a search for adult worms was conducted in 162 rats which were killed 7, 10, 12, 14, 16, 19, 37, and 42 days following infection. The worm burden in the untreated animals decreased rapidly after the seventh day of infection and reached zero by the sixteenth day. In the thymectomized animals the worms were eliminated somewhat more slowly but in a manner which was not significantly different from that of the untreated controls. In the animals receiving antilymphocytic globulin more worms were recovered in the intestine and a few of them persisted up to the end of the experiment 42 days after infection. In the group which was treated with thymectomy and antilymphocytic globulin the worms were eliminated from the intestine so

Table I Effect of Neonatal Thymectomy on Recovery of *T. spiralis* Adult Worms and Larvae

| Group | Treatment | No. of rats | Parasites recovered/ larvae given | | Larvae, day 40 |
| | | | Adult worms | | |
			Day 7	Day 12	
I	Thymectomized	45	0.52	0.15	75.0
II	Controls	51	0.48	0.044	67.0

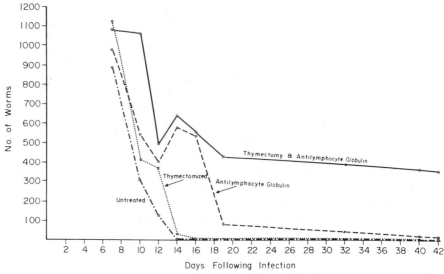

Figure 1 The effect of thymectomy and/or antilymphocyte globulin on *T. spiralis* worm burdens (162 rats).

slowly that at the end of the experiment a considerable number of adults could still be recovered from these animals. The effect of thymectomy and antilymphocytic globulin was also noticeable in the number of larvae recovered from the muscles of the rats in the various groups 37 and 42 days after infection (Table III). The animals which had been thymectomized and received antilymphocytic globulin harbored a significantly greater number of larvae than those receiving ALG only. These, in turn, had a significantly greater number of larvae than either the thymectomized or the untreated control animals.

Passive Transfer of Cells

Since these results raised the possibility of a role of cell mediated immunity in the elimination of worms from the intestine, attempts were made to passively transfer immunity to *T. spiralis* in rats by sensitized lymphoid cells. In the initial studies consisting of three separate experiments involving 137 rats, the thymus, lymph nodes and spleen were removed from donor animals 56 days after infection with *T. spiralis*. The lymphoid cells were obtained from these organs as described and the recipient animals were pretreated by injecting these cells intraperitoneally. Pretreatment control animals were injected with cells obtained from the thymus, lymph nodes, and spleen from uninfected rats. Eight or nine days after pretreatment all animals were challenged with *T. spiralis*. One-third of the animals were killed 7 days and one-third 13–14 days after infection. The intestines were examined for the presence of adults. The remaining animals

Table II Effect of Neonatal Thymectomy on Antibody Responses of Rats Infected with *T. spiralis*

Group	Treatment	No. of rats	Soluble antigen fluorescent antibody titer						Passive cutaneous antibody (% reactors)		
			7 Days		12 Days		40 Days		Day 7	Day 12	Day 40
			GMT[a]	% R[b]	GMT	% R	GMT	% R			
I	Thymectomized	45	1	3	37	100	90	100	25	77	83
II	Controls	51	<1	2	96	100	152	100	22	82	100

[a] GMT, Geometric mean of the titer.
[b] % R, Percent reactors.

Table III Effect of Thymectomy and/or Antilymphocyte Globulin (ALG) On Numbers of *T. spiralis* Larvae

Group	Treatment	No. of rats	Parasites recovered/ larvae given Day 37	Day 42
I	Thymectomy	9	Not done	79.0
II	Thymectomy + ALG	11	366.0	325.0
III	ALG only	10	141.0	181.0
IV	Controls	22	79.0	75.0

were killed 40 days after infection and the muscles were digested for counting the larvae. As indicated in Table IV no significant differences in the three groups were observed 7 days after infection. However, by the fourteenth day the rats receiving sensitized cells had fewer worms than those which received nonsensitized cells or those that received no cells at all. Similarly, a significant reduction in the number of larvae was observed in the group of animals receiving sensitized cells (Group I) as compared to the other two control groups (Groups II and III).

Serum was obtained from the 137 animals used in these experiments and tested for the presence of fluorescent antibodies and homocytotropic reaginic antibodies. The results summarized in Table V indicate that fluorescent antibodies were detectable at low titers in a few animals receiving sensitized cells 7 days after infection. No significant differences were observed in the three groups 13–14 and 40 days after infection. Seven days after infection anaphylactic antibodies were present in approximately one-third of the rats receiving sensitized cells. The number increased until eventually, 40 days after infection, all of the rats were positive for passive cutaneous anaphylactic antibodies. In the remaining two groups no reaginic antibodies were detected 7 days after infection. A few positive reactors were observed 2 weeks after infection and by the fortieth day after infection nearly all of the infected rats in Groups II and III were positive.

These results suggested that antigen might have been passed to the recipient animals by transferring spleen cells. Therefore, another series of experiments was set up in which lymphoid cells were obtained only from

Table IV Effect of Passive Transfer of Lymphocytes (Thymus, Spleen, and Lymph Nodes) on Number of *T. spiralis*

Group	Treatment	No. of rats	Parasites recovered/ larvae given Adult worms Day 7	Day 14	Larvae, Day 40
I	Sensitized cells	59	0.47	0.012	80.0
II	Nonsensitized cells	39	0.58	0.055	125.14
III	No cells	39	0.56	0.055	126.6

Table V Effect of Passive Transfer of Lymphocytes (Thymus, Spleen, and Lymph Nodes) on Antibody Responses of Rats Infected with *T. spiralis*

Group	Treatment	No. of rats	7 Days GMT[a]	7 Days % R[b]	14 Days GMT	14 Days % R	7 Days	12 Days	40 Days
							Passive cutaneous antibody (% reactors)		
I	Sensitized cells	59	2	30	125	100	31	79	100
II	Nonsensitized cells	39	<1	10	81	100	0	22	100
III	No cells	39	<1	10	149	100	0	9	90

[a] GMT, Geometric mean of the titer.
[b] % R, percent reactors.

the lymph nodes of rats previously infected with *T. spiralis* since it was considered that these organs would be less likely to contain larval debris. Comparable numbers of these cells were injected intraperitoneally into recipient animals 8 and 9 days before infection and the course of infection was followed. A total of 58 rats was divided into two groups and the animals were killed 7 and 14 days after infection. The results (Table VI) indicate once again that 2 weeks after infection the group of animals receiving sensitized cells had fewer worms than the control animals receiving no cells. The results of serologic tests are summarized in Table VII. Among the rats receiving sensitized cells fluorescent antibodies at a very low titer were detected in a few rats 7 days after infection. The sera of all of the animals were reactive 1 week later. Passive cutaneous anaphylactic antibodies were detected 7 days after infection in all of the rats of the group receiving sensitized cells but in none of the animals in the control group. Fourteen days after infection approximately one-half of all the rats showed anaphylactic antibodies.

The results of these experiments suggested the possibility that humoral factors may play some role in the expulsion of adults. In the groups in which expulsion of adult worms was delayed by neonatal thymectomy the antibody response measured by SAFA and PCA tests appeared to be somewhat suppressed. Conversely, in the groups which received sensitized cells the expulsion of worms and the humoral response were increased.

Table VI Effect of Passive Transfer of Lymphocytes (Lymph Nodes) on Numbers of *T. spiralis* in Rats

Group	Treatment	No. of rats	Day 7	Day 12
			Adult worms recovered/ larvae given	
I	Sensitized cells	29	0.53	0.002
II	No cells	29	0.65	0.010

Table VII Effect of Passive Transfer of Lymphocytes (Lymph Nodes) on Antibody Responses to *T. spiralis* in Rats

Group	Treatment	No. of rats	Soluble antigen fluorescent antibody titer				Passive cutaneous antibody (% reactors)	
			7 Days		12 Days		7 Days	12 Days
			GMT[a]	% R[b]	GMT	% R		
I	Sensitized cells	29	3	24	58	100	25	67
II	No cells	29	<1	3	46	100	0	42

[a] GMT, Geometric mean titer
[b] % R, Percent reacting

To determine whether or not this was a causal relationship another experiment was set up in an attempt to passively transfer resistance by humoral factors. A total of 90 animals were divided into three groups (Table VIII). Thirty rats of the first group received intraperitoneally 1 ml of globulin from rats which had been infected with *T. spiralis* on the day preceding the infection, on the day of infection and again 8, 9, and 10 days following infection. This globulin was both PCA and SAFA positive. Thirty rats of the second group received the same amount of normal globulin by the same route. The remaining animals received no globulin and served as additional controls. The number of adults recovered in the three groups 7 days after infection was not significantly different. However, on the twelfth day the control group receiving no globulin had a lighter worm burden. No significant difference was observed in the number of larvae digested from the muscles in the rats of the three groups 40 days after infection. These data indicate that passive transfer of large amounts of immune globulin failed to reduce the number of adult worms in the intestine or the number of larvae in the muscles.

Discussion

Neonatal thymectomy failed to affect the number of adult worms found in the rats one week following infection. These results are similar to those obtained in rats during the first week of infection with the rodent malaria *Plasmodium berghei* (Stechschulte, 1969). However, although there was no effect on the establishment of this nematode, thymectomy apparently interfered with the rate of expulsion of adult worms and a significant difference between the thymectomized and control animals was evident 13–14 days after infection. These results are also similar to those obtained in rats infected with *Nippostrongylus brasiliensis* (Wilson *et al.*, 1967; Ogilvie and Jones, 1967).

It is widely accepted that neonatal thymectomy inhibits cellular im-

Table VIII Effect of Passive Transfer of Serum on Numbers of *T. spiralis* in Rats

| | | | Parasites recovered/ larvae given | | |
| | | | Adult worms | | |
Group	Treatment	No. of rats	Day 7	Day 12	Day 40
I	Immune globulin	30	0.53	0.25	94.0
II	Normal globulin	30	0.46	0.18	111.3
III	Controls (no globulin)	30	0.55	0.11	111.3

munity as manifested by late skin homograft rejection and impaired delayed-type hypersensitivity reactions. This effect in the rat has been amply documented (Jankovic *et al.,* 1962; Arnason *et al.,* 1962). On the other hand antibody production to certain antigens also requires thymic participation (Arnason *et al.,* 1964; Azar *et al.,* 1964; Miller and Osoba, 1967). In our experiments, the time course of development of homologous anaphylactic and of fluorescent antibodies was not significantly different between the thymectomized rats and the controls, although the antibody response of both types seemed to be somewhat lower in the thymectomized group than in the controls. Lower PCA antibody titers after infection with *N. brasiliensis* were also observed in thymectomized rats (Wilson *et al.,* 1967; Ogilvie and Jones, 1967).

The exact mechanism by which thymectomy alters the host response to *T. spiralis* infection in the rat is not known. Although it is recognized that the techniques used to measure the antibody response in these studies might be unsatisfactory for the detection of a specific type of protective antibody, it seems unlikely that the decreased ability to dislodge adult worms from the intestine can be attributed to impaired antibody production. However, since quantitation of PCA antibody was not done, one cannot determine whether a reduction in titer occurred. The observation that passive transfer of large amounts of immune globulin failed to increase the rate of adult worm expulsion or the number of larvae recovered from the muscles provides additional evidence to this effect and supports the reported failure by Larsh and his co-workers to transfer resistance in mice by serum alone (Larsh *et al.,* 1970). Copro-antibodies of the IgA and IgE immunoglobulin classes would probably not be readily transferable by this method. Therefore, failure to dislodge adult worms by passive transfer of serum does not rule out the possibility of a humoral mechanism.

Although no direct measurement of cellular immunity was available in our experiments, neonatal thymectomy could have resulted in increased susceptibility to *T. spiralis* infection by an impairment of this segment of the immune response. However, thymectomy also would be expected to inhibit antibody production to at least some antigens. To further investigate the relative role of cells and serum, a series of experiments was undertaken to investigate the capacity of immune lymphoid cells to transfer protection to the recipient animals infected with *T. spiralis.*

The effect of immunosuppressive agents on the course of infection was measured by giving antilymphocyte globulin (ALG) 2, 1, and 0 days prior to infection. This caused a marked increase in the retention of adult parasites in the gut and of the number of larvae in the muscles. This increased susceptibility is quite consistent with observations in rodent malaria (Barker and Powers, 1971; Spira *et al.,* 1970; Lourie, 1972) and *Trichinella* infection in mice (Larsh *et al.,* 1972). Since the effects of ALG on the immune response are similar to those obtained with neonatal thymectomy it was not surprising to observe that in the animals which have been thymectomized and given ALG, the ability to dislodge worms from the intestine was even further impaired and that as late as 42 days after infection these rats still had a considerable number of adults in their gut. Similarly, these rats had a significantly higher number of larvae in the muscles as compared with any of the other group. Therefore, the expulsion of adult worms from the intestine was impaired by neonatal thymectomy and by antilymphocytic globulin and a passive transfer of immunity to *T. spiralis* was obtained with a lymphoid cell population but not with globulin from previously infected animals.

Lymphoid cells obtained from donor animals previously infected with *T. spiralis* were capable of transferring protection to recipient animals. Pools of lymphoid cells were initially obtained from a combination of lymph nodes, thymus, and spleen. When the experiments were repeated using lymphoid cells collected only from lymph nodes, similar but less striking results were obtained. It is possible that the observed protective effect could be the result of active immunization, since lymphoid cells obtained from previously infected animals could contain *Trichinella* antigen. This possibility could not be ruled out especially since the animals which received sensitized cells developed fluorescent and reaginic antibodies earlier than the animals receiving nonsensitized cells or those receiving no cells at all.

Recent studies by Larsh and his co-workers (1972) showed that sensitized mice developed an immunity which could be transferred to recipients by spleen cells. Conversely, injections of antithymocytic serum retarded the expulsion of the adult worms from the small intestine. These results, which are consistent with those observed in our experiments in rats, are compatible with the hypothesis that the mechanism for expulsion of adult *T. spiralis* in mice and rats has a cell-mediated basis. Although indirect evidence that cellular immunity contributes to the expulsion of worms from the gut has been obtained, further studies are necessary to definitely identify and characterize the role of cellular immunity in the development of resistance to *T. spiralis* and to distinguish between the time course development of immediate and delayed hypersensitivity reactions. Even the demonstration of elimination of adult worms from the host as a result of intestinal inflammation mediated by immediate or delayed hypersensitivity is no proof that a precise causal relationship exists.

Therefore, in spite of extensive experimentation, the mechanism of protection to *T. spiralis* in rats has still not been definitely characterized. The ability of transferred cells to produce antibody is well documented and some degree of enhanced antibody production seemed to occur in the pretreated animals. Some evidence of the enhanced antibody protection in rats pretreated with sensitized cells was obtained in our experiments. Humoral antibodies could have contributed to the acquired resistance to *T. spiralis* infection even though no such evidence was obtained by passive transfer of serum from infected animals. One must conclude, therefore, that the results obtained so far do not provide conclusive evidence which enables one to separate the effect of either humoral or cellular immunity in developing resistance to *T. spiralis* infection.

As recently reported by Kettman (1972), there is strong evidence that the same cell population may be involved in delayed hypersensitivity reactions and cell cooperation resulting in antibody synthesis. In such a case resistance to *T. spiralis* infection may be mediated by a single mobile population of cells.

Summary

Rats manifest a resistance to *Trichinella spiralis* by expelling adult worms from the intestinal tract after the seventh day of infection with consequent reduction in the number of larvae in the muscles. To test whether the worm expulsion may be primarily caused by a specific delayed hypersensitivity reaction, investigations were conducted to determine if (1) the highly specific resistance is significantly reduced by factors known to reduce the number of circulating lymphocytes and the degree of delayed hypersensitivity, i.e., neonatal thymectomy and the use of antilymphocytic globulin; (2) the resistance is significantly increased by passive transfer of washed sensitized lymphocytes, and (3) the resistance is not increased by passive transfer of immune serum.

In replicate experiments rats were subjected to neonatal thymectomy or sham operations within 24 hr after birth. All of the animals were infected with *T. spiralis* at approximately 2 months of age, and they were killed 1, 2, and 6 weeks after infection. Antibody levels to *T. spiralis* were determined by the soluble antigen fluorescent antibody (SAFA) technique and by the homologous passive cutaneous anaphylactic (PCA) test. Although neonatal thymectomy did not interfere with the production of fluorescent and homocytotropic reagin-like antibodies, the expulsion of adult worms from the intestine was delayed by 2 or 3 days. Injections with antilymphocytic globulin interfered with the ability of rats to eliminate the adult worm population in the intestine. The animals which were neonatally thymectomized and also given antilymphocytic globulin retained considerable worm burdens up to 6 weeks after inoculation. Consequently, the number of larvae recovered in the muscles of these animals was greater than that in the untreated controls.

Passive transfer of immunity to *T. spiralis* in rats was attempted by using sensitized lymphoid cells. Immunity in normal recipients could be transferred by $10 - 10^9$ mixed lymphoid cells of thymus, spleen, and lymph nodes from hyperinfected cell donors. One week after infection, the number of worms established in the intestines was similar in those animals that received cells from immunized donors, those that received cells from nonimmunized donors, and those that had not been given any cells. However, 2 weeks after infection fewer adult worms were found in the "immune" cell recipients and 6 weeks after infection fewer larvae were recovered. No difference was detected in the levels of antibodies by the SAFA test, but PCA antibodies occurred earlier in immune cell recipients. Passive transfer of large amounts of immune globulin failed to reduce the number of adult worms in the intestine or the number of larvae in the muscles.

Although these results suggest that lymphoid cells play an important role in the immune reaction to *T. spiralis* infections in rats, they do not provide conclusive evidence of the relative role of cellular or humoral factors.

Acknowledgments

The authors wish to express their appreciation to Mr. William Hildreth and SP-5 Robert Tomlinson for their competent technical assistance.

References

Arnason, B. G., Jankovic, B. D., Waksman, B. H., and Wennersten, C. (1962). Role of thymus in immune reactions in rats. II. Suppressive effect of thymectomy at birth on reactions of delayed (cellular) hypersensitivity and the circulating small lymphocyte. *J. Exp. Med.* **116,** 177–186.

Arnason, B. G., de Vaux St-Cyr, C., and Relyveld, E. H. (1964). Role of the thymus in immune reactions in rats. IV. Immunoglobulins and antibody formation. *Int. Arch. Allergy* **25,** 206–224.

Augustine, D. L., and Theiler, H. (1932). Precipitin and skin tests as aids in diagnosing trichinosis. *Parasitology* **24,** 60–86.

Azar, H. A., Williams, J., and Takatsuki, K. (1964). Development of plasma cells and immunoglobulins in neonatally thymectomized rats. *In:* V. Defendi, and D. Metcalf, (eds.), "The Thymus." Wistar Institute Press, Philadelphia, Pennsylvania, pp. 75–88.

Bachman, G. W. (1928). An interdermal test in experimental trichiniasis. *J. Prev. Med.* **2,** 513–523.

Barker, L. R. and Powers, K. G. (1971). Impairment of antibody response and recovery in malarial rodents by anti-lymphocyte serum. *Nature London* **229,** 429.

Briggs, N. T. (1963). Hypersensitivity in murine trichinosis: Some responses of *Trichinella*-infected mice to antigen and 5-hydroxytrytophan. *Ann. N. Y. Acad. Sci.* **113,** 456–466.

Briggs, N. T., and DeGiusti, D. L. (1966). Generalized allergic reactions in *Trichinella*-infected mice: The temporal association of host immunity and sensitivity to exogenous antigens. *Amer. J. Trop. Med. Hyg.* **15,** 919–929.

Catty, D. (1969). "Monograph in Allergy. The Immunology of Nematode Infections: Trichinosis in Guinea Pigs as a Model." S. Karger, New York and Basel.

Gore, R. W., and Sadun, E. H. (1968). A soluble antigen fluorescent antibody (SAFA) test for the immunodiagnosis of trichinosis in man and experimental animals. *Exp. Parasitol.* **23,** 272–279.

Gore, R. W., Burger, H. J., and Sadun, E. H. (1970). Mechanisms of immunity in rats infected with *Trichinella spiralis J. Parasitol.* **56,** (Abstr.) 122.

Jankovic, B. D., Waksman, B. H., and Arnason, B. G. (1962). Role of the thymus in immune reactions in rats. I. The immunologic response to bovine serum albumin: antibody formation, Arthus reactivity and delayed hypersensitivity in rats thymectomized or splenectomized at various times after birth. *J. Exp. Med.* **116,** 159–176.

Kettman, J. (1972). Delayed hypersensitivity: Is the same population of thymus derived cells responsible for cellular immunity reactions and the carrier effect? *Immunol. Commun.* **1,** 289–299.

Kim, C. W. (1966). Delayed hypersensitivity to larval antigens of *Trichinella spiralis. J. Infect. Dis.* **116,** 208–214.

Kim, C. W., Savel, H., and Hamilton, L. D. (1967). Delayed hypersensitivity to *Trichinella spiralis.* I. Transfer of delayed hypersensitivity by lymph node cells. *J. Immunol.* **99,** 1150–1155.

Kim, C. W., Jamuar, M. P., and Hamilton, L. D. (1970). Delayed hypersensitivity to *Trichinella spiralis.* III. Effect of repeated sensitizations in donors and recipients. *J. Immunol.* **105,** 175–186.

Larsh, J. E., Jr., Goulson, H. T., and Weatherly, N. F. (1964). Delayed hypersensitivity in mice infected with *Trichinella spiralis.* Transfer of peritoneal exudate cells. *J. Parasitol.* **50,** 496–498.

Larsh, J. E., Jr., Race, G. J., Goulson, H. T., and Weatherly, N. F. (1966). Studies on delayed (cellular) hypersensitivity in mice infected with *Trichinella spiralis.* III. Serologic and histopathologic findings in recipients given peritoneal cells. *J. Parasitol.* **52,** 156–166.

Larsh, J. E. Jr., Goulson, H. T., Weatherly, N. F., and Chaffee, E. F. (1970). Studies on delayed (cellular) hypersensitivity in mice infected with *Trichinella spiralis*. VI. Results in recipients injected with antiserum or "freeze-thaw" spleen cells. *J. Parasitol.* **56,** 1206–1209.

Larsh, J. E. Jr., Weatherly, N. F., Goulson, H. T., and Chaffee, E. F. (1972). Studies on delayed (cellular) hypersensitivity in mice infected with *Trichinella spiralis*. VII. The effect of ATS injections on the number of adult worms recovered after challenge. *J. Parasitol.* **58,** 1052–1060.

Lourie, S. H. (1972). The effect of *Plasmodium berghei* on the immune response in rats. *Proc. Helminthol. Soc. Wash.* **39,** 477–484.

Melcher, L. R. (1943). An antigenic analysis of *Trichinella spiralis*. *J. Infect. Dis.* **73,** 31–39.

Miller, J. F. A. P., and Osoba, D. (1967). Current concepts of the immunological function of the thymus. *Physiol. Rev.* **47,** 437–520.

Mota, I., and Wong, D. (1968). Homologous and heterologous passive cutaneous anaphylactic activity of mouse antisera during the course of immunization. *Life Sci.* **7,** 1289–1293.

Mota, I., Sadun, E. H., Bradshaw, R. M., and Gore, R. W. (1969a). The immunologic response of mice infected with *Trichinella spiralis*. Biological and physicochemical distinction of two homocytotropic antibodies. *Immunology* **16,** 71–81.

Mota, I., Sadun, E. H., and Gore, R. W. (1969b). Homocytotropic antibody response in mice infected with *Schistosoma mansoni:* Comparison with the response following *Trichinella spiralis* infection. *Exp. Parasitol.* **24,** 251-258.

Mota, I., Wong, D., and Sadun, E. H. (1969c). Separation of mouse homocytotropic antibodies by biological screening. *Immunology* **17,** 295–301.

Mota, I., Wong, D., Sadun, E. H., and Gore, R. W. (1969d). Mouse homocytotropic antibodies. Cellular and Humoral Mechanisms in Anaphylaxis and Allergy. Karger, Basel and New York, pp. 23-36.

Ogilvie, B. M., and Jones, V. E. (1967). Reaginic antibodies and immunity to *Nippostrongylus brasiliensis* in rats. I. The effect of thymectomy, neonatal infections and splenectomy. *J. Parasitol.* **57,** 335–349.

Sadun, E. H., Mota, I., and Gore, R. W. (1968). Demonstrations of homocytotropic reagin-like antibodies in mice and rabbits infected with *Trichinella spiralis*. *J. Parasitol.* **54,** 814–821.

Sharp, A. D., and Olson, L. J. (1962). Hypersensitivity responses in *Toxocara-, Ascaris-,* and *Trichinella*-infected guinea pigs to homologous and heterologous challenge. *J. Parasitol.* **48,** 362.

Spira, D. T., Silverman, P. H., and Craines, C. (1970). Anti-thymocyte serum effects on *Plasmodium berghei* infection in rats. *Immunology* **19,** 759.

Stechschulte, D. J. (1969). *Plasmodium berghei* infections in thymectomized rats. *Proc. Soc. Exp. Biol. Med.* **131,** 748–752.

Wilson, R. J. M., Jones, V. E., and Leskowitz, S. (1967). Thymectomy and anaphylactic antibody in rats infected with *Nippostrongylus brasiliensis*. *Nature London* **213,** 398–399.

Zvaifler, N. J., Sadun, E. H., and Becker, E. L. (1966). Anaphylactic (reaginic) antibodies in helminthic infections. *Clin. Res.* **14,** 336.

Part IV
Clinical and Diagnostic Aspects

The Soluble Antigen Fluorescent Antibody Test in Detecting Trichinellosis in Swine: Problems and Recent Progress

Robert S. Isenstein

Animal Parasitology Institute
Beltsville Agriculturual Research Center,
Agricultural Research Service,
U.S. Department of Agriculture
Beltsville, Maryland

Introduction

During the past several years our laboratory has been interested in developing and perfecting a soluble antigen fluorescent antibody test for trichinellosis in swine that would apply to industrial situations. The test itself has been used successfully in diagnosing parasitic infections, among those being human schistosomiasis (Toussaint, 1966) and trichinellosis (Gore and Sadun, 1968a). Our particular interest in this test rests on the assumption that the procedure will be rapid, inexpensive, and adaptable to automation.

In preliminary laboratory trials it was possible to detect infections of 100 or more larvae per animal and 0.9 or more larvae per gram of diaphragm tissue with an accuracy of 86% from 3 weeks postinfection to 91% from 6 weeks postinfection.

Because of these promising results with the test in experimentally infected laboratory-raised swine, we decided to find out how the procedure would perform under actual industrial conditions.

Materials and Methods

Assuming that we would be more likely to find *Trichinella* infections in garbage-fed pigs, we collected samples in an abattoir where garbage-raised pigs were regularly killed. The pigs are killed at a rapid rate—about 13/min—so the animals had to be randomly selected for tissue sampling. Blood, from each pig sampled, was collected in 40-ml centrifuge tubes

385

during exsanguination, and muscle tissue samples were taken from the diaphragm pillars, the base of the tongue, and the genioglossus muscle beneath the tongue as the carcasses were routinely processed. Each muscle sample weighing between 5 and 20 gm was mechanically blended with a small volume of saline and subjected to artificial peptic digestion for approximately 2 hr at 40° C in a solution of 2% pepsin–1.2% HCl per 10 gm muscle. Undiluted serum from the blood samples was tested using the soluble antigen fluorescent antibody technique essentially as described by Sadun and Gore (1967) and Gore and Sadun (1968b). This method employs the indirect fluorescent antibody procedure using a cellulose acetate matrix previously saturated with a lipid-free *T. spiralis* larval antigen. The results of the test were read with a fluorometer.

Results

Of 236 garbage-fed pigs sampled and tested in this manner, 17 or 7.2% were infected as determined by muscle digestion. Seven infected animals, or 3% of the total sample, were considered to be heavily infected and harbored between 4 and 1325 larvae per gram of tissue. Ten pigs or 4.2% were considered to be lightly infected and harbored an average of less than one larva per gram of muscle tissue.

A β-type II distribution was fitted to the data according to Kendall and Stuart (1963). A χ-square goodness of fit test was made which showed that the data fitted the distribution (Fig. 1).

From the relationships exhibited by the theoretical curve we can establish a critical point at a fluorometer reading of 58 such that 5% of all readings are contained in the tail of the distribution (Fig. 1). From readings taken on the sera from animals subsequently established as heavily infected it was found that 44% of single readings were lower than the critical value established and 56% fell in the critical area. Thus with three readings, which are routinely made on each serum, we have a probability of $(.44)^3 = .08$ of missing a heavily infected animal and thus a probability of .92 of detection. The type I error is then 5% and the type II 8%.

As progress is being made to refine and improve the test the above technique must be tested on an independent set of readings since these data were used to establish the method and cannot be used to continually test it.

Discussion

On the basis of tests completed on the limited number of animals available, the results of the soluble antigen fluorescent antibody testings are promising. However, at the present stage of our program, extreme

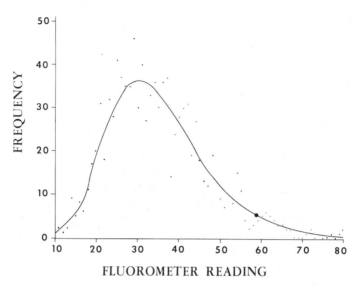

FLUOROMETER READING

Figure 1 Graph of calculated frequency curve and observed data points. The calculated curve follows

$$y = \frac{\Gamma(a+b)}{\Gamma(a)\Gamma(b)} \frac{\chi^a}{(1+\chi)^{a+b+1}}$$

a B-type II function with parameters $a = 11.099$ and $b = 32.682$, which were computed by the method of moments. • , Fluorometer reading of 58 or greater considered to be a positive reading.

caution should accompany interpretation of data until more data have been accumulated. This means that many more naturally infected pigs must be tested and a more efficient scheme must be devised to determine where these pigs can be found. A second interrelated problem is in determining the sensitivity of the test. In experimentally infected laboratory-raised pigs, infections of slightly less than one larva per gram of diaphragm tissue could be detected. However, naturally infected pigs had predominantly heavy infections, and thus far it has not been determined whether the threshold of detection in naturally infected pigs differs from that of pigs reared and infected in the laboratory.

Finally, a word or two about the origin of infected pigs. Owners of garbage feeding establishments naturally defend their product. They maintain that (1) the very nature of garbage has changed over the years, (2) the garbage is nutritionally well balanced, and (3) precautions are taken to insure that it is thoroughly cooked. Finally, they say that, since they are fully aware of the adverse publicity attendant with garbage feeding, they have a vested interest in insuring that such garbage is not the origin of infection for pigs. It is impossible to pass judgment on these claims with the limited knowledge at hand.

However, there is reason to believe that at least some pigs were infected before their arrival at garbage feeding farms. If so, then it is probable that some pigs thought to be non-trichinous because they were grain-fed may nonetheless be infected.

Summary

Garbage-raised swine were tested for trichinellosis using the soluble antigen fluorescent antibody procedure to determine test performance under actual industrial conditions. Of 236 garbage-fed pigs surveyed, 7 pigs (3%) were heavily infected; 10 pigs, (4.2%) were lightly infected as determined by peptic digestion of muscle tissue. Biometrical analysis of the data indicated that it would be possible to identify 92% of the heavily infected pigs with a false positive rate of 5%, using the soluble antigen fluorescent antibody technique.

Acknowledgment

The author expresses his appreciation to Dr. Judson McGuire, Biometrical Section, Northeastern Region, ARS, USDA, Beltsville, Maryland, for his assistance with the biometrical analysis.

References

Gore, R. W., and Sadun, E. H. (1968a). A soluble antigen fluorescent antibody (SAFA) test for the immunodiagnosis of trichinosis in man and experimental animals. *Exp. Parasitol.* **23**, 287–293.

Gore, R. W., and Sadun, E. H. (1968b). Development of a soluble antigen fluorescent antibody test (SAFA) for amebiasis. *Exp. Parasitol.* **22**, 316–320.

Kendall, M. G., and Stuart, A. (1963). "The Advanced Theory of Statistics," 2nd Ed., Vol. I: Distribution Theory. Griffin Ltd., London.

Sadun, E. H., and Gore, R. W. (1967). Relative sensitivity and specificity of soluble antigens (metabolic and somatic) and whole cercariae in fluorescent antibody tests for schistosomiasis in humans and rabbits. *Exp. Parasitol.* **20**, 131–137.

Toussaint, A. J. (1966). Improvement of the soluble antigen fluorescent antibody procedure. *Exp. Parasitol.* **19**, 71–76.

Clinical Pattern and Pathogenesis of the Abdominal Syndrome in Trichinellosis

N. N. Ozeretskovskaya and N. I. Tumolskaya

*E. I. Martsynovsky Institute of Medical Parasitology
and Tropical Medicine
Ministry of Public Health
Moscow*

Introduction

So far there are no sufficiently clear-cut data on the clinical and pathogenic characteristics of the abdominal syndrome in trichinellosis. In severe trichinellosis the abdominal syndrome may reach 42% of the patients (Kratz, 1866). In endemic foci of trichinellosis (United States, Poland, Byelorussia), irrespective of the severity of the disease, patients with the abdominal syndrome varies from 8.5 to 29% or more (Bogdanovich, 1938; Gancarz and Dymek, 1960; Shields *et al.,* 1961; Ozeretskovskaya, 1968).

Results

Among our 146 patients the abdominal syndrome was observed in 51 (34.9%), predominantly in moderately severe or severe trichinellosis (Table I). These were patients who had repeatedly ingested intensively infected meat; 39 patients belonged to the group with the most severe outbreaks of trichinellosis, including 27 patients with outbreaks caused by natural or "nonadapted" *Trichinella* strains, in the Bennet islands due to polar bear meat (1956), in the Komi A.S.S.R. (1959) and in Kamchatka (1967) due to brown bear meat, in the Leningrad region (1957) due to swine infected from the meat of caged fur animals, and in the Krasnodar region (1966) due to swine pastured in the wild (Table II).

Two types of abdominal syndrome have been established. Out of 51 patients 24 had diarrhea during the first 1–4 days of the disease, sometimes watery, numbering up to three to five times daily without noticeable

389

Table I   Frequency of Abdominal Syndrome in Trichinellosis of Varying Severity

| | Frequency according to severity | | | | |
Form of trichinellosis	Mild	Moderately severe	Severe	Highly severe	Total frequency
Total	47	63	28	8	146
Including patients with abdominal syndrome					
During incubation	1	2	2	–	5
Initial	5	10	8	1	24
Delayed	2	13	5	2	22
The percent of patients with abdominal syndrome	17.02	39.68	53.57	37.5	34.9

admixture of mucus and blood in the stool, accompanied by episodes of abdominal pains in half the cases. We called this type the "initial" abdominal syndrome. In five patients who repeatedly ingested intensively infected pork and bacon, diarrhea was observed during the incubation period from 7–10 days to 11–17 days after infection.

Irrespective of the severity of the disease, the initial abdominal syndrome developed and disappeared during the first week of clinical disease. It was found, however, that in mild forms of the disease the initial abdominal syndrome appeared late in the fourth week, in trichinellosis of moderate severity late in the third week (Table III, $P < .02$), and in severe trichinellosis early in the third week after infection (Table III, $P < .01$). The initial abdominal syndrome occurred more frequently in patients from an endemic focus of trichinellosis (Table II, $P < .05$).

In the second type, or the "delayed" abdominal syndrome, we classified abdominal pains and bowel disturbances observed in patients during the entire course of the disease. In contrast to the initial abdominal syndrome, the leading symptom here was not diarrhea, but abdominal pains

Table II   Frequency and Character of the Abdominal Syndrome in Trichinellosis Due to Synanthropic, "Nonadapted" or Natural *Trichinella* strains

| | | Patients with abdominal syndrome | | Character of the abdominal syndrome | |
Source of infection	Total	Number	Percent	Initial	Delayed
Pork in endemic areas	80	24	30.0	20	4
Meat of swine pastured in nature or fed with caged fur animals	53	21	39.6	6	15
Meat of wild animals	13	6	46.1	3	3
Total	146	51		29	22

Table III Day of Appearance and Cessation of Initial and Delayed Abdominal Syndromes[a] Depending on Severity of Trichinellosis in Patients Untreated or Treated with Steroids

Form of trichinellosis	Number of patients			Days of clinical disease					Days after infection					
	Total	With abdominal syndrome		Initial		Delayed			Initial		Delayed			
		Initial	Delayed	Onset	Cessation	Onset	Cessation in patients		Onset	Cessation	Onset	Cessation in patients		
							Treated	Untreated				Treated	Untreated	
Mild	47	5	2	1.2 ±0.1	4.0 ±0.49	10.0	14.5		27.2 ±0.59	30.0 ±0.64	30.5	35.0	
Moderate	63	10	13	1.7 ±1.17	4.5 ±0.53	6.2 ±2.34	22.4 ±3.24	14.8 ±3.03	21.0 ±1.99	23.6 ±2.06	30.8 ±2.88	45.2 ±1.7	39.4 ±2.83
Severe and highly severe	36	9	7	1.9 ±0.67	5.3 ±1.0	2.0 ±0.85	44.5 ±10.08	30 ±2.64	16.4 ±2.28	19.2 ±4.22	20.1 ±3.42	54.6 ±10.33	46.3 ±2.6

[a] There was short term diarrhea without abdominal pains during the incubation period in one mild, two moderate, and two severe cases of trichinellosis.

accompanied by diarrhea only in 9 out of 22 patients. In 18 out of 22 cases the infection was caused by "nonadapted" or natural *Trichinella* strain (Table II, $P < .002$). In mild cases of trichinellosis the delayed abdominal syndrome developed in the second week, in moderately severe ones by the end of the first week, and in severe cases during the first days of the disease (Table III) which corresponded to the beginning of the fifth day and end of the third week after infection (Table III, $P < .05$). Abdominal pains disappeared in the second to third and fifth weeks of the disease, respectively, which corresponded to the end of the fifth and eighth week after infection (Table III). The duration of the delayed abdominal syndrome was proportional to the severity of the disease (from 1–2 to 5 weeks). In one case of complicated trichinellosis, abdominal pains and diarrhea continued up to the seventy-fourth day of the disease. In patients treated by steroids the duration of the abdominal syndrome did not change significantly (Fig. 1). In four patients abdominal pains developed upon discontinuation of steroids.

In 15 patients, including seven with severe and very severe trichinellosis, abdominal pains developed in the first week and were accompanied by diarrhea. Such abdominal syndrome was observed in a child 8 years of age in a severe outbreak of trichinellosis in the foothill areas of Krasnodar region due to a pig fed on "free pasture." Despite intensive desensitization and cardiac therapy the patient died on the thirty-fifth day after infection. The larval count was 16.250–22,500/gm. Histologically diffuse myocarditis, hemorrhagic pneumonitis, diffuse-focal meningoencephalitis, erosive hemorrhagic enterocolitis with massive lymphoid infiltration and proliferative endovasculitis were found (Fig. 2).

Among 22 patients seven had paroxysmal pains. The paroxysms occurred from the first days of the disease. All these patients had maculopapulous or hemorrhagic eruptions. Three patients had diarrhea. The pains were localized in the epigastric region or in the right hypochondrium, and in two patients in the right ileocoecal region also. In five patients the abdominal paroxysms were resistant to steroids and disappeared only after treatment with hormones and large doses of novocaine. Two patients received no steroids.

One patient, 57 years of age, who consumed repeatedly the meat of a pig fed on meat of caged fur animals, had fulminating agues of such severity that she was twice prepared for surgical operation. Despite steroid therapy, the paroxysms continued for a month and stopped only after massive intravenous infusions of novocaine. The patient died on the fifty-seventh day of the disease exhibiting edema-hemorrhagic syndrome and pneumonitis. The density of larvae in this case was 4440/gm. The pathological findings consisted of systemic vasculitis of the hyperergic type (Ozeretskovskaya and Vikhert, 1960). Another patient with abdominal paroxysms (the same outbreak) was hospitalized for "biliary colic."

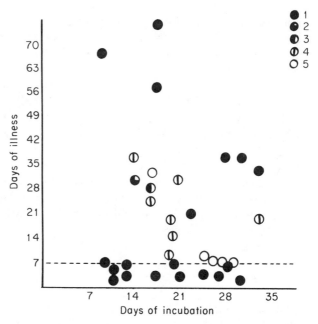

Figure 1 The action of steroids on the duration of abdominal syndrome in respect to the beginning of treatment in the first (5), second (4), third (3), or fourth (2) week after infection in patients with trichinellosis of different incubation periods (1 = untreated patients).

The third patient, 37 years of age, developed acute abdominal pains predominantly in the right part of the abdomen, exudative eruptions all over the body, marked muscle weakness, and fever up to 39°C on the forty-fourth day after he ingested polar bear meat. One week later he had myalgia, facial edema, and hemorrhagic eruptions. On the twelfth day of the disease eosinophilia was 88%, leukocytosis 28,200, ESR 15 mm/hr. This patient did not receive steroids. The disease ran a course of the abdominal form of Schöenlein-Henoch (Ozeretskovskaya, 1958). One month after the onset, there was leukocytosis (14,200), eosinophilia (29%), and the X-ray examination revealed gastroduodenitis and gall bladder dyskinesia. After intravenous infusions of novocaine, polyvitamins, antihistamines, and physiotherapy the pains were considerably relieved.

Of particular interest was the observation of a patient, 36 years of age, who contracted trichinellosis in August 1967, in Kamchatka from ingesting brown bear meat. During the first 2 weeks of the disease, the patient showed weakness, palpitations, myalgia, cough, fever up to 39°C, leukocytosis (32,000), and eosinophilia (70%). He was given prednisolon. Palpitations and myalgia did not disappear. He developed pains in the epigastric region and right hypochondrium. The X-ray examination showed a "niche" in the posterior wall of the duodenum. The steroids were discontinued. However, a remission occurred only after 4 months of active anti-ulcerosis therapy. During the subsequent 2 years, he was hospitalized four times with the same complaints and the ulcer was again detected. In May 1969, biopsy of the gastric mucosa was performed, and chronic atrophic gastritis with pronounced infiltrations of lymphoid-histocytic elements and eosinophils were established (Figs. 3 and 4). The ECG showed signs of metabolic disorders in the left ventriculum wall. In the next 2 years, myalgia, cardiac pains, weakness, ulcerous pains, and eosinophilia (6–16%) persisted.

A similar course of the disease was observed in a patient, 27 years of age, from an outbreak in the Leningrad region (see above). One year after infection, eosinophilia (6%) was present and the density of larvae in the brachialis was 510/gm. Relapses of the duodenal ulcer occurred during 2 years of the follow-up.

Discussion

The abdominal syndrome was associated with penetration by *Trichinella* larvae of the bowel mucosa, with mesadenitis, and abdominal paroxysms with infection of the diaphragm (Gould, 1945; Kaljus, 1952). The pathogenesis of the abdominal syndrome in trichinellosis, however, is much more complicated.

The development of the initial abdominal syndrome corresponding to the maximum levels of antibodies against adults (Oliver-González, 1941), its dependence upon the larval density and particular superinfection and its short duration and benign character show the protective nature of this syndrome and its association with the process of elimination of intestinal *Trichinella* via a "self-cure" phenomenon (Stewart, 1955). In our opinion, the initial abdominal syndrome in trichinellosis is one of clinical manifestations of the secondary immunological response—a rise in the levels of humoral and cytophilic antibodies and delayed hypersensitivity in response to the emergence of metabolic antigens by the worms during molting, leading to elimination of adults from the intestine. The protective immunological nature of the initial abdominal syndrome in trichinellosis is confirmed by its frequency in residents of endemic areas of trichinellosis (Table II, $P < .05$). Diarrhea in the incubation period in patients who had repeatedly ingested infected meat must be considered to be the response to a superinfection (Ozeretskovskaya, 1968).

Of special interest is the pathogenesis of the delayed abdominal syndrome in trichinellosis. Occurrence of abdominal pains relatively late in the disease, their paroxysmal character correlated with hypereosinophilia of the blood and skin lesions, frequently of the hemorrhagic type, and diffuse lymphohistiocytic and eosinophilic infiltrations of the intestinal

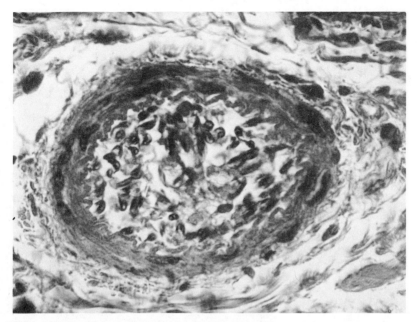

Figure 2 Proliferative endovasculitis in submucosa of the large intestine of patient who had severe trichinellosis and died 35 days after infection. H & E; × 587.

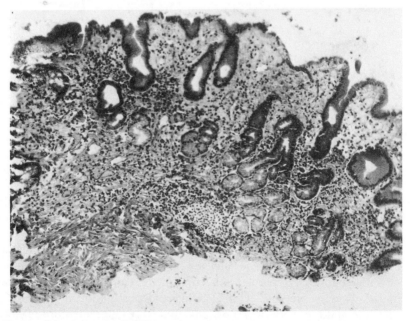

Figure 3 Trichinellosis from consumption of brown bear meat. Persisting duodenal ulcer. Atrophic gastritis with diffuse lymphohistiocytic and eosinophilic infiltrations. H & E; × 107.

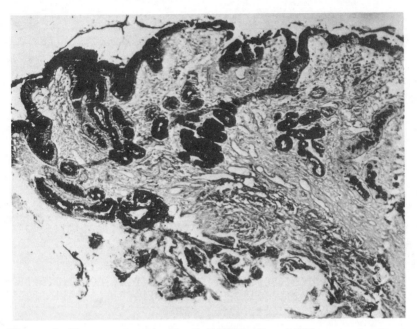

Figure 4   The same case as Fig. 3. PAS reaction; × 74.

mucosa suggest the immunopathological nature of the paroxysmal delayed abdominal syndrome and its pathogenic similarity with hemorrhagic vasculitis and analogous conditions in drug and serum diseases (Tareev, 1953; Ozeretskovskaya, 1958, 1968). The lack of effect in the treatment of the delayed abdominal syndrome with steroids is explained by the resistance of vasculitis to steroids as well as by the stimulation of mature parasites with steroids.

We found the possibility of development in opisthorchiasis and strongyloidiasis of the "secondary" or "symptomatic" duodenal and gastric ulcers with clear-cut clinicomorphological characteristics (Ozeretskovskaya and Karzin, 1971; Karzin, *et al.*, 1972). Their nonspecific nature is confirmed by the similar rate of development of gastroduodenitis in different infections, generalized allergic reactions in patients, tissue eosinophilia, and vasculitis in the mucosa of gastrointestinal tract (Figs. 2 and 3). The association between ulcerative lesions and sensitization by *Trichinella* antigens or antigen-antibody complexes is confirmed by the regular exacerbation of the ulcer, sometimes with bleeding and perforation after dehelminthization and recovery of the patients following complete cure of helminthic diseases (Ozeretskovskaya and Karzin, 1971).

The prospects of cure of the ulcer of the upper part of the gastrointestinal tract in trichinellosis seem to be less optimistic as shown by the above observations. Treatment with thiabendazole in the chronic phase of trichinellosis is quite risky (Kozar *et al.*, 1966). After infection with natural *Trichinella* strains the state of sensitization and ulcerative lesions are maintained by abnormal encapsulation of muscle larvae (Pereverzeva *et al.*, 1971) which determine long-time emergence of *Trichinella* antigens. The provocative role in two of our observations was probably played by steroid therapy which was an ulcerogenic factor on the one hand and an inhibitory factor in the formation of muscle larvae cysts (Ozeretskovskaya and Vikhert 1960) on the other. In any case, in the third patient receiving no steroid therapy, despite infection with the arctic *Trichinella* strain, gastroduodenitis ran a more favorable course.

Our observations indicate that, despite its doubtlessly nonspecific nature, the abdominal syndrome in trichinellosis is rather a contraindication to prescription of steroids. The most effective treatment is vigorous desensitization with novocaine, an antiserotinin agent.

Summary

Among 146 patients with trichinellosis the abdominal syndrome was observed in 51 (34.9%), mainly in moderately severe and severe trichinellosis. The "initial" abdominal syndrome of benign character is described; it is manifested during the first week of disease, and depending on its severity, in the third or fourth week after infection ($P < .01 - .02$), and is typical of trichinellosis in endemic areas. The "delayed" abdominal syndrome, depending on the severity of the disease, which develops in the third to fifth week after invasion ($P < .05$), is manifested predominantly by pains, and not infrequently is the leading symptom; it is typical of trichinellosis derived from meat of wild animals or of infection with "non-adapted" *Trichinella* strains from swine fed meat of wild or caged animals ($P < .02$). Abdominal paroxysms of seven patients are described which are accompanied by hemorrhagic or other eruptions, sometimes by hypereosinophilic leukocytosis. Two patients developed duodenal ulcer persistently relapsing during 2 and 4 years of follow-up. The "delayed" abdominal syndrome is resistant to steroids but yields to treatment with massive infusions of novocaine. The pathogenesis is discussed.

References

Bogdanovich, M. O. (1938). The complications in trichinellosis. *Med. Parazitol. Parazit. Bol.* **7**, 736–744.

Gancarz, Z, and Dymek, E. (1960). Clinical and epidemiological observations on an outbreak of trichinellosis in Bydgoszcz (Poland), 1959. *Wiad. Parasitol.* **6**, 334–335.

Gould, S. E. (1945). "Trichinosis." Thomas, Springfield, Illinois.

Kaljus, V. A. (1952). Trichinelloz cheloveka. *Medgiz, Mosk.,* 248 pp.

Karzin, V. V., Tumolskaya, N. I., and Ozeretskovskaya, N. N. (1972). Some clinico-morphological peculiarities of gastric and duodenal lesions at the acute phase of opistorchiasis. *Med. Parazitol. Parazit. Bol.* **41**, 387–391.

Kozar, Z., Jakowska-Klimowicz, J., and Sladki, E. (1966). Thiabendazole therapy in human trichinellosis. *Wiad Parasitol.* **12**, 605-617.

Kratz, F. (1866). Die Trichinenepidemie zu Hedersleben.

Oliver-Gonzalez, J. (1941). The dual antibody basis of acquired immunity in trichinosis. *J. Infec. Dis.* **69**, 254–270.

Ozeretskovskaya, N. N. (1958). On the pathogenicity of algic-syndrome in trichinellosis. *Sov. Med.* (6), 90–95.

Ozeretskovskaya, N. N. (1968). The clinico-epidemiological peculiarities of trichinellosis from the different regions of the U.S.S.R. *Med. Parazitol. Parazit. Bol.* **37**, 387–397.

Ozeretskovskaya, N. N., and Karzin, V. V. (1971). Some peculiarities of the clinical patterns of gastric and duodenal ulcer and the other lesions of gastrointestinal tract in the chronic opistorchiasis. *Sov. Med.* (10), 106–111.

Ozeretskovskaya, N. N., and Vikhert, A. M. (1960). The systemic vasculitis in trichinellosis. *Klin. Med.* **38**, 67–76.

Pereverzeva, E. V., Ozeretskovskaya, N. N., and Veretennikova, N. L. (1971). Histomorphological investigations on the polar bear strain of *Trichinella. Wiad. Parasitol.* **17**, 465–475.

Shields, L. H., Smith, D. A., Cook, R. W., Jr., Witte, E. J., and Lindsey, G. D. (1961). A local outbreak of trichinosis. *Ann. Intern. Med.* **54**, 734–744.

Stewart, D. F. (1955). Self-cure in nematode infestations of sheep. *Nature London* **176**, 1273–1274.

Tareev, E. M. (1953). V. A. Kaljus. Trichinelloz cheloveka. Recenzia. *Sov. Med.* (4), 46.

Elevated IgE Levels in Trichinellosis

Eugene B. Rosenberg,

Divisions of Nuclear Medicine and Oncology
University of Miami,
Miami, Florida

George E. Whalen,

Gastroenterology Section,
Veterans Administration Center,
Wood, Wisconsin

and Steven H. Polmar

Immunology Branch, National Cancer Institute,
National Institutes of Health
Bethesda, Maryland

Introduction

Elevated IgE levels have previously been reported in patients with hay fever (Berg and Johannson, 1969), allergic asthma (Juhlin *et al.,* 1969), atopic eczema (Berglund *et al.,* 1968), and parasitic diseases including ascariasis (Johansson *et al.,* 1968), capillariasis (Rosenberg *et al.,* 1970), and visceral larva migrans (Hogarth-Scott *et al.,* 1969).

These parasitic diseases were well established before serum IgE levels were measured, and therefore it was not possible to determine the exact time at which IgE levels became elevated. An opportunity for studying the time course of rising IgE levels was presented by a patient with acute trichinellosis. The development of elevated IgE levels in this patient was correlated with the patient's clinical course after ingestion of meat infected with *Trichinella spiralis.*

Materials and Methods

A 25-year-old law student was in excellent health until he ingested three "Saratoga lamb chops." This meat consists of a slice of lamb and

399

a slice of pork rolled together with the pork on the inside. He noted that the meat in the center was pink. Seven days after eating this poorly cooked pork he noted weakness and malaise. Sixteen days after ingestion he developed a temperature of 102°F, abdominal cramps, borborygmi, and diarhea. Eighteen days after eating the meat, he had generalized muscle stiffness, myalgia, scleral injection, periorbital edema, a rash, and an unremitting fever which rose to 105°F. Two days later, on admission to the hospital, he was unable to move without muscle pain. His facial features were distorted by chemosis and periorbital edema. All mucles were tender and those of his upper extremities appeared swollen.

On admission the patient had a WBC of 10,000 cells/cm^3 with 21% eosinophils. His hematocrit was 43%. Other laboratory values included: creatinine phosphokinase, 1,150 units; SGOT, 24 units; SGPT, 31 units; calcium, 8.2 mg%; total protein, 5.0 gm% with a normal electrophoretic pattern; Coombs test, negative; EKG, normal. A skin test for *Trichinella* was 3+ positive with 11 mm of induration and 15 mm of erythema at 20 min. A control skin test showed 2 mm of induration. A latex fixation test for *Trichinella* was negative. A muscle biopsy obtained on day 33 of illness contained encysted *Trichinella* larvae as shown in Fig. 1.

Immunoglobulin Studies

Serum IgE was quantitated by a solid phase radioimmunoassay using insoluble specific anti-IgE and purified radioiodinated IgE myeloma protein (Mann *et al.,* 1969; Polmar *et al.,* 1973). Serum IgA, IgD, IgG, IgM, κ, and λ levels were assayed by radial immunodiffusion.

A correlation of IgE levels with the patient's clinical course is presented in Fig. 2. Twenty-one days after pork ingestion, the patient's IgE level was 500 ng/ml (normal range 108–800 ng/ml). Twenty-seven days after exposure to *T. spiralis* larvae, the patient's IgE level increased threefold to 1600 ng/ml, and 4 days later, it was 1700 ng/ml. Six months after pork ingestion, his IgE level had decreased to 760 ng/ml, which is within normal range.

The increase of IgE occured along with an increase of IgG from 615 mg% to 1400 mg% and an increase of IgM from 188 mg% to 750 mg%. IgA and IgD levels were not significantly increased during this interval. The increase of IgG, IgM, and IgE heavy chains were accompanied by increases of both κ and λ light chains (Table 1).

The rise in IgE levels was preceded by clinical symptoms including diarrhea, high fever, myalgia, chemosis, and rash. An increase in circulating eosinophils accompanied the rise in IgE; high IgE levels persisted as eosinophilia diminished. Evidence of muscle damage was found 28 days after ingestion when CPK, SGOT, and SGPT levels were elevated. Following thiabendazole therapy and the rise of IgE levels, the patient's temperature, myalgia, and periorbital edema decreased, and he recovered completely.

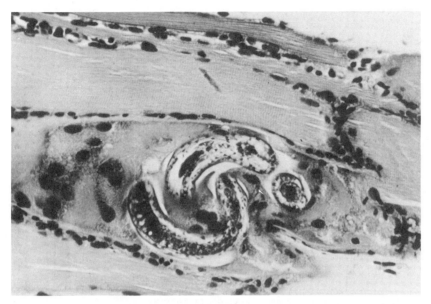

Figure 1   Encysted *Trichinella* larvae in muscle biopsy. H & E, × 450.

Discussion

This case history illustrates the rise of normal IgE levels to three times normal in a patient with trichinellosis 27 days after infection. The IgE level increased further between the twenty-seventh and thirty-first days and was normal 173 days postingestion.

Patients with diseases including hay fever, allergic asthma, atopic eczema, ascariasis, capillariasis, and visceral larva migrans have previously been reported to have elevated IgE levels. The parasitic disorders, especially capillariasis, have been associated with very high IgE concentrations. However, documentation of the time at which IgE levels increase was impossible because of the difficulty of ascertaining the onset of infection. This case of trichinellosis is unique because the exact time that the patient ate the contaminated meat and became infected with *T. spiralis* larvae is known. The rise of circulating IgE developed 22–27 days after exposure and returned to normal by 6 months after infection. When the rise of IgE occurred, the patient was being treated with thiabendazole. The IgE levels in patients with capillariasis were decreased after treatment with this anthelminthic (Rosenberg *et al.,* 1970). Because thiabendazole is effective in eliminating *T. spiralis* as well as *Capillaria p̓hilippinensis* parasites, treatment with thiabendazole may have limited the magnitude of the IgE response in this patient.

Levels of IgM and IgG have been shown to increase within 1 and 2

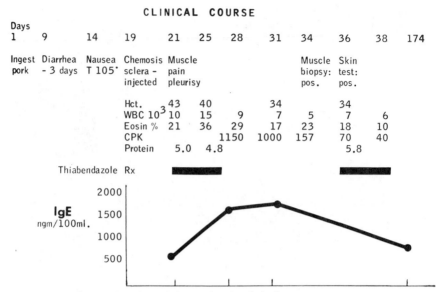

Figure 2   IgE levels and the patient's clinical course.

weeks, respectively, after antigenic stimulation (Fahey, 1965). The rise in IgE level between the third and fourth week after ingestion indicates that IgE production is a late component of the humoral immune response to *T. spiralis* in man. Zvaifler *et al.* (1966) studied reaginic antibody levels, by passive cutaneous anaphylaxis, in a patient with trichinellosis. These authors detected low levels of reaginic antibody after 2 weeks and found higher levels of reaginic antibody between the fourth and sixteenth weeks after infection. Similar observations have been made in animals experimentally infected with *T. spiralis.* Two biologically distinct homocytotropic antibodies appeared in mice 5 weeks after *T. spiralis* infection and reached peak levels at 9 weeks (Mota *et al.,* 1969). Homocytotropic antibodies, measured by passive cutaneous anaphylaxis, were found in rabbits 2 weeks after infection with *T. spiralis,* but these reactions did not reach their peak until 18 weeks after infection (Sadun *et al.,* 1968).

There are marked differences of the ability of *T. spiralis, Capillaria philippinensis,* and *Trichuris trichiura* to stimulate IgE production. These differences are of great interest because these three parasites belong to the same subfamily of nematodes. *Capilloria philippinensis* and *T. spiralis* appear to stimulate IgE production while *T. trichiura* does not. Although these three parasites are closely related taxonomically and morphologically, their life cycles and the severity of the diseases they produce vary considerably. *Capilloria philippinensis* and *T. spiralis* parasites both penetrate intestinal epithelium and migrate through host tissues. Tada and Ishizaka (1970) have shown that IgE producing plasma cells are present in

Table I Immunoglobulin Levels in Trichinellosis

Days after ingestion	IgA (mg%)	IgG (mg%)	IgM (mg%)	IgD (mg%)	IgE (ng/ml)	κ (mg%)	λ (mg%)
21	55	615	188	1.4	500	345	155
27	51	1060	555	1.4	1600	540	425
31	78	1400	750	1.5	1700	760	550
174	98	1310	300	4.2	716	680	345
Control	140	930	130	3	293	580	230
Mean	(70–280)[a]	(620–1400)	(70–250)	(0.2–30)	(108–800)	(350–980)	(130–420)

[a] Numbers in parenthesis indicate range.

peritoneal lymph nodes and in intestinal mucosa. Elevated IgE levels in patients with capillariasis and trichinellosis may be the result of the access of migrating worms or their products to peritoneal nodes, as well as to mucosal lymphoid tissue. *Trichuris trichiura* in asymptomatic cases, is usually restricted to the lumen of the cecum and colon. This pattern of organ involvement may be an important factor limiting IgE synthesis. Moreover, *T. trichiura* larvae do not penetrate intestinal mucosa. Therefore this parasite or its products would not be ordinarily expected to stimulate IgE production in peritoneal nodes. Infections with *T. trichiura* are occasionally severe, leading to bloody diarrhea and prolapse of the rectum. Studies of IgE levels in these symptomatic individuals would be of interest because in heavy infection *T. trichiura* worms can penetrate intestinal mucosa.

The route of antigenic challenge can determine whether antibodies will be synthesized systemically or in local secretions (Newcomb *et al.,* 1969). Immunoglobulin E has been found in nasal washings and bronchial secretions (Ishizaka and Newcomb, 1970). The high concentration of IgE in these secretions suggests that this immunoglobulin is produced locally by the plasma cells of mucous membranes. A local IgE response may be found in patients with trichinellosis, trichiuriasis, and other parasitic diseases and should be sought through studies of the IgE in their intestinal fluids.

This patient had severe symptoms before IgE levels rose. His clinical improvement was associated with anthelminthic therapy and a rise in circulating IgE. Immunoglobulin E mediates the Prausnitz-Kustner reaction (Stanworth *et al.,* 1967) and is commonly referred to as reagin or skin sensitizing antibody (Ishizaka *et al.,* 1969). Well controlled studies in animals have indicated that antibodies resembling human reagins develop in both the primary and secondary immune response to intestinal helminths and that high antibody titers correlate with reduction of worm burdens (Ogilvie, 1967). Studies of visceral larva migrans showed that all patients with high IgE levels had antibodies to *Toxocara* antigen determined by passive cutaneous anaphylaxis in monkeys (Hogarth-Scott *et al.,* 1969). It seems likely that the increased concentrations of IgE in our patient with trichinellosis reflected the amount of IgE antibody present and that IgE antibodies may be part of a protective immune response against *T. spiralis* parasites. On the other hand, IgE antibodies may be harmful in certain situations. IgE antibodies can sensitize a variety of cells (Lichtenstein and Osler, 1964; and Ishizaka, 1969) so that they release histamine and other vasoactive amines in the presence of anti-IgE antibodies (Ishizaka *et al.,* 1969). Animals with high reagin titers develop intestinal hemorrhages following injection of parasitic antigen suggesting that reagins may also sensitize cells in the intestine. The correlation of IgE concentration and severity of illness in patients with capillariasis suggests that IgE antibodies may contribute to the pathogenesis of diarrhea, malabsorption, and enteric protein loss in that parasitic disease (Rosenberg *et al*, 1970). Studies of additional patients with trichinellosis are necessary to determine the biological properties of the IgE antibodies synthesized in man following infection with *T. spiralis*.

Summary

A patient with trichinellosis was studied to determine the immunoglobulin response to infection with *Trichinella spiralis*. Of particular interest was a threefold increase of the patient's IgE level, which occurred 3 weeks after infection. IgE levels doubled and IgM levels tripled between the third and fourth weeks after infection. During the 4 weeks following infection IgA and IgD levels did not change.

Elevation of IgE was a late component of the humoral immune response to *T. spiralis* infection. Trichinellosis is the fourth parasitic disease to be associated with elevated IgE levels and first in which the time course of the IgE rise has been documented. The ability of *T. spiralis* to stimulate IgE production appears related to its penetration of intestinal epithelium and its migration through host tissues.

Acknowledgments

We appreciate the assistance of Miss Rita Grance in preparing this manuscript.

References

Berg, T., and Johansson, S. G. O. (1969). Concentration in children with atopic diseases: a clinical study. *Int. Arch. Allergy* **36**, 219–232.

Berglund, G., Finnstrom, O., Johansson, S. G. O., and Moller, K. L. (1968). Wiskott-Aldrich syndrome: a study of 6 cases with determination of the immunoglobulin A, D, G, M, and N. *Acta Paediat. Scand.* **57**, 89–97.

Fahey, J. L. (1965). Antibodies and immunoglobulins: Normal development and changes in disease. *J. Amer. Med. Ass.* **194**, 255–258.

Fahey, J. L., and McKelvey, E. M. (1965). Quantitative determination of serum immunoglobulins in antibody-agar plates. *J. Immunol.* **94**, 84–90.

Hogarth-Scott, R. S., Johansson, S. G. O., and Bennich, H. (1969). Antibodies to *Toxocara* in the sera of visceral larva migrans patients: The significance of raised levels of IgE. *Clin. Exp. Immunol.* **5**, 619–625.

Ishizaka, K. (1969). The identification and significance of gamma E. *Hosp. Prac.* **4**, 70–81.

Ishizaka, K., and Ishizaka, T. (1967). Identification of γE antibodies as a carrier of reaginic activity. *J. Immunol.* **99**, 1187–1198.

Ishizaka, K., and Newcomb, R. W. (1970). Presence of γE in nasal washings and sputum for asthmatic patients. *J. Allergy* **46,** 197–204.

Ishizaka, T., Ishizaka, K., Johansson, S. G. O., and Bennich, H. (1969). Histamine release from human leucocytes by anti-γE antibodies. *J. Immunol.* **102,** 884–892.

Johansson, S. G. O., Mellbin, T., and Vahlquist, B. (1968). Immunoglobulin levels in Ethiopean preschool children with special reference to high concentrations of immunoglobulin E (IgND). *Lancet* **1,** 1118–1121.

Juhlin, L., Johansson, S. G. O., Bennich, H., Hogman, C., and Thyresson, N. (1969). Immunoglobulin E in dermatoses: Levels in atopic dermatitis and urticaria. *Arch. Dermatol.* **100,** 12–16.

Lichtenstein, L. M., and Osler, A. G. (1964). Studies on the mechanisms of hypersensitivity phenomena: histamine release from human leukocytes by ragweed pollen antigen. *J. Exp. Med.* **120,** 507–529.

Mann, D., Granger, H., and Fahey, J. L. (1969). Use of insoluble antibody for quantitative determination of small amounts of immunoglobulin. *J. Immunol.* **102,** 618–624.

Mota, I., Sadun, E. H., Bradshaw, R. M., and Gore, R. W. (1969). The immunological response of mice infected with *Trichinella spiralis. Immunology* **16,** 71–81.

Newcomb, R. W., Ishizaka, K., and Devald, B. (1969). Human IgE and IgA diphtheria antitoxins in serum, nasal fluids, and saliva. *J. Immunol.* **103,** 215–224.

Ogilvie, B. M. (1967). Reagin-like antibodies in rats infected with the nematode parasite *Nippostrongylus brasiliensis. Immunology* **12,** 113–131.

Polmar, S. H., Waldman, T. A., and Terry, W. D. (1973). A comparison of three radioimmuno assay techniques for the measurement of serum IgE. *J. Immunol.* **110,** 1253–1261.

Rosenberg, E. B., Whalen, G. E., Bennich, H., and Johansson, S.G.O. (1970). Increased circulating IgE in a new parasitic disease—human intestinal capillariasis. *N. Eng. J. Med.* **283,** 1148–1149.

Sadun, E. H., Mota, I., and Gore, R. W. (1968). Demonstration of homocytotrophic reagin-like antibodies in mice and rabbits infected with *Trichinella spiralis. J. Parasitol.* **54,** 814–821.

Stanworth, D. R., Humphrey, J. H., Bennich, H., and Johansson, S.G.O. (1967). Specific inhibition of the Prausnitz-Küstner reaction by an atypical human myeloma protein. *Lancet* **ii,** 330–332.

Tada, T., and Ishizaka, K. (1970). Distribution of γE-forming cells in lymphoid tissues of the human and monkey. *J. Immunol.* **104,** 377–387.

Zvaifler, N. J., Sadun, E. H., and Beckler, E. L. (1966). Anaphylactic (reaginic) antibodies in helminthic infection (abstract). *Clin. Res.* **14,** 336.

A Rapid Screening Hemagglutination Test for the Diagnosis of Human Trichinellosis

Wojciech S. Plonka, Zygmunt Gancarz, and
Bozenna Zawadzka-Jedrzejewska

*Department of Medical Parasitology
National Institute of Hygiene,
Warsaw*

Introduction

Sadun and Allain (1957) described the slide hemagglutination test for detecting anti-*Trichinella* antibodies but its application as a screening procedure in the study of this infection in large patient groups is difficult because it requires inactivation of sera and daily, freshly prepared erythrocytes. A simple hemagglutination drop method was described by Garabedian *et al.* (1960) for the detection of specific antibodies in serum samples from patients with hydatid disease. This method was adopted for rapid testing of antibodies in sera of individuals with *Trichinella* infection.

Materials and Methods

Sera were obtained from patients ill or suspected of trichinellosos. All patients came from epidemic foci of trichinellosis. The sera were not inactivated or adsorbed with sheep red blood cells (SRBC).

One percent saline suspension of dried and powdered *T. spiralis* larvae was frozen and thawed 10 times, centrifuged, and after 24 hr was dialyzed lyophilized, and used as the antigen.

The procedure for the stabilization and sensitization of SRBC with tannic acid and antigen was carried out according to Stavitsky (1954). Briefly, it consists of treatment of washed and packed SRBC with a 1:20,000 dilution of tannic acid (Amend) at 37° C for 10 min and then washing them with buffered saline, pH 7.2. Coating of the tannic acid-treated SRBC was carried out by mixing 1 volume of 2% erthrocyte suspension with 1 volume of antigen and 4 volumes of buffered saline, pH 6.4. The amount of antigen was titrated before each sensitization procedure and usualy it was 0.5 mg of lyophilized per ml of buffered saline. This mixture was incubated at room temperature for 30 min with occasional shaking. It was then centrifuged and the packed, tannic acid-treated, antigen-coated erythrocytes were washed twice with normal rabbit serum (1:150 dilution in buffered saline, pH 7.2). Two percent saline suspension in 1:150 dilution of normal rabbit serum was prepared from the sensitized erythrocytes. One volume of this suspension was then mixed with an equal volume of 20% formalin (37% formaldehyde) in buffered saline, pH 7.2, resulting in a 1% suspension of formalinized erythrocytes. SRBC prepared in this manner could be kept at 4° C for 6 months. Washing out of formalin was not necessary.

Hemagglutination tests were run by adding to the wells in the metaplexi or Takatsy trays, or to small test tubes, successively, one drop of the serum to be tested (1:5 in saline), two drops of saline, and three drops of 1% formalinized-treated erythrocytes. The trays were shaken and left at room temperature for 60 min. Controls were included each time. These consisted of tannic acid–antigen-treated cells mixed with known positive and known negative sera, and tannic acid–saline-treated cells mixed with each tested serum and known positive and known negative sera, respectively.

Sera which appeared to be positive or doubtful in the screening procedure could then be tested quantitatively by the same method using the dilution method. This was done by preparing serial, twofold dilutions of the serum with saline in test tubes, and mixing three drops of each dilution with three drops of 1% suspension of formalinized SRBC.

A total of 215 human sera were tested. Of these, 77 were obtained from individuals ill or suspected of having trichinellosis, 60 normal sera from individuals with no complaints of any disease and 78 sera which were positive in serological tests for cysticercosis, echinococcosis, fascioliasis, toxoplasmosis, leptospirosis, syphilis, and typhoid and paratyphoid fevers. The latter group also included sera from individuals with tuberculosis and neoplastic disease.

Results and Discussion

In the group of 77 sera tested by the screening hemagglutination test a doubtful result was obtained in only one case, the serum from the patient with echinococcosis. The remaining sera were negative. All of the normal sera were negative.

All of the sera from individuals ill or suspected of trichinellosis were tested, in addition to the screening test, by indirect hemagglutination test (Stavitsky, 1954), indirect immunoflourescence test (Brzosko *et al.,* 1965), complement fixation test (Jezioranska, 1955) and ring precipitation test

(Bachman, 1928) routinely used in our laboratory. The results are presented in Table I.

In order to define the dynamics of the antibody titer in particular tests, a group of 20 sera chosen among 77 was tested several times at weekly intervals. The result obtained are summarized in Table II.

As can be seen from the tables on serologic tests in the diagnosis of trichinellosis in man, the most sensitive appeared to be the hemagglutination test. A complete convergence was found between results of the indirect hemagglutination and the screening hemagglutination tests. However, there is a relatively high percentage of doubtful results in the indirect hemagglutination test as compared to the screening test. This may be associated simply with the fact that in the indirect hemagglutination procedure nonformalinized erythrocyctes were used.

High sensitivity of the hemagglutionation test was emphasized by Kagan and Bargai (1956) and by Price and Weiner (1956) in the diagnosis of trichinellosis and by Zawadzka-Jedrzejewska *et al.* (1971) in the diagnosis of fascioliasis in cattle.

From the tables it can also be seen that the lowest percentage of positive results were obtained in the complement fixation test, which is known to be a sensitive test. The only explanation for this is the assumption that the greater part of the sera were from individuals in the initial phase of the disease, the period in which this test is, as a rule, negative. This may also account for the low percentage of positive results in the indirect immunoflourescence test.

In conclusion it can be stated that the screening hemagglutination test is characterized by high sensitivity and specificity. Moreover, it has other advantages, e.g., its performance is very simple, very small amount of material is needed for the test, the results can be obtained in a relatively short time, and the use of the formalinized SRBC makes it possible to perform the test under almost any conditions.

Table I A Comparison of the Results from 77 Sera Tested by Different Methods

	Positive		Negative		Doubtful	
Test	Number	Percent	Number	Percent	Number	Percent
Screening hemagglutination	45	58.4	28	36.4	4	5.2
Standard hemagglutination	45[a]	58.4	15	19.5	17	22.1
Indirect immunofluorescence	30	39.0	45	58.4	2	2.6
Complement fixation	11	14.3	65	84.4	1	1.3
Ring precipitation	17	22.1	56	72.7	4	5.2

[a] Titer 1:160 accepted as diagnostic.

Table II Results of Serological Tests in 20 Trichinellosis Patients in Relation to the Duration of Disease

| | Results after various weeks of disease | | | | | | | | | | | |
| Test | 4 | | 5 | | 6 | | 7 | | 8 | | 9 | |
	Number of positive	Percent	Number of positive	Percent	Number of positive	Percent	Number of positive	Percent	Number of positive	Percent	Number of positive	Percent
Screening hemagglutination	15	75	18	90	20	100	20	100	20	100	20	100
Indirect immunofluorescence	9	45	13	65	16	80	19	95	20	100	20	100
Complement fixation	1	5	5	25	10	50	14	70	16	80	20	100
Ring precipitation	5	25	8	40	15	75	19	95	20	100	20	100

Summary

A simple hemagglutination test is described for screening human trichinellosis in large population groups. Formalinized erythrocytes, which can be stored for at least 6 months, are used as a base for this test. Comparison of results obtained by the indirect and screening hemagglutination tests indicates that both tests have the same diagnostic value. Doubtful results may occasionally be obtained necessitating the use of the dilution method in these cases.

Acknowledgments

This work was supported in part by grant CDC-E-P-2 from the Centor for Disease Control, U.S. Public Health Service.
This work was published in part in the *Journal of Immunological Methods* Vol. 1, pp. 309–312, 1972.

References

Bachman, G. W. (1928). A precipitin test in experimental trichinosis. *J. Prev. Med.* **2**, 35–48.

Brzosko, W., Gancarz, Z., and Nowoslawski, A. (1965). Immunofluorescence in the serological diagnosis of *Trichinella spiralis* infection. *Exp. Med. Microbiol.* **17**, 355–365.

Garabedian, G. A., Malakian, A. H., and Matossian, R. M. (1960). A simple hemagglutination drop test for human hydatidosis. *Ann. Trop. Med. Parasitol.* **54**, 233–235.

Jezioranska, A. (1955). Diagnostic value of trichina antigens by trichinellosis. *Acta Parsitol. Pol.* **3**, 191–215.

Kagan, I. G., and Bargai, U. (1956). Studies on the serology of trichinosis with hemagglutination, agar diffusion tests and precipitin ring tests. *J. Parsitol.* **42**, 237–245.

Price, S. G., and Weiner, L. M. (1956). Use of hemagglutination in the diagnosis of trichinosis. *Amer. J. Clin. Pathol.* **26**, 1261–1269.

Sadun, E. H., and Allain, D. S. (1957). A rapid slide hemagglutination test for the detection of antibodies to *Trichinella spiralis*. *J. Parasitol.* **43**, 383–388.

Stavitsky, A. B. (1954). Micromethods for the study of proteins and antibodies. I. Procedures and general applications of hemagglutination and hemagglutination-inhibition reaction with tannic acid and protein-tested red blood cells. *J. Immunol.* **72**, 360–367.

Zawadzka-Jedrzejewska, B., Gancarz, Z., and Plonka, W. S. (1971). Application of serological tests in the diagnosis of invasion of *Fasciola hepatica*, Linne 1758. *Exp. Med. Microbiol.* **23**, 267–275.

Electrocardiographic Changes in Trichinellosis. Experimental Studies in Rabbits

Leon Chodera and Zbigniew Pawłowski

Clinic of Parsitic Diseases
Medical Academy of Poznán
Poznán

Introduction

The pathogenesis of the changes in the bioelectric myocardial activity in acute trichinellosis has not been satisfactorily elucidated to date (Chodera, 1969; Gould, 1945; Parrisius *et al.,* 1942; Wołoszczuk and Malik, 1969). The hypothesis generally accepted is that toxic changes and/or eosinophilic myocarditis found in trichinellosis are responsible for them (Gould, 1945; Parrisius *et al.* 1942; Wołoszczuk and Malik, 1969). However, the eosinophilic myocarditis, very often focal and limited to the connective tissue, does not account for deviation in the depolarization and repolarization of myocardial cell membranes. There are discrepancies between clinical symptoms and quickly changing patterns of electrocardiographic curves, as well as between the latter and the histopathological picture in fatal cases (Gould, 1945). Our observations of the electrocardiographic curves in cases of severe human trichinellosis in several epidemics, including one fatal case, confirms the existence of such discrepancies. Systemic studies were carried out during an epidemic and included 15 cases which were in several instances severe. Observation of the patients from the onset of acute symptoms gave rise to the conviction that disturbances in potassium and/or protein metabolism may play an important, if not the main, role in the development of pathological bioelectric activity of the myocardium during the acute phase of trichinellosis (Chodera, 1969).

This chapter attempts to evaluate in animals the influence of metabolic potassium and/or protein changes on the pathogenesis of the abnormal pictures of electrocardiographic recordings.

413

Materials and Methods

The study was carried out on six adult rabbits with an average body weight of 3 kg. They were infected orally with encapsulated *Trichinella spiralis* larvae of the Krotoszyn strain (1960) with a dose of 5000/kg body weight. The infected rabbits were observed for 2 months. The following examinations were carried out before infection and then twice weekly for 5 weeks and on day 59 after infection: leukocyte and eosinophil counts, anal temperature, body weight, serum potassium and protein levels, electrocardiographic recordings (one lead apparatus Simplicard 2 with paper transport of 50 mm/sec). After the appearance of distinct symptons of acute trichinellosis, such as fever up to 40° C, rise in leukocytes per cubic millimeter, loss of appetite and body weight, and the presence of very significant electrocardiographic changes, a solution containing potassium ions (dilution 3:10 of Elkinton II solution containing 3 gm KCl/20 ml) was slowly injected intravenously into the marginal ear vein of the rabbits. These experiments were carried out once during the fourth and/or fifth week of infection (one rabbit), repeated once after 3 or 4 days in three animals, and repeated twice after 7 and additional 4 days (one rabbit). In one rabbit an undiluted Elkinton II solution was used. Electrocardiographic recordings were made before and during the infusion of potassium ions, as well as after stopping the injection.

Results

The electrocardiographic changes in the course of the acute phase of trichinellosis in rabbits concerning heart rate, voltage $R_{I^{00}III}$ peaks, the behavior of ST interval and T-wave as compared with the same parameters before the potassium ions injection are presented in Table I.

In all the rabbits the heart rate rose from about 250–280/min to about

Table I Character of Electrocardiographic Changes in Acute Trichinellosis in the Rabbit

Rabbit	Heart rate per minute	R_{I-III}	ST_I	$ST_{II/III}$ aVF	T_{I-III} aVF	$ST_{V\ apex}$
1	↑	↓	—	↓	↓	—
2	↑	↓	±	↓	↓	↓
3	↑	↓	±	↓	↓	↓
4	↑	↓	±	↓	↓	↓
5	↑	↓	—	↓	↓	↓
6	↑	↓	—	↓	↓	—

[a] ↑, Acceleration of heart rate; ↓, diminution of R peak voltage flattening or inversion of T-wave; ±, slight changes; —, no changes.

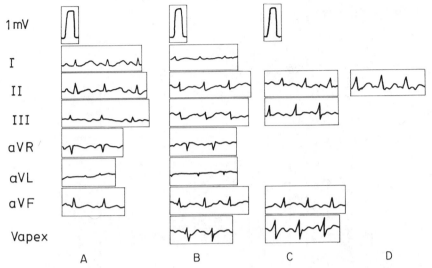

Figure 1 Electrocardiographic tracings in rabbit 1. A, Before infection; B, 5 weeks after infection with distinct changes in several parameters; C, like B—normalization of the electrocardiographic tracings after injection of diluted Elkinton II solution (K^+ ions); D, like B and C—EKG tracing typical for hyperkalemia after overdosage of Elkinton solution.

330/min. Generally a diminution in the R peak voltage, at least in one lead runs parallel with the increased heart rate. Very significant depression of the ST interval below the diastolic isoelectric level was noted in all the recordings II, III, and aVF throughout the observation but to a lesser degree in other leads, too (I and V apex). The T-wave, as a rule, exhibited a flattening following infection. In some instances it was negative in one or more leads. The electrocardiographic changes began as early as the fifth day of infection (three rabbits), and were present in all the rabbits on the twelfth day becoming most intensive during the fourth and fifth week of infection. This is illustrated in Table II.

Table II illustrates the instability of the changes in the electrocardiographic recordings. Their intensity changed temporarily from examination to examination in four rabbits. A slow intravenous infusion of 3:10 dilution of Elkinton II solution performed 10 times in five rabbits at 3- to 7-day intervals always reduced almost completely all electrocardiographic changes noted before beginning the infusion, but the changes reappeared within a few minutes after stopping the infusion. In one rabbit undiluted Elkinton solution led to the disappearance of the EKG changes due to trichinellosis, while continuation of the infusion led to the death of the animal. The intravenous infusion of potassium ions reduced the depression of the ST interval, normalized the T-wave and the R peak, but did not change the increased heart rate. The electrocardiographic changes described above are, by way of example, presented in Fig. 1.

Table II Intensity of Electrocardiographic Changes in the Course of Acute Trichinellosis in the Rabbit

Rabbit	Intensity of electrocardiographic changes at progressive days of infection[a]										
	0	5	12	14	19	21	25	28	32	35	59
1	−	±	++	++	++	+++	+++	++ / +++	+++ Elk +	+++ / ++ Elk +	+
2	−	−	++	+	++	++ / ++	++	+++ Elk +	+++ / ++ Elk +	+++ Elk +	exit.
3	−	++	++	+	++	+++ Elk +	+++	+++ / ++ Elk +	+++ / ++ Elk +	++++ / +++	+++ / +++
4	−	±	++	±	+++	+++	++	+++	++ Elk +	++ / +++ .Elk +	+
5	−	±	++	++	+++	+++	++++ / +++ Elk +	++++ / +++ Elk +	+++	+++	±
6	−	−	++	+++	++ Elk +	exit.					

[a]The symbols ±, +, ++, +++, and ++++ represent the intensities of electrocardiographic changes; Elk, intravenous injection of diluted Elkinton II solution; Elk +, intravenous injection of undiluted Elkinton II solution.

As compared with the recordings made before the infection (Fig. 1A), the electrocardiograms made during acute trichinellosis (Fig. 1B) exhibit distinct changes in several parameters. The influence of potassium ions infusion is represented by the recordings of Figure 1C. When K^+ ions infusion was accelerated, the EKG recordings resulted in a pattern typical of hyperpotassemia (Fig. 1D).

Table III presents some of the laboratory findings which may be interesting in the interpretation of the experiment. There was a significant drop in the serum protein level beginning the second week of infection with a tendency toward normal in the weeks following. The lowest values are presented in Table III. The serum potassium exhibited fluctuations in a wide range, The lowest values were generally noted at the peak of the disease, but in one case only the K^+ ion concentration dropped distinctly below 4 mEq/liter. In all the cases a slight elevation in leukocyte and eosinophil counts was noted.

Discussion

The results obtained in experimental trichinellosis in rabbits confirm earlier findings in human trichinellosis suggesting an influence of disturbances in protein and potassium metabolism found in this disease on the EKG recordings (Chodera, 1969). This is evident from the reversibility of the EKG changes during K^+ ion infusion and their lability in the course of the disease. Their reappearance after stopping this K^+ ion infusion gives rise to the conviction that a gradient mechanism of these ions through the myocardial cell membranes may be responsible for the pattern of the actual EKG recordings. The lesion of semipermeability of myocardial cell wall may be of toxic character, as well as protein depletion found as a rule, in severe actue trichinellosis (Rachoń et al., 1965; Chodera, 1969), may play an important role in the potassium loss of muscle cells (Busila et al., 1968). Other metabolic changes, such as tissue enzyme leakage (Boczon et al., 1969), disturbed carbohydrate metabolism (Pawlowski, 1967), closely linked to kaliemia (Chodera et al., 1957), may be additional causes of K^+ ion depletion. This, in turn, at the level of myocardial cell membranes, leads to disturbances of the repolarization and/or depolarization processes of the myocardium. The wide range of potassium levels in the blood serum generally showed a tendency toward lower values, but, it did not, as a rule, run parallel to the actual state of the infection and EKG changes. One reason for this seems to be the vegetarian nutrition of rabbits. Nevertheless, our impression is that the EKG changes in trichinellosis do not depend so much upon the actual serum potassium level but rather upon the direction of K^+ ion transport through the myocardial cell wall. A K^+ ion gradient mechanism seems to be at work in trichinellosis at the level of

Table III Some Laboratory Findings in the Course of Acute Trichinellosis in the Rabbit

Rabbit	Serum protein (gm %) mean and range		Lowest K$^+$ level (mEq/liter)	Highest body temperature (°C)	Highest count/mm^3 leukocytes	eosinophils
1	5.9	4.3–5.4	4.4	40.2	10,400	3800
2	5.4	3.4–6.9	4.3	40.3	11,200	3600
3	5.9	4.4–6.2	3.5	39.3	11,000	3600
4	5.3	5.2–5.8	4.0	39.6	13,200	5600
5	5.2	3.5–5.8	4.5	39.2	13,200	4800
6	4.9	3.7–4.8	5.0	30.0	12,600	3400

damaged cell membranes, which leads to a leakage of different substances, one of them certainly being kalium ions.

Summary

The experiment was undertaken to confirm the clinical suggestion concerning the pathogenesis of electrocardiographic changes often found in human trichinellosis (Chodera, 1969).

Six adult rabbits were infected with *Trichinella spiralis* larvae (5000/kg body weight). Electrocardiographic recordings, serum protein and serum potassium level estimations, and leukocyte and eosinophil counts were made twice a week. Electrocardiographic changes in the R peak, the T-wave and the ST interval were observed in all the animals as early as the fifth day of infection and were most distinct in the fourth and/or fifth week of trichinellosis. In individual animals the electrocardiographic changes were unstable and transient as was the serum potassium level and the tendency to lower values was evident. The serum protein level dropped rather early. In the fourth and fifth week of infection the animals with evident electrocardiographic changes were treated with K^+ ions. During the intravenous infusion of potassium ions the electrocardiographic changes disappeared almost completely in all the rabbits and reappeared within a few minutes after the end of the infusion. This phenomenon was noted when the experiment was repeated after 3–7 days.

The experiments on rabbits confirm the clinical suggestion that the changes in the bioelectric activity of the heart muscle in trichinellosis depend on a gradient mechanism in potassium turnover linked to protein depletion.

Acknowledgments

This study was supported by grant CDC-E-2, Center for Disease Control, U.S. Public Health Service.

References

Boczon, K., Chodera, L., Gerwel, C., Michejda, J., and Wisniewska, M. (1969). Changes in enzymatic activity in course of human trichinellosis. *Wiad. Parazytol.* **15**, 707–710.

Busila, V. T., Dragomirescu, M., Dragomirescu, L., and Maager, P. (1968). Functional and metabolic alterations in human trichinellosis. *Wiad. Parazytol.* **14**, 195–200.

Chodera, L, (1969). Electrocardiographic changes and potassium metabolism in the course of acute phase of trichinellosis. *Wiad. Parazytol.* **15,** 731–732.

Chodera, L., Mazurowa, A., and Smarsz, C., (1957).. Badania nad wspózależnościa przemian metabolicznych w zakresie elektrolitów i weglowodanów oraz żamian electrokardiograficznych pod wplywem leczniczych dawek adrenaliny. *Pol. Archi. Med. Wewn.* **27,** 1319–1333.

Gould, S. E. (1945). "Trichinosis." Thomas, Springfield, Illinois.

Parrisius, W., Lampe, G., Romer, W., and Hönighaus, L. (1942). Erfahrugen während einer Trichinose-Epidemie. *Deut. Militaraerztl.* **7,** 198–209.

Pawłowski, Z. (1967). Adrenal cortex hormones in intestinal trichinellosis. III. Effect of adrenalectomy and hydrocortisone, insulin, alloxan and glucose treatment on elimination of *Trichinella spiralis* adults in hooded rats. *Acta Parasitol. Pol.* **15,** 179–189.

Rachoń, K., Januszkiewicz, J., and Wehr, M., 1965. Uwagi o gospodarce bialkowej w przebiegu wlosnicy u ludzi. *Przeg. Epidemiolo.* **21,** 417–425.

Woloszczuk, J., and Malik, A., (1969). Polycardiographic evaluation of the heart muscle condition in the patients and persons with trichinellosis. *Wiad. Parazytol.* **15,** 733–737.

Diagnosis of Trichinellosis by Hemagglutination with a Purified Larval Antigen

Omar O. Barriga
and Diego Segre

*Department of Pathobiology, School of Veterinary Medicine
University of Pennsylvania, Philadelphia
College of Veterinary Medicine, University of Illinois
Urbana, Illinois

Introduction

Accurate diagnosis of human trichinellosis rests mainly on the detection of specific immune responses of the host. Although many procedures have been proposed to detect these responses (see Kagan and Norman, 1970; Barriga, 1973), the techniques most commonly used in clinical practice are cutaneous tests and bentonite agglutination. Indirect fluorescent antibody tests are becoming important in the detection of light infections, and complement fixation tests are usually employed as a reference for comparison with other tests. Cutaneous tests are positive in only about 60% of the cases (Schenone et al., 1970) and frequently yield false positive reactions (Kagan and Norman, 1970). Bentonite agglutination is a simple procedure but not sensitive enough to detect light or recent infections and may persist positive for several years (Schultz et al., 1967). The indirect fluorescent antibody test is sensitive and specific (Sadun et al., 1962; Crandall et al., 1966) but rather involved to perform in nonspecialized laboratories. The complement fixation test is only moderately sensitive and specific (Kozar and Kozar, 1968). Although Labzoffsky et al. (1964) reported positive indirect fluorescent antibody reactions with serum of patients taken during the first week of disease, most authors have found that the tests usually become positive in man after the third week of disease (Gancarz, 1964; Labzoffsky et al., 1964; Kozar and Kozar, 1966, 1968; Jezyna et al., 1967; Kagan and Norman, 1970; Kassur and Woloszczuk, 1970).

The sensitivity and specificity of a given test is strongly influenced by the procedure used to prepare the antigen (Sleeman and Muschel, 1961; Maynard and Kagan, 1964; Ivey and Slanga, 1965; Adonajlo et al., 1967;

421

Hacig *et al.,* 1967; Gancarz, 1968; Subbotin, 1968). Kagan (1965), Kozar and Kozar (1968), and Bessonov and Volfson (1970) recommended that several tests be performed simultaneously with the same serum to over-come this difficulty.

Delay in diagnosis of human trichinellosis extends the hospitalization . period, precludes an early and more effective treatment, increases the likelihood of complications and sequelae, prevents one from obtaining reliable information about the possible origin of the infection, limits the findings of atypical cases associated with the reference case and retards or negates the condemnation of the infective meat to prevent further cases. A sensitive, specific, and reproducible method for the early diag-nosis of human trichinellosis is therefore highly desirable.

The purpose of this investigation was to develop a test with these char-acteristics which would be simple enough to be employed in any diagnostic laboratory. The first step was to purify a highly active antigenic com-ponent from larval extracts of *Trichinella*. This component was used later in hemagglutination (HA) tests with sera from infected rabbits to find its efficacy in detecting early antibodies and with sera from human patients to compare its sensitivity with those of an antigen and test in current use.

Materials and Methods

Infection

Larva-donor rabbits, rats, and mice were infected orally with about 10 *Trichinella* larvae per gram of body weight. Serum-donor rabbits were infected in the same manner with four larvae per gram of body weight. The original larvae were obtained by pepsin–HCl digestion of infected mouse carcasses, separated from the detritus in a Baermann apparatus (Beaver, 1953), washed five times in 0.15 M NaCl solution by centrifuga-tion at 156 g for 5 min, washed once in 10% petroleum ether in 0.15 M NaCl solution (v/v), and washed two more times in 0.15 M NaCl. The larvae from the larva-donor animals were recovered by the same procedure on the thirtieth day of infection.

Crude Extract

Since rabbit and rodent larvae vary markedly in size and wet weight was not regarded as an accurate measurement, the quantification of larvae for extraction was done on the basis of their packed volume in 15 ml, 120×17 mm, long conical glass tubes, after centrifugation at 156 g for 10 min. When convenient, the volume was converted to weight on the as-sumption that the specific weight of a *Trichinella* larva is approximately 1.069 (Barriga, 1971). The recovered larvae were resuspended in 0.0175 M phosphate buffer, pH 6.8, and homogenized at 45,000 rpm for nine periods of 1 min each in a VirTis "45" homogenizer, maintaining the flask in an ice bath. The homogenate was centrifuged at 28,000 g for 30 min at 2°C. The supernatant fluid was regarded as the crude extract and the sediment was extracted with the same buffer at 4°C for 24 hr. A similar centrifugation yielded a supernatant fluid that was considered the second extract, and a sediment that was extracted again in the same manner. This procedure was repeated until a seventh extract was obtained. On one occasion the sediment of the homogenate was lyophilized and extracted as described above. The crude extract for the experiments reported here was obtained from rabbit parasites. Protein measurements on the crude extract and on all the fractions were performed according to the Folin-Lowry technique (Lowry *et al.*, 1951) using twice crystallized ovalbumin as standard.

Fractionation of the Crude Extract

Fractionation was attempted by salt precipitation, Sephadex filtration, and DEAE-cellulose chromatography.

Salt Precipitation   Three 2-ml aliquots of crude extract were mixed with 2.0 ml, 3.0 ml, and 4.66 ml, respectively, of saturated ammonium sulfate solution to bring the final concentration to 50%, 60%, and 70% saturation. The tubes were allowed to stand at room temperature for several minutes and were centrifuged at 1400 g for 15 min. The supernatant fluids and sediments were dialyzed against 0.0175 M phosphate buffer before estimating protein and performing immunological analysis.

Sephadex Filtration   An aliquot of crude extract was dialyzed against 0.32 M NaCl solution containing 10^{-3} M sodium borate buffer and was passed through a Sephadex G-200 column (59 cm in height and 1.0 cm in diameter) equilibrated previously with the same buffer. Ninety 3-ml fractions were collected and their protein content was monitored by optical density at 280 nm wavelength (OD_{280}). Those fractions that appeared to constitute a single peak were pooled together and concentrated before measuring protein and performing immunological analysis. A similar procedure was performed using a Sephadex G-150 column with the same dimensions.

DEAE-Cellulose Chromoatography   A DEAE-cellulose column (45 cm in height and 2.5 cm in diameter) was equilibrated with 0.0175 M phosphate buffer, pH 6.8, and loaded with an aliquot of crude extract. The column was washed successively with the same buffer at 0.0175 M, 0.07 M, 0.14 M, 0.2 M, and 0.3 M, and the materials eluted at every molarity were collected separately. The molarities higher than 0.0175 M were obtained by adding appropriate amounts of NaCl to the original 0.0175 M buffer. The fractions were concentrated before antigenic analysis.

Antigenic Analysis

The crude extract and the different fractions were analyzed by gel double diffusion and by immunoelectrophoresis against sera from an infected rabbit and from a rabbit hyperimmunized with the crude extract. Double diffusion tests were run with 1.5% Noble Agar containing 0.01% sodium azide in 0.0175 M phosphate buffer, pH 6.8, and incubated up to 7 days at room temperature. Immunoelectrophoresis was performed on microscope slides covered with 4.0 ml of 1.5% Noble Agar in 0.075 M barbital buffer, pH 8.6. All the fractions were previously dialyzed against the same buffer and electrophoresed for 90 min at room temperature with a constant current of 7.5 mA per slide. The slides were incubated for 48 hr at room temperature and the results were recorded photographically.

Sera

The sera utilized in the antigenic analysis were obtained from a rabbit infected with *Trichinella* larvae 60 days earlier (SI) and from a rabbit hyperimmunized with the crude extract emulsified with Freund's complete adjuvant (SH). The rabbit sera for HA tests were obtained at different times up to 30 days after infection (see Table II). Serum from an infected rabbit hyperimmunized with the fraction obtained by elution of the DEAE-cellulose column with 0.07 M buffer (0.07 M fraction) (anti-0.07 M serum) was used as a positive control and to run HA inhibition tests. Human sera were obtained from 41 trichinellosis patients which had been previously tested by bentonite agglutination (BA) with acid soluble protein antigen (Melcher, 1943) and from 50 clinically healthy persons. Rabbit sera taken before infection were used as negative controls. All sera utilized in HA and HA inhibition tests were inactivated at 56° C for 30 min and absorbed with normal sheep red blood cells (SRBC).

Hemagglutination (HA) Tests

HA tests were performed with the optimal dilution of the 0.07 M fraction coupled to SRBC by glutaraldehyde (Avrameas *et al.,* 1969). Five volumes of 2.5% washed SRBC in 0.15 M phosphate buffered saline (PBS), pH 7.2, were mixed with five volumes of 0.07 M fraction containing 0.2 mg of protein ml, and with one volume of 1% gluteraldehyde, and stirred at room temperature for 2 hr. After this period the SRBC were washed five times in PBS and resuspended at 2.5% in 1% inactivated and adsorbed normal rabbit serum in PBS (1% NRS). HA tests were run ·in Kahn tubes containing 0.5 ml of the sera diluted in twofold steps in 1% NRS and 1 drop (approximately 0.05 ml) sensitized SRBC. Sedimentation patterns were regarded as positive when the SRBC formed perfect shields or large shields with ragged edges.

Aliquots of sensitized SRBC were frozen and stored at −15° C, stored at 4° C in liquid form, or lyophilized and stored at 4° C, to find their shelf life.

HA Inhibition Tests

The end-point dilution of the anti-0.07 M serum was considered to contain 1 HA unit of antibody. Dilutions (0.25 ml) of this serum containing 16 HA units were incubated for 15 min with serial dilutions (0.25 ml) of the crude extract and of different fractions and sensitized SRBC were added to the mixtures. HA inhibition was indicated by settling of the SRBC in a tight button. Similar HA inhibition tests were performed with the early negative serum of infected rabbits but using only 4 HA units of antibody.

Results

Crude Extract

The crude extract did not show a lipid layer after high-speed centrifugation at 2° C. Homogenization and centrifugation (first extraction) of the larvae recovered over 72% of all the protein obtained by seven successive extractions (Table I). Immunoelectrophoresis of a crude extract containing 8.2 mg of protein/ml revealed 11 precipitin bands against SI and 21 against SH (Fig. 1). The first band to appear and the one that yielded the most intense line both by gel double diffusion and by immunoelectrophoresis was designated antigen A. Immunoelectrophoresis with a crude extract containing 1.4 mg of protein/ml revealed four bands against SI and 12 against SH. Antigen A was always present.

Table I Protein Contents of Seven Successive Extractions on a 5-ml and on a 10-ml Sample of *Trichinella* Larvae

Extractions	Protein content			
	5-ml sample		10-ml sample	
	(mg)	(%)	(mg)	(%)
First	213	72.7	354	79.5
Second	28	9.4	45	10.0
Third	25	8.4	16	3.6
Fourth	15	5.1	10	2.2
Fifth	5	1.7	9	2.0
Sixth	6	2.0	7	1.6
Seventh	5	1.7	5	1.1
Total	297	100.0	446	100.0

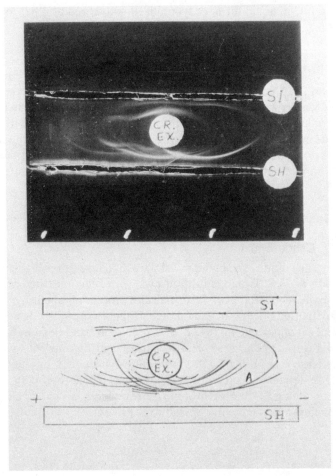

Figure 1 Immunoelectrophoresis of the crude extract (CR. EX.) with sera from an infected rabbit (SI) and from a hyperimmunized rabbit (SH). The crude extract contained 8.24 mg of protein/ml.

Fractions Obtained by Salt Precipitation

Ammonium sulfate at 50%, 60%, and 70% saturation precipitated 35.4%, 54.5%, and 75.8% of the protein in the crude extract, respectively. Immuno-electrophoresis of the fractions obtained at 50% saturation against SH revealed three bands in the supernatant fluid and in the sediment (Fig. 2). Both fractions contained antigen A. Precipitation at 60% saturation yielded a supernatant fluid with traces of antigen A and a sediment with a larger amount of antigen A and a contaminant component. Immunoelec-trophoresis with the supernatant fluid of precipitation at 70% saturation showed no bands but five antigens, including A, appeared with the sediment (Fig. 3).

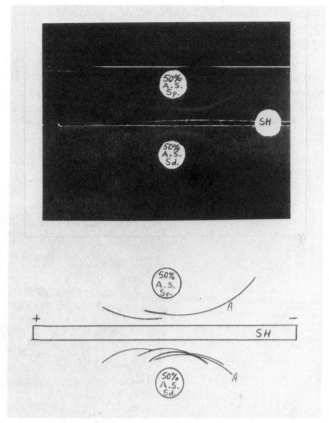

Figure 2 Immunoelectrophoresis of the supernatant (A.S. Sp.) and the sediment (A.S. Sd.) obtained by ammonium sulfate precipitation at 50% saturation with serum from a hyperimmunized rabbit (SH).

Fractions Obtained by Sephadex Filtration

Two peaks were obtained either with Sephadex G-200 or G-150. The ratio of the protein in the first and second peak was 1:1.57 in the eluate from Sephadex G-200 and 1:1 in the eluate from Sephadex G-150, as measured by OD_{280}. Immunoelectrophoresis with SH revealed antigen A and three other antigens in the second peak from Sephadex G-200. After filtration of the crude extract through Sephadex G-150 antigen A was found in both peaks, although it appeared more concentrated in the second peak, which contained two other antigens.

Fractions Obtained by DEAE-Cellulose Chromatography

Seventy-five to 80% of the protein applied in the column was recovered in the eluate. The distribution of the protein was 59.6%, 14.7%, 9.8%, 8.8%, and 6.7% as measured by the Folin-Lowry technique, in the fractions eluted with 0.0175 *M,* 0.07 *M,* 0.14 *M,* 0.2 *M,* and 0.3 *M* buffer, respectively. The fraction eluted with 0.0175 *M* buffer came out in the four peaks, all the other fractions came out as single peaks.

Although all the peaks of the 0.0175 *M* fraction had some antigenic activity, none of them contained antigen A (Figs. 4 and 5). Immunoelectrophoresis of the 0.07 *M* fraction revealed antigen A and a weak contaminant band with SI and antigen A with three faint contaminant lines with SH (Fig. 6). Fractions 0.14 *M* and 0.2 *M* showed several antigens but no A (Figs. 6 and 7). Fraction 0.3 *M* revealed only a faint band.

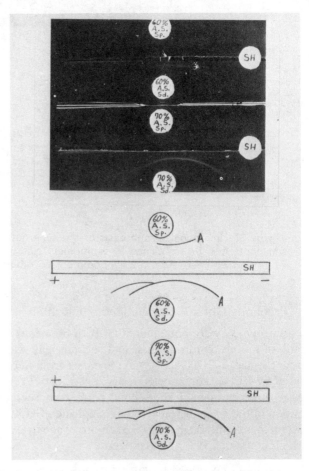

Figure 3 Immunoelectrophoresis of the supernatants (A.S. Sp.) and the sediments (A.S. Sd.) obtained by ammonium sulfate precipitation at 60% and at 70% saturation with serum from a hyperimmunized rabbit (SH).

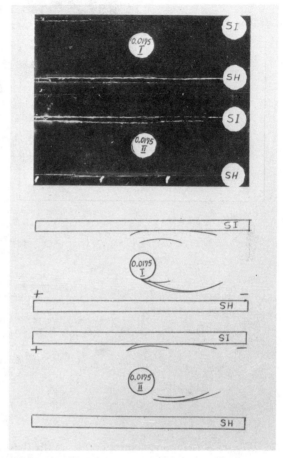

Figure 4 Immunoelectrophoresis of the first (0.0175 I) and the second (0.0175 II) peaks obtained by elution of a DEAE-cellulose column with 0.0175 *M* buffer against sera from an infected rabbit (SI) and from a hyperimmunized rabbit (SH).

Serology

Sensitization of the SRBC under the stated conditions yielded very reproducible results. However, slight variations in gluaraldehyde concentration or in the time of incubation resulted in marked differences in titers: although some of these titers were very high, they were very difficult to reproduce. Antigen derived from rabbit parasites was used in all the tests; antigen from rodent parasites was used on a few occasions but the end points were less sharp than those obtained with antigen of rabbit origin. Otherwise, they yielded similar results.

HA tests with the sera of eight infected rabbits yielded the results shown

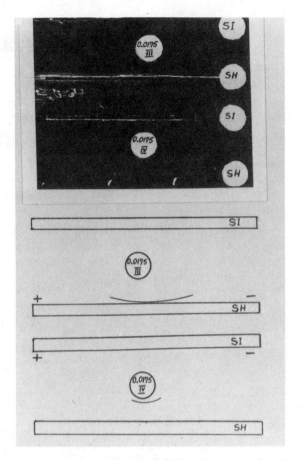

Figure 5 Immunoelectrophoresis of the third (0.0175 III) and the fourth (0.0175 IV) peaks obtained by elution 'of a DEAE-cellulose column with 0.0175 *M* buffer against sera from an infected rabbit (SI) and from a hyper-immunized rabbit (SH).

in Table II: two of eight tested rabbits became positive on the fifth day of infection and a third one became positive on the sixth day. All the six rabbits tested were positive on the seventh day and two additional rabbits tested on the tenth day were also positive. Table III presents the HA and the BA titers obtained with sera from 41 human patients. The correlation between these titers is shown in Fig. 8. All 50 sera from healthy persons were negative by HA.

HA inhibition tests with the crude extract and its fractions (Table IV) revealed a 45-fold increase of antigen A specific activity in the 0.07 *M* fraction over the crude extract. No other fraction showed comparable results. HA inhibition tests with early negative sera from infected rabbits yielded inconclusive results. Sensitized SRBC yielded the same titer with

Table II Hemagglutination Titers[a] of Sera from *Trichinella* Infected Rabbits at Different Times after Infection

Rabbits	Larvae per gm of muscle	Results at different days after infection[b]														
		1	2	3	4	5	6	7	9	10	11	12	13	14	15	30
R1	10,000	-	-	-	-	0	-	-	-	10	-	-	-	-	160	1280
R2	40	-	-	-	-	0	-	-	-	320	-	-	-	-	640	1280
R3	3,000	-	-	-	-	0	-	160	160	-	320	-	160	-	320	1280
R4	1,000	-	-	-	-	0	-	10	40	-	80	-	320	-	640	-
R5	500	0	0	0	0	0	80	80	160	-	-	160	-	80	-	1280
R6	2,400	0	0	0	0	10	80	320	640	-	-	320	-	320	-	1280
R7	110	0	0	0	0	10	80	640	640	-	-	640	-	1280	-	2560
R8	435	0	0	0	0	0	0	10	10	-	-	20	-	40	--	40

[a]Expressed as the reciprocals of the end-point serum dilutions.
[b]-, Not done; O, negative.

Table III Anti-*Trichinella* Titers[a] of 41 Sera from Human Patients, Tested by Bentonite Agglutination and by Hemagglutination

Sera	Bentonite titers	Hemagglutination titers
1379	2,560	10,240
3519	1,280	20,480
2296	1,280	81,920
1087	1,280	10,240
4137	1,280	5,120
4577	1,280	10,240
5402	640	5,120
5403	640	2,560
2397	640	10,240
2004	640	40,960
3966	320	2,560
2525	320	10,240
4148	320	1,280
Lot 10	320	5,120
2265	320	20,480
2040	320	10,240
2412	320	2,560
1321	160	5,120
4485	80	160
4145	80	5,120
3692	40	320
3693	40	320
3871	40	160
4165	40	320
2990	40	640
2987	40	320
2208	40	1,280
Lot 11	40	2,560
4143	40	5,120
2573	40	320
2043	40	80
1595	20	160
0710	20	320
7879	20	160
6550	20	320
2546	20	2,560
4114	10	80
1504	10	10,240
4149	10	320
2271	5	40
2157	5	320

[a] Expressed as the reciprocals of the end-point serum dilutions.

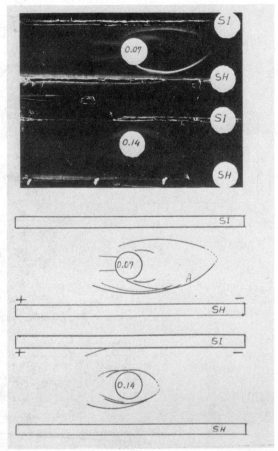

Figure 6 Immunoelectrophoresis of the fraction obtained by elution of a DEAE-cellulose column with 0.07 *M* (0.07) and with 0.14 *M* (0.14) buffers against sera from an infected rabbit (SI) and from a hyperimmunized rabbit (SH). The anodic lines with 0.07 fraction were considered nonspecific precipitates.

the positive control serum after 3 months when lyophilized and stored at 4°C. Frozen sensitized SRBC also maintained their sensitivity for at least 3 months but positive reactions did not yield perfect shields. Storage at 4°C for 3 months reduced the sensitivity by 32-fold.

Discussion

The results obtained with the extraction procedure described suggest that treatment of the suspension of larvae with petroleum ether prior to the extraction eliminates most of the lipids without affecting the infectivity

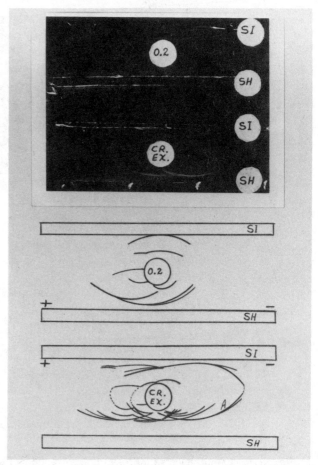

Figure 7 Immunoelectrophoresis of the fraction obtained by elution of a DEAE-cellulose column with 0.2 *M* buffer (0.2) and of the crude extract (CR. EX.) against sera from an infected rabbit (SI) and from a hyperimmunized rabbit (SH).

of the parasites or reducing the immunogenicity of the antigenic extract. This simple method may make unnecessary more elaborate delipidation procedures. The routine performance of repeated extractions does not seem justified since the protein yield of the second and further extractions was very low compared to that of the first extraction (Table I). The protein recovered in the first extraction from a 5-ml and a 10-ml sample of larvae were 4% and 3.3%, respectively, of the estimated larval wet weight. These percentages compare well with the recoveries of 3.5% by Melcher (1943), 3% by Sleeman and Muschel (1961) and 2% (for *Toxocara canis*) by Jeska (1967).

The number of antigen–antibody systems found in the crude extract

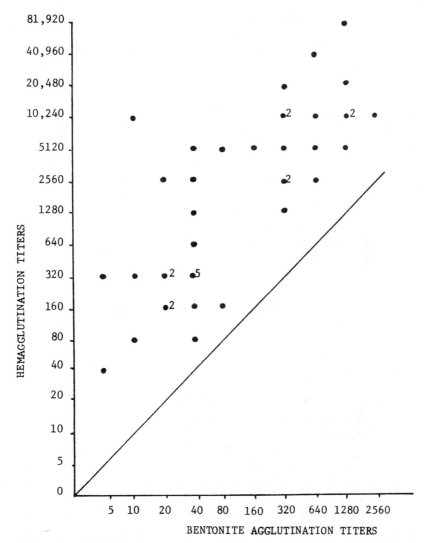

Figure 8 Correlation between hemagglutination and bentonite agglutination titers (expressed as the reciprocals of the end-point serum dilutions) in patients of trichinellosis. The bisector represents a correlation −1.0 and the numbers accompanying some dots represent the number of sera that yielded that correlation.

was 11 with SI and 21 with SH. This compares to a maximum of 19 bands found with serum from infected rabbits by Ermolin (1969) and of 19 bands found with serum of hyperimmunized rabbits by Biguet *el al.* (1965). Although part of the discrepancies between the results reported by different authors must be due to different abilities of individual rabbits to produce antibodies against the same antigenic complex (Tanner and Gregory,

Table IV Hemagglutination Inhibition by Crude Larval Extract and its Fractions

Fraction	Micrograms of protein needed to inhibit 16 HA units
Crude extract	0.24
Extract of lyophilized sediment	2.0
50% salt precipitation:	
Supernatant fluid	≤ 0.34 [a]
Sediment	≤ 0.56 [a]
60% salt precipitation:	
Supernatant fluid	1.3
Sediment	0.07
70% salt precipitation:	
Supernatant fluid	8.6
Sediment	0.09
0.0175 M—I	>172.0 [b]
0.0175 M—II	>107.0 [b]
0.0175 M—III	>80.0 [b]
0.0175 M—IV	>42.0 [b]
0.07 M	0.0054
0.14 M	7.6
0.2 M	22.0
0.3 M	50.0

[a] Lesser quantities not tried.
[b] No inhibition at the highest concentration tried.

1961), there is a decisive influence of the concentration of the extract on the number of antigenic systems detected. Unfortunately this information is not always provided in the literature.

Antigen A was selected to develop a diagnostic test because it was the first and strongest to react by precipitation in gel and because Van Peenen (cited by Kent, 1963), Dymowska *et al.* (1967), and Kagan (1967) found a cathodic band, in the same region of the immunoelectropherogram as antigen A, by reacting extracts of *Trichinella* with sera of human patients.

Lyophilization does not seem to improve the yield of antigen A, since its specific activity in an extract of lyophilized sediment was over eight times lower than in the crude extract (Table IV). We frequently found an insoluble precipitate after freezing and thawing fraction 0.07 M. These two observations suggest that antigen A might be partially denatured by freezing and thawing. In any case, these results do not justify the routine use of lyophilization to obtain antigen A.

Fractionation of crude extract by salt precipitation did not prove useful since antigen A was either present in both supernatant fluid and sediment or it was contaminated with considerable amounts of other antigens (Figs. 2 and 3 and Table IV). Sephadex filtration suggested that antigen A must be a very large molecule. The presence of other antigenic components of similar molecular size in the larval extract limited the usefulness of Sephadex filtration for purification of antigen A. Elution from DEAE-cellulose with 0.0175 M buffer eliminated about 60% of the protein in the column. Subsequent elution with 0.07 M buffer yielded the bulk of antigen A although elutions with higher molarities of buffer demonstrated that small amounts of this antigen remained in the column (Table IV).

The location of antigen A and of the contaminant antigens in the immunoelectropherogram of the 0.07 M fraction (Fig. 6) suggests that this antigen may be further purified by methods based on electric charge. However, since fraction 0.07 M had 45 times more antigen A specific activity than the crude extract (Table IV), since the contaminant bands were very weak (Fig. 6), and since the protein yield of fraction 0.07 M was only 4.5% of the protein applied on the DEAE-cellulose, due mainly to its long tailing, further purification was not attempted. Antigenic components of *Trichinella* larvae with characteristics similar to those of antigen A have been described. Mills and Kent (1965) isolated a component similar to antigen A by DEAE-Sephadex chromatography of a preparation containing three to four antigens. Tanner (1970) isolated a band with the same electrophoretic mobility as antigen A by continuous electrophoresis of Sephadex G-200 eluates of a larval extract containing 11 antigens. These preparations were not available to us for direct comparison, but their identity with antigen A may be safely assumed.

Since the infective *Trichinella* larvae get into the intestinal mucosa a few hours after infection (Gursch, 1949; Shanta, 1967) and molt there (Ali Khan, 1966; Kozek, 1971), an early immune response against antigens derived from that parasitic stage should be expected. The results of HA tests with serum from infected rabbits (Table II) showed that antigen A detected antibodies between the fifth and the tenth day of infection and that the antibody response does not appear to be related to the intensity of the muscular infection within the range observed by us. It is worth noticing that rabbit R8, which never produced high-titered antiserum, and rabbit R, which had a critical infection, yielded positive HA tests on the seventh and the tenth day of infection, respectively.

HA titers of sera from 41 human patients averaged 3.7 twofold dilutions higher than the corresponding BA titers. The correlation coefficient between the titers by the two tests was +0.76. However, the correlation coefficients were +0.23 when only the 23 sera with BA titers of 80 or lower were considered and +0.44 when only the 18 sera with BA titers of 160 or higher were included. These differences strongly suggest that the two tests detect different antibodies. Since the sera came from patients with overt disease, one could assume that early infections were more abundant among the sera with lower BA titers. Considering the greater discordance between the two tests at the lower BA titers and the results obtained with sera from infected rabbits, it may be expected that the HA tests with antigen A is more efficient in detecting early anti-*Trichinella* antibodies than the BA test. The negative results of HA tests with 50 normal human sera suggest that the specificity of this test is high in the absence of other conditions.

Although as little as 1.35 ng of fraction 0.07 M protein was expected to neutralize 4 HA units, HA inhibition tests with early negative sera from infected rabbits did not reveal the presence of antigen A in the blood of the animals.

Some HA tests with nonadsorbed positive sera yielded exactly the same titers as the respective adsorbed sera suggesting that adsorption of the test sera may not be necessary. The marked variations in the titers deteced by the sensitized SRBC depending on slight modifications in glutaraldehyde treatment point to some degree of denaturation of the specific antigen during the sensitization procedure. However, the results reported here indicate that HA with antigen A is a sensitive and simple means for detection of early *Trichinella* infections, and that it may be useful as a routine diagnostic aid.

Summary

A crude saline extract of *Trichinella* larvae was analyzed by immunoelectrophoresis against serum from an infected rabbit (SI) and serum from a rabbit hyperimmunized with the same extract (SH). Eleven bands developed with SI and 21 with SH. A band with the mobility of γ-globulin (antigen A) was the earliest to react and produced the heaviest band. Fractionation of the crude extract was attempted by ammonium sulfate precipitation, Sephadex filtration and DEAE-cellulose chromatography. Elution of the DEAE-cellulose column with 0.07 M phosphate buffer, pH 6.8, after washing with 0.0175 M buffer, produced a fraction in which antigen A specific activity was increased 45-fold over the crude extract. This fraction contained antigen A plus three very faint contaminant bands when tested against SH.

The 0.07 M fraction coupled to sheep red blood cells (SRBC) by glutaraldehyde was used in hemagglutination (HA) tests with sera from eight infected rabbits, from 41 trichinellosis human patients, and from 50 healthy persons. All rabbits yielded positive HA reactions between the fifth and the tenth day of infection, with titers up to 640. All sera from human patients were positive by HA with an average titer 3.7 twofold dilutions higher than those detected by bentonite agglutination (BA) tests. The correlation coefficient between HA and BA titers was $+0.76$: it became a $+0.23$ when only 23 sera with BA titers of 80 or lower were considered, and a $+0.44$ when only 18 sera with BA titers of 160 or higher were included. This and other considerations suggest that the HA test with antigen A detects different and earlier antibodies than the BA test. All sera from healthy persons were negative by HA.

HA inhibition tests did not reveal antigen A in early negative sera from infected rabbits. However, only 5.4 ng protein of the 0.07 M fraction were required to inhibit 16 HA units. Sensitized SRBC yielded unchanged titers for at least 3 months when lyophilized and stored at 4° C. The HA test with antigen A is proposed for routine detection of early *Trichinella* infections.

Acknowledgments

We wish to thank Dr. N. D. Levine, College of Veterinary Medicine, University of Illinois, Urbana, Illinois, whose support made this work possible; Dr. N. F. Weatherly, Department of Parasitology, School of Public Health, University of North Carolina, Chapel Hill, North Carolina, for furnishing the parasites; Dr. I. G. Kagan, Center for Disease Control, Atlanta, Georgia; Dr. F. Knierim, Departamento de Microbiología y Parasitología, Universidad de Chile, Santiago, Chile; Dr. R. J. Martin, Illinois State Department of Public Health, Springfield, Illinois; and Dr. E. H. Sadun, Walter Reed Army Institute of Research, Washington, D.C., for providing the human serum samples; and Mr. Rolando Ramírez, Departamento de Microbiología y Parasitología, Universidad de Chile, Santiago, Chile, for performing the statistical calculations.

This work was supported in part by the grant AI-00033 from the National Institute of Allergy and Infectious Diseases, National Institutes of Health. A portion of this research was supported by funds from the Illinois Agricultural Experiment Station.

References

Adonajlo, A., Gancarz, Z., Dymowska, Z., and Zapart, Z. (1967). Intradermal tests and serological reactions with antigens of *Trichinella spiralis* in persons infested by different forms of parasites. *Helminthologia* **8**, 23–30. (In Russian; English summary.)

Ali Khan, Z. (1966). The post embryonic development of *Trichinella spiralis* with special reference to ecdysis. *J. Parasitol.* **52**, 248–259.

Avrameas, S., Taudou, B., and Chuilon, S. (1969). Glutaraldehyde, cyanuric chloride and tetraazotized-*o*-dianisidine as coupling reagents in the passive hemagglutination test. *Immunochemistry 6*, 67–76.

Barriga, O. O. (1971). Analysis and isolation of antigenic fractions of *Trichinella spiralis* larval extracts. M.S. thesis. University of Illinois, Urbana, Illinois.

Barriga, O. O. (1973). Serologic diagnosis of trichinosis with a purified larval antigen. Ph.D. Thesis. University of Illinois, Urbana, Illinois.

Beaver, P. C. (1953). Persistence of hookworm larvae in the soil. *Amer. J. Trop. Med. Hyg.* **2**, 102–108.

Bessonov, A. S., and Volfson, A. G. (1970). The use of an immunological survey method of the Chukotsk population for trichinellosis studies. *Wiad. Parazytol.* **16**, 24–33. (In Russian; English summary.)

Biguet, J., Tran Van Ky, P., Moschetto, Y., and Gnamey-Koffy, D. (1965). Contribution à l'etude de la structure antigenique des larves de *Trichinella spiralis* et des precipitines experimentales du lapin. *Wiad. Parazytol.* **11**, 299–315.

Crandall, R. B., Belkin, L. M., and Saadaliah, S. (1966). Complement staining with fluorescent antibody for detection of antibody in experimental trichinosis. *J. Parasitol.* **52**, 1219–1220.

Dymowska, Z., Aleksandrowicz, J., and Zakrzewska, A. (1967). Antigens of *Trichinella spiralis*. II. Serological tests. *Acta Parasitol. Pol.* **15**, 203–211.

Ermolin, G. A. (1969). Antigenic structure of decapsulated larvae of *Trichinella spiralis*. *Wiad. Parazytol.* **15**, 599–600.

Gancarz, Z. (1964). Studies on the efficacy of serological tests with *Trichinella spiralis* antigens in the diagnosis of cases of trichinellosis on epidemic foci. *Acta Parasitol. Pol.* **12**, 441–454.

Gancarz, Z. (1968). Immunobiological methods in diagnosis of trichinosis in man and animals. *Excerpta Med., Sect. 4 Microbiol.* **22** (201), 36.

Gursch, O. F. (1949). Intestinal phase of *Trichinella spiralis* (Owen, 1835) Railliet, 1895. *J. Parasitol.* **35**, 19–26.

Hacig, A., Solomon, P., Ianco, L. and Smolinski, M. (1967). Valeur de quelques antigenes standardises de *Trichinella spiralis* apprecies par le test de l'intradermoreation. *Arch. Roum. Pathol. Exp. Microbiol.* **26**, 273–278.

Ivey, M. H., and Slanga, R. (1965). An evaluation of passive cutaneous anaphylactic reactions with *Trichinella* and *Toxocara* antibody–antigen systems. *Amer. J. Trop. Med. Hyg.* **14**, 1052–1056.

Jeska, E. L. (1967). Antigenic analysis of a metazoan parasite, *Toxocara canis*. I. Extraction and assay of antigens. *Exp. Parasitol.* **20**, 38–50.

Jezyna, C., Tomaszko, H., and Zaborowska-Sulkowska, A. (1967). Complement fixation, ring precipitation and microprecipitation tests in 74 patients with trichiniasis. *Wiad. Parazytol.* **13**, 237–241. (In Polish English summary.)

Kagan, I. G. (1965). Evaluation of routine serologic testing for parasitic diseases. *Amer. J. Pub. Health* **11**, 1820–1829.

Kagan, I. G. (1967). Characterization of parasite antigens. *In:* "Immunological aspects of Parasitic Diseases," Scientific Publication No. 150, Pan American Health Organization, Washington D.C., pp. 25–36.

Kagan, I. G., and Norman, L. G. (1970). The serology of trichinosis. *In:* S. E. Gould (ed.), "Trichinosis in Man and Animals," Thomas, Springfield, Illinois, pp. 222–268.

Kassur, B., and Wołoszczuk, I. (1970). The usefulness of serological tests in the diagnosis of trichiniasis during the years 1953–1968. *Trop. Dis. Bull.* **67**, (2897), 1509.

Kent, N. H. (1963). Fractionation, isolation and definition of antigens from parasitic helminths. *Amer. J. Hyg. Monogr. Ser.* (22), 30–46.

Kozar, Z., and Kozar, M. (1966). Evaluation of the charcoal card test, as compared with other serological tests in the diagnosis of trichinellosis. *Wiad. Parazytol.* **12**, 629–635.

Kozar, Z., and Kozar, M. (1968). Dynamics and persistence of antibodies in trichinellosis. *Wiad. Parazytol.* **14**, 171–185.

Kozek, W. J. (1971). The molting pattern in *Trichinella spiralis*. I. A light microscope study. *J. Parasitol.* **57**, 1015–1028.

Labzoffsky, N. A., Baratawidjaja, R. K., Kuitunen, E., Lewis, F. N., Kavelman, D. A., and Morrissey, L. P. (1964). Immunofluorescence as an aid in the early diagnosis of trichinosis. *Can. Med. Ass. J.* **90,** 920–921.

Lowry, O. H., Rosengrough, N. J., Fair, L., and Randall, R. J. (1951). Protein measurements with the Folin-phenol reagent. *J. Biol. Chem.* **193,** 256–261.

Maynard, J. E., and Kagan, I. G. (1964). Intradermal tests in the detection of trichinosis. Further observations on two outbreaks due to bear meat in Alaska. *N. Eng. J. Med.* **270,** 1–6.

Melcher, L. R. (1943). An antigenic analysis of *Trichinella spiralis. J. Infec. Dis.* **73,** 31–39.

Mills, C. K., and Kent, N. H. (1965). Excretions and secretions of *Trichinella spiralis* and their role in immunity. *Exp. Parasitol.* **16,** 300–310.

Sadun, E. H., Anderson, R. I., and Williams, J. S. (1962). Fluorescent antibody test for the serological diagnosis of trichinosis. *Exp. Parasitol.* **12,** 424–433.

Schenone, H., Roos, L., Rojas, A., and Ramirez, R. (1970). Tendencia epidemiologica de la triquinosis en Santiago de Chile. *Bol. Chil. Parasitol.* **25,** 46–51.

Schultz, M. G., Kagan, I. G., and Warner, G. S. (1967). Card flocculation test in the field diagnosis of trichinosis. *Amer. J. Clin. Pathol.* **47,** 26–29.

Shanta, C. S. (1967). The life cycle of *Trichinella spiralis.* I. The intestinal phase of development. *Can. J. Zool.* **45** (Suppl.), 1255–1260.

Sleeman, H. K., and Muschel, L. H. (1961). Studies on complement fixing antigens isolated from *Trichinella spiralis.* I. Isolation, purification and evaluation as diagnostic agents. *Amer. J. Trop. Med. Hyg.* **10,** 821–833.

Subbotin, N. F. (1968). Efficiency of immunological reactions for the diagnosis of trichinelliasis. *Helminthol. Abstr.* **38,** 65.

Tanner, C. E. (1970). Immunochemical study of the antigens of *Trichinella spiralis* larvae. IV. Purification by continuous-flow paper electrophoresis and column chromatography. *Exp. Parasitol.* **27,** 116–135.

Tanner, C. E., and Gregory, J. (1961). Immunochemical study of the antigens of *Trichinella spiralis* larvae. I. Identification and enumeration of antigens. *Can. J. Microbiol.* **7,** 473–481.

In Pursuit of a Vanishing Disease: Clinical and Epidemological Experience with Trichinellosis in New York City, 1944–1971

Howard B. Shookhoff

Division of Tropical Diseases
Bureau of Infectious Disease Control
Department of Health
City of New York
New York

The number of cases of trichinellosis reported annually to the Department of Health of the City of New York has declined from an average of 150 in the period 1945 through 1949 to an average of 9 in the period 1967 through 1971. The prevalence of *Trichinella spiralis* infection as determined by routine examination of muscle tissue from human diaphragms obtained at autopsy declined from 22 out of 100 in 1937 to 11 out of 309, or 3.5% in 1959–1961 (Most and Helpern, 1941; Most, 1965). Parallel observations have been reported from other parts of the United States (Most, 1965).

There seems little doubt that the incidence of this infection has been on the wane for many years. Since the identification of the organism and the determination of the life cycle in the middle of the nineteenth century, cases of trichinellosis have apparently become less prevalent and less severe. This is due in part to public health measures related to the raising of pigs and the processing of meat and in part to the education of the public to the danger of eating raw or insufficiently cooked pork. Until the end of the nineteenth century, many Europeans ate raw chopped pork deliberately. Severe infections were frequent and there were epidemics in which the mortality was as high as 30%. In this century, epidemics have most often been due to food in which the infected porcine muscle is diluted. In sausage, there is a mixture of fat, blood and other uninfected tissue. In commercial sausage, dilution further occurs because the tissues of several animals are combined. Consequently, as in the epidemic reported by the writer and co-workers (Shookhoff *et al.*, 1946), outbreaks tend to be of milder cases with little or no mortality. The 1944 epidemic involved 84 cases with no deaths. It is generally accepted that the severity of the disease is closely correlated with the number of larvae ingested. The other

443

major source of outbreaks in New York City in recent years has been the accidental mixing of pork with beef in the butcher's grinder. This also leads to light infections by virtue of the dilution of the infectious meat. In New York, we have had only one reported fatal case since 1951. The fatality in 1951 occurred in the father of a family which ate homemade sausage from a single pig bought and slaughtered privately. All five members of the family were sufficiently ill to be hospitalized.

The latest fatal case occurred in 1971 in a woman from Thailand who ate raw marinated pork. A brief summary of the last fatal case is as follows: Two women and a man from Thailand had been in New York City for a very few months when they prepared a pork loin by marinating it for 2 days in lemon and pepper. They then consumed it without cooking. Most of the pork was eaten by the two women. Two days later all three suffered abdominal pain, diarrhea, fever, and malaise. Ten days after eating the pork they all had periorbital edema and cough. One woman, 45 years of age, developed high fever, prostration, dysarthria, dysphagia, and trismus. She died 15 days after eating the pork in cardiac arrest despite administration of steroid therapy and emergency treatment of the complication.

A case of the moderately sereve trichinellosis typical of those seen in present-day hospital practice is that of a man of 34 years, born in the Dominican Republic. He had lived in New York City for 1 year. Five days before he was admitted he noticed that his eyes were red and painful. The next day he developed fever and shaking chills. Three days before admission, his temperature was 41° C. He was found to have hemorrhages in the conjunctivas of both eyes. There was swelling of the face in the area of the parotid glands suggesting to some members of the staff that he had mumps. A transient eruption was noted on his trunk.

His total leukocyte count varied from 9000 to 6200/mm^3. On the day of admission, there were 7% eosinophils. This gradually increased to 26% 8 days after admission. The sedimentation rate of erythrocytes was 12 mm in 1 hr (normal) on admission. It increased to 24 mm on the fourth day and 25 mm on the fifth day. The serum transaminase (SGOT) was 95 units (slightly elevated.) A muscle biopsy was done on the fifth hospital day, the tenth day of illness. A crush preparation failed to show larvae but they were found after digestion in artificial gastric juice. They were also seen in histological sections. A flocculation test for trichinellosis was negative 14 and 23 days after the onset of illness but the complement fixation test was positive on the thirteenth day of illness. On the same day the intradermal test with *Trichinella* antigen was positive.

The patient's fever remained between 40° and 41° C for 2 days and then became remittent and gradually subsided becoming normal on the ninth hospital day. No specific treatment was given although the use of thiabendazole was discussed. The source of the infection was sausage purchased in a Hungarian meat market and eaten uncooked.

A relatively mild case of trichinellosis is exemplified by that of a 36-year-old woman whose presenting symptom was muscle pain for 4 days, mainly in the neck, shoulders, and legs. One day before the onset she noted swelling of her eyelids and congestion of the scleras. She was not aware of fever and had no gastrointestinal disturbances. Physical examination showed periorbital edema with subconjunctival hemorrhages. Leukocytes were 5500/mm^3 with 30% eosinophils. An attempt at demonstrating larvae in the circulating blood was unsuccessful. Intradermal test with *Trichinella* antigen was negative at 20 min but there was a delayed positive reaction at 24 hr. The precipitin test was positive (no other serologic tests were being done at the time). She was not hospitalized but was seen periodically as an outpatient. She did have slight fever the day after she was first seen, or the sixth day of illness, but was apparently afebrile within the next 2–3 days. She was given Hetrazan which had no definable effect. Periorbital edema and subconjunctival hemorrhages cleared within the first week but muscle aching was a persistent and troublesome complaint. On the fifteenth day of illness an intradermal test with *Trichinella* antigen gave an immediate positive reaction, the precipitin test was positive at the same titer as previously, and the leukocytes were 7700/mm^3 with 28% eosinophils. After 4 weeks she was lost to follow-up. This case illustrates the persistence of muscle pain in a patient who continued physical activity during the illness. It is my impression that this is less troublesome in patients who are forced by the severity of the illness to go to bed. The epidemiology of this case was interesting. At first she insisted that she had been infected from Virginia ham which was the only form of pork she ate. Since this product is already cooked when purchased, another source was sought. She denied eating raw chopped meat but 2 weeks later when she was questioned again she stated (1) that she and her son frequently nibbled raw chopped meat when she was preparing meat loaf and (2) that she periodically purchased raw chopped pork from the same butcher for a neighbor and the butcher had only one grinder.

Reporting of trichinellosis cases is far from complete and this is due in part to failure of diagnosis. The type of case that must usually go unrecognized and would explain the higher prevalence of infection in autopsy specimens than is suggested by reported cases is exemplified by that of a 58-year-old man whose wife and two children were the first three cases reported in the 1944 outbreak referred to above (Shookhoff et al., 1946.) When I investigated the illnesses in the family, I found that the mother and children had all eaten mettwurst sausage repeatedly for luncheon. The father triumphantly stated that he was fine, having abstained from the ill-fated sausage. Several days later I received a report of a positive precipitin reaction with his name on it. I visited his home again and found that, shortly after my earlier visit, he had developed a backache and slight fever lasting less than 2 days. He consulted his family physician who would ordinarily have considered him to have mild influenza. However, because of the illness of the other members of the family, the physician ordered a blood count which showed an eosinophilia of 24%. Upon reconsideration, the father remembered that he had indeed eaten a small amount of the mettwurst.

At times even more clear-cut cases are not diagnosed. In 1945 I was asked to investigate a case of trichinellosis in a business man who insisted it was due to a Virginia ham sandwich eaten at a roadside restaurant during a business trip. Since he was quite ill, I did not press him with my epidemiological doubts. Three days later he telephoned me to say that his wife was also ill with trichinellosis and that she had not accompanied him on the trip. He recalled an earlier picnic at which his wife and another family ate chopped meat grilled over an open fire. Contact with the other family revealed that the father was well but his wife and two children were ill with what was termed a peculiar type of "grippe." The peculiarity was periorbital edema. Blood counts revealed eosinophilia except in the father who had cooked at the picnic, had courteously taken his hamburgers last so that they were well-cooked and thus had escaped infection. Without the epidemiological investigation, his family would have recovered without the correct diagnosis.

Discussion

The second case described above represents the general characteristics of trichinellosis as it appears in New York City. The onset is usually with manifestations referable to the eyes. Fever of varying degree and muscle pain or weakness or both follow within a very few days. The classically described prodromal gastrointestinal symptoms are usually absent, but vomiting or diarrhea or both may accompany the other manifestations of dissemination of the larvae. Eosinophilia is a constant finding but the increase may be very slight in the early days of illness. The erythrocyte sedimentation rate is usually normal at the onset, and later is elevated.

Muscle biopsy may fail to demonstrate larvae in the milder cases and immunological tests are of great importance to the clinician, although they may not establish the diagnosis early in the illness. The writer is not convinced that any of the specific therapies proposed is effective under clinical conditions, possibly because a really early diagnosis is not achievable. The use of steroids as palliative therapy is indicated in moderately severe or severe infections, especially when there is involvement of the heart or central nervous system. They are very effective in mitigating the symptoms and controlling the life-threatening complications.

Summary

Trichinellosis has declined in frequency and severity in New York City. Most of the cases being seen are due to sausage-type products or to accidental admixture of pork with chopped beef. Cases of varying degree of severity are described. Epidemiological investigation has turned up very mild and even moderately severe cases which would otherwise have not been recognized.

References

Most, H. (1965). Trichinellosis in the United States; Changing epidemiology during the past 25 years. *J. Amer. Med. Ass.* **193,** 871–873.

Most, H., and Helpern, M. (1941). Incidence of trichinosis i;n New York City. *Amer. J. Med. Sci.* **202,** 251–257.

Shookhoff, H. B., Birnkrant, W. B., and Greenberg, M. (1946). An outbreak of trichinosis in New York City; with special reference to the intradermal and precipitin tests. *Amer. J. Pub. Health* **36,** 1403–1411.

Antibody Response to *Trichinella spiralis*

Inger Ljungström

Department of Parasitology
National Bacteriological Laboratory
Stockholm, Sweden

Introduction

The development and persistence of antibodies to *Trichinella spiralis* have been extensively studied in laboratory animals (Tanner, 1968; Crandall and Crandall; 1972), but very few such studies have been reported in human patients (Kagan *et al.,* 1968; Clark *et al.,* 1972; Rosenberg *et al.,* 1971).

In 1969 two small outbreaks of trichinellosis occurred in Sweden. In all, 25 clinical cases were detected. The age of the patients, 9 men and 16 women, varied between 14 and 60 years of age. The disease was, in general, mild or of moderate severity (Odelram, 1973). Nine patients were hospitalized for periods not exceeding 2 weeks. No deaths occurred.

These outbreaks provided the opportunity to follow the antibody response from only a short time after the onset of the clinical illness and over a comparatively long period, which in some cases exceeded 2 years. That intradermal administration of antigen may influence the antibody response has been demonstrated both with tuberculin (Waksman, 1958), toxoplasmin (Huldt, personal communication), and echinococcus antigen (Huldt *et al.,* 1973). For this reason skin tests were not performed on the group of people examined in this evaluation.

Materials and Methods

Sera

In the first outbreak eight cases of trichinellosis occurred and in the second 17 cases. Sera were obtained every 2–4 weeks over a period of 6 months and then at longer intervals for another 18 months.

Antigens

Trichinella larvae were obtained from infected white Sprague-Dawley rats. Infected rat muscle was digested in a solution of 1% pepsin (Difco 1:3000) in tap water containing 0.5% HC1. The proportion of infected muscle to digestion medium was about 75 gm/1000 ml of solution.

The free, washed larvae were used for antigen and prepared according to Bozicevich *et al.* (1951). The larvae were homogenized in saline and extracted for 24 hours at 4° C. To remove the largest particles the preparation was centrifuged twice at 3000 *g* for 15 min and 25,000 *g* for 15 min. One batch of antigen was used for passive hemagglutination and one batch for radioallergosorbent test. The results from the chemical analysis of the antigen batches are shown in Table I. The total nitrogen content of the preparations was determined by the micro method of Kjeldahl and the protein content according to Folin-Ciocalteu with the modification of Lowry. Bovine serum albumin (BSA), fraction 5 (Armour Pharmaceutical Company, Ltd.) was used as a standard. Diaphragms from *Trichinella*-infected rats, heavily infected 6–8 weeks earlier, were used as antigen in the indirect immunofluorescence test. The diaphragms were cut into 5-mm wide strips which were then rolled and frozen at −70° C. Frozen sections of the rolls were prepared and fixed in acetone for 10 min at room temperature.

Passive Hemagglutination (PA)

The test was performed according to Boyden (1951) with tanned sheep erythrocytes (dilution of tannic acid 1:120,000) using the micro modification described by Takatsy (1955).

Indirect Immunofluorescence (IFL)

Seven preparations of fluorescein-labeled anti-γ-globulin were used. Data concerning these preparations are given in Table II. All sera from each patient were tested at the same time with the same batch of conjugate.

Table I Chemical Data on Two Batches of Antigen

Antigen [a]	Total N (mg/ml) [b]	Protein N (mg/ml) [b]	Protein (mg/ml) [c]
I	0.14	0.08	1.1
II	2.02	1.50	9.36

[a] Antigen I used for PA, antigen II for RAST.
[b] Micro method of Kjeldahl.
[c] Folin-Ciocalte u method, modification of Lowry. As standard: BSA, fraction V (Amour Pharmaceutical Company, Ltd.).

Table II Chemical Data and Specificity of the Conjugates Used for IFL [a]

Fluorescein conjugated immunoglobulin [b]	Working dilution	Weight F/P_{10}^{-3}	Mol F/P	Ab P (mg/ml)	PA			Precipitations titer		
					IgG	IgM	Ig A	IgG	IgM	IgA
I. Sheep antihuman polyvalent SBL	1:8-1:20	3.7-8.0	2.9-3.6	-	-	-	-	-	-	-
II. Rabbit antihuman IgG SBL	1:8	6.3	-	-	120,000	160	80	8	<1	<1
III. Sheep antihuman IgG 1005^{II}A SBL	1:10	7.7	3.1	1.4	-	-	-	-	-	-
IV. Sheep antihuman IgG (lot 3541 Wellcome)	1:30	4.3	1.02		-	-	-	-	-	-
V. Sheep antihuman IgM (lot K 1387 Wellcome)	1:16	9.6	3.6	-	40	12,800	40	-	-	-
VI. Sheep antihuman IgA (lot 4293 Wellcome)	1:2	2.4	-	-	-	-	-	-	-	-
VII. Swine antihuman IgA (lot 0170 Wellcome)	1:4	10.3	-	-	<10	<10	64,000	<1	<1	2

[a] All sera from each patient were tested at the same time with the same batch of conjugate.

[b] I, II, V, VII, used for testing whole sera; III, IV, V, VI, used for testing sucrose gradient fractions.

The antibody titer and specificity of the conjugates were tested either by double diffusion in gel (Beutner *et al.,* 1968) or by determining antibody protein per milliliter by using reverse Mancini technique. For monospecific conjugates PA using tanned cells coated with IgM, IgG, and IgA was also performed. The IFL staining was performed the conventional way with incubation at each step for 30 min at room temperature. As a diluent and for rinsing, isotonic phosphate buffered saline (PBS), pH 7.4, was used. In order to avoid nonspecific staining the slides were immersed for 13 min in Evans' blue, diluted 1:500 in PBS, pH 7.4. The slides were mounted in buffered 90% glycerin, pH 7.4.

The preparations were examined in a Zeiss binocular fluorescence microscope, equipped with a HBO 200 mercury vapor light, BG III exciter filter, 44/50 barrier filter, and ordinary light condenser. Figure 1 shows a positive reaction with specific staining of the cuticle and the stichosome.

Sucrose Gradient Centrifugation

A gradient of sucrose ranging from 10 to 37% was prepared. One-tenth of heat-inactivated serum, diluted 1:4, was layered on top of the gradient, to a total volume of 5 ml. Centrifugation was carried out with the use of a Spinco ultracentrifuge, rotor SW 50, 35,000 rpm for 18 hr at 4° C. Serial fractions of 0.4 ml were collected dropwise from the bottom of the tubes. All fractions from each serum were tested for antibody activity at the same time.

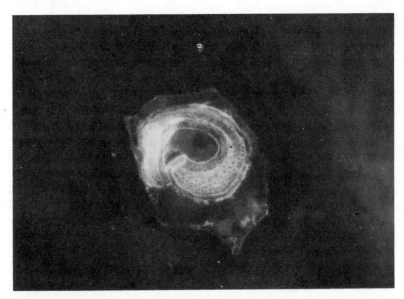

Figure 1 IFL staining of Trichinella-infected rat diaphragm. X 322.5

Radioimmunosorbent Test (RIST)

The test used for quantitation of IgE (Johansson *et al.*, 1968a) was the Phadebas IgE test (Pharmacia, Uppsala). In RIST specific anti-IgE (anti-FcND) was coupled to CNBr-activated Sephadex R particles. The IgE concentration of a serum was evaluated from its capacity to inhibit the binding of ^{125}I-labeled IgE to particle bound antibodies as compared to a standard.

In 1971, 20 sera were tested using IgND (Johansson and Bennich, 1967) as the standard and the results were expressed in nanograms per milliliter. Since 1972 a reference serum made available by WHO (prep. 68/341) and designated to contain 10,000 units (Rowe *et al.*, 1970) was used for standardization. Fifty sera were tested in 1972 using this standard. To express earlier data in units per milliliter a conversion factor of 0.5 was used (Johansson, personal communication).

Radioallergosorbent Test (RAST) (Wide *et al.,* 1967)

This test was used for the estimation of IgE antibodies essentially as described by Johansson *et al.* (1971). The *Trichinella* antigen was coupled to 100 CNBr-activated filter paper (Munktells 00H) discs with a diameter of 5 mm. A volume of 0.1 ml of a reference reaginic serum in suitable dilutions of the serum samples was incubated with one allergen-paper disc for 3 hr at room temperature. After washing five times with saline containing 0.1% Tween 20, 0.2 ml of ^{125}I-labeled anti-IgE representing ap-

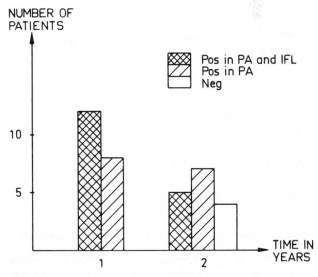

Figure 2 Number of sero-positives and sero-negatives as measured by PA and IFL 1 and 2 years after onset of disease.

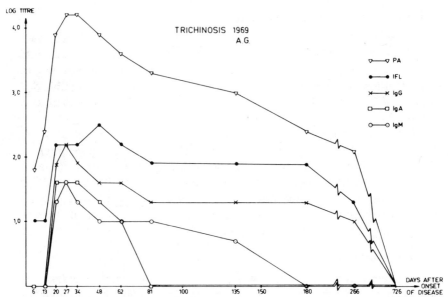

Figure 3 Antibody response in one case of trichinosis as measured by PA and IFL. The representation of Ig classes in the antibody population, tested by IFL using class specific conjugates.

proximately 80,000 cpm was added for another incubation period over-night at room temperature. The excess of labeled anti-IgE was then washed away and the radioactivity bound to the paper discs was measured in a γ-scintillation detector.

Results

Development and Persistence of Antibodies

In all 25 cases antibodies were demonstrated by both PA and IFL within 2–3 weeks after the onset of clinical symptoms. After a rapid rise, titers remained at the same high level for about 1 month, whereafter they slowly decreased. From Fig. 2 it can be seen that after one year all 20 patients tested still had antibodies demonstrable by PA, and that 12 were also sero-positive by IFL. After 2 years 12 of 16 patients were still positive by PA and five by IFL. Figure 3 shows the antibody response in a representative case.

Representation of Ig Classes in the Antibody Population

The presence of specific IgM, IgA, and IgC antibodies was determined by IFL on unfractionated serum using class specific conjugates. In all, sera from thirteen cases were tested. It should be noticed that in the case

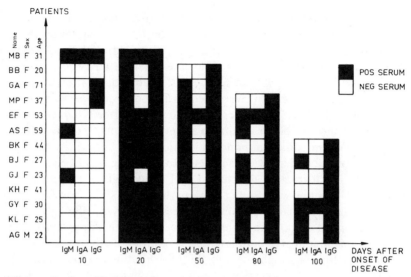

Figure 4 Specific IgM, IgA, and IgG antibodies to *Trichinella* larvae demonstrated by IFL in thirteen cases of trichinellosis. Sera taken at different times after onset of disease.

demonstrated in Fig. 3, both IgM and IgA antibodies were present in rather high titers during the first 6 weeks of infection and that IgM peristed for more than 4 months. Figure 4 shows the presence of different Ig classes in the antibody population at various periods after the onset of illness.

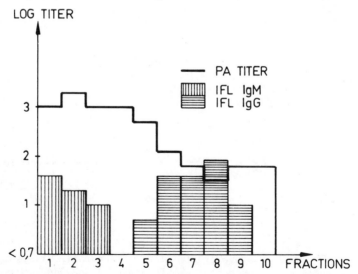

Figure 5 Distribution of IgM and IgG antibodies to *T. spiralis* in density gradient centrifugation fractions of sera from a case of trichinellosis. The fractions were collected from the bottom of the centrifuge tube.

Ten days after the onset of the disease IgM, IgA, and IgG antibodies were demonstrated in only one case and IgM or IgG in four different cases. At 20 days IgM and IgG antibodies were demonstrated in all cases and IgA in nine. At 50 days IgG was demonstrated in all twelve cases, IgM in ten, and IgA antibodies in four cases. Eighty days after the onset of illness, IgG antibodies still were demonstrated in all cases, IgM in 70% and IgA only in 20%. The last column shows that after 100 days antibodies were still demonstrable in sera from all seven patients tested and that four still had IgM antibodies and one had antibodies of IgA class.

Sera from 12 patients were subjected to sucrose gradient centrifugation, whereafter each fraction was tested by PA and IFL, using class specific conjugates reacting with either IgM or IgG. All sera showed the same antibody pattern. Figure 5 shows the presence of specific IgM and IgG in the serum of one of the patients. As can be seen the serum contained considerable amounts of both IgM and IgG antibodies most clearly demonstrated by IFL. The high titers in the IgM fractions as demonstrated by PA reflects the enhanced capacity of this technique to detect such antibodies. It has been calculated that PA is 200–500 times more effective in determining IgM antibodies than antibodies of the IgG class (Greenbury et al., 1963).

IgE assays were performed by Dr. Johansson, Uppsala. The mean level of total IgE was tested by RIST. In all 70 sera from 11 patients, obtained at different stages of the disease, were examined. The results are demonstrated in Fig. 6. The mean level of IgE in healthy blood donors was found

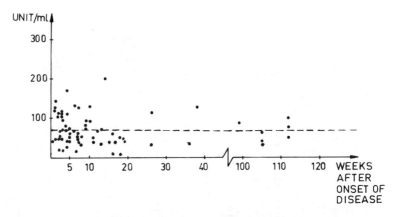

Figure 6   The level of total IgE in 70 sera from 11 cases of trichinellosis measured as unit per milliliter. The mean 71 units/ml for the total IgE level in healthy blood donors is represented by a dotted line. The range in the same material was 10-506 units/ml.

to be 71 units/ml and the range 10–506 units/ml (Johansson, personal communication). As can be seen in Fig. 6 in all sera tested the total IgE level was within the range of the normal controls.

Four sera obtained from two patients at 11, 20, 21, and 95 days after the onset of the disease were tested by RAST and they gave 359, 408, 402, and 470 cpm, respectively. The corresponding counts for a negative control was 354. These results do not indicate the presence of specific IgE.

Discussion

Two methods, PA and IFL, were used for antibody detection. Both techniques seem to be reasonably sensitive as judged by the time for earliest demonstration of antibody and the overall reactivity of sera from patients with clinical symptoms. In a statistically randomized normal sample consisting of 467 healthy Swedes, 22.7% were positive with a titer of 1:32 and 7% with 1:64 (Ljungstrom, unpublished data). Trichinellosis is a comparatively rare disease in Sweden since Swedish legislation demands that diaphragams from all slaughtered swine be examined by trichinoscopy. It is, therefore, unlikely that the low titer reactivity in this sample indicates specific antibodies. The high efficiency of PA to detect IgM antibodies suggests that reactions in low titers with this technique often may be due to heterophilic antibodies.

The specificity of IFL probably is higher than PA. However, as the larvae contain carbohydrate determinants (Tanner, 1963; Dirk van Peenen and Kent, 1960) low titers with this test might also represent cross reactions.

Circulating antibodies against *Trichinella* were first demonstrated at a time when they could be expected, judged by data obtained from experimental trichinellosis (Kagan, 1960; Ljungstrom, unpublished data). During the initial months of the disease the antibody moiety contained considerable amounts of IgM and IgA antibodies. There is reason to believe that IgA antibodies initially are formed locally in the intestine in connection with the localization of the *Trichinella* larvae within the mucosa. It has been shown that when large amounts of such secretory IgA are formed, a part of the antibody pool may pass over into the circulation where the IgA appears in monomeric form (Heremans and Vaerman, 1971). It has been suggested that IgA producing cells in the lamina propria may recirculate and later appear in lymphoid organs (Heremans and Bazin, 1971). One may, therefore, assume that later in the infection circulating IgA is formed in part by such recirculating cells. The pool of IgA-producing cells in lymphatic tissue probably also is stimulated in connection with the migration and encapsulation of the larvae.

The comparatively long-lasting persistence of IgM and IgA indicates continuous presence of the antigen. This raises the question whether and to what extent during this period the antigen is present in the form of immune complexes. Local deposition of such complexes around the encysted larvae in the muscles has been demonstrated by Novoslawski *et al.* (1969). However, little is known about the possible appearance of circulating immune complexes and their deposition in glomeruli and blood vessels.

A number of helminthic infections are accompanied by the production of reaginic antibodies which may appear in large amounts (Johansson *et al.,* 1968b; Hogarth-Scott *et al.,* 1969; Rosenberg *et al.,* 1970; Huldt *et al.,* 1973). The rather long-lasting intestinal phase suggests that such antibodies may be formed in *Trichinella* infections. Immediate reactions to intradermally administered *Trichinella* antigens have been reported and summarized by Fife (1971). A recent study of one human case of trichinellosis also showed increased level of total IgE during the fourth week after infection (Rosenberg *et al.,* 1971). It is, therefore, somewhat surprising that in 70 sera from 11 of our cases no increase in total IgE level was demonstrated. The fact that IgE antibodies were not demonstrated by RAST in four sera tested does not necessarily mean that these sera did not contain any specific IgE. As a crude antigenic preparation was used for RAST it cannot be excluded that only a small proportion of the CNBr-coupled material represented relevant antigen. Studies are in progress by using a purified antigenic preparation to investigate further the possible occurrence of specific IgE in sera from patients with trichinellosis.

Summary

Two small outbreaks of trichinellosis occurred in Sweden in 1969. In all, 25 clinical cases were detected. Sera from the infected persons were collected every 2–4 weeks over a period of 2 years. With the aid of passive hemagglutination (PA) and indirect immunofluorescence (IFL) tests, the development and persistence of antibodies were followed.

Antibodies were demonstrated as early as 11–20 days after the onset of clinical symptoms and the titers reached a peak 4–7 weeks later. Decrease in antibody levels usually occurred 2–3 months after the peak was reached. One year after the onset of clinical illness, sera from 12 of 20 patients were still reactive in the serologic tests and after 2 years five patients were seropositive in both tests. The representation of Ig classes in the antibody population was studied on whole serum with the aid of IFL using class specific conjugates. Determination of IgM and IgG antibodies also was performed on sucrose gradient fractions. Both PA and IFL with class specific conjugates were used for this purpose. Antibodies of IgM and IgA classes were found in high titers and also for comparatively long periods. The total IgE level, tested by radioimmunosorbent test (RIST) was not significantly elevated, nor could specific IgE be demonstrated by radioallergosorbent test (RAST).

Acknowledgments

I wish to express my gratitude to Dr. S. G. O. Johansson, Uppsala, for the help with the IgE measurements and also for valuable discussions. The skillful technical assistance of Miss Elisabeth Ericsson and Mrs. Maria Karpinska is gratefully acknowledged.

References

Beutner, E. H., Sepulveda, M. R., and Bernett, E. V. (1968). Quantitative studies of immunofluorescent staining. III. Relationships of characteristics of unabsorbed antihuman IgG conjugates to their specific and non-specific staining properties in an indirect test for antinuclear factors. *Bull. WHO* **39**, 587-606.

Boyden, S. V. (1951). The adsorption of proteins on erythrocytes treated with tannic acid and subsequent hemagglutination by antiprotein sera. *J. Exp. Med.* **93**, 107-200.

Bozicevich, J., Tobie, J. E., Tomas, E. L., Hoyem, H. M. and Ward, S. B. (1951). A rapid floccalation test for the diagnosis of trichinosis. *Pub. Health Rep.* **66**, 806-814.

Clark, P. S., Brownsberger, K. M., Saslow, A. R., Kagan, I. G., Noble, G. R., and Maynard, J. E. (1972). Bear meat trichinosis epidemiologic, serologic, and clinical observations from two Alaskan outbreaks. *Annu. Intern. Med.* **76**, 951-956.

Crandall, R. B., and Crandall, C. A. (1972). *Trichinella spiralis:* Immunologic response to infection in mice. *Exp. Parasitol.* **31**, 378-398.

Fife, E. H., Jr. (1971). Advances in methodology for immunodiagnosis of parasitic diseases. *Exp. Parasitol.* **30**, 132-163).

Greenbury, C. L., Moore, D. H., and Nunn, L. A. C. (1963). Reaction of 7 S and 19 S components of immune rabbit antisera with human group A and AB red cells. *Immunology* **8**, 421-433.

Heremans, J. F. and Bazin, H. (1971). Antibodies induced by local antigenic stimulation of mucosal surfaces. *Ann. N.Y. Acad. Sci.* **190**, 268-275.

Heremans, J. F., and Vaerman, J. P. (1971). Biological significance of IgA antibodies. *In:* B. Amos (ed.), "Progress in Immunology," Academic Press, New York, pp. 884-885

Hogarth-Scott, R. S., Johansson, S. G. O., and Bennich, H. (1969). Antibodies to Toxocara in the sera of visceral alrva migrans patients: the significance of raised levels of IgE. *Clin. Exp. Immunol.* **5**, 619-625.

Huldt, G., Johansson, S. G. O., and Lantto, S. (1973). Echinoccocosis in Northern Scandinavia. Immune Reactions to *E. granulosus* in Kautokeino Lapps. *Arch. Environ. Health* **26**, 36-40.

Johansson, S. G. O., and Bennich, H. (1967). Immunological studies of an atypical (myeloma) immunoglobulin. *Immunology* **13**, 381–394.

Johansson, S. G. O., Bennich, H., and Wide, L. (1968a). A new class of immuno-globulins in human serum. *Immunology* **14**, 265–272.

Johansson, S. G. O., Mellbin, T., and Wahlquist, B. (1968b). Immunoglobulin levels in Ethiopian preschool children with special reference to high concentrations of immunoglobulin E (IgND). *Lancet* **1**, 1118–1121.

Johansson, S. G. O., Bennich, H., and Berg, T. (1971). *In vitro* diagnosis of atopic allergy. III. Quantitative estimation of circulating IgE antibodies by the radio-allergosorbent test. *Int. Arch. Allergy Appl. Immunol.* **41**, 443–451.

Kagan, I. G. (1960). Trichinosis: A review of biologic, serologic and immunologic aspects. *J. Infec. Dis.* **107**, 65–93.

Kagan, I. G., Maddisson, S. E., and Norman, L. (1968). Reactivity of human im-munoglobulin in echinococcosis and trichinosis. *Amer. J. Trop. Med. Hyg.* **17**, 79–85.

Novoslawski, A., Brzosko, W. J., and Gancarz, Z. (1969). Immunopathological aspects of experimental trichinellosis. *Wiad. Parazytol.* **5/6**, 642–643.

Odelram, H. (1973). A trichinosis epidemic. *Scand. J. Infec. Dis.* **128**, 273.

Rosenberg, E. B., Whalen, G. E., Bennich, H., and Johansson, S. G. O. (1970). Increased circulating IgE in a new parasitic disease-human intestinal capil-lariasis. *N. Eng. J. Med.* **283**, 1143–1149.

Rosenberg, E. B., Polmar, S. H., and Whalen, G. E. (1971). Increased circulating IgE in trichinosis. *Ann. Intern. Med.* **75**, 575–578.

Rowe, D. S., Tackett, L., Bennich, H., Ishizaka, K., Johansson, S. G. O., and An-derson, S. G. (1970). A research standard for human serum immunoglobulin E. *Bull. WHO* **43**, 609–611.

Takatsy, G. (1955). The use of spiral loops in serological and virological micro-methods. *Acta Microbiol. Acad. Sci. Hung.* **3**, 191–202.

Tanner, C. E. (1963). Immunochemical study of the antigens of *Trichinella spiralis* larvae. III. Enzymatic degradation of the major precipitating antigen. *Exp. Parasitol.* **14**, 346–357.

Tanner, C. E. (1968). Relationship between infecting dose, muscle parasitism, and antibody response in experimental trichinosis in rabbits. *J. Parasitol.* **54**, 98–107.

Van Peenen, P. F. D., and Kent, N. H. (1960). Extraction of immunologically ac-tive protein complexes from *Trichinella spiralis* larvae. *J. Parasitol.* **46** (Suppl.), 23.

Waksman, B. H. (1958). Cell lysis and related phenomena in hypersensitive reac-tions, including immunohematologic diseases. *Progress Allergy* **5**, 349–458.

Wide, L., Bennich, H., and Johansson, S. G. O. (1967). *In vitro* diagnosis of allergy by an *in vitro* test for allergen antibodies. *Lancet* **II**, 1105.

Part V

Treatment

An Analysis of Approximately 150 Reports of Compounds Tested for Efficacy in Clinical or Experimental Trichinellosis

William C. Campbell and Lyndia S. Blair

Merck Institute for Therapeutic Research, Rahway, New Jersey

Introduction

The literature on trichinellosis is replete with reports of the efficacy of various preparations in reducing the intensity of the infection. These reports stem from both the clinic and the laboratory; they deal with cursory observation as well as rigorous experimentation, and with crude natural products as well as refined synthetic chemicals. In the English language there have been two major reviews of the chemotherapy of trichinellosis. Gould's review of 1945 is a mine of information on the older reports (from the beginning of the century to 1943). Zaiman's review of 1970 is both recent and comprehensive; it presents an excellent evaluation of the significance of the reports, especially in relation to clinical medicine. In other languages the most comprehensive review known to us is that of Lupascu *et al.,* in Rumanian, published in 1970.

Despite the excellence of earlier reviews there seems to us to be a need for a critical appraisal and classification of the 145 compounds that have been reported as effective or as ineffective in the treatment of trichinellosis. The physician confronted with clinical trichinellosis is generally interested only in the safest and most effective drug available at the time. Those interested in controlling transmission of trichinellosis, or in the experimental chemotherapy of the infection, are interested in the broadest range of active drugs (while the medicinal chemist may be interested not only in these but also in related compounds known to be inactive). In the present paper we have dismissed those compounds which we consider to have no significance in experimental or clinical trichinellosis and we have attempted to summarize very briefly the efficacy of those drugs we consider to be of special significance either in the treatment or the study of the infection.

463

References have been kept to a minimum because it is intended to publish the approximately 250 pertinent references elsewhere (Campbell and Blair, 1974).

Drugs That Are Probably Inactive

It can at once be said that the great majority (127) of reported compounds are of little consequence, since they must be labeled "probably inactive." The term "inactive" is used herein to mean devoid of selective toxicity to the parasite. Compounds that appear to be toxic to the parasite and the host at approximately the same dosage are thus considered inactive, since selective toxicity has not been demonstrated. On the other hand, for the information to be of value to the synthetic chemist a compound should not be labeled inactive unless it has been tested reasonably well at reasonably high dosage. If these criteria of activity and inactivity have not been met, it makes little difference whether certain compounds have been reported in the literature as active (36 compounds) or as inactive (81 compounds). All such compounds must be considered either inactive or, at best, slightly active at barely tolerated dosages. For all practical purposes they can be dismissed as "probably inactive."

The 127 compounds listed as "probably inactive" fall into several categories (Table I). They include the following natural products: camphor, oil growth substance, oil of turpentine, papain, mexicaina (plant enzyme), pomegranate rind, corn oil, garlic, milk, pilzfutter. Also included are 16 miscellaneous chemicals that have no obvious unifying characteristic (e.g., chloroform, aminopyrine, glycerol, benzene). There are also salts or organic compounds of the following metals: arsenic, antimony, mer-

Table I   Types and Numbers of Compounds Reported in the Literature with Respect to Chemotherapy of Trichinellosis

| | Probably inactive | | |
| | Reported | Reported | Clearly |
Type of compound	inactive	active	active
Natural products	6	4	0
Miscellaneous chemicals	35[a]	6	0
Metal salts and organometallics	13[b]	8	0
Antibiotics	11	9	0
Sulfonamides	8	0	0
Other non-metallic drugs	8	9	28
	81	36	28

[a] Includes seven naphthoquinones, and 18 benzimidazoles some of which may be partially active.
[b] Antimonials grouped as single entity.

cury, silver, copper, magnesium. There are 20 antibiotics and five sulfon-amide drugs. Finally among the 127 "probably inactive" compounds, is a group of 17 compounds generally regarded as drugs, but not of the metal-lic, antibiotic, or sulfonamide type. Because these compounds include several classic antimicrobial or antiparasitic agents they are itemized here-with: acridine, aspidium extract, emetine hydrochloride, gentian violet, kousso, monomycin, pyrimethamine, rivanol, acriflavine, p-benzylphenyl carbamate (Butolan), coumaphos, hexylresorcinol, 8-hydroxyquinoline-7-sulfonic acid salt with aminopyrine (Causyth), metronidazole, pheno-thiazine, tetrachlorethylene, thymol.

Drugs Active in the Enteral Phase

The 28 drugs that are considered active in any phase of trichinellosis are listed in Table II. With the exception of the three antimitotic drugs, these drugs have all been reported active against *Trichinella spiralis* in the intestinal tract of the host. In the case of piperazine and diethylcarbama-zine the reports of efficacy have been so equivocal that these drugs should be considered as being, at best, marginally active in enteral trichinellosis. (Indeed piperazine might well be relegated to the category of drugs "prob-ably inactive" in any phase of trichinellosis.)

Some compounds are highly active against newly ingested *Trichinella* larvae but are either less active or inactive against the adult worms. Such compounds are cambendazole, parbendazole, thiabendazole, cadmium oxide, and ethanol. Other compounds show good activity against adult *Trichinella* but little or no activity against the developing worm in the gut; examples are methyridine, pyrantel tartrate, dithiazanine, tetramizole, famaphos, and ruelene.

Inhibition of larviposition in trichinellosis can be of obvious practical importance even in the absence of a vermifugal or vermicidal action. Most drugs have not been examined for this type of activity, but the effect is known to occur with cambendazole and thiabendazole (at dosages less than those required to remove the adult worms) and is known not to occur in the case of phthalophos.

Drugs Active in the Parenteral Phase

Because of the special importance of drugs effective against *Trichinella* larvae in the most musculature, these drugs are itemized below with notes on their actions and effective dosages.

Cambendazole is active against the migrating larvae in mice at 0.025% in the feed, and against the encysted larvae at 50 mg/kg daily for 7 days.

Table II Drugs Active in Trichinellosis, with Indication of Whether Activity is Exerted on Enteral or Parenteral Phase of Infection

Drug	Enteral	Parenteral	Reference
Benzimidazoles			
Cambendazole	+	+	Campbell and Yakstis, 1970; Duckett and Denham, 1970
G572, G581	+	+	Konovalova *et al.*, 1966
Mebendazole	+	+	Thienpoint *et al.*, (in Part V, this volume)
Parbendazole	+	+	Theodorides and Laderman, 1969
Thiabendazole	+	+	Campbell, 1961; Cuckler, 1961
Organophosphates			
Bayer 9018	+	+	Lamina (in Part V, this volume)
Bromophos	+	−	Fitzner, 1967
Dimethoate	+	−	Zimmermann, 1964
Famophos	+	−	Weissenburg, 1963; Zimmermann, 1964
Fenthion	+	+	Meilinger, 1964
Haloxon	+	−	Martinez *et al.*, 1966
Phthalophos	+	−	Campbell and Cuckler, 1967
Ruelene	+	−	Janitschke, 1962
Trichlorphon	+	+	Schoop and Lamina, 1959
Antimitotics			
Daunomycin	No test	+[a]	Gretillat, 1970
Methotrexate	No test	+[a]	Gretillat, 1970
Thiotepa	No test	+[a]	Gretillat, 1970
Miscellaneous			
Cadmium oxide	+	−	Larsh and Goulson, 1957
Diethylcarbamazine	+(?)	+[a]	Oliver-Gonzalez and Hewitt, 1947
Dithiazanine	+	−	McCowen *et al.*, 1958
Ethanol	+[b]	−	Kestner, 1864
Methyridine	+	−	Janitschke, 1962
Phytohemagglutinin	+[a]	−	Pereverseva *et al.*, (in Part II, this volume)
Piperazine	+(?)	−	Chan and Brown, 1954
Pyrantel tartrate	+	−	Howes and Lynch, 1967
Rotenone	+	No test	Guerra, 1946
Tetramisole	+	+	Thienpont *et al.*, 1966

[a] Effect seems to be primarily immunological (nonspecific).
[b] Effective only if given close to time of inoculation and in sufficient concentration (as distinct from dosage).

Larvae that survive treatment have been reported to retain infectivity for other hosts.

G572 and G581 designate 2-(2′chlorophenyl)benzimidazole and 2-(2′pyridyl)benzimidazole, respectively. These appear to be the most efficacious members of a series of novel benzimidazoles tested in mice by workers in Moscow, who concluded that they were similar in potency to thiabendazole and that G572 was less toxic than thiabendazole and cheaper to produce.

Mebendazole is active against migrating larvae in rats at 0.01% in the feed, and against encysted larvae at 0.05%. Although this drug has been tested against other helminthoses in man, there are at present no reports of trials in human trichinellosis.

Parbendazole is active against migrating and encysted larvae in mice at 0.05%. By analogy with other benzimidazoles, this is probably not the minimum effective dosage for efficacy against the migrating larvae.

Thiabendazole is active against migrating larvae in mice at 0.05% in feed, and against encysted larvae at 0.5%. Even frequent treatment by gavage is unlikely to yield efficacy as good as that obtained by continuous dietary medication. It is variably active against migratory larvae in pigs at 50 mg/kg two times per day for 10 days and active against encysted larvae at 75 mg/kg two times per day for 14 days. In man the efficacy of thiabendazole has not been clearly defined. Favorable, sometimes dramatic, clinical response has followed the use of conventional clinical dosages (25 mg/kg two times per day for 2 or 3 days). In some instances the duration of infection at time of treatment was unknown, but in other cases it was known to be as long as 6 weeks. Biopsy evidence of destruction of larvae has not been obtained in the few instances in which it was sought, but this finding is of limited significance because of the inadequate sampling inherent in the method. On the other hand, when larger dosages were used (50 mg/kg once daily for 10 days) there was evidence of dead larvae as well as clinical amelioration of the disease. Because of the sporadic nature and limited size of trichinellosis outbreaks, a definitive assessment of the value of thiabendazole (or any other drug) in clinical trichinellosis will probably take many years to complete.

Bayer 9018 is an organic phosphate that is active against migratory and encysted larvae in mice at the somewhat toxic dosage of 500 mg/kg daily for 3 days.

Fenthion is an organophosphate that is slowly metabolized in mammals and thus does not have to be administered repeatedly at short intervals. In mice, an oral or intraperitoneal treatment at a dosage of 150 mg/kg, repeated after 5 days, is active against the encysted and migratory phases.

Trichlorphon, an organophosphate, is active against the migratory and encysted larvae in mice. The dosage required for good efficacy against the latter (300 mg/kg daily for 5 days) needs the conjoint administration of antidotes to offset the toxic effect of acetylcholinesterase inhibition in the host.

The antimitotic drugs thiotepa, methotrexate, and daunomycin have been reported to damage the *Trichinella* capsule in the musculature of laboratory animals and so cause the death of the encysted larva. To achieve this effect thiotepa was given as multiple intraperitoneal doses to rats (0.5–3.0 mg/animal) and guinea pigs (1.0 mg/animal) and rabbits (5.0 mg/animal). Methotrexate was given as multiple intramuscular doses to guinea pigs (2.0 mg/animal) and rabbits (5 mg/animals). Daunomycin was given as multiple intravenous doses to rabbits (5 mg/kg).

Diethylcarbamazine has been tested against parenteral *Trichinella* in laboratory animals and in man, with apparently conflicting results. The inconsistency may be due to failure to detect a slow indirect action in which the host's immunological attack on the larva is enhanced. Dosages of 6 mg/kg daily for 10 days (rats) and approximately 1 mg/kg four times per day (man) have been considered effective by some authors.

Tetramisole, at 0.5% in feed, is moderately effective against encysted *Trichinella* in mice. A high degree of efficacy cannot be attained at safe dosages.

Nonspecific Treatment

The symptomatic treatment of clinical trichinellosis is beyond the scope of this brief review. Corticosteroids have long been the mainstay of such treatment. It is now becoming evident that the distinction between specific and nonspecific effect is not absolute. Drugs such as antimitotic agents or phytohemagglutinin may exert a secondary antiparasitic effect resulting from a primary pharmacological or immunological action; while others, such as thiabendazole and diethylcarbamazine may have both specific and nonspecific primary effects.

Summary

Of almost 150 compounds reported in the literature as either active or inactive in *Trichinella spiralis* infections, only 28 were considered to have a substantial degree of efficacy. Many of the modern broad-spectrum anthelmintics are active against the enteral phase of trichinellosis in laboratory animals. Only 14 compounds were rated active against *Trichinella* in host musculature; these were certain benzimidazoles, certain organophosphates, tetramisole, diethylcarbamazine, and certain antimitotic agents (methotrexate, thiotepa, and daunomycin).

References

Campbell, W. C. (1961). Effect of thiabendazole upon infections of *Trichinella spiralis* in mice, and upon certain other helminthiases. *J. Parasitol.* **47** (Suppl.), 37.

Campbell, W. C., and Cuckler, A. C. (1967). Comparative studies on the chemotherapy of experimental trichinosis in mice. *Z. Tropenmed. Parasitol.* **18,** 408–417.

Campbell, W. C., and Yakstis, J. J. (1970). Efficacy of cambendazole against *Trichinella spiralis* in mice. *J. Parasitol.* **56,** 839–840.

Campbell, W. C. and Blair, L. S. (in press). Chemotherapy of *Trichinella* infections (a review). *Exp. Parasitol.*

Chan, K. F., and Brown, H. W. (1954). Treatment of experimental trichinosis in mice with piperazine hydrochloride. *Amer. J. Trop. Med. Hyg.* **3,** 746–749.

Cuckler, A. C. (1961). Thiabendazole, a new broad spectrum anthelmintic. *J. Parasitol.* **47** (suppl.), 36–37.

Duckett, M. G., and Denham, D. A. (1970). The effect of cambendazole on *Trichinella spiralis* infections in mice. *J. Helminthol.* **44,** 211–218.

Fitzner, J. (1967). Uber die Wirkung von Bromophos (Cela) auf die verschiedenen Entwicklungsstadien von *Trichinella spiralis* (Owen) bei experimentell infizierten Mausen. Dissertation, Hochschule, Hanover. (Cited in *Vet. Bull.,* 1968, *Abstr.* No. 4646.)

Gould, S. E. (1945). "Trichinosis." Thomas, Springfield, Illinois, p. 356.

Grétillat, S. (1970). Contribution a l'etude du traitement de la trichinose experimentale. Action de trois antimitotiques sur les larves de *Trichinella spiralis.* *Bull. Soc. Pathol. Exot.* **63,** 696–709.

Guerra, F. (1946). La accion de la rotenona y de la mexicaina en la triquinosis experimental de la rata. *Rev. Inst. Salub. Enferm. Trop.* **7,** 57–61.

Howes, H. L., Jr., and Lynch, J. E. (1967). Anthelmintic studies with pyrantel. I. Therapeutic and prophylactic efficacy against the enteral stages of various helminths in mice and dogs. *J. Parasitol.* **53,** 1085–1091.

Janitschke, B. (1962). Untersuchungen an Meerschweinchen uber. die Wirkung von Promintic und Ruelene auf Larven von *Trichinella spiralis* und *Toxocara canis.* Dissertation, Free University, Berlin.

Kestner, H. (1864). "Etude sur le *Trichina spiralis."* J. B. Bailliere et Fils, Paris. (Cited by Gould, 1945, *loc. cit.*)

Konovalova, L. M., Ozeretskovskaya, N. N., and Kolosova, M. O. (1966). [Search for the specific therapy for trichinellosis. III. Derivatives of benzimidazole-2-(3′-pyridyl)benzimidazole and 2-2-(2′nitrophenyl)-benzimidazole in experimental trichinellosis in white mice]. (In Russian.) *Med. Parazitol. Parazit. Bol.* **35,** 551–556.

Larsh, J. E., Jr. and Goulson, H. T. (1957). The effectiveness of cadmium oxide against *Trichinella spiralis* in mice. *J. Parasitol.* **43,** 440–445.

Lupascu, G., Cironeanu, I., Hacig, A., Pambuccian, G., Simionescu, O., Solomon, P., and Tintareanu, J. (1970). "Trichineloza." Editura Academiei Republicii Socialiste, Romania, 246 pp.

Martinez, A. R., Cordero, M. C., and Aller, B. G. (1966). Ensayos sobre la eficacia del haloxon contra *Trichinella spiralis Anal. Fac. Vet. Leon* **12,** 251. [Cited from Martinez, A. M., Cordero, M. C., and Aller B. G. (1968). The prophylactic effect of haloxon against experimental *Trichinella spiralis* infections in rats. *Ann. Trop. Med. Parasitol.* **62,** 63–66.]

McCowen, M. C., Callender, M. E., Brandt, M. C., Gossett, F. O. Gregory, R. P., and Shumard, R. F. (1958). Dithiazanine iodide, an effective broad-spectrum anthelmintic for small animals. *J. Parasitol.* **44** (Suppl.), 39.

Meilinger, W. (1964). Prufung eines Phosphonsaureesterpraparates (S.1752 Bayer) auf seine Wirksamkeit gegenuber Trichinellen bei der experimentell infizierten Maus. Dissertation, Johan Wolfgan Goethe University, Frankfurt, 49 pp.

Oliver-González, J., and Hewitt, R. I. (1947). Treatment of experimental intestinal trichinosis with 1-diethylcarbamyl-4-methylpiperazine hydrochloride (Hetrazan). *Proc. Soc. Exp. Biol. Med.* **66,** 254–255.

Schoop, G., and Lamina, J. (1959). Uber die Wirkung von Neguvon auf *Trichinella spiralis* in experimentell infirierten Mausen. *Monatsch. Tierheilk.* **11,** 167–171.

Theodorides, V. J., and Laderman, M. (1969). Activity of parbendazole upon *Trichinella spiralis* in mice. *J. Parasitol.* **55,** 678.

Thienpont, D., Vanparijs, O. F. J., Raeymaekers, A. H. M., Vandenberk, J., Demeon, P. J. A., Allewijn, F. T. N., Marsboom, R. P. H., Niemgeers, C. J. E., Schellekens, K. H. L., and Janssen, P. A. J. (1966). Tetramizole (R8299), a new, potent broad spectrum anthelmintic *Nature London* **290,** 1084–1086.

Weissenburg, H. (1963). Untersuchungen uber die Wirksamkeit von Famophos auf Magendarmwurmer bei Schafen. Dissertation, Free University, Berlin. 36 pp.

Zaiman, H. (1970). Drug Treatment of trichinosis. *In:* S. E. Gould (ed.), "Trichinosis in Man and Animals," Thomas, Springfield, Illinois, pp. 329–347.

Zimmermann, W. J. (1964). Efficacy of selected drugs against *Trichinella spiralis J. Parasitol.* **50,** 415–420.

Probable Sterilization of *Trichinella spiralis* by Thiobendazole: Further Clinical Observation of Human Infections

Czesław Gerwel, Zbigniew Pawłowski,
Wanda Kociecka, and Leon Chodera

Clinic of Parasitic Diseases
Medical Academy of Poznah
Poznań

Introduction

Thiabendazole was found able to prevent human symptomatic trichinellosis when used in the first week following consumption of infected meat (Gerwel, Kocięcka and Pawłowski, 1970). Clinical observations made on a group of seven patients heavily infected with *Trichinella spiralis* have lately given some new information and suggestions concerning thiabendazole action on adults.

Materials and Methods

A group of 23 people ate heavily infected raw and/or cooked pork before trichinoscopy was performed. The average number of *Trichinella* larvae, found by digestion method, in 1 gm of meat was 23. Seven patients, four females and three males, 12–37 years of age, ate raw meat. The calculated infective dose was between 1500 and 11,500 larvae.

Thiabendazole (TBI), 50 mg/kg body weight, was administered orally for 5 days following the fourth day after infection. All seven patients were admitted to our clinic in the first, second, fourth or fifth week of trichinellosis and observed up to 42, 51, or 56 days after infection. The routine laboratory tests, including complement fixation (CF) test with *Trichinella* antigen were performed. Five patients (numbers 1–5) with fever episodes were given corticosteroid treatment (Prednisonum, 30 mg daily). In two patients (numbers 1 and 4) biopsy of the deltoid muscle was performed on the forty-seventh day of trichinellosis. The muscle tissue was examined in part histopathologically, in part trichinoscopically, after cutting the specimen up into small pieces and repeatedly pressing the 'separated muscle fibers.

Results

The following criteria were adopted for the evaluation of intensity of clinical trichinellosis: rise in body temperature, periorbital edema, white blood cell, and eosinophil count, positive CF test, serum protein level and proteinogram, and in two cases, presence of larvae in muscle tissue (Fig. 1). In two patients (numbers 6 and 7) no clinical symptoms were observed, except for a short rise in the number of white blood cells (numbers 6 and 7) and eosinophils (number 6). They were infected with about 1500 larvae. Four other patients developed subclinical (numbers 2 and 3) or light (numbers 1 and 5) trichinellosis with fever episodes, transient periorbital edema, and muscle pain, leukocytosis, eosinophilia, and positive CF test. The estimated infective doses in these patients were 2500 larvae (numbers 2, 3, and 5) or 4500 larvae (number 1). The symptoms appeared as late as 26–28 days after infection. The first positive CF tests were observed 45 days after infection. Biopsy of patient 1 revealed 66 larvae in 1 gm of deltoid muscle tissue. A light trichinellosis also occurred in the last patient (number 4). He was hospitalized and treated with thiabendazole again on 14–18 days after infection because of fever which occurred on the fourteenth day. This patient developed very high leukocytosis and eosinophilia, but otherwise felt rather well. Only 33 *Trichinella* larvae in 1 gm of deltoid muscle were found on the forty-seventh day although the patient ate a pound of raw pork, i.e., about 11,500 infective larvae. It is important to note that in the two biopsies performed on day 47 after ingestion of raw meat, seven larvae were not yet encapsulated and only three larvae were encapsulated. Histopathologically (L. Gustowska) there were basophilia of muscle fibers in both specimens and an intense cellular infiltration around the nests of larvae in one patient (number 4).

Discussion

The results of prolonged and detailed clinical observations made on seven patients infected with a high number of *T. spiralis* larvae enriched and further developed our previously published opinion on the prevention of human symptomatic trichinellosis with thiabendazole (Gerwel *et al.,* 1970). The opinion was based on the observations of seven patients infected with relatively low doses and treated with thiabendazole in 1966 and 1968. Our unpublished observations (Gerwel *et al.,* 1972) made late in 1971 on a group of five patients infected with a dose of less than 1000

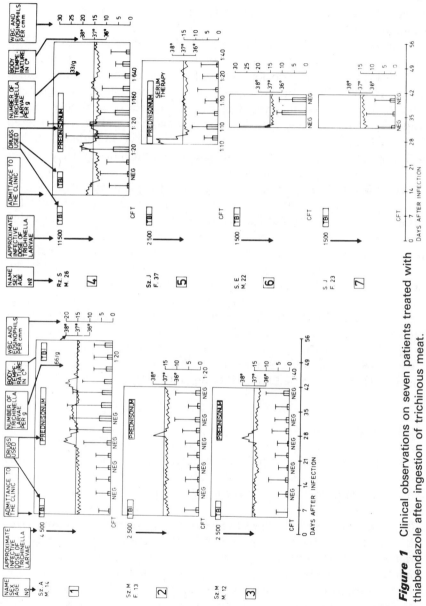

Figure 1 Clinical observations on seven patients treated with thiabendazole after ingestion of trichinous meat.

larvae and treated with thiabendazole from the second day after meat consumption, confirmed our views that thiabendazole treatment in the first week following ingestion of trichinous meat prevents symptomatic trichinellosis.

Now we are able to state that a 5-day thiabendazole treatment, instituted on the fourth day after infection, may not prevent symptomatic trichinellosis if the infective dose is high. But even in such cases the clinical picture is mild or light and completely out of proportion to the high number of infective larvae ingested. Our past and recent clinical observations lead to the practical suggestion that thiabendazole should be administered for a longer period (twice for 5 days with a 5-day break) in patients infected with more than 2000 larvae and treated not earlier than the fourth day after consumption of infected raw meat.

Detailed clinical observations and parasitological examinination of human trichinellosis have theoretical aspects as well. They confirm the results of the experiments of Blair and Campbell (1971) on the reversibility of thiabendazole-induced sterilization of *T. spiralis*. The experiments of Blair and Campbell (1971) were performed on mice, which were given feed containing 0.05% thiabendazole beginning on the third day of trichinellosis. When thiabendazole was given at 3–7 days of infection, no larvae were found in females on the seventh and the tenth day, but they were observed on the fourteenth day again. In the human cases presented, the late appearance of symptoms on 26–28 days and the lack of encapsulation in most muscle larvae on the forty-seventh day of infection (7 out of 10) strongly suggest the same temporary sterilization of *T. spiralis* females as that observed in mice by Blair and Campbell (1971).

Summary

Seven patients were given thiabendazole, 50 mg/kg body weight daily, between the fifth and ninth day after infection with *Trichinella*. The calculated infective doses were between 1500 and 11,500 larvae. Two patients showed eosinophilia and positive CF test only. Four patients developed subclinical or light trichinellosis as late as 26–28 days after infection. Light trichinellosis occurred in one patient who ate a pound of raw meat with 23 *Trichinella* larvae per gram. The conclusion is that thiabendazole treatment for 5 days is not able to prevent symptomatic trichinellosis when the infective dose is high and treatment is not possible before the fourth day following consumption of trichinous meat. But even in those cases the clinical picture is mild and out of proportion to the high infective dose. The late appearance of symptoms and the lack of encapsulation in most muscle larvae on the forty-seventh day of infection confirm the suggestion that thiabendazole induces a temporary sterilization of *Trichinella* females.

Acknowledgments

This study was supported by the grant CDC-E-2, Center for Disease Control, U.S. Public Health Service.
We thank the staff of the Provincial Sanitary-Epidemiological Station Wolsztyn, Poland, for organizing help in the *Trichinella* focus.

References

Blair, L. S., and Campbell, W. C. (1971). Reversibility of thiabenbazole-induced sterilization of *Trichinella spiralis. Wiad. Parazytol.* **17,** 641–644.
Gerwel, C., Kociecka, W., and Pawlowski, Z. (1970). Thiabendazole as a drug preventing human trichinosis. *Epidemiol. Rev.* **24,** 56–59.
Gerwel, C., Pawłowski, Z., Kociecka, W., and Chodera, L. (1972). Thiabendazole v profilaktike klinichieskogo trichinelloza. *Vses. Konf. Trikhinelloze. Vilinius, U.S.S.R.*

Search for Trichinellocides: The Relationship between the Structure and Activity of Benzimidazoles

M. O. Kolosova and N. N. Ozeretskovskaya

*E. I. Martsinovsky Institute of Medicinal Parasitology
and Tropical Medicine, Moscow*

In the treatment of trichinellosis the targets for chemotherapy are the muscle and the intestinal *Trichinella*. It is known that imidazoles which contain the dipeptides anserine and carnosine are specifically associated with muscle tissues while the anomalous histidine metabolism is characteristic of tissues affected by the disease. On the other hand, benzimidazole derivatives are supposed to be potential competitors with imidazoles of vital importance for the living cell. The benzimidazole series has therefore been selected as a promising area of search for trichinellocides.

The objective was to synthesize and test benzimidazole derivatives against experimental trichinellosis in mice, to determine the structure–activity relationships and to elucidate the mode of action of the drugs on *Trichinella spiralis*. The test results of selected benzimidazole derivatives against *T. spiralis* in white mice are presented in Table I. Other benzimidazoles are omitted.

A high activity of thiabendazole (Kolosova and Gein, 1965) against experimental trichinellosis (Frol'tsova *et al.*, 1966) prompted us to synthesize the isomeric 2-pyridylbenzimidazoles (G-514, G-581, G-582) which could be considered as isoelectronic analogs of thiazolylbenzimidazole. A number of 2-arylbenzimidazoles having various substituents in different positions of the 2-phenyl residue has also been prepared in order to judge the effect of the substituents on trichinellocidal properties. All the compounds synthesized were tested against immature and mature intestinal *Trichinella* as well as against muscle larvae. The results show that of the 2-heteryl- and 2-arylbenzimidazoles the most active ones are thiabendazole (G-491), 2-(2'-pyridyl)benzimidazole (G-581), and 2-(2'-chlorophenyl)-benzimidazole (G-572), i.e., those compounds in which a substituent in 2-aryl or a heteroatom in 2-heteryl residue is in the *ortho* position with respect to benzimidazole ring. Among the 2-amino derivatives the most effective was methoxycarbonylaminobenzimidazole (G-665). These drugs

477

Table I   Trichinellocidal Activity of 2-Substituted Benzimidazoles

Compound	R	Activity[a] at various days after infection (%)		
		2–4	7–14	25–30
G-491	4'-Thiazolyl	100	80	50
G-581	2'-Pyridyl	91	80	72
G-514	3'-Pyridyl	0	68	28
G-582	4'-Pyridyl	0	0	+39[b]
G-572	2'-Chlorophenyl	94	78	66
G-573	3'-Chlorophenyl	0	51	–
G-577	4'-Chlorophenyl	32	+44	–
G-571	2',4'-Dichlorophenyl	43	25	–
G-551	3'-Tolyl	0	0	–
G-552	3'-Nitrophenyl	0	0	–
G-620	2'-Aminophenyl	58	48	–
G-666	3'-Aminophenyl	70	64	–
G-660	4'-Aminophenyl	60	55	–
G-641	2'-Bromophenyl	36	40	–
G-665	Methoxycarbonylamino	81	96	89
G-756	Ethoxycarbonylamino	99	–	72

[a] Reduction of number of the larvae per 1 gm of tissue as compared with control.
[b] Increase of number of the larvae.

and 2-(3'-pyridyl)benzimidazole (G-514) which were active against mature intestinal *Trichinella* were tested against all stages of the parasite development. The 2-pyridylbenzimidazoles displayed a rather strong effect, thus verifying the possibility of substitution of the pyridine ring for the thiazole ring. The mode of action of the drugs was found to depend on the position by which the pyridine ring is attached to the C-2 atom of the benzimidazole moiety (Ozeretskovskaya *et al.*, 1969b). Thus, the 2-(2'-pyridyl)benzimidazole (G-581) is similar to thiabendazole in the intensity and mode of its action, whereas the 4'-pyridyl analog (G-582) is devoid of trichinellocidal activity and the 3'-pyridyl analog (G-513) exhibits a marked effect on mature intestinal *Trichinella* (Konovalova *et al.*, 1966). Among isomeric 2-chlorophenylbenzimidazoles the *ortho* compound (G-572) is most effective (Ozeretskovskaya *et al.*, 1971). The corresponding bromo derivative (G-641) has but low activity. No effective drugs were found among 2-aminophenylbenzimidazoles. Methyl- and ethylbenzimidazole-2-carbamates (G-665 and G-756) were the only two representatives of the large group of 2-acylaminobenzimidazoles and N_3-substituted benzimidazolylureas, which possessed considerable trichinellocidal activity. A special group consists of S-substituted derivatives of 2-mercapto- and 2-mercaptomethylbenzimidazoles. These compounds (not listed in table) displayed unusual activity resulting in intensive calcification of the larva, of its capsule, and of the sarcoplasm, suggesting changes in the metabolism of the larva and muscle tissue under the influence of the drugs. A detailed study of their mode of action is now in progress.

The activity of the compounds G-491, G-572, and G-581 was supposed to be associated with a planar conformation of their molecules provided by strong intramolecular hydrogen bonds. This conformation is apparently significant for effective interaction of the drug with a substrate (by superimposing) and chelation with appropriate groups of enzymes.

Further studies revealed that modification of G-491, G-572, and G-581 by substitution of methyl for benzimidazole imino hydrogen decreased the activity of the drugs by at least 50% (Kolosova et al., 1970). The effect is probably due to the disturbance of the coplanarity of the drug molecule and to the loss of its ability to react with nucleophilic groups of substrates, since the second (pyridine-like) nitrogen of benzimidazole can bind only electrophilic reagents. The importance of nucleophilic interactions for manifestation of activity by thiabendazole is borne out by the data of Prichard (1970).

It appeared reasonable to increase the lipophilic properties of the active drugs, since lipophilic nonionized anthelmintics penetrate through the gastrointestinal barrier better than ionized compounds (McManus et al., 1966). Therefore the N-acetyl and N-carbomethoxyl derivatives of G-491, G-572, and G-581 were prepared and their physicochemical and biological properties were studied. The compounds were found to hydrolyze easily to the parent drugs even in neutral media at room temperature. Due to the lower polarity they were expected to provide higher concentrations of the drugs in the organism. At the same time the ability of these compounds, unlike the aforementioned N-methyl derivatives, to generate the parent drugs by splitting off the acyl groups made it possible to retain the trichinellocidal activity.

The data presented in Table II demonstrate that introduction of the acetyl or carbomethoxyl group may have a different effect on the pharmacological properties of the preparations. With thiabendazole the activity is not affected noticeably on acetylation or carbomethoxylation, while with 2-(2'-pyridyl)benzimidazole it is somewhat reduced. An especially marked decrease in activity (approximately 90%) and an increase in toxicity was observed with N-carbomethoxy-2-(2'-chlorophenyl)benzimidazole (G-728) (Kolosova et al., 1971).

The effect of N-acylation on the biological properties of the drugs was found to correlate with the strength of the linkage between the acyl group and the cyclic nitrogen. It was established by chemical evidences and by ultraviolet (UV) spectroscopy that N-acetyl derivatives (G-719, G-726, and G-725), which are more similar to the parent drugs by their activity, are

Table II Effect of Substitution at N_1 on the Activity of Benzimidazole Derivatives

Compound	R	R_1	Activity (%)[a] at various days after infection		
			2–4	7–14	25–30
G-491	4'-Thiazolyl	H	100	80	50
G-491M	4'-Thiazolyl	CH_3	52	53	–
G-719	4'-Thiazolyl	$COCH_3$	94	89	–
G-669	4'-Thiazolyl	$COOCH_3$	72	90	–
G-572	2'-Chlorophenyl	H	94	78	66
G-572M	2'-Chlorophenyl	CH_3	35	32	–
G-726	2'-Chlorophenyl	$COCH_3$	62	16	32
G-728	2'-Chlorophenyl	$COOCH_3$	7	+8	+20
G-581	2'-Pyridyl	H	91	80	72
G-581M	2'-Pyridyl	CH_3	22	18	–
G-725	2'-Pyridyl	$COCH_3$	8	62	56
G-673	2'-Pyridyl	$COOCH_3$	39	12	16

[a] See footnote to Table I

hydrolyzed in neutral media at a faster rate than the corresponding carbomethoxyl derivatives (G-669, G-728, and G-673), the most slow being cleavage of carbomethoxyl group from G-728. The UV spectra of these compounds indicated that N-acylation resulted in a disturbance of the coplanarity of the molecule, the maximum divergence being also for G-728.

The information so far available is certainly insufficient for any positive conclusion about the mechanism of action of benzimidazole drugs in trichinellosis. It appears to be varied at different stages of trichinellosis. A steady increase of nonspecific histidine decarboxylase and accumulation of histamine in blood, liver, and muscle tissue is characteristic of trichinellosis (Bekish, 1972). We therefore suggest that competitive inhibition of histidine decarboxylase (Mardashov et al., 1967) is essential for the action of benzimidazoles at the muscle stage of trichinellosis (Ozeretskovskaya et al., 1969a).

Summary

About 60 benzimidazole derivatives have been synthesized and tested, among which are 2-aryl, 2-heteryl, 2-amino, and 2-mercapto-substituted compounds. Six of the preparations were found to be potent trichinellocides. Some structure–activity relations have been elucidated, in particular the effect of substituents in the positions 1 and 2 of the imidazole moiety upon trichinellocidal properties of the drugs. A mechanism is proposed to account for this effect.

References

Bekish, O. J. L. (1972). The metabolism of histamine in experimental trichinellosis in rats. *Mater. Dokl. Vses. Konf. Cyi Probl. Trichinellesa Cheloveka Zhivotnych Vilnus,* pp. 77–82.

Froltsova, A. E., Ozeretskovskaya, N. N., Konovalova, L. M., and Kolosova, M. O. (1966). Search for the specific therapy for trichinellosis. II. Thiabendazole in experimental trichinellosis of rats. *Med. Parazitol. Parazit. Bol.* (1), 102–106.

Kolosova, M. O., and Gein, O. N. (1965). Preparation of the 2-(4'-thiazolyl)-benzimidazole. *Med. Prom. S.S.S.R.* (10), 14–15.

Kolosova, M. O., Ozeretskovskaya, N. N., Gein, O. N., and Tchernyaeva, A. I. (1970). Search for the specific therapy for trichinellosis. VI. Chemical structure and antitrichellosis activity of benzimidazole derivatives. *Med. Parazitol. Parazit. Bol.* (5), 528–531.

Kolosova, M. O., Pereverzeva, E. V., Ozeretskovskaya, N. N., Gein, O. N., and Pudel, M. E. (1971). Search for the specific therapy for trichinellosis. VII. Effect of acylation on the activity of benzimidazole preparations in experimental trichinellosis in white mice. *Med. Parazitol. Parazit. Bol.* (5), 540–542.

Konovalova, L. M., Ozeretskovskaya, N. N., and Kolosova, M. O. (1966). Search for the specific therapy for trichinellosis. III. 2-(3'-pyridyl)benzimidazole in experimental trichinellosis in white mice. *Med. Parazitol. Parazit. Bol.* (5), 551–556.

McManus, E. C., Washko, F. V., and Tocco, D. J. (1966). Gastrointestinal absorption and secretion of thiabendazole in ruminants. *Amer. J. Vet. Res.* **27,** 849–855.

Mardashov, S. R., Dabagov, N. S., and Gonchar, N. A. (1967). The inhibitors of microbal histidine decarboxylase. *Vop. Med. Khim.* **13,** 78–82.

Ozeretskovskaya, N. N., Kolosova, M. O., Tchernyaeva, A. I., Pereverzeva, E. V., Tumol'skaya, N. I., and Bekish, O. J. L. (1969a). Benzimidazoles and steroid hormones in the therapy of experimental trichinellosis. *2nd Int. Conf. Trichinellosis Wroclaw,* pp., 77–80.

Ozeretskovskaya, N. N., Tumolskaya, N. I., and Kolosova, M. O. (1969b.) Search for the specific therapy for trichinellosis. IV. Pyridyl derivatives of benzimidazole in experimental trichinellosis in white mice. *Med. Parazitol. Parazit. Bol.* (2), 186–190.

Ozeretskovskaya, N. N., Tchernyaeva, A. I., Kolosova, M. O., and Kriventsova, T. D. (1971). Search for the specific therapy for trichinellosis. V. Chlorophenyl derivatives of benzimidazole in experimental trichinellosis in white mice. *Med. Parazitol. Parazit. Bol.* (4), 411–416.

Prichard, R. K. (1970). Mode of action of the anthelminthic thiabendazole in *Haemonchus contortus. Nature London* **228,** 684.

Chemotherapeutic Results in Experimental Trichinellosis

J. Lamina

Department of Parasitology and Zoology,
Technological University,
Munich-Freising

Introduction

The chemotherapy of trichinellosis is still unsatisfactory. It is true that intestinal and perhaps early migrating stages are relatively well influenced by numerous drugs, but these remedies almost completely fail to fight parasites which have already migrated into the muscle or are even encapsulated.

Normally, trichinellosis, which can be sometimes quite dangerous for human beings, is not diagnosed until the parasites have migrated into the muscular system. The hitherto existing chemotherapeutic methods are of doubtful success, as reported by Corridan (1969), Hall and McCabe (1967), Hennekeuser *et al.* (1968), Lapszewicz *et al.* (1969), and Thibaudeau and Gagnon (1969), to name just a few of the more recent investigations on this subject. It is therefore understandable that many parasitologists in the world are still trying to find a suitable therapy for trichinellosis in experiments with laboratory animals. More recent studies have been published, especially by Campbell (1961, 1970), Campbell and Cuckler (1962, 1963, 1964, 1966), Campbell and Hartman (1968), Campbell *et al.* (1963), (1970), Chan and brown (1954), Denham (1965), Duckett and Denham (1970), Froltsova *et al.* (1965), Gretillat (1970), Ivey and DeFeo (1963), Kozar *et al.* (1963, 1966a, b), Krupa *et al.* (1967), Lamina (1963, 1970), Lamina and Schoop (1966), Magath and Thompson (1952), Martinez *et al.* (1968), Minning and Ding (1951), Oliver-González and Hewitt (1947), Ozeretskovskaya *et al.* (1969a, b), Pambuccian *et al.* (1966, 1969), Schanzel and Hegorova (1964a, b), Schoop and Lamina (1959, 1962a, b, 1965) Schoop *et al.* (1964), Simionescu *et al.* (1969), Stone *et al.* (1964), Theodorides and Laderman (1969), Warda (1960), Wilson (1967), and Yushko (1962).

In nearly all these studies it is expressed that a successful therapy,

483

especially against encapsulated parasites, is seldom possible. In our own investigations therefore, eight different drugs were tested for efficacy on various stages of development of the parasite. For the most part the data have been published previously by the present author and his colleagues *(vide supra)* and are reviewed herein. These medicaments are: (1) piperazine (hexahydropyrazine); (2) dekelmin [2-(β-methoxyethyl)pyridine]; (3) Bromophos: (O,O-dimethyl-O,2,5-dichloro-4-bromophenyl thionophosphate); (4) Asuntol (3-chlor-4-methyl-7-oxycumarin-O,O-diethylthiophosphoric acid ester); (5) Bayer 9018 (3,5-dimethyl-4-methylmercaptophenyl-dimethylthionophosphoric acid ester); (6) Neguvon (trichlorphon; O,O-dimethyl-2,2,2-trichloroxyethylphosphoric acid ester); (7) Tiguvon [fenthion; O,O-dimethyl O-(4-methylmercapto-3-methylphenyl) thionophosphoric acid ester; Bayer S 1752]; and (8) thiabendazole [2-(4'-thiazolyl)-benzimidazole].

The experiments were designed to detect and measure the efficacy of the drugs on intestinal, migrating and encapsulated *Trichinella.*

Materials and Methods

Infective material was gained from mice and rats, which had been infected with *Trichinella spiralis* about 3 months before. To obtain the respective infective doses, small portions of muscle from the diaphragm, the tongue, or the chewing muscles were squashed in the compressorium and counted out into portions of 100 *Trichinella* each. With a small curved pincette the pieces of meat were pushed down the throat of the mice, which weighed approximately 23–25 gm. After that, the animals were put separately into jars to make sure that parts of the meat were not brought up unnoticed.

The drug was administered either orally with a blunt cannula deep down the throat or by a subcutaneous, intraabdominal, or intravenous injection.

A certain period of time after the treatment, the mice were killed with chloroform and the results of the test were taken. Hereby the same proportion of 300 mg muscle of the hindlegs were pressed in the compressorium and the *Trichinella* were counted.

In order to obtain the most reliable results possible of the efficacy of the drugs, one test group was formed of at least 10 mice. A corresponding number of animals served as a control: partly only the mean values of this group were reckoned, partly the relevant variances were taken into account. The relations of the upper variance of the treated animals and the lower variance of the untreated ones was decisive: if the values overlapped, there was no significant efficacy. The mean variance is obtained from following formula:

$$S = \pm \frac{(a_1 - m)^2 + (a_2 - m)^2 + \ldots + (a_n - m^2)}{n - 1}$$

a_1 is the value of the first test mouse, a_2 is the value of the second test-mouse, a_n is the value of each of n tested mice, n is the number of tested mice, m is the mean value. To obtain the mean value of *Trichinella* in 1 gm muscle, the values of each test were added up, multiplied by 3.33 and divided by the number of the examined animals.

Results

Effect of Piperazine (Hexahydropyrazine) on Various Stages of Development of *Trichinella*

In three test series of 50 mice each, the drug was tested on intestinal, migrating, and encapsulated *Trichinella*. The remedy was administered *per os*. In each series five groups of 10 mice were at our disposal. The first group was left untreated as a control. Twenty-four hours post-infection the second group received 2000 mg piperazine/kg body weight on 4 successive days, the third group received the same dosage eight times, the fourth group 12 times and the fifth group 16 times. The migrating stages were treated in the same way. Here the therapy started on the seventh day post infection. Whereas again 10 control animals (first group) were not treated, the medicine was given to the other groups four times, eight times, 12 times, or 16 times. Finally the same scheme of treatment was carried out for the third test series beginning on the thirty-sixth day post infection. All the animals were examined about 4 weeks after the last treatment. The results of each group (mean values of 10 animals) are compiled in Table I.

The results show that hexahydropyrazine has no influence at all on freshly encapsulated *Trichinella*. The treatment of the migrating stages of the parasite reduced the number of *Trichinella* encapsulated in the thighs by 33%. The highest, but by no means satisfying, antiparasitic effect was shown against intestinal *Trichinella*. Therefore this drug is without question not suitable for a practicable application on an infection with *Trichinella*.

Effect of Dekelmin [Methyridine; 2-(β-Methoxyethyl) pyridine] on Various Stages of Development of *Trichinella spiralis*

The test animals were again divided into three series of 60, 70, and 60 mice. In each series one group was left untreated. In the other groups of 10 mice each the drug was administered subcutaneously on 3 successive days in a dosage of 0.018 gm dissolved in 0.2 cm^3 *aqua dest*. The first group was treated on the second day post infection, the second group was

Table I The Effect of Piperazine (Hexahydropyrazine) on Various Stages of Development of *Trichinella spiralis*

Treatment against *Trichnella* stage	*Trichnella* per gram muscle of the thighs				
	Controls	Treated 4 times	Treated 8 times	Treated 12 times	Treated 16 times
Intestinal	1413.1 S ±502	1324.2 S ±571	884.5 ±488	709.2 ±169	987.6 ±309
Migrating	1770.1 S ±768.4	818.0 S ±189	1212 ±635	1289 ±493	1285 ±399
Encapsulated	1934.3 S ±906	1796.2 S ±705	1743.3 ±666	1870.1 ±754	1596.2 ±555

treated on the fourth day post-infection, the third group on the sixth day post-infection, and so on, until the last group was treated on the thirty-second day. Six weeks after the infection, all the experiments, the controls included, were evaluated. The results are compiled in Table II.

The results show that this drug has proven trichinocidal activity. The intestinal stages of the parasite are influenced very well, although the migrating and encapsulated larvae are not affected as well as should be expected from a good remedy.

Effect of Bromophos (*O, O*-Dimethyl-*O*,2,5-dichloro-4-bromophenyl thionophosphate) on the Various Stages of Development of *T. spiralis*

A 0.2-ml suspension contained the dosage of the medicine (30 mg bromophos). The drug was given orally and tested on intestinal, migrating, and encapsulated *Trichinella*. At least five weeks after infection and 8 days after the last rreatment, the mice were killed (at a time therefore, when the muscle stages of *Trichinella* were sure to be encapsulated as we know from experience).

In the first test series the drug was tested for its efficacy on intestinal *Trichinella*. For this, 100 mice were divided into four groups of 25. Whereas the first group was left untreated as a control, the other animals were treated for a period of 5 days, from days 3–7, 5–9, and 10–14 post-infection. The second test series for which there were also 100 mice at our disposal, was carried out in the same way. Here again one group remained untreated,

Table II The Effect of Dekelmin on Various Stages of Development of *Trichinella spiralis*

Treatment against *Trichinella* stage	Days of Treatment	*Trichinella* per gram thigh muscle	
		Treated group	Controls
Intestinal	2–4	0	1432.7
	4–6	0	
	6–8	3.4	
Migrating	8–10	173.1	1093.0
	10–12	516.5	
	12–14	1,115.5	
	14–16	1,221.3	
	16–18	1,632.0	
	18–20	978.6	
	20–22	736.8	
	22–24	1,070.3	
Encapsulated	24–26	237.6	364.4
	26–28	374.6	
	28–30	233.1	
	30–32	289.1	
	32–34	293.1	

whereas the medicine was administered to the other groups from days 13–17, 19–23, and 15–20 post infection. Unfortunately the last group of this series could not be evaluated due to a technical failure.

The last test series was directed against already encapsulated *Trichinella*. Here also 25 mice were left untreated. Three further groups were again treated for 5 days, starting on days 23, 27, and 31. The results of all three test series are compiled in Table III.

From these results one can, without doubt, say that Bromophos has a considerable effect on intestinal *Trichinella*. Migrating or already encapsulated forms were much more difficult to influence. In some groups there was a reduction of the number of parasites, but it was not significant enough for the drug to be applicable in trichinellosis.

Effect of Asuntol (3-Chlor-4-methyl-7-oxycumarin-*O,O*-diethylthiophosphoric acid ester) on Various Stages of Development of *T. spiralis*

The medicine was at our disposal in the form of a 16% Asuntol formulation and of Asuntol powder. In order to administer the appropriate amount of the compound, the drug was diluted with *aqua dest.* and given subcutaneously, intraabdominally, and *per os.*

Experiments designed to determine the lethal dosage of Asuntol powder, showed that for mice of a weight of about 25 gm, the following doses were definitely lethal: per os and intraperitoneslly 10–12 mg, and subcutaneously 50–60 mg. However, medication with the drug was possible with the following formulation.

Effective Nonlethal Dose (mg)

Asuntol formulation	Asuntol powder
per os 0.3	1–5
intraperitoneal 0.1–0.2	1–3
subcutaneous 0.3–0.4	4–8

By premedication with atropine and PAM, it was possible to double the first dosage of Asuntol formulation.

There were 80 mice at our disposal for the treatment of intestinal trichinellosis with Asuntol formulation. Ten animals were left as a control, the others were treated *per os,* subcutaneously, or intraabdominally for a few days, beginning on the first or the second day post-infection. The success of the treatment varied greatly, and a few animals were killed by the medication.

Similar observations were made in the second test series with 60 mice, where the treatment was carried out betwee the seventh and ninth day post-infection. Here mortality amounted to 20%.

Therefore, the treatment of the encapsulated parasites in a third test series was carried out under antidote premedication; 10 min before treat-

Table III The Effect of Bromophos on Various Stages of Development of *Trichinella spiralis*

Treatment against *Trichinella* stage	Treatment in days post-infection	*Trichinella* per gram thigh muscle	
		Treated group	Controls
Intestinal	3–7	83 S ±83	1276 S ±179
	5–9	337 S ±337	
	10–14	857 S ±148	
Migrating	13–17	1453 S ±221	1803 S ±368
	19–23	1375 S ±244	
Encapsulated	23–27 (5 deaths)	1497 S ±151	1480 S ±244
	27–31 (10 deaths)	765 S ±169	
	31–35 (2 deaths)	1075 S ±114	

ment, 100 mg PAM and 10 mg atropine were dissolved in 10 ml *aqua dest.* and 0.2–0.3 ml was given subcutaneously. Here also the effect was so variable and included again many casualties that no precise statement was possible. Also repeated experiments, in which the antidote was used on intestinal and migrating stages, were not as successful as expected in spite of higher dosage of medicine.

In summary this drug can be described as possessing a certain efficacy on *T. spiralis*. However, the toxic dosage and lethal dosage could not be determined exactly, obviously due to its poor solubility, so that many casualties occurred, which made a final statement impossible.

Effect of Bayer 9018 (3,5-Dimethyl-4-methylmercaptophenyl-dimethylthionophosphoric acid ester) on Various Stages of development of *T. spiralis*

The preparation was in the form of a powder containing 25% of the compound and was given to the animals in an amount of 50 mg of a suspension of 0.3 ml glycerin on 3 successive days. Here also the treatment was carried out in groups of 25 animals each against intestinal, migrating, and encapsulated *Trichinella* larvae. The results are summarized in Table IV.

The results show that this medicine has without doubt a good efficacy on all larval stages, although only intestinal *Trichinella* were destroyed completely. One should emphasize however, that the administered dosage was very near to the lethal dosage, as far as this could be observed with the help of the clinical picture of the test animals.

Effect of Neguvon (*O,O*-Dimethyl-2,2,2-trichloroxyethyl-phosphoric acid ester) with and without the Protection of Antidotes on Various Stages of Development of *T. spiralis*

In the first experiment we could ascertain that, without causing a toxic reaction, the water-soluble phosphoric acid ester Neguvon (trichlorphon) could be injected subcutaneously and intraabdominally in a daily dosage

Table IV   The Effect of Bayer 9018 on Various Stages of Development
of *Trichinella spiralis*

Treatment against *Trichinella* stage	Treatment in days post-infection	*Trichinella* per gram thigh muscle	
		Treated group	Controls
Intestinal	3–5	0	977.4 S ±695
	6, 6, 7	43.3 S ±41.8	
	10–12	232.8 S ±234.4	
Migrating	13–15	47.9 S ±44.1	1049.2 S ±645.3
	16, 16, 17	17.9 S ±18.9	
	19–21	48.2 S ±36.3	
Encapsulated	23–25	126.8 S ±103.3	1171.0 S ±433.2
	27–29	50.5 S ±43.2	
	31–33	60.7 S ±66.0	

of 4 mg on 4 successive days to mice weighing approximately 25 gm. If
the drug was given only every second day, the administered total dose
could be increased considerably. Hereby we succeeded in eliminating
97.5–100% of intestinal *Trichinella* in 70 mice by subcutaneous medication,
and 91.4–100% in 90 mice by intraabdominal medication. If the mice were
treated five times between the seventh and twentieth day post-infection
at the earliest, the drug succeeded in eliminating only 63.9–85.5% by subcutaneous administration. Encapsulated *Trichinella* were influenced with
this drug as well, if the medication was carried out after the twentieth day
post-infection, 14 doses being given on alternate days. In this case, in 30
mice, still 83.6–93.3% of the *Trichinella* could be destroyed compared with
the control animals.

The frequent medication however caused considerable stress for the
test animals. As a higher dosage was not possible without administering
antidotes before hand, atropine, PAM and Toxogonin were used as
premedication in new experiments. In the first experiment 0.2–0.3 ml
PAM + atropine (see above), that is, 2.5 mg PAM and 0.5 mg atropinum
sulfuricum, were given subcutaneously 10 min before treatment. By this
the preparation could be increased to 8 or 10 mg/animal on 5 successive
days.

In groups of 10 animals the treatment was carried out for 5 days against
intestinal, migrating, and encapsulated *Trichinella*, and against encapsulated trichinella on 8 successive days. The results show (Table V) that
higher dosing of the preparation under protection of antidotes considerably improves the results in combating trichinellosis against all stages of
development of the parasite. These good results were reproduced in a
further experiment with a total of 60 mice, in which Toxogonin (bis-4-
hydroxyiminomethyl pyridinum-(1)-ethyl) ether in combination with
atropine was used as an antidote and the phosphoric acid ester Neguvon

Table V The Effect of *Neguvon* with and without the Protection of Antidotes on Various Stages of Development of *Trichinella spiralis*

Treatment against *Trichinella* stage	Treatment in days post-infection	Number of *Trichinella* per gram	Controls *Trichinella* per gram
Medication repeated five times			
Intestinal	5–9	0	1453 S ±523
	7–11	0	
	9–13	8.7	
	11–15	18.7	
Migrating	13–18	153	1303 S ±411
	17–21	62	
	19–23	12	
Encapsulated	21–25	57	1271 S ±319
	23–27	59	
	25–29	80	
	40–44	135	
Medication repeated 10 times			
Migrating	9–18	25	1393 S ±401
Encapsulated	45–55 (30 mice)	12.5	

was administered only on 5 successive days. Here again the elimination especially of muscular *Trichinella* was 95% successful.

Effect of Tiguvon [*O,O*-Dimethyl *O*-(4-methylmercapto-3-methylphenyl)-*m*-thionophosphoric acid ester] on Various Stages of Development of *T. spiralis*

Whereas Neguvon has the quality of being decomposed in the organism and secreted quickly, Tiguvon was known to stay in the blood longer. Initial experiments eventually showed that this effective systemic preparation in the form of an oily 2% formulation stayed in the body of the animals for up to 4 days after administration. Consequently, the medicine had the advantage that it did not need to be applied as often as Neguvon. If a dosage of 0.2 ml (0.4 ml effective substance) was given orally or intraabdominally as a first application, the next treatment could then be carried out after the fifth day.

On a total of 60 mice (in groups of 10 animals) the per oral treatment was carried out twice daily every fifth day against intestinal, migrating and encapsulated *Trichinella*. The results of these test series, compiled in Table VI, show that if medication starts early enough, 100% of the *Trichinella* can be eliminated. If the treatment is carried out later, then, in spite of the fact the medicine is only given twice (that means a much smaller dosage of effective substance) at least 90% of the parasites are destroyed.

Table VI The Effect of Tiguvon on Various Stages of Development of *Trichinella spiralis*

Treatment against *Trichinella* stage	Controls *Trichinella* per gram	Treatment in days post-infection	Number of *Trichinella* per gram
Intestinal	1310 S ±272	1 + 5	0
		3 + 8	0
		5 + 10	0
		7 + 12	22
		9 + 14	46
Migrating	1778 S ±401	11 + 16	188
		13 + 18	97
		15 + 20	187
		17 + 22	125
		19 + 24	63
Encapsulated	1276 S ±212	21 + 26	58
		23 + 28	79
		25 + 30	61
		27 + 32	83
		29 + 34	123
		31 + 36	145

Effect of Thiabendazole [2-(4'-Thiazolyl)benzimidazole] on Various Stages of Development of *T. spiralis*

In our last test series the effect of thiabendazole on experimental trichinosis in mice was tested. The preparation was administered to the animals in a dosage of 10 mg in 0.2 cm^3 glycerin *per os*. The animals were treated in groups of 10, beginning on the first day post-infection until the twenty-third day post-infection, on 4 successive days. Then the therapy was started on the 32, days 32, 33, 34, and 38 post-infection (four or six times) in order to ascertain the effect of the medicine on already encapsulated *Trichinella*.

The result was that the intestinal *Trichinella* were eliminated completely if the therapy was started before the fifth day postinfection. If it was started later, there was still a distinct reduction of the parasites, of varying degrees among the groups. In the groups in which the medicine was tested on encapsulated *Trichinella*, there was also a certain perceivable effect compared with the controls. The drug's effect, especially on encapsulated *Trichinella*, was examined once again, in a larger scale test series, in which the dosage and the length of treatment were varied. The results are compiled in Table VII.

This last test series fails to show a regular effect on encapsulated *Trichinella*. It may be assumed that thiabendazole is not completely inactive against muscle *Trichinella*. The large variance in some groups, however, may be due to a difference in resorption of the preparation.

Table VII The Effect of Thiabendazole on Various Stages of Development of *Trichinella spiralis*

Test group	Number of animals	Post-infection treatment (days)	Dose (mg/day)	Number of encapsulated *Trichinella* per gram
1	50	34–39	5	924.9 S ±429.7
2	49	Controls	–	879.1 S ±525.1
3	50	33–42	5	856.4 S ±428.0
4	50	Controls	–	795.87 S ±474.3
5	50	56–61	10	572.16 S ±502.3
6	50	Controls	–	802.73 S ±429.7
7	46	54–63	10	250.08 S ±236.3
8	50	Controls	–	1,061.4 S ±626.8
9	50	103–108	10	712.35 S ±556.0
10	20	Controls	–	657.84 S ±571.0
11	48	101–110	5	932.6 S ±630.1
12	49	101–110	–	532.5 S ±357.7
13	29	Controls	–	970.89 S ±504.0

Therefore, the medicine does not seem to be appropriate for routine use until the factors for the varying effectiveness can be controlled.

Discussion

The present extensive examinations for solving therapeutic problems with the help of experimental trichinellosis in mice have shown in our own investigations, as well as in those of many other authors, that with numerous drugs it should not be difficult to eliminate trichinella from the gut of the host. As human trichinellosis is however often only diagnosed in the migrating stage of the parasites or in the early muscular stage, drugs are necessary which display a systemic effect. Hereby many difficulties occur. The preparations which show no, or very little toxicity, mostly display no, or only an unsatisfying effect on muscle *Trichinella*. Other preparations, as for example the group of phosphoric acid esters, which have (at least some of them) a systemic effect, are so toxic for the patient that the desired effect is only attainable with the help of antidotes, which have to be given before medication.

There seem to be differences in toxicity among the phosphoric acid esters. Some are decomposed and excreted very quickly, for example, the water-soluble Neguvon. This necessitates frequent administration, which understandably goes hand in hand with considerable stress for the organism for a long period after administration. On the other hand, Tiguvon administered only two times and at a much lower dosage than Neguvon was just as successful. Tiguvon has proved itself an effective systemic antiparasitic drug in the pour-on-method in veterinary medicine, especially against hypodermatinae. Even if this medicine, and perhaps the whole group of phosphoric acid esters, shows too many deficiencies for use in human trichinellosis, there seems to be at any rate a possibility of influencing and eliminating the parasite in all stages. According to my knowledge of the relevant literature, there is no better and more effective substance. Of course many experiments will be necessary before a human infection can and should be treated with such a drug. Thiabendazole, which is today often recommended and used against infection, only shows a good effect on the intestinal stages of the parasite, whereas encapsulated *Trichinella* are removed poorly and inconsistently. An explanation for the different effectiveness was unfortunately not found in our own investigations.

Summary

Eight different preparations were tested in experimentally infected mice on intestinal, migrating, and encapsulated *Trichinella* stages, partially under the protection of antidotes. Most of the drugs were more or less effective on the intestinal stages of the parasite. The migrating of encapsulated stage, however, was far less affected. The best results on encapsulated parasites were achieved with trichlorphon (Neguvon; *O,O*-dimethyl-2,2,2-trichlorxyethylphosphoric acid ester) under the protection of pyridine-2-alsoxine-*N*-methyliodide plus atropine sulfate as antidote by treating intraperitoneally 5 to 10 times, and with fenthion [Tiguvon; *O,O*-dimethyl-*O*-(4-methylmercapto-3-methylphenyl) thionophosphate] without the protection of an antidote by treating orally twice. Thiabendazole [2-4'-(thiazolyl)benzimidazole] given perorally also killed numerous encapsulated trichinella in a few test groups, but the results were not uniform and could not be reproduced. No reason for this was found.

References

Campbell, W. C. (1961). Effect of thiabendazole upon infections of *Trichinella spiralis* in mice, and upon certain other helminthiases. *J. Parasitol.* **47**, 37.

Campbell, W. C. (1970). Specific therapy of the muscle phase of Trichinellosis. *J. Parasitol.* (2nd Int. Congr. Parasitol.), **56** (Sect. II, Part 1), 47.

Campbell, W. C., and Cuckler, A. C. (1962). Effect of thiabendazole upon experimental trichinosis in swine. *Proc. Soc. Exp. Biol. Med.* **110**, 124–128.

Campbell, W. C., and Cuckler, A. C. (1963). The evaluation of anthelmintic efficacy in experimental trichinellosis. *Proc. Symp. Evaluation Anthelmintics*, Hannover, pp. 154–157.

Campbell, W. C., and Cuckler, A. C. (1964). Effect of thiabendazole upon the enteral and parenteral phases of trichinosis in Mice. *J. Parasitol.* **50**, 481–488.

Campbell, W. C., and Cuckler, A. C. 1966. Further studies on the effect of thiabendazole in swine, with notes on the biology of the infection. *J. Parasitol.* **52**, 260–279.

Campbell, W. C., and Hartman, R. K. (1968). Changes in the efficacy of three anthelmintics during the maturation of a nematode *(Trichinella spiralis). J. Parasitol.* **54**, 112–116.

Campbell, W. C., and Hakstis, J. J. (1970). Efficacy of cambendazole against *Trichinella spiralis* in mice. *J. Parasitol.* **56**, 839–840.

Campbell, W. C., Hartman, R. K., and Cuckler, A. C. (1963). Effect of certain anthihistamine and antiserotonin agents upon experimental trichinosis in mice. *Exp. Parasitol.* **14**, 23–28.

Chan, K. F., and Brown, H. W. (1954). Treatment of experimental trichinosis in mice with piperazine hydrochloride. *Amer. J. Trop. Med.* **3**, 746–749.

Corridan, J. P. (1969). Therapy in trichinosis with observations on the use of thiabendazole. *Irish J. Med. Sci.* **2**, 535–537.

Denham, D. A. (1965) Studies with methyridine and *Trichinella spiralis.* I. Effect upon the intestinal phase in mice. *Exp. Parasitol.* **17**, 10–14.

Duckett, M. G., and Denham, D. A. (1970). The effect of cambendazole on *Trichinella spiralis* in mice. *J. Helminthol.* **44**, 211–218.

Froltsova, A. E., Astafi'ev, B. A., and Konovalova, L. M. (1965). Poiski specificeskoj terapii trichinelleza. Sooscemie 1. Akrichin, clorofos, monomicin i preparat NRV pri eksperimental'nom trichinelleze krys. *Med. Parazitol. Parazit. Bol. Mosk.* **43**, 387–389.

Grétillat, S. (1970). Remarques sur l'action de deux antimitotiques sur les kystes larvaires de *Trichinella spiralis* et leur application dans le traitement de la trichinose experimentale. *C. R. Acad. Sci. Ser. D* **271**, 873.

Hall, W. J., and McCabe, W. R. (1967). Trichinosis. Report of a small outbreak ith observations of thiabendazole therapy *Arch. Int. Med.* **119**, 65–68.

Hennekeuser, H. H., Pabst, K., Poeplan, W., and Gerok, W. (1968) Zur Klinik und Therapie der Trichinose. *Deut. Med. Wochensch.* **93**, 867–873.

Ivey, M. H., and DeFeo, T. C. (1963). The effect of dithiazanine, given at various intervals after infection of *Trichinella spiralis* in mice. *Amer. J. Trop. Med. Kyg.* **12**, 62–64.

Kozar, Z., Sladki, E., and Kozar, M. (1963). Etudes sur la possibilite pharmacologiques d'azulenes pour le traitement de la trichinellose aique et chronique (chez la souris et chez l'homme). *Wiad. Parazytol.* **9**, 419–434.

Kozar, Z., Zarzycki, J., and Kozar, M. (1966a). Morphologic observations of *Trichinella*-infected muscles in mice treated with thiabendazole and Neguvon. *Wiad. Parazytolo.* **12**, 589–604.

Kozar, Z., Jackowska-Klimowicz, J., and Sladki, E. (1966b), Thiabendazole therapy in human trichinellosis. *Wiad. Parazytol.* **12**, 605–617.

Krupa, P. L., Hamburgh, M., and Zaiman, H. (1967). Effect of Hypothyroidism on resistance of mice to infection with *Trichinella spiralis. J. Parasitol.* **53**, 126–129.

Lamina, J. (1963). Die Weltverbreitung der Trichine und Moglichkeiten einer chemotherapeutischen Bakampfung. *Wien. Tierarztl. Wochenschr.* **50**, 981–995.

Lamina, J. (1970). Das Schicksal der Trichinen im Tierexperiment nach Abtotung durch Trichlorphon. III. Mitteilung. *Zentralbl. Bakteriol. Parasitenk. Infektionskr. Hyg. Abt. 1. Orig.* **214,** 272–280.

Lamina, J., and Schoop, G. (1966). Die Wirkung von Thiabendazol auf die verschiedenen Entwicklungsstadien einer experimentellen Mäusetrichinose. *Berlin. Muench. Tierarztl. Wochenschr.* **79,** *34–37.*

Lamina, J., Meilinger, W., and Schoop, G. (1966). Uber die trichinozide Wirksamkeit des Phosphorsaureesterpraparates S 1752 (Bayer) auf *Trichinella spiralis* bei experimentell infizierten Mausen. *Zentralbl. Bakteriol., Parasitenk. Infektionskr. Hyg. Abt. 1. Orig.* **200,** 124–131.

Lapszewicz, A., Pawlowski, Z., and Gabryel, P. (1969). Thiabendazole in human trichinosis, *Wiad. Parazytol.* **15,** 759–760.

Magath, T. B., and Thompson, J. H. (1952). Diethylcarbamzine in experimental trichinosis. *Amer. J. Trop. Med. Hyg.* **1,** 307–313.

Martinez, A., Cordero, M., and Aller, B. (1968). Versuche über die Wirksamkeit von Pyranteltartrat gegen *Trichinella spiralis. Berlin. Munchen, Tierarztl. Wochenschr.* **81,** 223–225.

Minning, W., and Ding, P. C., (1951). Hetrazan-Wirkung bei Mäusetrichinose. *Z. Tropinmed. Parasitol.* **3,** 103–108.

Oliver-González, J., and Hewitt, R. I. (1947). Treatment of experimental Intestinal trichinosis with 1-diethylcarbamyl-4 methylpiperazine hydrochloride (Hetrazan) *Proc. Soc. Exp. Biol. Med.* **66,** 254-255.

Ozeretskovskaya, N. N., Tumolskaya, N. I., and Kolosova, M. O., (1969a). Search for a specific therapy of trichinelliasis of white mice. *Med. Parazitol.* **38,** 521-528.

Ozeretskovskaya, N. N., Pereverzeva, E. V., Kolosova, M. O., Chernyaeva, A. A., and Rimalis, B. T. (1969b). Mechanism of chemotherapeutic activity and side effects of benzimidazole derivatives in trichinelliasis. *Wiad. Parazytol.* **15,** 682–684.

Pambuccian, G., Cironeanu, I., and Braunstein, I. (1966). The corticotherapy in experimental trichinellosis. *Wiad. Parazytol.* **12,** 571–582.

Pambuccian, G., Simionescu-Cracium, O., Cironeanu, I., and Braunstein, I. (1969). Host parasite relations in experimental trichinellosis in the course of various treatments. *Wiad. Parazytol.* **15,** 755–756.

Schanzel, H., and Hegerova, E. (1964a). The use of methyridine against the intestinal trichinellosis in white mice. *Sb. Vys. Sk. Zemed. Brne Rocnik XII (XXXIII)* **619,** 4.

Schanzel, H., and Hegerova, E. 1964b. Einfluss von Methyridin auf die Muskellarven von *Trichinella spiralis* bei künstlich invadierten Mäusen. *Angew. Parasitol.* **5,** 163–166.

Schoop, G., and Lamina, J. (1959). Uber die vermizide Wirkung von Neguvon auf *Trichinella spiralis* in experimentell infizierten Mäusen. *Monat. Tierheilk.* **11,** 167–171.

Schoop, G., and Lamina, J. (1962a). Uber die Wirkung eines wasserloslichen Phosphorsäureesters auf Trichinellen. I. Beeinflussarkeit von Darm—und Wandertrichinellen bei experimentell infizierfen Mäusen. *Zentralbl. Bakteriol. Parasitenk. Infektionskr. Hyg. Abt. 1. Orig.* **186,** 562–573.

Schoop, G., and Lamina, J. (1962b). Uber die Wirkung eines wasserloslichen Phosphorsäureesters auf Trichinellen. II. Die Auswirkung erhohter Dosierung unter dem Schutz von Antidoten. *Zentralb. Bakteriol. Parasiten., Infaktionskr. Hyg. Abt. 1 Orig.* **187**, 391–406.

Schoop, G., and Lamina, J. (1965). Die trichinozide Wirkung von Methyridin. *Deut. Tierärztl. Wochenschr.* **72**, 319–321.

Schoop, G., and Lamina, J., and Wunderlich, G. (1964). Die Wirkung von Piperazine (Hexahydropyrazon) auf die verschiedenen Entwicklungsstadien der *Trichinella spiralis* (owen) bei experimentell infizierten Mäusen. *Zentralbl. Bakteriol. Parasitenk. Infektions-kr. Hyg. 1 Orig.* **193**, 272–281.

Simionescu, O., Dumitrescu, S., and Mandache, E. (1969). Action of diethylcarbamazine) on the *Trichinella spiralis* larvae. Electronoptical studies (Abstr.). *Wiado. Parazytol.* **15**, 680–681.

Stone, O. J., Stone, C. T., and Mullins, J. F. (1964). Thiabendazole—probable cure for trichinosis. *J. Amer. Med. Ass.* **187**, 536–538.

Theodorides, V. J., and Laderman, M. (1969). Activity of parbendazole upon *Trichinella spiralis* in mice. *J. Parasitol.* **55**, 678.

Thibaudeau, Y., and Gagnon, J. J. (1969). Trichinosis—thiabendazole in the treatment of 11 cases. *Can. Med. Ass. J.* **101**, 533–536.

Warda, L. (1960). Dzialanie preparatow piperazynowych na jelitowe posacio wlosni. *(Trichinella spiralis)* (The action of piperazine preparations in intestinal forms of *Trichinella spiralis*). *Arch. Immunol. Ter. Dosw.* **8**, 327–346.

Wilson, R. (1967). Bear meat trichinosis. Profound serum protein alterations, minor eosinophilia and response to thiabendazole. *Ann. Int. Med.* **66** 965–971.

Yushko, A. V. (1962). Prednisolon in therapy of trichinellosis. Zdrawoochr. Belorussii, No. 1, pp. 52, *Wiad. Parazytolo.* (1), 147.

The Effect of Thiabendazole and Methotrexate or Phytohemagglutinin on Experimental Trichinellosis

N. N. Ozeretskovskaya, E. V. Pereverzeva, and
N. L. Veretennikova

*E. I. Martsynovsky Institute of Medical Parasitology
and Tropical Medicine,
U.S.S.R. Ministry of Public Health, Moscow*

Introduction

Thiabendazole is a highly effective trichinellocide which acts predominantly on the enteral phase of the infection (Campbell and Cuckler, 1964, 1966; Ozeretskovskaya *et al.,* 1969a). In the muscle phase the impaired metabolism and death of larvae due to medication increase the sensitization of the host (Kean and Hoskins, 1964; Kozar *et al.,* 1966; Ozeretskovskaya *et al.,* 1969a, 1972). The reduction of its trichinellocidal effect by glucocorticoids in the parenteral phase appears to be associated with inhibition of the activity of lymphoid tissue contributing to the death of muscle larvae (Ozeretskovskaya *et al.,* 1969a, b). In order to test this assumption we studied how the trichinellocidal activity of thiabendazole is modified by methotrexate, an antifolic factor, which selectively inhibits cell division, in particular of the lymphoid tissue (O'Brien, 1962). Methotrexate increases the percentage of implanted intestinal *Trichinella,* their survival, larval production, and larval density in the muscles (Pereverzeva *et al.,* 1972). The immunosuppressive effect of the drug disturbs the encysting of larvae and leads to their massive loss (Pereverzeva *et al.,* 1972).

In a second series of experiments we studied the effect of phytohemagglutinin (PHA), a nonspecific stimulant of lymphocytes, on the action of thiabendazole. PHA reduced markedly the adult count, changed the larval production, and disturbed the development and encapsulation of muscle larvae promoting their massive loss (see chapter by Pereverzeva *et al.,* Part II, this volume).

Materials and Methods

In the experiments with methotrexate 300 albino mice weighing 18–20 gm were divided into nine groups depending on the drugs given [methotrexate (M), thiabendazole (T), or methotrexate and thiabendazole (T-M)] and on the time of the treatment (2–4, 7–14, and 25–30 days of infection). Untreated mice were used as controls.

Groups of 30 mice each received the drugs (T, M, or T-M) at 2–4 or 7–14 days of infection. Groups of 20 mice each were treated at 21–25 days. Each animal was given 80 1.5-month-old decapsulated larvae of the Martsinovski laboratory *Trichinella* strain (Ozeretskovskaya *et al.,* 1969b). The infectivity of this strain changes with the age of muscle larvae from 16000 larvae/gm (1.5-2-month-old larvae) to 7000–6000 larvae/gm (3.5- to 4-month-old larvae). Larvae were decapsulated by the standard method (digestion with 0.3% pepsin solution in a 0.4% HC1 in proportion of 250 gm of muscles/3000 ml). Larvae were injected in a salt solution via a gastric tube. T was given as a starch paste in a single dose per day at 100 mg/kg. M was injected parenterally into paws as a salt solution at 5 mg/kg of body weight.

Three animals of each subgroup were killed 7, 15, 21, and 35 days after infection for counting of adult worms in the intestines and for histological, histochemical, and parasitological examinations, and for differential cell counts (per 100 cells in Romanovsky-Giemsa stained preparations). At day 35 and 60 of infection not less than five to six mice of each subgroup were killed. Diaphragm muscle of each animal was digested for larvae counting. The significance of the results was statistically evaluated. Masseter and gastrocnemius muscles were histologically examined (see Pereverseva *et al.,* Part II, this volume).

In experiments with PHA 400 mice were divided into nine groups in the same manner depending on the drugs given (PHA, T, or T-PHA) and time of the treatment (2–4, 6–11, and 25–30 days after invasion). But *Trichinella* larvae taken for invasion in these series were 3.5 months old and the last group of animals was sacrificed at day 90 of infection. The methods of histological and histochemical examinations and differential cell counts were the same (see Pereverseva *et al.,* Part II, this volume).

Results

Thiabendazole and Methotrexate

The percentage of implanted intestinal parasites in animals treated with M was markedly higher than in those that received T (Table I). In animals treated with T-M as compared with T groups the percentage of implanted intestinal parasites increased from 2.5 to 15% (2–4 days) and from 15 to 25% (6–11 days). The adults survived longer (Table I).

Table I Implantation of *Trichinella* in the Intestine of Mice Treated with Thiabendazole or Thiabendazole and Methotrexate

Treatment	Days of treatment	Implanted parasites as percent of larvae given on day:				
		7	15	21	35	60
Thiabendazole	2–4	2.5	0	0	0	0
Methotrexate	2–4	44	33	6	0	0
Thiabendazole +methotrexate	2–4	15	0	0	0	0
Thiabendazole	7–14	26	15	0	0	0
Methotrexate	7–14	30	28	28	3	0
Thiabendazole +methotrexate	7–14	28	25	7.5	5	0
Thiabendazole	25–30	24	21	6.5	0	0
Methotrexate	25–30	–	–	–	3	2
Thiabendazole +methotrexate	25–30	30	22	9	1	0
Control		32	30	10	0	0

In mice, treated with T at 2–4 days post-infection, no larva or morphological changes were found in the muscles during the first 2 weeks. On the twenty-first day a single young larva and affected fibers surrounded by massive granulation appeared. On the thirty-fifth day disturbances in the encystation of muscle larvae reached their maximum (Fig. 1) and the intensity

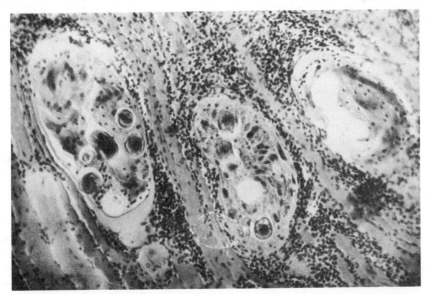

Figure 1 Encapsulated *Trichinella* larvae 35 days after invasion in mouse treated with thiabendazole on the days 7–14. Picrofuchsin after Romeis, × 140.

of invasion was 94% lower ($P < .001$) than in the control (Table II). On the sixtieth day the larval density was 84% lower ($P < .001$) than in the controls (Table II). Occasional larvae were found in well-formed cysts; no inflammatory reaction was observed.

The density of muscle larvae on the thirty-fifth day in animals treated with M at the early enteral phase (2–4 days) of infection was the same as in the control (Table II), but on the sixtieth day it was reduced by 26% ($0.001 < P < .01$) of the control (Table II). Given at 7–14 days and in particular at 25–30 days post-infection, M significantly increased the larval density as compared to the control, $0.001 < P < .001$, respectively (Table II).

In animals, treated on the days 2–4 with T-M, and in the controls, single muscle fibers with loss of the striations surrounded by lymphoid infiltrations extending 63–225 μm were observed on the seventh day of infection. No larvae were found in these fibers. By 15 days the destructive process was more extended. Part of the larvae was surrounded by massive cellular infiltration. On the day 21 spiral-shaped larvae were found but fewer than in the controls and the inflammatory reaction subsided. On the day 35 the muscle larval density was reduced by 48% ($P < .01$) of the control (Table II). The cysts were surrounded by massive granulations. Nonencysted larvae underwent lysis and resorption. On the day 60 the larval count was diminished by 50% ($P < .001$) of the control (Table II). Cysts were well formed; however, the encysted sarcoplasm was vacuolated, in some areas hyalinized, and retained only as a thin layer. Cysts were surrounded by massive infiltrates consisting of up to 72% of lymphoid cells. Most larvae lost their spiral form, their cuticle and hypoderm were detached, and many showed lysis.

In animals treated with T on days 7–14 post-infection, there were few spiral-shaped larvae, and the cyst walls had no hyaline layer by day 21. Infiltration occurred only around a few dead larvae. On the day 35 the larval density was reduced by 70% ($P < .001$) of the control (Table II). The remaining larvae were encysted, but the encapsulated sarcoplasm showed vacuolization and hyalinization. By day 60 the larval density was reduced only by 36% ($P < .001$), but the remaining larvae were destroyed despite scanty cell infiltration (Table II). In a single granuloma, larval remnants were found.

If the mice were treated with T-M on days 7–14 post-infection, the destructive changes in the muscle tissue were much more marked on day 15 than in animals treated with T alone, and in the controls. Infiltrations around the larvae were, however, less extensive. Larvae up to 219 microns in size have clear internal structure. On the contrary, on day 21 large cellular infiltrates were found around the dying larvae. These measured 315×126 to 1680×84 μm consisted of 21% neutrophils, 43% lymphoid cells, 26% plasma cells and 10% monocytes. By day 35 the larval density

Table II Density and Loss of Larvae on the Thirty-fifth and Sixtieth Day after Invasion in Mice Treated with Thiabendazole (I), Methotrexate (II), or Thiabendazole and Methotrexate (III) at Different Stages of Infection

Day of sacrifice after infection	Larvae per gram	Number of larvae at different days of treatment (after invasion)									Control
		2–4			7–14			25–30th			
		I	II	III	I	II	III	I	II	III	
35th	Average number	1100 ±233.5	15,450 ±259.1	8856 ±142.6	5550 ±397.3	14,250 ±237.3	7694 ±246.4	6800 ±221	12,307 ±264	12,020 ±185	16,975 ±197
	Reduction as percent of control	94	10	48	70	17	55	60	28	30	100
60th	Average number	1263 ±27	5849 ±392	4020 ±77	5104 ±159	10,660 ±258	11,025 ±114	2780 ±136	21,430 ±491	12,281 ±303	7950 ±215
	Reduction as percent of control	84	26	50	36	+34[a]	+38[a]	65	+170[a]	+54[a]	100

[a] Increased larval count.

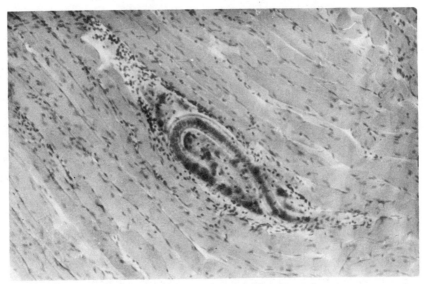

Figure 2 Encapsulating larvae 35 days after invasion in mouse treated with thiabendazole and methotrexate on days 7–14. H&E, × 56.

was reduced to 55% ($P < .01$) of control (Fig. 2, Table II). There were many spindleshaped, U-shaped, and even young larvae with undifferentiated structures (Fig. 3). Initial signs of fiber destruction and extensive hemorrhages appeared. In the infiltrates lymphoid cells made up only 39% (in controls 66%), neutrophils 30%, and plasmocytes 25%. By day 60 the intensity of invasion exceeded by 38% the control value ($P < .001$, Table II). The cyst-walls were 13–45 μm thick. A marked process of hyalinization of encysted sarcoplasm, starting from the periphery, was observed. Cysts were surrounded by abundant infiltrates. However, in contrast to animals receiving T alone, very few larvae were dying.

In mice treated with T at 25–30 days of infection, larval density was reduced to 60% ($P < .001$) of control (Table II) by day 35. As compared to the control, there was more vacuolated and hyalinized encapsulated sarcoplasm, the larvae formed no tight spirals (Fig. 4), and they were dying within limited cellular infiltrations. By day 60 the larval density was reduced to 65% ($P < .001$) of control (Table II). Cellular infiltration was moderate but many larvae were dying or resorbed (Figs. 5 and 6).

In animals, treated by T-M on days 25–30, the density of larvae at day 35 was reduced only by 30% ($P < .001$, Table II). Most larvae were encysted, but occasionally some were found whose development corresponded to that seen in the controls on day 15 after invasion (Figs. 7 and 8). Cellular infiltrates were scanty, comprising up to 62% lymphocytes, 26% neutrophils, and 12% plasma cells. By day 60 the larval density exceeded

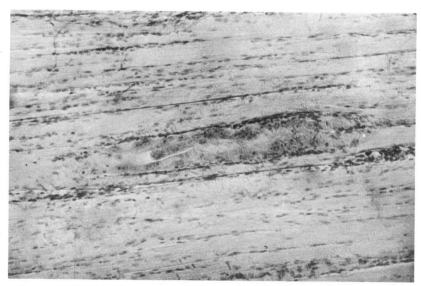

Figure 3 The same group of animals. Undifferentiated *Trichinella* larva 35 days after invasion. H & e, × 140.

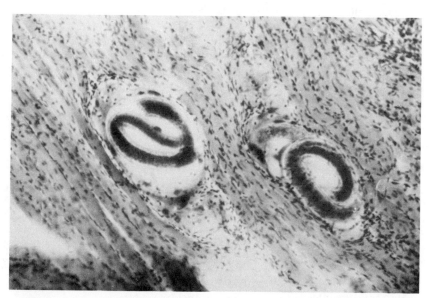

Figure 4 Dying larvae 35 days after invasion in mouse treated with thiabendazole at 25–30 days. H & E, × 140.

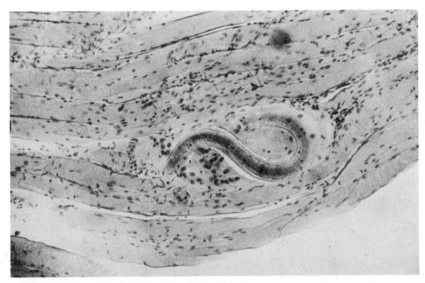

Figure 5 A larva which lost its S form 60 days after invasion in mouse treated with thiabendazole at 25–30 days. Picrofuchsin after Van Gieson, × 140.

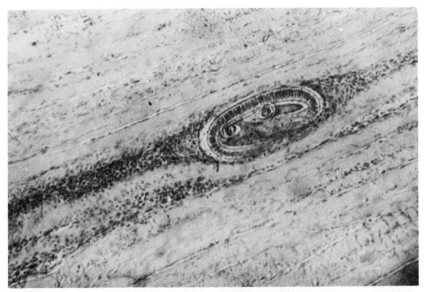

Figure 6 The same group of animals. A larva with destroyed inner structure 60 days after invasion. H&E, × 140.

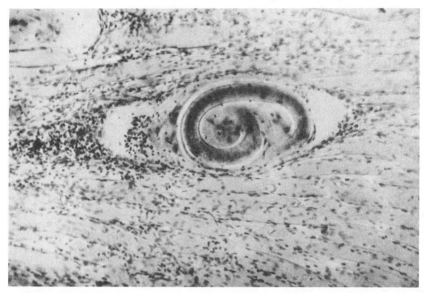

Figure 7 Encapsulated larvae 35 days after invasion in mouse treated with thiabendazole and methotrexate at 25–30 days. Picrofuchsin after Van Gieson, × 140.

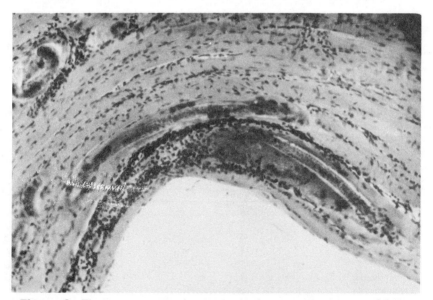

Figure 8 The same group of animals. Nonencapsulated larvae 35 days after invasion. H&E, × 140.

the control value by 54% ($P <$ .001, Table II). The morphological findings were similar to those in mice treated with T alone at the same period of time.

Thiabendazole and PHA

The effect of PHA on the development of *Trichinella* has been described by Pereverzeva *et al.,* in Part II, this volume. In mice treated with T-PHA on days 2–4 of infection, implantation and survival of the larvae were slightly higher than after T or PHA alone (Table III). When the drugs were given on days 6–11 the percentage of implanted larvae was much lower. No adults were found on day 35 in mice treated on days 25–30.

Given at 2–4 days of infection, PHA reduced the larval density in the muscles by 99% ($P <$ .001) of the control (Table IV). The PHA treatment during days 6–11 of infection diminished the larval counts to 53% of the control ($0.001 < P <$ .01). But if mice were treated with PHA 25–30 days post-infection the larval count increased up to 239% ($P <$ .001, Table IV).

In mice treated with T-PHA at 2–4 and 7–11 days, no trichinellocidal activity was observed on day 35 (Table III). On day 90 after invasion in the first variant of the experiment (treatment on day 2–4), the trichinellocidal effect of T-PHA was equal to that of T alone and only slightly exceeded that of PHA alone, but the difference was significant (474 $\pm$19.01 and 1293 $\pm$22.4, $P <$ .001, Table IV). In the second variant of the experiment (treatment on days 6–11), the treatment with T-PHA rather increased the intensity of invasion by day 35. On day 90 reduction of the invasion was similar in all three groups (Table IV). However, in the third variant of the experiment (treatment on days 25–30), the trichinellocidal effect of T-PHA at day 35 reached 88% ($P <$ .001), whereas PHA alone increased the inten-

Table III   Implantation of *Trichinella* in the Intestine of Mice Treated with Thiabendazole, PHA, or Thiabendazole and PHA

Treatment	Days of treatment	Implanted parasites as percent of larvae given on day: (%)			
		7	15	21	35
Thiabendazole	2–4	2.5	6.3	0	0
PHA	2–4	0	0	0	0
Thiabendazole + PHA	2–4	10	6.5	0	0
Thiabendazole	6–11	–	16	0	0
PHA	6–11	–	14	8	0
Thiabendazole + PHA	6–11	–	7.5	3.7	0
Thiabendazole	25–30	–	–	–	0
PHA	25–30	–	–	–	0
Thiabendazole + PHA	25–30	–	–	–	0
Control		42	30	21	0

Table IV Density and Loss of Larvae on the Thirty-fifth and Ninetieth day after Invasion in Mice Treated with Thiabendazole (I), PHA (II), or Thiabendazole and PHA (III) at Different Stages of Infection

Day of sacrifice after infection	Larvae per gram	Days of treatment (after infect)									Control
		2-4			6-11			25-35			
		I	II	III	I	II	III	I	II	III	
35th	Average number	204 ±14.4	11 ±1.05	1,070 ±66.3	556 ±18	626 ±15.4	1,580 ±59.0	–	5,035 ±156	148 ±10	1,280 ±92.5
	Reduction, as per cent of control	84	99	16	57	53	+23[a]	–	+239[a]	88	100
60th	Average number	596 ±26.1	1,293 ±22.4	474 ±19.1	572 ±14.6	417 ±14.6	734 ±12.1	1,924 ±55.5	1,155 ±42.4	1,829 ±56.5	3,726 ±63.2
	Reduction, as per cent of control	84	65	87	85	89	80	49	69	50	100

[a] Increased larval count.

sity of invasion by 239% (*P* < .001, Table IV). On day 90 the effect of T-PHA treatment did not differ from those obtained with either drug alone (Table IV).

In animals treated with T-PHA at 2–4 and 7–11 days post-infection, only a single *Trichinella* larva appeared in the muscles by day 15. The destruction of the affected muscle fibers measured only 300–400 μm as compared to the controls which measured to 1500 μm. At the same time marked cellular infiltrations appeared consisting of 60–70% lymphoid cells. *Trichinella* larvae were only 70 μm in length and showed no differentiation. By the twenty-first day the internal structure of worms became more distinct, but, as in the animals treated with PHA alone, the larvae were far from encysting which could be noted only at day 35 of infection and was continuing up to day 90. Encystation was constantly accompanied by active cellular infiltration with predominantly lymphoid cells. Increasing vacuolation and hyalinization of the encysted sarcoplasm and gradual loss of the larvae were observed.

In mice treated with T-PHA on day 25–30, as compared with those treated with T alone (Fig. 9), there was marked enhancement of cellular infiltration around the larvae and in the intramuscular connective tissue on the thirty-fifth day. As compared to PHA-treated animals, the cyst formation was delayed (Fig. 10). On day 90 an active cellular infiltration and different stages of the death and resorption of *Trichinella* larvae were observed, whereas in the animals treated with T alone, the cellular infil-

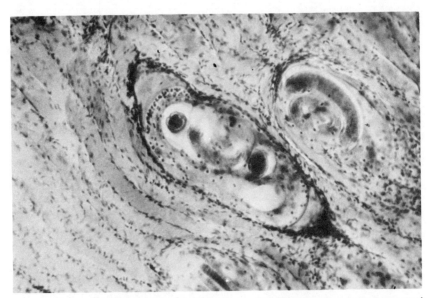

Figure 9 Encapsulated larvae 35 days after invasion in mouse treated with thiabendazole at 25–30 days. H&E, × 140.

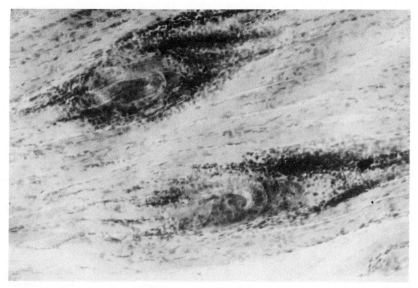

Figure 10 Nonencapsulated larvae 35 days after invasion in mouse treated with thiabendazole and PHA. H&E, × 140.

tration was moderate and the larvae showed terminal stages of destruction (Figs. 5 and 6), and in the animals treated with PHA alone infiltration persisted only around a few dying larvae.

Discussion

Our experiments demonstrate that the addition at any stage of *Trichinella* infection of an immunosuppressive drug (methotrexate) to thiabendazole reduces the immediate trichinellocidal action by a factor of 1.5–2 ($P < .01$ for the subgroup 2–4 days, $P < 0.05$ for subgroup 25–30 days, Table II). Two months later the intensity of invasion increases significantly in animals treated with T-M on days 7–14, and particularly on days 25–30 post-infection ($P < .001$ for all subgroups, Table II).

Higher larval count in the T-M subgroups treated during days 7–14 and 25–30 of infection as compared with animals treated with T alone is due to an increase in the number of implanted *Trichinella* and their survival, and to the production of larvae. In the third experimental variant (25–30 days) inhibition of the lymphoid tissue activity and some increase in the survival of adults and their larval production lead to a significantly enlarged larval count on day 60 as compared with the group of animals treated with T alone (Tables I and II; Figs. 4 and 5).

There may be another aspect to the inhibitory effect of methotrexate.

The immunosuppressive action of the drug is enhanced by the ability of thiabendazole to activate the hormone production of the adrenal cortex (Bekish, 1972a). This effect may be more important at the late muscle phase when the adult parasites disappear, but the increase of larval density reaches 54% ($P < .001$) as compared with T subgroup (Table II).

PHA produces a prominant trichinellocidal effect if given in the early enteral phase of *Trichinella* infection. This action is significantly higher on day 35 of infection and is not markedly less than the effect of T alone at day 90 ($P < .001$, Table IV). The effect is due to the activation of lymphoid tissue by PHA (Nowell, 1960; Marshall and Roberts, 1963 [see Pereverseva *et al.*, Part II, this volume]). The addition of PHA to thiabendazole in early stages of infection (days 2–4 and 6–11), contrary to our expectations, inhibited the effect of T considerably on the intestinal *Trichinella* and on the larval production (Tables III and IV; $P < 001$ in both variants). However, stimulation of lymphoid tissue and disturbances of encapsulation of larvae by day 90 caused death of 87 and 80% of the larvae, (in both variants $P < .001$, Table IV). Thus, the action of PHA at the early enteral phase of infection reduces the immediate effect of thiabendazole but does not affect the final result.

The action of PHA upon the enteral and parenteral parasites resembles the action of glucocorticoids, although the latter first stimulate the enteral phase and then cause destruction of the muscle larvae (Coker, 1956; Ozeretskovskaya *et al.,* 1966; Pawlowski, 1967; Campbell, 1968) whereas PHA inhibits the enteral parasites, but then, after a definite period of time, leads to increased larval density in the muscle. This stimulation may be due to the intensive infiltrations by lymphoid cells, to the activation of immunological responses, and to the increase of the histamine level in the muscle tissue. Recent experiments of Bekish (1972b) show that the density of muscle larvae correlates positively with the level of the induced and mast cell-produced histamine.

Possibly the striking increase (239%) of larval density on the thirty-fifth day in the subgroup treated with PHA during days 25–30 infection ($P < .001$, Table II) is due to the activated inflammation, the increased permeability of the vessels and the biochemical changes in muscle tissue produced by histamine, which favor the implantation of larvae. But, finally, the active immune reactions lead to the reduction of larval count, which is significantly higher than the reduction produced by thiabendazole (1155 ± 42.4 and 1924 ± 55.5, $P < .001$, Table IV).

Quite probably it is the same mechanism, together with the increased larval productivity, which produce the very high larval density on day 35 and its significant reduction on day 90 ($P < .001$, Table II) in controls, invaded with 1.5-month-old larvae. Methotrexate inhibits the inflammation (immune response) and increases the larval count on day 90 of infection to 170% ($P < .001$, Table II).

The lower infectivity of 3.5-month-old larvae leads to inactive inflammatory processes and immune responses which result in a larger percentage of implanted intestinal larvae, in a lower period of larval production (Table III) and in a significant increase of the larval density from the thirty-fifth to the ninetieth day of infection ($P < .001$, Table IV). PHA, provoking an active immune response, by the ninetieth day of infection significantly decreases the density of larvae in all groups of animals as compared to the control ($P < .001$, Table IV).

Thiabendazole and PHA given together (T-PHA) are most active at 4–5 weeks of infection (Table IV)—a period which is of great interest from a medical point of view. In respect to the stimulation of larval production by PHA given alone at this period, perhaps it would be more effective to start the treatment with thiabendazole and then successively give PHA or some other immunostimulant.

These experiments are being continued. Our results confirm the important role of the lymphoid tissue in the pathogenesis of trichinellosis and in its treatment with thiabendazole. Further experiments concerning action of lymphoid tissue stimulants on the trichinellocidal effect of benzimidazoles in the muscle phase of infection are of great interest.

Summary

Thiabendazole-T (100 mg/kg), methotrexate-M (5 mg/kg), and phytohemagglutinin-PHA (25 mg/kg) or thiabendazole with methotrexate (T-M) or PHA (T-PHA) were given at the enteral and parenteral stages of experimental trichinellosis.

Albino mice were invaded by decapsulated larvae, and were divided into 18 groups depending on the drug given and the period of treatment.

The animals were examined with histological, histochemical, and parasitological techniques on days 7, 14, 21, and 35, post-infection. The density of muscle larvae was determined by digestion on days 35 and 60 (T-M) or on days 35 and 90 (T-PHA) of the infection.

The immunosuppressant methotrexate increased the number and life span of the intestinal worms and the extent and duration of the production of larvae. Given with thiabendazole, M reduces the immediate and delayed trichinellocidal activity of thiabendazole at all stages of the infection, but especially in the period of the twenty-fifth to thirtieth days. Methotrexate seemed to intensify the side effects of the T treatment.

PHA, a nonspecific stimulant of the lymphoid tissues, if given in the early parenteral phase of infection, inhibits the intestinal parasites and decreases the density of muscle larvae by 99% of the control value ($P < .001$) by day 35 of infection. The surviving parasites reduce this effect to a value of 65% of the control ($P < .001$) by day 90 of infection, however.

Given during the period of early enteral phase or of the migration of larvae, PHA did not alter the chemotherapeutic effect of T but given during 25–30 days did decrease the larval density by 88%. This fact is of great interest since thiabendazole given alone at this stage of infection is less effective.

References

Bekish, O. J. L. (1972a). Biochemical aspects of the host–parasite adaptation in trichinellosis. Doctoral thesis, Minsk.

Bekish, O. J. L. (1972b). The histamine system of the host in *Trichinella* infection. *Zdravookhr. Beloruss.* **9**, 89–90.

Campbell, W. C. (1968). Effect of antiinflammatory agents on spontaneous cure of *Trichinella* and *Trichuris* in mice. *J. Parasitol.* **54**, 452–456.

Campbell, W. C., and Cuckler, A. C. (1964). Effect of thiabendazole upon the enteral and parenteral phases of trichinosis in mice. *J. Parasitol.* **50**, 481–488.

Campbell, W. C., and Cuckler, A. C. (1966). Further studies on the effect of thiabendazole on trichinosis in swine with notes on the biology of the infection. *J. Parasitol.* **52**, 269–279.

Coker, C. M. (1956). Cellular factors in acquired immunity to *Trichinella spiralis,* as indicated by cortisone treatment of mice. *J. Infec. Dis.* **98**, 187–197.

Kean, B. H., and Hoskins, D. W. (1964). Treatment of trichinosis. *J. Amer. Med. Ass.* **190**, 852–853.

Kozar, Z., Jakowska-Klimowicz, J., and Sladki, E. (1966). Thiabendazole therapy in human trichinellosis. *Acta Parasitol. Pol.* **12**, 605–607.

O'Brien, J. S. (1962). The role of the folate coenzymes in cellular division. A review. *Cancer Res.* **22**, 267–281.

Ozeretskovskaya, N. N. (1970). The formation of pathological process in the acute and chronic phases of helminthiases. *Med. Parazitol. Parasita. Bol.* **39**, 515–525.

Ozeretskovskaya, N. N., Kolosova, M. O., Tschernyaeva, A. I., Pereverseva, E. V., Tumolskaya, N. I., and Bekish, O.-J. L. (1969a). Benzimidazoles and steroid hormones in the therapy of experimental trichinellosis. *2nd Int. Conf. Trichinellosis Wroclaw,* pp. 77–80.

Ozeretskovskaya, N. N., Pereverzeva, E. V., Kolosova, M. O., Tschernyaeva, A. I., and Himalis, B. C. (1969b). On the mechanism of chemotherapeutical activity and side effects of benzimidazole derivatives in trichinellosis. *Wiad. Parasitol.* **15**, 682–684.

Ozeretskovskaya, N. N., Pereverzeva, E. V., Kolosova, M. O., Klein, U. S., Bekish, O.-J. L., and Veretennikova, N. L. (1972). The problems of the therapy of trichinellosis in men and animals. *Mater. Dokl. Vses. Konf. Prob. trichinelleza Czeloveka Zchevotnykh Vilnius,* pp. 111–115.

Pawlowski, Z. (1967). Hormones of adrenal cortex in experimental trichinellosis in rat. I. Effect of prednisone on the number of mature and larval forms. *Acta Parasitol. Pol.* **15**, 163–172.

Pereverzeva, E. V., Ozeretskovskaya, N. N., and Veretennikova, N. L. (1972). The action of methotrexate on the development and encapsulation of *Trichinella* larvae in experimental animals. *Mater. Dokl. Vses. Konf. Probl. Trichinelleza Czeloveka Zchivotnykh, Vilnius,* pp. 115–119.

Anthelmintic and Histopathological Effects of Mebendazole on *Trichinella spiralis* in the Rat

D. Thienpont, O. F. Vanparijs, and R. Vandesteene

Janssen Pharmaceutica
Beerse, Belgium

Introduction

Studies in turkeys and pheasants have shown that whereas single doses of mebendazole (methyl 5-benzoylbenzimidazole-2-carbamate, original synthesis of Janssen Pharmaceutica, Beerse, Belgium) were almost inactive against *Syngamus trachea,* medicated treatment for 5 consecutive days was extremely effective. A 100-mg standard dose of mebendazole twice a day for 3–4 consecutive days was almost 100% effective against mono- and polyinfections with *Ascaris lumbricoides, Necator americanus, Ancylostoma duodenale,* and *Trichuris trichiura* (Brugmans *et al.,* 1971; Chaia and Da Cunha, 1971; Gatti *et al.,* 1971; Vandepitte *et al.,* 1973).

Only a few drugs are active on the different phases of *Trichinella spiralis* in laboratory animals (Campbell and Cuckler, 1964; Campbell and Yakstis, 1970). Thiabendazole and cambendazole are the most active. In this study we wish to report the activity of mebendazole against the enteral, migrating, and encysting phases of *T. spiralis* in rats and to study the influence of the drug from the histopathological pictures of the larvae in the rat muscle.

Materials and Methods

All experiments were performed on male Wistar rats, 5 weeks old and weighing about 150 gm. The animals were housed in individual cages and fed on a commercial rat feed plus water *ad libitum.*

They were inoculated by stomach tube with approximately 4000 L_4 larvae each. Larvae for inoculation were obtained from ground rat muscle in digestion fluid containing 2% pepsin and 1% hydrochloric acid. The mixture was stirred constantly for 4–5 hr at 37° C. The digest was passed through a 50 mesh sieve to remove the larger particles of undigested material. Larvae were washed and collected on a 200 mesh sieve (pore width, 74 μm) and were then resuspended in 0.8% saline and counted by sampling. The same method was used in all experiments to detect the efficacy of mebendazole on larvae in the migrating and encysted phases.

For the enteral phase of *T. spiralis* the entire small intestine was opened, cut in segments of 10–20 cm and incubated at 37° C in 90 ml warm 0.8% saline for about 2 hr. Ten ml of 0.4% sodium hydroxide were added and the mixture was refrigerated for 4–5 hr. The preparation was then passed through a 10-mesh sieve to remove gut fragments. The collected worms were concentrated by sedimentation and decantation before counting.

The medicated feed was prepared by mixing the pure substance of mebendazole in the rat feed at concentrations varying from 10 to 1000 ppm and fed *ad libitum* for 7–14 days as indicated in Table I. Autopsy and postmortem examination were performed at day 1 to 7 after the end of treatment. Untreated controls were also autopsied at the same times as the treated animals.

Histopathology

For the histopathological studies, a total of 36 infected rats were used and divided into three groups as follows: the first group received mebendazole in the diet at a concentration of 125 ppm from day 17 to 21 post-infection. Mebendazole at a concentration of 500 ppm was administered through the diet of a second group of animals from day 55 to 70 post-infection. A third group of untreated infected rats served as controls (Table I).

For the first group autopsy was performed on days 18, 19, 20, 21, and 22 post-infection, for the second group on days 58, 60, 63, 65, 67, and 70 post-infection during treatment and also on days 3, 5, and 8 after the end of mebendazole treatment. Control animals were autopsied on days 17 and 55 post-infection.

Animals were killed by decapitation. Suitable histological preparations stained with hematoxylin and eosin (H&E) after Carazzi, and periodic acid Schiff (PAS) after Hotchkiss—McManus, were made from the following organs: tongue, diaphragm, and psoas muscle. The specimens were preserved in 10% buffered neutral formalin. Immediately after autopsy fresh preparations of the same organs were examined by trichinoscopy.

Table I Experimental Design

Mebendazole treatment (ppm)	Intestinal Phase Schedule (days)	Intestinal Phase Number of animals	Migrating Phase Schedule (days)	Migrating Phase Number of animals	Encysted Phase Schedule (days)	Encysted Phase Number of animals	Histo-pathology Number of animals
1000	−2 to 7	2	7–14	2	21–28	4	
500					28–35	2	
					21–35	6	
					34–48	5	
					55–70		18
250					21–35	2	
125					17–21		10
100	−2 to 7	2	7–14	4	21–25	4	
			14–21	4			
32	−2 to 7	4	7–14	3			
	−0 to 7	4					
	−2 to 21	5					
10	−2 to 21	1					
Total number of treated animals		18		13		23	28
Total number of controls		6		13		16	8

Results

Efficacy on the Enteral Phase

The early intestinal phase of *Trichinella* can be eliminated by continuous medication from day 2 to day 7 by 100 ppm as well as by 1000 ppm of mebendazole in the diet (Table II). At 32 ppm in the feed from day 2 to day 7 or from day 0 to day 7 no adult worms were recovered at necropsy on the eighth day. In some animals only a few juveniles with or without sexual differentiation were found. At 32 ppm from day 2 to day 21, no juveniles or adult worms were found in the intestine. The same treatment schedule at 10 ppm is suggested to be the end point of activity since at this dose level, 1 mg/kg/day, 420×10^3 larvae were counted.

Efficacy on the Migrating Phase

When autopsy was performed on day 15 or day 22 after infection a few adult worms were recovered in the intestines of the control rats, but not when autopsy was performed on days 28 to 35.

At a concentration of 1000 ppm, mebendazole eliminated all larvae when fed from day 7 to day 14 after infection (Table III).

A drug concentration of 100 ppm or 32 ppm was 100% effective against adult worms and larvae when fed either from day 7 to day 14 or from day 14 to day 21 after inoculation (Table III).

Efficacy on the Encysting Phase

In the encysting phase the duration of medication seems important. A concentration of 1000 ppm of mebendazole in the diet given for 1 week failed to kill all *T. spiralis* larvae. If the medicated feed was given from day

Table II Autopsy Results of Infected Rats After Dietary Administration of Mebendazole on the Intestinal Phase of *T. spiralis*.

Dose (ppm)	Day dosage schedule	Day of autopsy	Number of animals	Organ	Number of adults or muscular larvae $\times 10^3$ per rat					
1000	−2 to 7	8	2	Intestine	0	0				
100	−2 to 7	8	2	Intestine	0	0				
32	−2 to 7	8	4	Intestine	0.002[a]	0.11[a]	0	0		
	−0 to 7	8	4	Intestine	0.014[a]	0.004[a]	0	0		
	−2 to 21	22	5	Intestine	0	0	0	0	0	
10	−2 to 21	22	1	Intestine	0					
				Muscles	420					
Controls		8	6	Intestine	0.92	2.14	2.35	3.2	1.5	0.6
		15	4	Intestine	3.5	2.2	0.04	0		
		22	5	Intestine	0.5	0.05	0.12	0	0	
				Muscles	542	612	428	344	270	

[a] Only juveniles or larvae in intestines

Table III Autopsy Results of Infected Rats after Dietary Administration of Mebendazole on the Migrating and Encysting Phases of *T. spiralis*

Dose ppm	Day dosage schedule	Day of autopsy	Number of animals	Organ	Number of adults or muscular larvae $\times 10^3$ per rat					P
I. Migrating phase										
1000	7–14	28	2	Muscles	0	0				
100	7–14	15	2	Muscles[a]	0	0				
	14–21	22	6	Muscles[a]	0	0	0	0		
32	7–14	15	6	Muscles[a]	0	0	0	0		
Controls		28	2	Muscles[a]	419	207				
		22	5	Muscles	542	612	428	344	270	
				Intestine	0.5	0.05	0.12	0	0	
II. Encysting phase										
1000	21–28	35	4	Muscles	.75	13.9	12.0	34.7		0.029
	28–35	42	2	Muscles	1.6	1.8				
500	21–35	42	6	Muscles	5.6	0.2	0	0		0.001
	34–48	56	4	Muscles	9.6	1.0	35.2	6.4	59.2	0.004
250	21–35	42	2	Muscles	40.4	118				
125	25–35	42	4	Muscles	120	108	0	0		0.002
Controls		35	5	Muscles	354	674	808	207	340	
		42	8	Muscles	200	240	400	132	260	
					396	232			172	
		56	5	Muscles	135	127	186	176		

[a] No. *T. spiralis* adults in the intestine

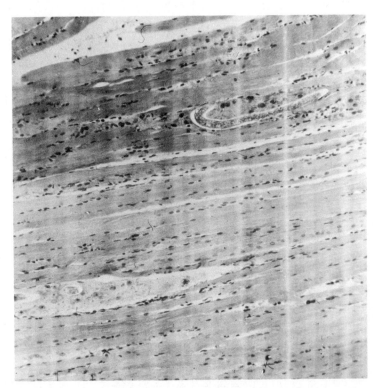

Figure 1 Psoas control rat 17 days post-infection, stretched larvae; a parasitized fiber with an intact portion and a swollen migration track with hypertrophied muscle nuclei and lytic sarcous material (H&E, × 100).

21 to day 28, a 96% reduction was obtained, and from day 28 to day 35 after infection a 99% reduction. At 500 ppm fed for 14 days from day 21 to 35, the results were better and complete cure was noted in four out of six animals. When treatment started 14 days later, from day 34 to day 48 after infection, all animals were positive in the digestion technique but the number of larvae was significantly lower in the treated rats ($P = .004$) than in the controls. At 250 ppm and 125 ppm given from day 21 to day 35 after infection a marked reduction and even complete cure was observed (Table III).

Histopathology

No difference could be observed as to the degree of infection between the animals of each group, although the infestation in the migratory phase was higher than in the encapsulated phase. The sequence of observed effects and their timing were similar in all the animals and very constant, which suggests that the adult worms void their larvae in a very short lapse of time.

The highest infection rate was found in the tongue (mean 60 parasites in one 4-μm thick transverse section) followed by the diaphragm and the psoas. In the diaphragm the progress of the lesions seemed 24–48 hr in advance of that of the lesions in the tongue.

Treatment with mebendazole at 125 ppm for 5 consecutive days during the migratory phase produced a tremendous and fast larval mortality. During this treatment period one can observe in control animals a gradual coiling up from stretched form to S or 8 forms, together with a progressive regeneration of the altered fiber portions, due to larval migration (Fig. 1). In the treated animals a reduction in PAS positivity of the parasite was noticeable even after 1 day and became more striking as treatment continued. Starting on day 2 of treatment, an increasing inflammatory reaction developed about the thickened portion of the sarcolemma which enveloped the parasites. This reaction mainly consisted of proliferating histiocytes together with infiltration of lymphoid cells and eosinophils. On day 5 of treatment a reduction in the number of coiled larvae and the appearance of macrophages and even giant cells forecast the death of the larvae (Fig. 2). The latter observations coincide with those of trichinoscopy.

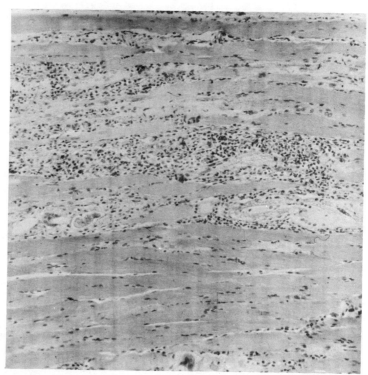

Figure 2 Psoas 17 days post-infection and 5 days mebendazole, 125 ppm; striking inflammatory reaction about killed larvae; note reduced staining affinity of the larvae and presence of a mild number of giant cells (H & E, × 100).

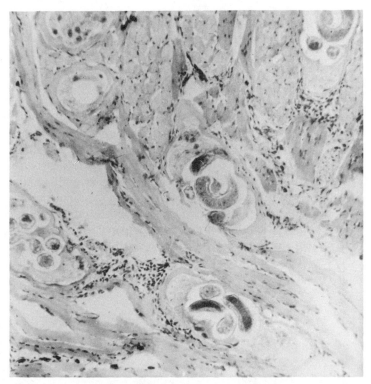

Figure 3 Tongue control rat 55 days post-infection, full encapsulated coiled larvae with occasional accumulation of lymphoid cells at the poles (H&E, × 100)

The sequence of changes during the encapsulated phase with treatment at 500 ppm for 15 days could be followed easier in the tongue and diaphragm sections than in the psoas sections. An active proliferation of histiocytes and macrophages about the capsules, faint on day 3 (day 58 post-infection) became prominent with numerous mitotic figures from day 5 and reached its maximum around day 8 in the diaphragm (Fig. 6) and day 10 in the tongue (Figs. 4 and 7). Later on this feature subsided and infiltration of polymorphonuclears supervened.

Starting on the fifth day of treatment, the PAS reactivity of the larvae themselves revealed a gradual depletion of the reacting substances; concomitantly, the capsule gradually disappeared (Figs. 5 and 6).

While the capsule was delacerated and digested one could observe wandering cells crossing the capsule. Ultimately these cells surrounded the parasite or fragments of it. Giant cells appeared at this site about the tenth day (Fig. 7) of treatment. It is likely that the ensuing regressive changes (Figs. 8 and 9) will be comparable to the tissue response around dead larvae

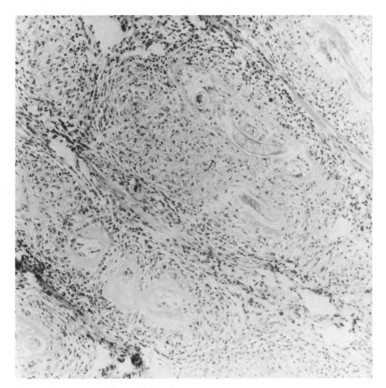

Figure 4 Tongue 55 days post-infection and 10 days mebendazole, 500 ppm; totality of the inflammatory reaction (H&E, × 100).

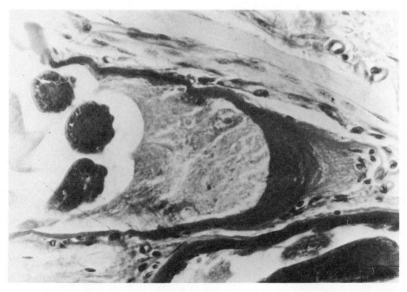

Figure 5 Tongue control rat 55 days post-infection; half of lemon-shaped cyst; strong postive reaction of capsule and and of coiled parasite (PAS, × 500).

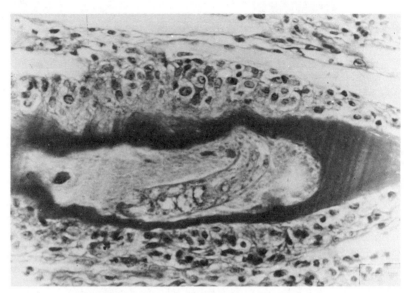

Figure 6 Diaphragm 55 days post-infection and 8 days mebendazole, 500 ppm; macrophagic activity; reduced PAS positivity of the larvae (PAS, × 500).

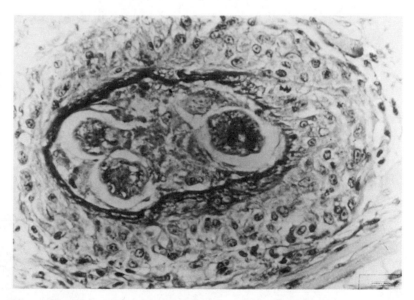

Figure 7 Tongue 55 days post-infection and 8 days mebendazole, 500 ppm; severe macrophagic proliferation; note mitotic figures, dilacerated capsule, distorted contours of the parasite (PAS, × 500).

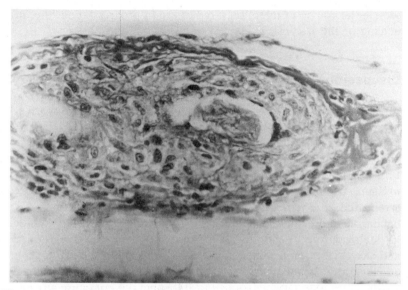

Figure 8 Diaphragm 55 days post-infection—15 days mebendazole, 500 ppm; autopsy 8 days post-treatment; barely recognizable parasite fragments on the way to disappearance (PAS, × 500).

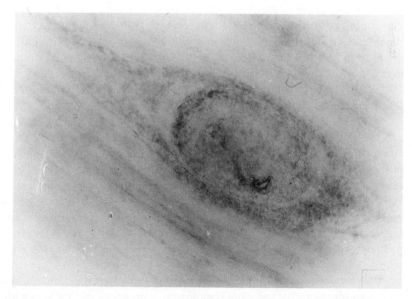

Figure 9 Psoas 55 days post-infection; 15 days mebendazole, 500 ppm; autopsy 15 days post-treatment; parasite as viewed by trichinoscope; lytic larva and filling up of cyst with wandering cells (× 150).

seen in the course of infection. Studies are in progress about the ultimate healing of the lesions.

Discussion

The efficacy of modern anthelmintics against trichuroid worms, given in a single dose is poor, except for methyridine against *Trichuris* spp., *Capillaria* spp., and intestinal *T. spiralis* adults, for dichlorvos against *T. vulpis,* and for tetramisole against intestinal *Capillaria* spp. of the chicken. From studies on mebendazole in man and in animals infected with *Trichuris* spp., *Capillaria* spp. and also with hookworm it may be concluded that a repeated dose is necessary to reach high to 100% cure rates. For thiabendazole and cambendazole similar observations have been made.

Mebendazole is generally poorly absorbed, the blood level is rather low, and the rhythm of feeding of the parasite is insufficiently known. The administration of medicated feed with mebendazole for 7 days or 14 days at concentrations varying from 10 to 1000 ppm did not cause any mortality although the daily feed consumption per rat slightly decreased at 1000 ppm.

The juvenile and adult *T. spiralis* of the intestinal phase are sensitive to mebendazole at 100 ppm. At 32 ppm, given for 8–10 days, a very limited number of juveniles were detected in the intestine of isolated rats. Prophylactic treatment of mebendazole, at 32 ppm cleared all juveniles as well. The optimal results against the muscular larvae were obtained during the migrating and the early encysting phase. After a 7-day treatment, starting at days 7 and 14 post-infection at 1000 or 100 ppm and at 32 ppm starting at day 7 post-infection all animals were negative for muscle larvae.

The larvae in the encysted phase are the most resistant and higher dose levels are needed to reach a 100% cure.

With 500 ppm of mebendazole in the rat diet, which corresponds to an average of 50 mg/kg/day, the best results are obtained. It seems that the larvae present at day 7 after the end of the treatment are still under the influence of mebendazole which reached the larvae and stays there for relatively longer periods than in the blood and muscle of the rat host. Within a few weeks all the larvae will die under the influence of a decreased glucose uptake and an increased glycogen depletion induced by mebendazole (Van den Bossche and de Nollin, 1972). Work is in progress to find out whether the larvae found at autopsy in the treated rats are still viable.

The process of histological changes of the migrating and encysting larvae under the influence of mebendazole is progressive. It starts with the degeneration of the larvae and it is followed by cellular invasion which is massive during the migrating phase.

Summary

The activity of mebendazole was tested against the enteral, migrating, and encysted muscular phase of *Trichinella spiralis* in rats.

Mebendazole was administered on medicated feed. A 100% activity was reached at 32 ppm against the enteral phase and the migrating phase. A 14-day treatment at 125–500 ppm gave a 100% reduction of live larvae of the encysted phase.

The histopathological evolution of the *T. spiralis* infection was followed in treated and untreated controls. The effect of mebendazole can be observed from day 3 by reduction of PAS positive material of capsule of the cyst. At day 8 the depletion of PAS materials is definite. At day 10 starts the formation of the granuloma, the invasion of the wandering cells within the cysts, and phagocytosis.

References

Brugmans, J. P., Thienpont, D., Van Wijngaarden, I., Vanparijs, O. F., Schuermans, V. L., and Lauwers, H. L. (1971). Radiochemical and pilot clinical study in 1278 subjects. *J. Amer. Med. Ass.* **217**, 313–316.

Campbell, W. C., and Cuckler, A. C. (1964). Effect of thiabendazole upon the enteral and parenteral phase of trichinosis in mice. *J. Parasitol.* **50**, 481–488.

Campbell, W. C., and Yakstis, J. J. (1970). Efficacy of cambendazole against *T. spiralis* in mice. *J. Parasitol.* **56**, 839–840.

Chaia, G., and Da Cunha, A. S. (1971). Therapeutic-action of mebendazole against human helminthiasis. *Folha Med.* **63**, 843–852.

Gatti, F., Krubwa, F., Lontie, M., Vandepitte, J., and Thienpont, D. (1971). Proc. VIIth Intern. Congr. Chemotherapy, Prague, August 26, 1971.

Gould, S. E. (1945). "Trichinosis." Thomas, Springfield, Illinois.

Van den Bossche, H., and De Nollin, S. (1972). Effects of mebendazole on the absorption of low molecular weight nutrients by *A. suum. Int. J. Parasitol.* **3**, 401–407.

Vandepitte, J. Gatti, F., Lontie, M., Krubwa, F., Nguete, M., and Thienpont, D. (1973). Le mebendazole, un nouvel anthelminthique a large spectre tres actif contre le trichocephale. *Bull Soc. Pathol. Exotique* **66**, 165–178.

Part VI
Epidemiology and Control

Trichinellosis in British Columbia: Eight Incidents Traced to Pork and Bear Meat

Ernest J. Bowmer

Division of Laboratories
Vancouver, British Columbia, Canada

As trichinellosis is a foodborne disease often presenting with all the abrupt drama of food poisoning, you will, I trust, forgive me for the following droll tale.

> "I was married twice," the man explained, "and I'll never marry again. My first wife died after eating poisonous mushrooms and my second wife died of a fractured skull."
> "That's a shame," said his friend. "How did it happen?"
> "She wouldn't eat her mushrooms."

This is a brief account of the occasions when people have unwittingly ingested, in their pork or bear meat, as a viable protein supplement, the cysts of *Trichinella spiralis,* the garbage worm.

Since 1949, eight trichinellosis incidents have been reported from British Columbia. Pork was the vehicle in four episodes with 34 persons ill, bear meat in three episodes affecting 21 persons, while the vehicle was not recorded in one incident affecting four persons. Table I shows the geographic distribution of these incidents.

Incident 1

We have been unable to uncover any details of this incident.

Table I Trichinellosis in British Columbia: Eight Incidents Traced to Pork and Bear Meat (1949–1971)

| | | No. of Patients | | | | |
| | | Male | Female | Total | | |
Incident	Year	Male	Female	Total	Location	Vehicle
1	1949	?	?	4 [a]	Prince Rupert	Uncertain, probably bear
2	1949	1	0	1	North Vancouver	Bear
3	1958	1	0	1	Vancouver	Pork
4	1958	0	2	2	Duncan	Pork
5	1960	3	4	7	Vancouver	Pork
6	1960	3	0	3	Kamloops	Bear
7	1961	12	12	24	Abbotsford	Pork
8	1971	10	7	17	West Kootenays	Bear
Total	1949–1971	30	25	59		

[a] Sex of patients not known, probably all male hunters

Incident 2

A 39-year-old hunter shot a bear and ate a bear steak rare in the mountains of British Columbia. One week later he complained of head cold and developed generalized pains in muscles of arms and legs, periorbital edema, and swelling of tongue, cheek, and floor of mouth. On admission to hospital 2 weeks after the meal, he was seriously ill with temperatures ranging from 38.3° to 40.0° C. The white cell count was 11,000/mm^3 with 21% eosinophilia. Biopsies of sartorius and gastrocnemius muscles revealed numerous encysted larvae of *Trichinella spiralis*. During the fourth week he developed cyanosis and pain in his right foot due to an embolus. After embolectomy, the patient made an uneventful recovery and was free from symptoms when discharged from hospital in the sixth week. Samples of bear meat revealed numerous encysted larvae of *T. spiralis*.

Incident 3

This 30-year-old Portuguese immigrant developed typical symptoms of trichinellosis, so severe that he was admitted to the hospital. Muscle biopsy revealed cysts of *T. spiralis*. Although he regularly ate pork, it was usually well cooked.

Incident 4

Two women from Germany had a habit of eating undercooked pork products; both had typical symptoms.

Incident 5

During September 1960 three men and four women, 20–39 years old, acquired trichinellosis after eating raw or undercooked pork from a Vancouver sausage manufacturer. Three victims were employees at two delicatessen stores; four were customers. The diagnosis was confirmed by muscle biopsy in two; by skin test, in five.

Incident 6

Three men went into the hills north of Kamloops, shot a black bear, and ate rare bear steaks. Two developed typical symptoms; one who did not like the flavor of rare bear meat ate less and was less ill.

Incident 7

In 1961 British Columbia's largest outbreak was traced to ingestion of uncooked farmer's sausage containing meat from a locally slaughtered hog. Twenty-four persons fell ill with diarrhea, fever, muscle pains, and periorbital edema. After the index case had been diagnosed by muscle biopsy, subsequent cases were confirmed by intradermal sensitivity and serologic tests.

By patient inquiry and energetic leg work the Medical Health Officer and his Public Health Inspectors established the wholesalers and retailers who had sold the trichinous meat to the afflicted. The patients were not all local residents and included travelers who had stopped and purchased the widely acclaimed farm sausage.

Incident 8

After a decade of low incidence, trichinellosis now appeared as a large outbreak in British Columbia (Schmitt *et al.*, 1972). During November and December 1971, epidemiological investigation revealed patients with trichinellosis in five areas of the Province.

Index Cases

This epidemic came to the attention of the West Kootenay Health Unit on November 10, 1971, when a family physician reported an unexplained illness in a patient from Castlegar. When admitted to a hospital on October 29, 1971, this 56-year-old woman had fever, sore muscles, diarrhea and periorbital edema, associated with 55% eosinophilia. She had been ill for 4 weeks and, after some imporvement, had returned to work, but she relapsed the same day. Her 69-year-old friend developed similar but milder symptoms. The diagnosis of trichinellosis was made on November 15 by skin tests and confirmed on November 16 by biopsy of the deltoid muscle of the younger woman.

On October 7 both women had eaten cuts of smoked meat at a West Kootenay inn where they also purchased homemade smoked sausages. A few days later they became ill.

Epidemiological Investigation

By alerting the Medical Health Officers of British Columbia, 15 more persons with trichinellosis were discovered. All were linked, directly or indirectly, to the same inn where the two Castlegar women (numbers 1 and 2) had eaten. One man and four women employees (numbers 3–7) regularly ate at the inn. One man, a local resident (number 8) ate smoked bear meat and salami sausage from the inn. A man from California brought smoked bear meat and smoked sausage from the inn to a Chilliwack home. The Chilliwack couple (numbers 9 and 10) and the Californian (number 11) ate smoked sausage uncooked and bear meat cooked, while the son-in-law (number 12) of the Chilliwack couple, visiting from North Vancouver, just ate smoked sausage uncooked. All four became ill. The wife of the Californian and the daughter of the Chilliwack couple ate no meat and were not ill. A second Chilliwack couple took the rest of the smoked sausage on a protracted camper trip to Mexico. It is to be hoped that they cooked it well before eating it. After returning home, the Californian (number 11) suffered from severe "stomach flu" but did not consult a physician. Two men from Victoria (numbers 13 and 14) and two men from Kelowna (numbers 15 and 16) ate smoked meat and sausage while visiting the inn. Another man from Kelowna (number 17) ate bear meat, from a hunter, presumably smoked at the inn.

Source of Infection

Around mid-September this hunter had killed a large American black bear within 1 mile of the local open-faced garbage dump. He then asked a relative of the innkeeper to process it, in return for a 20-kg cut of the smoked meat. Inspection of the inn revealed no trace of bear meat. On November 17 the proprietor stated that the cold plate and smoked sausages contained only beef and pork products. He produced sales slips to show that he bought the pork from a federally inspected meat processing plant in Vancouver. Later, it was discovered that during September bear meat was smoked at the inn in a homemade cold smoker by hanging large steaks, roasts, and hams over sawdust fires in the smokehouse for 12–14 hr. Before smoking, sausage meat was immersed in "hot" water for 15–20 min. The findings strongly support the epidemiological conclusion that bear meat and salami or smoked sausage containing bear meat transmitted trichinellosis to at least 17 persons who ate meat from the inn during September and October.

Clinical Features (Table II)

So protean were the initial symptoms that the preliminary diagnosis was usually "stomach flu." In one patient appendicitis was suspected; in another, cholecystitis. A third patient with prominent periorbital edema was treated for sinusitis. To combat severe fatigue, two young women took iron pills. One woman with stiff jaw muscles was investigated for tetanus.

Table II Clinical Features of 17 Patients, Trichinellosis Outbreak, British Columbia, 1971

Signs and symtoms	Number	Percent
Myalgia	17	100
Fever	14	82
Diarrhea	13	76
Fatigue	11	65
Periorbital edema	8	47
Abdominal cramps	6	35
Visual disturbances	6	35
Nausea, vomiting	5	29
Skin lesions	3	18
Dyspnea	2	12

Laboratory Investigations (Table III)

1. Serial total and differential white cell counts.
2. Biopsies of deltoid or gastrocnemius muscle.
3. Bachman intradermal test.
4. At the Institute of Parasitology, Macdonald College, McGill University, sera were tested for *Trichinella* precipitation, agglutination, and hemagglutination reactions.
5. At the Center for Disease Control, Atlanta, Georgia, sera were tested for *Trichinella* bentonite flocculation.
6. Meat products including bear meat and sausages were examined by the digest-compressorium technique of Simon and Stovell (1972).
7. Using specific animal antisera in precipitation tests, the Royal Canadian Mounted Police Crime Laboratory determined the species of these meat and sausage samples.

Bear Meat and Sausages

In November 1971 bear meat and sausages were found to contain non-viable larvae of *T. spiralis.* Larvae were seen in samples of smoked sausage

Table III Results and Dates of Skin Tests and Laboratory Findings of 17 Patients, Trichinellosis Outbreak, British-Columbia, 1971

Case	Skin test	White blood count	Eosinophils (%)	Date	P[a]	AG[b]	BF[c]
1	15 Nov; Pos	2 Nov; 16,350	2 Nov; 55	15 Nov	Pos	8	Neg
				7 Dec	Pos	8	40
2	15 Nov; Pos	9 Nov; 13,150	9 Nov; 31	15 Nov	Pos	4	Neg
				7 Dec	Pos	4	40
3	17 Nov; Pos			17 Nov	Pos	Pos[d]	10
				9 Dec	Pos	Pos[d]	5
4	17 Nov; Pos			17 Nov	Pos	128	80
5	17 Nov; Pos			17 Nov	Pos	64	160
6	17 Nov; Pos			17 Nov	Pos	128	320
				9 Dec	Pos	8	80
7	9 Dec; Pos			9 Dec	Pos	32	320
8	9 Dec; Pos			9 Dec	Pos	64	5120
9		5 Nov; 8,200	5 Nov; 45	20 Nov	Pos	64	10
				11 Jan			160
10		27 Nov; 11,760	1 Nov; 36	15 Jan	Pos	4	40
				17 Feb	Pos	4	20
11							
12	8 Dec; Pos	8 Nov; 10,400	29 Nov; 42	8 Dec	Pos	16	320
				4 Jan	Pos	16	160
13	19 Nov; Pos	15 Nov; 14,900	15 Nov; 50	19 Nov	Pos	4	80
14	19 Nov; Pos	15 Nov; 23,250	15 Nov; 51	12 Nov	Pos	2	
				19 Nov	Pos	4	80
15	10 Dec; Pos	14 Nov; 23,100	14 Nov; 52	23 Nov	Pos	64	160
				29 Nov	Pos	64	1280
16	10 Dec; Pos	15 Nov; 11,400	15 Nov; 32	21 Nov	Pos	8	80
				4 Jan	Neg	16	640
17	23 Nov; Neg	15 Nov; 16,800	16 Nov; 44	22 Nov	Pos	8	80

[a] Precipitation test.
[b] Reciprocal of dilution giving standard agglutination.
[c] Reciprocal of dilution giving standard bentonite flocculation.
[d] Weakly reactive.

from the home of the two Castlegar women (numbers 1 and 2); in a sample of salami obtained from patient number 8; in remnants of bear meat eaten by the Chilliwack couple and their son-in-law (numbers 9, 10, and 12) and in remnants of bear meat eaten by one of the Kelowna men (number, 17).

In bear muscle, trichinellae appeared as coiled larvae within thick-walled cysts. The concentration of larvae per gram ranged from 12 in smoked sausage to 150 in salami and to 575 in bear meat. To make inspection of the blended meat products for trichinellae more sensitive, individual fragments of each sample were separated by color and consistency and examined. To identify the animal species in such meat, the balance of each trichinous sample was sent for serologic examination to the Crime Laboratory. The smoked sausage was found to contain meat of deer family and pig family origin; the salami, of bear family and pig family origin.

Unconfirmed Trichinellosis

Since 1961, some 40 other patients have been investigated for trichinellosis; they have had doubtful reactions in skin tests or serologic tests. Trichinellosis was considered in the differential diagnosis because of eosinophilia, muscle pain, fever, periorbital edema, or history of eating raw pork sausage.

Discussion

In closing I would like to pose a few questions.

1. Are we going to have to amend the late Ogden Nash's (1959) statement on trichinellosis? Copyright 1942 by Ogden Nash.

> "The hog converted into pork
> Puts trichinosis on your fork."

2. How many missed cases are there?
3. Specifically, what is the reservoir of ursine and therefore human trichinellosis? Is it bears eating pork at poorly maintained garbage dumps?
   Or bears eating rats?
   Or bears eating bear remnants?
   Or maybe some so far undisclosed sylvatic cycle?
4. In Incident 8, were the pork and the salami in fact adulterated by bear meat? If so was the adulteration accidental or on purpose?
5. Are surveys of incidence of trichinous cysts in wild animals warranted?
6. How can we educate the public about avoiding ursine trichinellosis?
7. Should we issue a written warning to hunters when they buy their hunting licenses?

As illustrated in a famous limerick, ingestion is what trichinellosis is all about.

> There was a young lady from Niger,
> Who smiled as she rode on a tiger,
> They came back from the ride
> With the lady inside,
> And the smile on the face of the tiger.

Acknowledgments

Many physicians and public health officials participated in collecting clinical, epidemiological, and investigational data on these outbreaks of trichinellosis. I would particularly like to acknowledge the contribution of Dr. G. D. M. Kettyls in Incident 7; the work of Drs. N. Schmitt, P. C. Simon, P. L. Stovell, A. S. Arneil, and D. A. Clark during the study of Incident 8; the attending physicians of patients in all incidents; and the diagnostic serologic tests performed by Dr. C. E. Tanner and Dr. I. G. Kagan.

References

Nash, O. (1959). A Bulletin Has Just Come In. *In* "Verses from 1929 On." Little, Brown & Co., Boston, Massachusetts.

Schmitt, N., Bowmer, E. J., Simon, P. C., Arneil, A. S., and Clark, D. A. (1972). Trichinosis from bear meat and adulterated pork products: A major outbreak in British Columbia, 1971. *Can. Med. Ass. J.* 107, 1087–1091.

Simon, P. C., and Stovell, P. L. (1972). A digest compressorium technique for detection of *Trichinella spiralis* larvae. *Can. J. Comp. Med.* **36,** 178–179.

Trichinella spiralis Infections in the Netherlands

E. J. Ruitenberg and J. F. Sluiters

*Laboratory of Pathology, National
Institute of Public Health,
Bilthoven, the Netherlands*

Trichinella spiralis infections have not occurred in human beings or animals in the Netherlands during the last 40 years. This statement is based on the results of the examination of over 1000 human diaphragms in 1941 and again in 1966 (Kampelmacher *et al.,* 1966). Further evidence may be found in the negative results of the examination of 773 wild boars in 1961 through 1963. Negative results were also obtained in the examination of 100 wild rats caught in or in the neighborhood of slaughterhouses in 1962. In 1965 another 100 rats were shot at a rubbish dump; examination of them also yielded negative results. All these investigations were carried out by means of trichinoscopy and digestion of the diaphragm (Ruitenberg *et al.,* 1968).

When pork is imported, various countries require a declaration stating that the meat concerned has been examined for *Trichinella* or that *Trichinella* does not occur in swine in the exporting country. In countries where trichinellosis is a public health hazard, this inspection is carried out by means of trichinoscopic examination of the diaphragm. As this method is only reliable with highly infected animals, however, it does not meet the requirements in countries where *Trichinella* infections occur only sporadically and where the pigs are only very slightly infected. If the animals are infected with a small number of larvae, trichinoscopic examination of the diaphragm is usually negative.

In the Netherlands trichinoscopic examination was carried out until 1962. No infected pigs have been found since 1926. These data would seem to indicate that *Trichinella* infections do not occur either in pigs or in wildlife reservoir. In contrast to our own reassuring results there was a

539

communication made by Kabatnik in 1958 and repeated by Lehmensik in 1964 that in the Federal Republic of Germany *Trichinella* had been found 10 times in 654,603 pigs imported from the Netherlands.

In order to obtain more information on the present state of affairs, it was decided to study the situation in detail using three methods.

1. Trichinoscopy. The advantage of this method is the possibility of examining each pig presented for slaughter. The major drawback is the low reliability.
2. Digestion method. This is the most reliable method. Even a small number of *Trichinella* larvae is detected. For routine examination of slaughter animals, however, it is very time consuming. This method was advocated by Zimmerman (1967) in the United States. He proposed to examine groups of 20 pigs from one farm together. Each sample included 20 x 5 gm of diaphragm.
3. Serologic methods. Although various serologic methods have been used experimentally, the immunofluorescence technique seemed to be the most promising. Sadun *et al.* (1962) described this method for the serodiagnosis of trichinellosis in man. Later, Scholtens and his co-workers (1966), Sulzer and Chisholm (1966), and Ruitenberg and his co-workers (1968) applied this method on sera from pigs experimentally infected.

In this last study the results from the immunofluorescence method, trichinoscopy, and the digestion method in experimentally infected pigs were compared (Table I). It should be pointed out that in the pigs infected with 5000 larvae the first positive titer in the immunofluorescence test was observed 26 days after infection in three out of four animals. In the pigs infected with 500 larvae the immunofluorescence test showed a positive titer 33 days after infection in two out of four animals, and in the pigs infected with 250 and 100 larvae the first titer was detected at 40 days after infection. The animals were slaughtered 100 days after infection, which was the normal slaughter age. It may be concluded from the data presented in this table that trichinoscopy yielded positive results in the animals infected with 5000 larvae and in two out of four animals infected with 500 larvae. The immunofluorescence test gave positive results in all animals, except in one animal infected with 100 larvae and the group infected with 50 larvae. The digestion method yielded positive results in all infected animals except in the same animal infected with 100 larvae. The negative results in both the immunofluorescence test and the digestion method with the one animal infected with 100 larvae were due to the fact that difficulties were encountered in administering the larvae to this pig.

The results of this investigation were rather promising, especially since the immunofluorescence test was negative in 1000 healthy control animals.

The immunofluorescence test was both very sensitive and specific.

Table I Immunofluorescence Test, Trichinoscopy, and Digestion Method in Pigs (20 kg) 100 Days after Infection with Various Numbers of *T. spiralis* Larvae

Pig	Number of larvae	Immunofluorescence test	Results Trichinoscopy	Digestion method
1	5000	+	+	+
2	5000	+	+	+
3	5000	+	+	+
4	5000	+	+	+
5	500	+	+	+
6	500	+	+	+
7	500	+	−	+
8	500	+	−	+
9	250	+	−	+
10	250	+	−	+
11	100	+	−	+
12	100	−	−	−
13	50	−	−	+
14	50	−	−	+
15	0	−	−	−
16	0	−	−	−

With regard to the sensitivity it may be concluded that when the pigs were infected with 100 or more larvae, antibodies were produced above the detection level. In the two pigs infected with 50 larvae the immunofluorescence test failed to detect any. Although antibodies are probably formed, they were not detectable with the immunofluorescence test.

The sensitivity of the immunofluorescence test was further examined in rats experimentally infected with various numbers of *T. spiralis* larvae: (1000, 500, 250, 100, 50, 25, 10, 5, and 0) (Ruitenberg *et al.,* 1972). In this experimental model, 25 larvae proved to be the smallest number which gave rise to a detectable amount of antibodies in all three animals in the group (Fig. 1).

One of the problems in using a serologic test for *Trichinella* infections in pigs is the possibility of cross reactions with other worm infections, especially *Ascaris lumbricoides.* The antigenic relationship between *Trichinella* and *Ascaris* has been pointed out by several authors (Kent, 1963; Tanner and Gregory, 1961, 1963a, b).

Using the complement fixation test, Ruitenberg and his co-workers (1968) observed cross reactions in sera from rabbits which had been immunized with both male and female *Ascaris lumbricoides* and with their metabolic products. These cross reactions were, however, not encountered when the immunofluorescence test was used.

A drawback of the immunofluorescence test is that it is possible for it to be negative while the digestion method is positive. This was the case from the very onset of a *Trichinella* infection (Ruitenberg *et al.,* 1972).

Groups of two adult rats were infected with 1000 *T. spiralis* larvae.

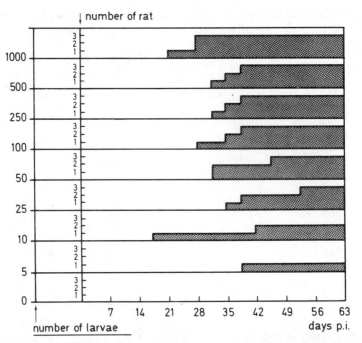

Figure 1 Results of immunofluorescence test in groups of three rats, infected with various numbers of *T. spiralis* larvae (dose–time relationship). Crosshatched blocks show number of rats of each group with positive immunofluorescence tests from a particular post-infection time.

Up to 15 days after infection both the immunofluorescence and the digestion method were negative. At 17 days and thereafter the digestion was positive in all the animals while the immunofluorescence test yielded consistently positive results from day 27 (Table II).

The basic purpose of this investigation was to develop a rapid, specific, and sensitive test for detecting *Trichinella* infections in pigs. Mainly because it was impossible to detect slight infections by trichinoscopy the

Table II Results of Studies Using the Immunofluorescence Test and the Digestion Method in Two Groups of Rats Infected with 1000 *T. spiralis* Larvae

| Portmortem examination | Results | |
(days after infection)	I.F. test	Digestion method
3–15	−, −	−, −
17	−, −	+, +
20	+, +	+, +
22	−, −	+, +
24	+, −	+, +
27–43	+, +	+, +

prospects for the immunofluorescence test seemed very good. This is particularly true in countries where *Trichinella* infections in pigs do not occur at all, or in areas where the infections are only slight. In countries where the infections have not been detected for a long time, such as the Netherlands, the immunofluorescence test seemed a good method for keeping a permanent check on the absence of antibodies against *Trichinella* in pigs and possibly in other animals by means of examining statistically valid random samples.

For this purpose, 5000 sera from healthy pigs were examined annually from 1967. This number should be regarded as a representative sample from the total number of slaughtered pigs in those years (4.5–5 million).

However, after examination of 10,000 sera, one serum showed a titer of 1:4 (Ruitenberg and Kampelmacher, 1970). On the basis of this observation further investigations were carried out on the farm where the pig originated. It appeared that this farm, with over 100 pigs, was rather unhygienic. Furthermore, a high number of rats was present. Pigs from this farm were examined by means of trichinoscopy, the immunofluorescence test, and the digestion method (Table III).

From 44 pigs examined, 11 were positive with the digestion method, while all animals were negative with trichinoscopy and the immunofluorescence test. In examining nine sera from sows, three were positive with the immunofluorescence test. Twenty-nine rats from the farm which were examined with the digestion method yielded positive results in only three animals.

At that moment the situation with regard to *Trichinella* infections in the Netherlands had to be reevaluated. Although the conditions on this farm were rather unhygienic, it seemed possible that *Trichinella* infections could occur elsewhere in the country as well. Therefore, the immunofluorescence test was dropped and attention was focused on the digestion method. In order to obtain more information on the situation at hand the following procedure was adopted.

Table III Examination for the Presence of *Trichinella* Infection in Pigs and Rats from One Farm

| | | Number of animals | | |
| | | Positive with | | |
	Examined	Immunofluorescence test	Trichinoscopy	Digestion method
Routine sera	3	1	N.d.[a]	n.d.
Pigs	44	0	0	11
Sows	9	3	n.d.	n.d.
Rats (*Rattus norvegicus*)	29	n.d.	n.d.	3

[a] N.d., Not done.

Table IV Prevalence of *T. spiralis* Larvae in Pigs in the Netherlands from April 1969–1971

		Number of lots[a]	
Year	Number of animals	Examined[b]	Positive
April 1969–1970	2869	337	23
1971	2419	501	23

[a] All animals from one lot originated from one farm.
[b] Pooled sample from each lot included 20 gm of tongue and 20 gm of diaphragm
from each animal.

Since most information seemed to be obtained when farms could be
examined, a modified pooled sample digestion method as proposed by
Zimmermann (1967) was adopted. Animals from one farm were preferably
examined when they were presented for slaughter in lots of at least 10
animals. From each animal 20 gm of tongue musculature and 20 gm of
diaphragm were examined. The results from these investigations from
April 1969 to April 1971, are presented in Table IV. It is clear from these
results that *T. spiralis* infections in pigs occur in the Netherlands.

The actual numbers of larvae, which were found in the pooled samples
from the positive lots are presented in Table V. In this table the number
of larvae per total amount of material per farm, i.e., 400 gm, is listed. In
the majority of the lots only 1–10 larvae were present.

Farms from which the positive lots originated were mainly localized in
the southern and eastern part of the Netherlands (Fig. 2). This could
suggest that the infected animals are predominantly present in those
regions. However, the samplings included particularly those slaughterhouses important for export. These slaughterhouses are mainly localized
in those regions. In these areas the large pig farms are concentrated as
well.

Since the rat *(Rattus norvegicus)* is regarded as an important source

Table V Number of *T. spiralis* Larvae Present in
Pooled Samples from 23 Positive Lots in April
1969–1970, and from 23 Positive Lots in 1971

	Number of positive lots	
Number of larvae per 400 gm	April 1969–1970	1971
1–10	15	20
11–20	2	1
21–30	3	2
31–40		
41–50	1	
51–60		
61–70	1	
71–80		
81–90		
91–100	1	

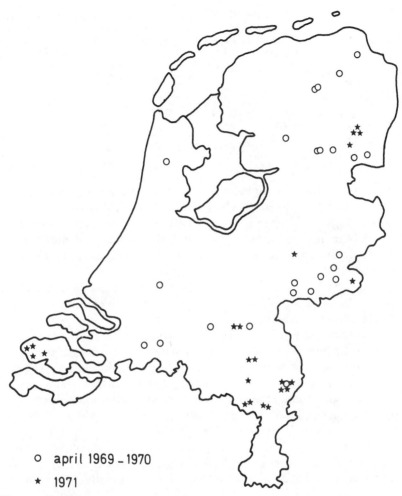

○ april 1969 – 1970

★ 1971

Figure 2 Prevalence of *T. spiralis* larvae in pigs in the Netherlands (April 1969–1971).

of infection for pigs a number of these animals was also examined. From the results presented in Table VI it may be concluded that *Trichinella* infections do occur in wild rats as well. These animals may play a role as a wildlife reservoir of *T. spiralis*. The number of larvae found indicates, however, that the infection in those animals is only minor. Light infections were also found in other wildlife (Table VII).

Since the fox *(Vulpes vulpes)* is at the end of a food chain it may serve as an indicator for the presence of *T. spiralis* in a certain area. From 96 foxes examined in the period from April 1969 to 1971, three animals proved to be slightly infected. The black rat *(Rattus rattus)* also proved to be infected.

Table VI Prevalence of *T. spiralis* Larvae in Rats *(Rattus norvegicus)* in the Netherlands from April 1969–1971

	Number of animals	
Year	Examined[a]	Positive
April 1969–1970	247	6
1971	351	13

[a]Samples included tongue and diaphragm per animal.

In conclusion one might speculate about the sudden reappearance of *Trichinella* infections in the Netherlands. Redetection seems, however, a more suitable term since it is very likely that a low level of infection has always been present. Due to the application of the immunofluorescence technique, the first positive case was found, albeit after the examination of about 10,000 sera over a period of 2 years.

A thorough investigation of pooled samples by means of the digestion method finally led to the conclusion that *Trichinella* infections occurred throughout the Netherlands.

One final question remains to be answered. What are the consequences of these findings for public health in general and for meat inspection in particular? As has been stated above, trichinoscopy is very effective in detecting *Trichinella* infections in pigs, which are high enough to cause trichinellosis in man. However, trichinoscopy would never have revealed the low infection levels present in our country. The highest number of larvae detected was 97 larvae per 400 gm tissue. In experimentally infected pigs, trichinoscopy yielded positive results only if the diaphragm contained at least three larvae per gram (Ruitenberg and Kampelmacher, 1970). This would have meant 1200 larvae per 400 gm. Consequently, reintroduction of

Table VII Prevalence of *T. spiralis* Larvae in Wildlife in the Netherlands from April 1969–1971

	Number of animals			
	Examined[a]		Positive	
Species	April 1969–1970	1971	April 1969–1970	1971
Fox *(Vulpes)*	69	27	2	1
Badger *(Meles)*	2	0	0	
Wild boar *(Sus scrofa)*	77	58	0	0
Black rat *(Rattus rattus)*	0	25		12

[a]Samples included tonque and diaphragm per animal.

trichinoscopy, including inspection of all slaughtered pigs, would not seem to be appropriate. Moreover, there is no reason to believe that the present level of *Trichinella* found in pigs has any consequence to human infections.

However, in the scope of health protection of man it is necessary to check continuously for a possible build-up of *Trichinella* infections. In our opinion this permanent check should be performed by means of the digestion method of pooled samples since this is the most sensitive diagnostic method (Fig. 3).

Finally, it seems appropriate to verify the results of this check by examining the human population. For this purpose the examination of human diaphragms as performed from 1964 to 1966 (Kampelmacher *et al.*, 1966) should be repeated.

SCHEMATIC REPRESENTATION OF THE DETECTION LEVELS OF 3 DIAGNOSTIC METHODS FOR TRICHINOSIS

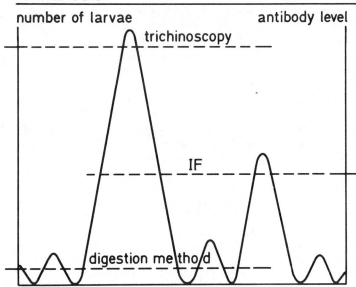

Figure 3 Schematic representation of the detection levels of three diagnostic methods for trichinellosis.

References

Kabatnik, J. (1958). Trichinenfunde bei inländischen Schlachtschweinen. *Deut. Schlacht und Viehhof Zeitung 9,* 12.

Kampelmacher, E. H., Ruitenberg, E. J., and Berkvens, J. M. (1966). Onderzoekingen naar het voorkomen van *Trichinella spiralis* bij de mens in Nederland. *Ned. Tijdschr. Geneesk.* **110,** 1927–1929.

Kent, N. H. (1963). Isolation of specific antigens from *Ascaris lumbricoides var. suum. Exp. Parasitol.* **14**, 296–303.

Lehmensick, R. (1964). Trichinellosis in Europe. *Proc. 1st Int. Congr. Parasitol. Rome* **2**, 661.

Ruitenberg, E. J., and Kampelmacher, E. H. (1970). Diagnostische Methoden zur Feststellung der Invasion mit *Trichinella spiralis. Fleischwirtschaft* **50**, 42–44, 47.

Ruitenberg, E. J., Kampelmacher, E. H., and Berkvens, J. M. (1968). The indirect fluorescent antibody technique in the serodiagnosis of pigs infected with *Trichinella spiralis. Neth. J. Vet. Sci.* 1, 143–153.

Ruitenberg, E. J., Duyzings, M. J. M., and Kampelmacher, E. H. (1972). Studies on the reliability of the fluorescent antibody technique in the serodiagnosis of trichinosis. *Neth. J. Vet. Sci.* **4**, 141–149.

Sadun, E. H., Anderson, R. I., and Williams, J. S. (1962). Fluorescent antibody test for the serological diagnosis of trichinosis. *Exp. Parasitol. 12,* 423–433.

Scholtens, R. G., Kagan, I. G., Quist K. D., and Norman, L. G. (1966). An evaluation of tests for the diagnosis of trichinosis in swine and associated quantitative epidemiologic observations. *Amer. J. Epidemiol.* **83**, 489–500.

Sulzer, A. J., and Chisholm, E. S. (1966). Comparison of the I.F.A. and other tests for *Trichinella spiralis* antibodies. *Pub. Health Rep.* **81**, 729–734.

Tanner, C. E., and Gregory, J. (1961). Immunochemical studies of the antigens of *Trichinella spiralis* I. *Can. J. Microbiol.* **7**, 473–481.

Tanner, C. E., and Gregory, J. (1963a). Immunochemical studies of the antigens of *Trichinella spiralis* II. *Exp. Parasitol.* **14**, 337–345.

Tanner, C. E., and Gregory, J. (1963b). Immunochemical studies of the antigens of *Trichinella spiralis* III. *Exp. Parasitol.* **14**, 346–357.

Zimmermann, W. J. (1967). A pooled sample method for post-slaughter detection of trichiniasis in swine. *Proc. 71st Annu. Meet. U.S. Livestock Sanit. Ass. Phoenix, Arizona, Oct. 16–20,* pp. 358–366.

Trichinellosis in Domestic and Wild Animals in Rumania

I. Cironeanu

Food Industry Department
Bucharest

Introduction

Animal trichinellosis in Rumania continues to draw the attention of experts in parasitology and meat inspection. Many investigations carried out in this area, particularly since 1956, were aimed at assessing the epizootiologic situation in both domestic and wild animals, so as to adopt control measures against this helminthic zoonosis.

Trichinellosis in Swine

The first information regarding the existence of trichinellosis in swine in this country goes as far back as 1868, when *Trichinella spiralis* larvae were detected in a hog from a locality in the southeast section of the country (Cironeanu, 1961). Subsequently, in 1874, the parasite was identified in pork, when six people in the town of Jassy fell ill (three died). Five years later, the parasite was found in the carcass of another hog in the town of Focsani (Cironeanu, 1963). Although these cases were sporadic, they demonstrated unquestionably the presence of trichinellosis in the hog population. Despite this fact, cases of human trichinellosis were relatively infrequent due to the fact that people here like pork thoroughly boiled or roasted.

A trichinoscopic examination was introduced and improved, first at the Bucharest slaughterhouse in 1913, and then in the other slaughterhouses throughout the country, hence greater numbers of *T. spiralis* infected hogs were detected.

On the average, 0.077% of infected hogs were identified at the Bucharest slaughterhouse over the 1913–1952 period (Cristescu *et al.,* 1958). In the ensuing years, this rate decreased significantly to 0.013% in 1961 and

0.002% in 1971. This significant drop was due to the slaughter of an increased number of hogs from state owned swine-breeding farms, particularly large-scale fattening farms with more than 100,000 animals, where sanitary measures are strictly observed.

The average prevalence of infected animals found at the major slaughterhouses in Rumania over the 1932–1939 period was 0.055% (Lupu and Cironeanu, 1960). During this period the highest prevalence of trichinellosis (more than 0.06% was recorded in the former Bacau, Tutova, and Covurlui districts, in Moldavia, Mehedinti, and Vlasca in Muntenia, and in Tulcea and Constanta in Dobrogea.

Subsequently, during the 1956–1971 period, the prevalence of *Trichinella*-infected hogs varied between 0.071% in 1956, and 0.020% in 1970 (Fig. 1). Mention should be made of the fact that more than 20% of the cases detected had massive infection. In some cases, especially in sows, the larval count per gram of diaphragm surpassed 4000. The highest incidence was recorded in the middle region of Moldavia, in Oltenia, and in a few areas in Transylvania. In other regions of the country, hog infection was sporadic, and in Banat it was almost nonexistent.

The course assumed by hog trichinellosis during the 1956–1971 period in the north of Moldavia, a region investigated thoroughly for several consecutive years, is shown in Fig. 1. During this period, 0.024% of hogs were infected. As a result of the prophylactic measures adopted here, the prevalence of trichinellosis was maintained under this limit, reaching 0.002% in 1971. Most of the infected hogs (0.034%) originated from individual farms, and only 0.001% came from state farms. Monthly analyses (1964–1970) regarding this infection indicated that 88% of the positive animals were detected during the second half of the year.

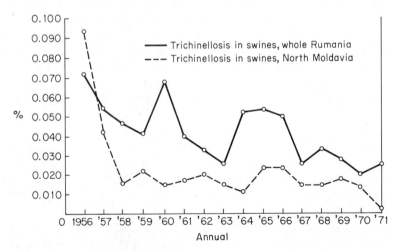

Figure 1 Annual dynamics of trichinellosis in swine in Rumania (1956–1971).

Trichinellosis in Game

Trichinellosis in Wild Boars *(Sus scrofa ferus)*

Trichinella spiralis was detected in 24 of the 12,000 wild boar carcasses examined over the 1956–1967 period (Cironeanu *et al.,* 1965b, Cristescu *et al.,* 1958; Lupascu *et al.,* 1970; Lupu and Cironeanu, 1960). Another 7744 animals were examined during the 1968–1971 period; 22 positives (0.286%) were detected. Most of the infected animals came from the northern parts of Moldavia and Transylvania.

Trichinellosis in Bears *(Ursus arctos)*

Of the 98 bears examined between 1958 and 1967, 10 (10.2%) were positive (Lupascu *et al.,* 1970). The examination of carcasses of another 306 bears shot in the Carpathians during the 1968–1971 period led to the detection of another 20 positives. The infected animals had been shot in the Rodnei, Bistrita, Caliman, Vrancea, Retezat, and Apuseni Mountains.

The prevalence of trichinellosis in dogs and cats examined since 1956 never surpassed 3.4%, while in the 12 wild species of Carnivora and small rodents, all over the country, it reached 13.5% (Cironeanu, 1963, 1964; Lupascu, *et al.,* 1970; Lupu and Cironeanu, 1960). Table I shows the prevalence of trichinellosis in some wild and domestic animals in the north of Moldavia.

Observations Regarding the Epizootiology of Trichinellosis

Recent investigations have pointed out several ecological factors which favor the occurrence of sporadic cases of trichinellosis, and even outbreaks in hogs and other animals (all references).

These observations showed that individually raised hogs were infected

Table I Trichinellosis in Domestic and Wild Animals in North Moldavia (1956–1970)

	Number of Animals		
Species	Tested	Infected	%
Dogs *(Canis familiaris)*	234	21	8.17
Cats *(Felis domestica)*	57	8	14.03
Wild boars *(Sus scrofa ferus)*	48	1	2.08
Bears *(Ursus arctos)*	11	2	18.18
Wolves *(Canis lupus)*	2	2	100.00
Foxes *(Vulpes vulpes)*	102	23	22.55
Martens *(Martes martes)*	10	1	10.00
Wild cats *(Felis silvestris)*	12	1	8.33
Polecats *(Putorius putorius)*	27	5	18.51
TOTAL	503	64	12.72

particularly in the summer and in the fall, when they were left free, in some areas, to feed on the gardens or on pastures near forests, rivulets, and floodland. In these places they could find remnants of rat carcasses or carcasses of domesticated or wild carnivores left on the ground. *Trichinella*-infected hogs were sometimes found near the houses of hunters or of foresters. Sows, particularly those over 2 years of age were more frequently parasite-carriers and to a higher degree than males; this may be due to their higher protein requirements during gestation or nursing period, which induces them to look for meat scraps or to hunt for rats.

The fact that trichinoscopic examination in hogs slaughtered in the rural area was not performed favored the dissemination of this disease in the biotopes incriminated.

Trichinella infection within hog-breeding farms was invariably induced by rats *(Rattus norvegicus)*. It seems that *T. spiralis* strains isolated from rats have a high infectivity for hogs; in some rats the larval density was as high as 1000 parasites per 1 gm muscle (Gherman *et al.,* 1959). The observations showed that once trichinellosis occurred on a hog-breeding farm, with the rat as host, the extent and intensity of the infection increased in both animal species, and could not be eradicated except by total elimination of the rat and hog population.

Trichinellosis infection in rats since 1956, recorded in various areas of the country, reached an average of 5.56%, the highest ratio being registered in rats from slaughterhouses, flaying-houses, rat skin processing plants, or in those captured near animal cemeteries, or even on some hog-breeding farms (Lupu and Cironeanu, 1960). On such farms where intense trichinellosis of hogs assumed a circumscribed character, rodent dynamics were observed over a period of time through caudal markings. It was observed that the rats continued to live in their environment in well-defined colonies, hence the insular aspect of the infection both in rats and hogs. The elucidation of this phenomenon particularly allowed for the complete eradication of trichinellosis outbreaks (Marches, 1972).

Trichinellosis in registered dogs and cats sometimes paralleled infection in the hog population. This phenomenon was more obvious in areas situated in the middle of Moldavia.

The major and permanent reservoir of trichinellosis in Rumania is in the field and forest animals, particularly the Carnivora, in which the prevalence sometimes exceeds 20% (Lupu and Cironeanu, 1960). The examination of the gut contents of 14 wild animal species—Carnivora, Omnivora, Insectivora—showed a very close relationship between the type of feeding and the prevalence of trichinellosis (Almasan *et al.,* 1965). Thus, the carcasses of wild animals shot and left in the fields after skinning, and the remarkable resistance of *Trichinella* in adulterated meat or meat that is submitted to only a mild cold temperature, result in the maintenance and dissemination of trichinellosis outbreaks in nature during the cold season when food is diminished. The presence of the parasite in some small field rodents (up to 12.9% in *Microtus arvalis* and *Pitymys subterraneus*) (Lupu and Cironeanu, 1960), which are assiduously hunted by every domestic and wild Carnivora, contributes to a large extent to the natural dissemination of this disease.

Considering all the ecological factors favoring the maintenance and spreading of trichinellosis in the sensitive animal species, we have constructed the cycle of *T. spiralis* under the natural conditions existing in this country (Fig. 2). In the ruthless fight for life between the various animals, where an endless row of "eaters" and "eaten individuals" are a matter of fact, each parasite-carrier constitutes a link in the epizootiological chain of trichinellosis infection.

The knowledge of the epizootiological situation of trichinellosis allows us to better and more rationally orient ourselves to future measures that would more effectively control this helminthic zoonosis. With this aim in view, the large-scale application of the trichinoscopic examination in rural areas, the introduction of the digestion method using peptone broth for

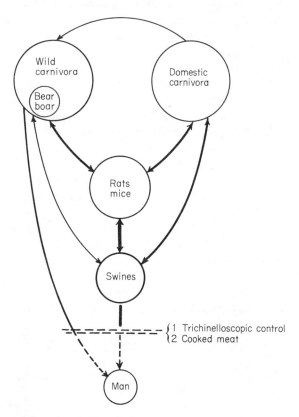

Figure 2 Epizootiological cycle of *T. spiralis*.

hogs slaughtered in large slaughterhouses, and the sanitary education of the population are essential factors of the eradication program.

Summary

Investigations carried out during the last few years (1956–1971) resulted in the accurate assessment of the extent and intensity of trichinellosis in various domestic and wild animal species.

Subsequent to 1956, the prevalence of trichinellosis in hogs diminished to 0.077%, reaching only 0.026% in 1963; after that period the prevalence has remained about the same (0.020%) in 1970, although varying from one zone to another. The monthly data for infected hogs showed a much higher prevalence in the second half of the year. More than 20% of the cases showed massive larval infections. In some mature sows, 4000 larvae were detected per gram of diaphragm muscle. Most of the infected hogs had been bred individually on farms. Rats are the major source of infection, but carcasses of other animals sensitive to *Trichinella spiralis* are also an important source. State farms, and particularly large-scale fattening units with a population of more than 100,000 were generally free from trichinellosis. Hog control within slaughterhouses has been carried out since 1913 through adequate trichinoscopic examinations, while on large-scale units the peptone digestion method is used (tested by I. Cironeanu and M. Cristescu).

Trichinella-induced infections in wild boars assumed a prevalance of 0.2%, while in bears the prevalence of trichinellosis was 6.5%.

In domestic dogs and cats, the prevalence of trichinellosis was not higher than 3.4%, while in another 12 wild carnivorous species as well as in small rodents examined since 1956 (foxes, wolves, wild cats, martens, polecats, badgers, minks, otters, rats, hamsters, and field mice), the prevalence was 13.5%.

These investigations give us a better picture of the distribution of trichinellosis in animals in Rumania, and hence allow us to adopt the best control measures.

References

Almasan, H. *et al.* (1965). Contributii la cunoasterea infestarii animalelor salbatice cu *T. spiralis* in legatura cu hrana consumata. *Microbiol. Parazitol. Epidemiol.* **3**, 267.

Cironeanu, I. (1961). Istoricul si combaterea trichinelozei in tara noastra. *Microbiol. Parazitol. Epidemiol.* **5**, 317–407.

Cironeanu, I. (1963). Factorii care conditioneaza epidemiologia si epizootologia trichinelozei in regiunea Arges. *Microbiol. Parazitol. Epidemiol.* **4**, 345–350.

Cironeanu, I. (1964). The epizootology of trichinellosis in swine and other domestic and wild animals in Romania. *Proc. 1st Int. Congr. Parasitol. Rome* **II**, 664–665.

Cironeanu, I. (1971). Certaines particularites epizootologiques concernant l'infestation a *Trichinella spiralis* chez les porcs. *C. R. 1ᵉʳ Multicolloque Eur. Parasitol. Rennes* **1–4**, 26.

Cironeanu, I. (1972). Some observations on the incidence and intensity of trichinellosis in pigs and edible wild animals. *1st Nat. Conf. Parasitol. Bucharist*, *5–6,* 329.

Cironeanu, I., and Tomutia, H. (1967). Sur un foyer de trichinellose porcine aux implications epidemiologiques. *Helminthologia* **8**, 71–74.

Cironeanu, I., Pitei, G., Sindilaru, F., Calancea, I., Presbitereanu, L., and Vladeanu, I. (1965a). Unele aspecte privind focalitatea trichinelozei la porci si consideratii asupra corelatiei cu focarele naturale. *Microbiol. Parazitol. Epidemiol.* **3**, 266.

Cironeanu, I., Schram, C., Nan, T., and Muica, P. (1965b). Trichineloza la mistreti in Transilvania. *Microbiol. Parazitol. Epidemiol.* **3**, 266 (abstracts).

Cristescu, M., Nistor, T., and Popescu, C. (1958). Frecventa trichinozei la porcii sacrificati in abatorul Bucuresti. *Microbiol. Parazitol. Epidemiol.* **7**, 63–66.

Gherman, I., Marches, G., Popescu, C., Trocan, M., and Sendroiu, I. (1959). Frecventa trichinozei la sobolani. *Prob. Zootech. Vet.* **3**, 57–60.

Lupascu, G., Cironeanu, I., Hacig, A., Pambuccian, G., Simionescu, O., Solomon, P., and Tintareanu, J. (1970). "Trichineloza." *Edit. Acad. Republ. Socialis Romania,* 246 pp.

Lupu, A., and Cironeanu, I. (1960). Ancheta asupra frecventei si raspindirii parazitului *T. spiralis* la animalele domestice si salbatice din Romania. *In.* S.S.M. (ed.), *Zoonoze"* Bucharest, pp. 337-366.

Marches, G. (1972). Contributions to the knowledge of the maintenance bioecological characteristics of the trichinellosis foci by rats. *1st Nat. Conf. Parasitol. Bucharest* **5–6**, 327.

Epizoology and Epidemiology of Trichinellosis in the *U.S.S.R.:* Prospects for Eradication of the Infection

A. S. Bessonov

*The All-Union K.I. Skryabin Institute of
Helminthology, Moscow*

Introduction

Numerous reviews on epizootiology and epidemiology of trichinellosis in the USSR (Koryazhnov, 1948; Kalyus, 1952; Merkushev, 1955, 1965; Berezantsev, 1956, 1963, attempted to give an objective evaluation of the existing situation in this helminth disease. New data were utilized to develop concrete proposals for intensifying prophylaxis and control of trichinellosis.

The above-mentioned reviews resulted in a revision of existing ideas concerning the primary modes of transmission and sources for the distribution of trichinellosis, and the leading role of wild animals, especially carnivores, as reservoirs of trichinellosis (Koryazhnov, 1938, 1948). Former theories on the pathogenesis of the disease were revised and the allergic concept of pathogenesis was substantiated (Kalyus, 1952). It was established that in different zones of the country the main source of infection varied depending on the animals and the factors of transmission (Merkushev, 1955). These theoretical considerations suggested practical measures which brought about a revision of the instructions for the control of trichinellosis.

The latest analysis of the epizootic and epidemiological situation of trichinellosis in the USSR was made by the present author, but the results were only partly published (Bessonov, 1970a, b, c, 1972). The chapter is a short account of the main data on the above-mentioned problem.

Materials and Methods

The material for general conclusions and analyses consisted of published reports and data from veterinary and medical accounts on trichinellosis in the USSR.

Published Reports

More than a thousand published reports from 1865 to 1970 were ana-lyzed in relation to the distribution of trichinellosis among animals (more than 100 species), the incidence of the disease among humans, the dy-namics of the infection rate in man and animals, the sources of infection, and the ways of distribution of *Trichinella spiralis*. Data on the postmortem examinations of human cadavers for trichinellosis were also included.

Veterinary and Medical Accounts

The veterinary and medical accounts on trichinellosis were analyzed for each year during the last 15–20 years. A more precise definition of these data was made by circulating a questionnaire with a request to an-swer a number of specific questions.

Statistical Analysis

A statistical analysis of the data included the calculation of the mean and the mean-quadratic deviations and the significance of differences. The value $P = .05$ was taken as a significant level. The value t_B was calculated according to the student's tables with $N_1 + N_2 - 2$ as the degree of free-dom and $P = .05$. If $t > t_B$, then the mean difference was considered as significant (Kaminsky, 1964).

Results

As a result of examining more than 150,000 animals (excluding pigs), trichinellosis in the USSR was reported in 57 species of wild and domestic animals, including 34 species of carnivores, 14 species of rodents, five species of insectivores, two species of sea mammals, and two species of artiodactyls. The highest intensity of infection was noted among carnivores (51 ±1.24% in *Canis lupus,* 36.58 ±4.34% in *Canis aureus,* 23.7 ±0.959% in *Nyctereutes procyonoides,* 36.26 ±5.04% in *Felis silvestris,* 27.73 ±4.28% in *Martes foina,* 18.4 ±0.430% in *Vulpes vulpes,* and others). The results of examinations of 23,611 domestic dogs *(Canis familiaris)* and 8958 domestic cats *(Felis catus)* demonstrated that they were infected with trichinellosis up to 2.67 ±0.105% and 7.67 ±0.281%, respectively. A cer-tain threat as a source of infection for man and animals is present in the meat of some sea mammals (0.8 ±0.55% of 254 *Odobenus rosmarus* ex-amined, 1.48 ±0.55% of 473 *Phoca groenlandica* examined), and of artio-dactyls (1.3 ±0.214% of 2815 *Sus scrofa* examined).

The highest foci of trichinellosis in pigs were recorded in the Byelo-russian SSR, where more than half of all infected animals were found each year, followed by the Ukrainian SSR and the Russian SFSR (Fig. 1).

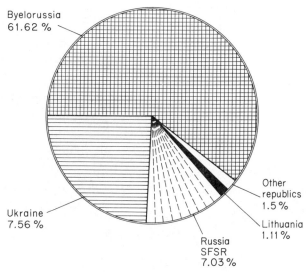

Byelorussia
61.62 %

Other
republics
1.5 %

Lithuania
1.11 %

Ukraine
7.56 %

Russia
SFSR
7.03 %

Figure 1 Comparative data on cases of trichinellosis (percent) in swine in the USSR for 1958–1967

A steady decline in the incidence of infection in pigs in a number of districts of the USSR which were previously considered as very unsafe (Voronezh, Lipetsk, Volgograd, Astrakhan, Kharkov, Zaporozhie, Donetsk, Voroshilovgrad, and other districts) was observed during the last 20–30 years, and in some of them it is not reported at present. This tendency is due to the advances in animal husbandry, a decrease in the wild animal territory, and other social and cultural changes.

The incidence of trichinellosis in man in the USSR was caused in most cases (92.4 ±0.258%) by consumption of pork from pigs slaughtered at home and rarely (2.9 ±0.15%) by consumption of meat from wild animals. More than 80% of the clinical cases of trichinellosis in man were reported from Byelorussia (Fig. 2) which may be explained by the customs and habits of the local population to consume raw, smoked and raw, jerked sausages and ham, to graze pigs in forests, and to slaughter them at home. Three and four-tenths ±0.175% of all trichinellosis cases were derived from consumption of pork imported from other districts with a high incidence of pig trichinellosis.

The above-mentioned sources of infection of man (home slaughter of local pork, imported pork, and meat of wild animals) indicate three seasons of trichinellosis outbreaks in the USSR: winter (the main one), spring–summer (imported pork) and summer–autumn (meat of wild animals).

According to the data from examinations of human cadavers, the infection rate with *Trichinella* larvae was 1.51 ±0.117%. Taking into account the examinations of human cadavers made by the compressor

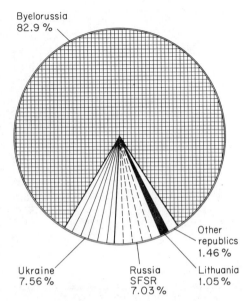

Figure 2 Comparative data on the incidence of trichinellosis (percent) among the population in USSR for 1946–1967

slide method only, the infection rate decreased from 1.5% in 1952 (Kalyus, 1952) to 1.145 ±0.102% in 1969, or by 20%.

The progress in the control of trichinellosis in the USSR may be explained primarily by the fact that the antitrichinellosis measures have a planned and complex character. These measures include the compressor trichinelloscopy of all slaughtered pigs and the technical utilization of *Trichinella*-infected carcasses irrespective of their infected rate and the viability of larvae, the creation of industrial-type farms which practice year-round housing of animals, a reliable thermal decontamination of foodstuffs, and also a wide propaganda program for individual and public prophylactic measures.

Many foci of trichinellosis in Byelorussia, Ukraine, Russian SFSR, and Lithuania have been completely eradicated. The number of *Trichinella*-infected pigs in the USSR in 1971, when compared to 1966, decreased twice (the ratio of infected pigs to total number slaughtered was 1:30,000), in Byelorussia nearly six times (1:10,000) and in Lithuania more than three times (1:300,000).

Discussion

During the last 15–20 years the situation concerning trichinellosis in the USSR was characterized by the following changes. The incidence of pig trichinellosis steadily decreased in Byelorussia, Ukraine, southern Russian SFSR, particularly in Lithuania. The incidence in human infection was decreased. This was confirmed by the examination of human cadavers which were infected during 1952–1969 by 0.355% less than during the preceding 15 years. At the same time isolated outbreaks of trichinellosis in humans occurred more often during the last years because of the consumption of meat from wild animals (wild boars, bears, badgers, and others), particularly in the northern and southern regions of the USSR, and by consumption of imported pork or pork products. This is explained by a significant increase in tourism, amateur hunting, and long distance travel (motor transport, aircraft, and others). The last two factors have lengthened the traditional winter season of trichinellosis outbreaks prolonging it until spring and summer, and in regions of mass tourism, until the end of summer and even autumn. Undoubtedly all this complicates the control of trichinellosis.

An essentially new moment in epizootiology was the rise of the role of caged fur animals and sea mammals in the distribution of trichinellosis. The fur animal husbandry and the sea animal hunting industry are rapidly progressing branches of the USSR national economy. Thus, it is necessary to intensify veterinary and sanitary control on fur animal farms and ships practicing sea animal hunting.

It is evident that the eradication of trichinellosis is possible in densely populated regions because of a sharp limitation in the circulation of *T. spiralis* in nature. This can be accomplished by the regulation of species and population of animals, by supplemental feeding of animals, and by the introduction of several sanitary measures, such as clearing of forests, removal of carcasses, transformation of forests into forest parks and reserve territories, and other methods.

Summary

The incidence of trichinellosis in man and animals and the mode of infection with *Trichinella spiralis* in the USSR have been studied for the last 15–20 years. Trichinellosis has been recorded in 57 species of wild and domestic animals and in man. The highest incidence of infection was found in large carnivores (51% in wolves, and 18.4% in foxes).

Trichinellosis in man and pigs were observed mainly in Byelorussia, where more than half of all the cases of infection in pigs and more than 80% of all the cases of infection in man were recorded. Of the human cases 92.4% were caused by consumption of meat from pigs slaughtered at home and only 3.4% by consumption of meat from wild animals. Three seasons for outbreaks of human trichinellosis were observed: winter (fresh pork after home slaughter), spring–summer (imported pork), and summer–autumn (meat of wild animals). The incidence of trichinellosis in man and pigs has steadily decreased, in cadavers it has decreased by 0.355% during the last 10 years, or by one-fifth when compared with the preceding decade. Some increase in the role of caged fur animals and sea mammals as a source of infection for man and animals is underlined in the present paper. The prospects for eradication of trichinellosis in the USSR are discussed.

References

Berezantsev, Y. A. (1956). "Epidemiology of Trichinellosis." Leningrad.

Berezantsev, Y. A. (1963). "Human Trichinellosis." Leningrad.

Bessonov, A. S. (1970a). Trichinellosis of wild and synanthropic animals in the U.S.S.R. *Tr. Vses. Inst. Gelmintol. Imeni K. I. Skrjabina* **16,** 35–41.

Bessonov, A. S. (1970b). Some problems in epizootiology and prophylaxis of trichinellosis at present. *Tr. Vses. Inst. Gelmintol. Imeni K. I. Skrjabina* **16,** 25–33.

Bessonov, A. S. (1970c). Materials on epizootiology of trichinellosis in USSR. *Byull. Vses. Inst. Gelmintol. Imeni Skrjabina* **4,** 17–20.

Bessonov, A. S. (1972). The peculiarities of zonal distribution of pig trichinellosis in the USSR. *Mater. Dokl. Vses. Konf. Prob. Trichinelleza Tcheloveka Zhivotnykh* (May 30–June 1, 1972), 18–22. *Vilnyus.*

Kalyus, V. A. (1952) "Human Trichinellosis." Moscow.

Kaminsky, L. S. (1964) "Statistical Analysis of Laboratory and Clinical Data." Moscow.

Koryazhnov, V. P. (1938). To the epizootiology of trichinellosis. *Sov. Vet.* (2), 70–71.

Koryazhnov, V. P. (1948). The scientific basis of control of trichinellosis. Tezisy dissertatsii na soiskanie utchenoi stepeni doktora veterinarnykh nauk. *Tr. Gelmintol. Lab. Akad. Nauk SSR* (3), 278–281.

Merkushev, A. V. (1955). The circulation of *Trichinella* infection in nature and in its natural foci. *Med. Parazitol. Parazit. Bol.* **24,** 125–130.

Merkushev, A. V. (1965). 100-th anniversary of examinations for trichinellosis in USSR. *Wiad. Parazytol.* **11,** 229–231.

The Electrohydraulic Effect on *Trichinella spiralis* Larvae in Muscle Tissue

A. S. Bessonov

The All-Union K. I. Skryabin Institute of Helminthology,
Moscow

L. A. Yutkin

The Electrohydraulic Effect Problem Laboratory,
Agrophysical Institute, Leningrad

Introduction

Electric discharges in liquids (EHE) are widely used in industry for processing hard materials (Yutkin, 1955). Positive results with EHE were also demonstrated by the decontamination of helminth eggs and larvae in liquid manure (Tcherepanov, 1971). Although the effect of the EHE on *Trichinella spiralis* larvae in muscle tissues had not been studied previously, one can suppose that it can be destructive. Therefore, the purpose of the present investigation was to study the possibilities of using EHE for decontamination of meat slaughter wastes and animal carcasses used for food for pigs and caged fur animals.

Materials and Methods

The EHE action was studied in two trials on carcasses of rats and cats experimentally infected with *T. spiralis*. Samples of infected muscles each weighing 25 gm (trial 1) were taken from a white rat 3 months after its infection with 2000 *Trichinella* larvae of VIGIS laboratory strain. About 700 encapsulated larvae were found in each gram of muscle tissue. Two samples were divided into pieces (1 × 1 cm) and were treated by EHE. The third sample was left as an untreated control.

Two cats were infected with 4000 *Trichinella* larvae each and were killed 3 months later. The incidence of infection in the carcasses was 1 and 1.5 larvae, respectively, per gram of muscle tissue. These carcasses weighing 550 and 700 gm, respectively (trial 2), were also cut into pieces (1 × 1 cm) and then treated by EHE; 100-gm samples from each carcass were left as untreated controls.

The EHE experimental chambers (reactors) were 5 liters (trial 1) and 9 liters (trial 2) in volume with electrodes in the vertical position.

Treatment Regimes

A regime of 50 kV, 0.1 μF and 1000 or 2000 electric impulses was used in trial 1, and of 50 kV, 1 μF and 2000 or 3000 impulses was used in trial 2. The ratio between muscle volume and liquid volume was 1:50 and 1:8, respectively.

Control Analyses

The sediment collected after EHE was screened under a microscope and the visually undamaged *Trichinella* larvae were counted. The control untreated muscle samples were digested in artificial gastric juice (Bessonov, 1964) and the recovered larvae were counted under a microscope.

To test the infectivity, the visually undamaged larvae from trial 1 were administered to white mice (one mouse for each tested sample); 200 larvae recovered from the control sample were given to the third mouse. All mice were killed 5 days later and their intestines were examined for sexually mature *T. spiralis* by the method of Bessonov (1964).

Results

After the treatment with 1000 impulses in trial 1 a foamy suspension with a temperature of 40° C was formed in the reactor. In the sediment 343 visually undamaged larvae were found, of which 39 had a spiral form and 12 were encapsulated.

After 2000 impulses in trial 1, the suspension was more uniform, the temperature reached 60° C, and the visually undamaged larvae numbered only 122, including six spiral and encapsulated ones. In the control sample in trial 1, 17,265 larvae were recovered of which 45 had a sickle form and were motile after heating (Table I).

Thr treatment of cat carcass with 2000 impulses in trial 2 raised the temperature to 64° C in the reactor. Spirally formed larvae were not recovered in the sediment (only three were undamaged visually and had a sickle form), whereas 98 larvae of which 95 had a spiral form and were motile after heating were recovered in the 100-gm control sample. After 3000 impulses in trial 2 the temperature in the reactor reached 72° C and no undamaged larvae were recovered; 151 larvae of which 149 were motile were recovered in the 100-gm control sample (Table I).

A study of the infectivity of visually undamaged larvae demonstrated that they could not establish themselves in mice intestines, i.e, the mice did not harbor any sexually mature worms at necropsy. However, 36 males and 48 females of adult worms were recovered from the intestine of the control mouse.

Table I Action of EHA on *Trichinella spiralis* Larvae in Muscle Tissue

Weight (gm) of sample (carcass)	EHE treatment regime	Muscles/liquid phase ratio	Duration of EHE treatment	Temperature in the reactor after treatment	Number of larvae after EHE treatment	
					Total of visually undamaged	Spiral forms
Trial 1 (rat carcasses)						
25	50 kV, 0.1 μF, 1000 impulses	1:50	4 min, 35 sec	40°C	343	39
25	50 kV, 0.1 μF, 2000 impulses	1:50	8 min, 50 sec	60°C	122	6
25[a]	–	–	–	–	17,265	17,220
Trial 2 (cat carcasses)						
550	50 kV, 1 μF, 2000 impulses	1:8	8 min, 15 sec	64°C	3	0
100[a]	–	–	–	–	98	95
700	50 kV, 1 μF, 3000 impulses	1:8	13 min, 23 sec	72°C	0	0
100[a]	–	–	–	–	153	149

[a] Control samples, not treated with EHE.

Discussion

The EHE treatment regime used in trial 1 destroyed most *Trichinella* larvae in muscle tissues and those which appeared to be visually undamaged were unable to establish themselves in mice intestines.

EHE exerts its action on live objects in many ways. Besides powerful waves and cavitation these objects are subjected to intimate contacts with discharge plasma, to high temperatures in the discharge canal, to ultraviolet irradiation, and to other factors. Apparently, the action of these complex factors on the *Trichinella* larvae can account for the loss of their infectivity despite their undamaged appearance.

The regimes tested in trial 1 were hardly optimal in respect to their power, number of electric impulses, and the ratio between treated samples and liquid phase (1:50). This was confirmed by the better results with practically all larvae destroyed in trial 2 in which the mass of muscles and bones was considerably greater (22 and 28 times) and the ratio between the mass and liquid phase was smaller (1:8). Moreover, the longer periods of treatment (8 min, 15 sec and 13 min, 23 sec) and the higher temperatures in the reactor (64° and 72° C) guaranteed a reliable killing of morphologically undestroyed larvae.

A valuable quality of EHE is its powerful and destructive action on solid objects such as bones. In all tested regimes the bones were destroyed faster and more completely than soft parts of the carcasses; they were transformed into the finest sandlike particles.

Our trials demonstrated that EHE can be used for decontamination of *Trichinella*-infected meat, slaughter and kitchen meat scraps. The advantage of this method over the present chemical methods (treatment with acid and alkaline solutions) and physical methods (treatment with high and low temperatures, vacuum drying, and others) is in the rapidity of decontamination (a few minutes) and in the fact that the resulting product retains the valuable properties of raw meat important for use as food for caged fur animals.

References

Bessonov, A. S. (1964). A trial of artificial immunization of animals against trichinellosis and the use of precipitating sera for diagnosing this helminthosis by Ascoli's method. *Wiad. Parazytol.* **10,** 691–715.

Tcherepanov, A. A. (1971). A study of electrohydraulic effect on helminth eggs and larvae. Theses of reports on the symposium of young scientists in agriculture. *Anim. Husb. Vet. Sci. Leningrad Oct. 1971,* pp. 63–65.

Yutkin, L. A. (1955). "Electrohydraulic Effect." Mashgiz, Moscow–Leningrad.

The Importance of Differentiating *Trichinella spiralis* for the Prophylaxis of Trichinellosis

V. A. Britov

Division of Regional Epizootiology
Far-Eastern Research Institute of Veterinary Science
Blagoveshchensk

Introduction

During the last decade, the problem of *T. spiralis* strains was widely discussed in the world literature, but no convincing diagnostic criteria were available. This hampered the understanding of the fact that trichinellosis in wild carnivores was found everywhere and in swine only in certain places.

For the identification of *Trichinella* species we used the method of interbreeding of *Trichinella* larvae in white mice and we also studied their specificity in relation to the host.

Materials and Methods

For interbreeding purposes we used *Trichinella* recovered from wild and domestic animals from Eurasia, Africa, and North America. Twenty-three strains were examined: two from *Nyctereutes procyonides* from Amur district, one from *Alopex lagopus* from Magadan district, two from *Gulo gulo* from Kamtchatka district, one from *Ursus (Thalarctos) maritimus* from Canadian Arctic region, one from *Ursus arctos* from Primorye province, five from *Vulpes vulpes* from the Sakhalin and Kunashir Islands, Mordevia, Tataria, and Odessa district, two from the domestic cat and dog from the Primorye province, two from *Vulpes corsac* from Kazakhstan, one from *Crocuta crocuta* from South Africa, five from domestic pigs from Primorye and Krasnodar provinces, Byelorussia, United States, and Canada, and one from a man from the Primorye province. The interbreeding procedure has been published earlier (Britov, 1971a).

Furthermore white mice, white rats, rabbits, guinea pigs, cats, dogs, and domestic pigs were infected with *Trichinella* recovered separately from wild animals and domestic pigs.

Results

All strains recovered from a man and domestic pigs interbred successfully and produce a fertile progeny: these strains did not interbreed with *Trichinella* recovered from wild and other domestic animals. *Trichinella* from a spotted hyena from South Africa and from a fox from the Odessa district interbred and produced a fertile progeny; these strains did not interbreed with *Trichinella* recovered from other wild animals, but ocassionally interbred with those from domestic pigs and produced a small number of larvae which were partly or completely infertile.

All strains recovered from wild and domestic animals, except domestic pigs, a spotted hyena from South Africa, and a fox from the Odessa district, interbred successfully and produced a fertile progeny.

During host-specificity studies of different *Trichinella* strains, it was established that *Trichinella* from wild animals from Eurasis and North America had a low virulence rate in pigs and rats and a high one in carnivores. *Trichinella* from a wolf from Mordovia, a raccoon dog from the Amur district, and a polar fox from Magadan district were administered to 14 pigs with a dose of 10–20 specimens per gram of live weight. Six pigs did not become infected and the other 8 had a weak infection of 1–60 larvae per gram of muscle tissue. In muscles of infected pigs all the *Trichinella* larvae perished quite quickly from cellular reaction and phagocytic resorption. Most larvae perished during the second month after the infection. Ninety to 130 days after infection no larvae could be found in the pig muscles. In rabbits the death and phagocytosis of all larvae took place during 1½ years after infection and in rats it took less time. However, in dogs the larvae were viable and infective for more than 7 years.

Trichinella from South African hyena administered to domestic pigs, rats, rabbits, and dogs produced approximately the same host–parasite relationship. The host–parasite relationships were entirely different in animals administered with *Trichinella* recovered from domestic pigs. All 12 pigs administered larvae from domestic pigs from Byelorussia, Krasnodar province, and Canada with a dose of 10–20 larvae per gram of live weight became infected. The incidence of infection was high (1000–12,000 larvae per gram of muscle); the larvae developed unhindered in the pig muscle and preserved their infectivity for 2 years and 9 months (period of our observation). Rabbits, cats, mice, and rats became severely infected with this strain and the infective larvae were viable in them during practically the entire life of the host.

On the basis of these data on the interbreeding studies of different *Trichinella* strains and studies of host–parasite relationships, we concluded that in nature there exist at least three biological units of *Trichinella*, named at first as varieties (Britov, 1971b), and later raised to the species rank (Britov and Boev, 1972).

Discussion

In our studies we started with the data of Nelson *et al.* (1963), Zimoroi (1963) and Kruger *et al.* (1969) which demonstrated that *Trichinella* larvae recovered from various animal species from different geographic zones had different virulence for laboratory animals and pigs. This fact gave grounds to suppose the presence of different genotypes in *Trichinella*. The method of interbreeding of *Trichinella* larvae recovered from different animal species has made it possible to discover the genetic isolation of three *Trichinella* units. At present there are enough data to assume the existence of at least three species in the genus *Trichinella*. *Trichinella spiralis* (Owen, 1835) is peculiar to domestic pigs and also to some synanthropic animals. *Trichinella nativa* (Britov and Boev, 1972) parasitizes mainly wild carnivores of the northern hemisphere higher than 40° north latitude. *Trichinella nelsoni* (Britov and Boev, 1972) is widely distributed in wild carnivores of Africa and Asia to the south of 40° north latitude.

From the evolutionary aspect, *T. spiralis* is the youngest species of *Trichinella*. If the appearance of *T. nativa* is dated as Miocene during the flourishing of Carnivora, and of *T. nelsoni* a little later in Pleiocene, *T. spiralis* became isolated about 6000–7000 years ago after the domestication of wild pigs. The isolation and stabilization of *T. spiralis* as a separate species in pigs could not take place spontaneously in nature because the speciation required numerous passages through pigs only. This became possible only after the domestication of wild pigs and intensive pig breeding in pig breeding areas. The synanthropic foci of trichinellosis appeared and still exist. The development of exchange and trade favored further distribution of locally stabilized *T. spiralis* all over the world in pigs and pig products. It took root only in those places where there was a direct transmission of infection from pig to pig through products of slaughter or kitchen wastes. Such conditions were available and are now present in Byelorussia, the Ukraine, the southern part of Krasnodar province, and also in Poland, the United States, Canada, and several other countries with intensive pig breeding.

Pigs were brought to the New World from Eurasia, and with the pigs *T. spiralis* was transported also. The factors of transmission of trichinellosis remained the same as in Europe since the immigrants arrived with their old habits and traditions. In this regard the greatest attention must be paid to synanthropic foci by finding *T. spiralis,* destroying it, and publicizing the scientific information on factors of transmission of this helminth.

The wild carnivores infected with *T. nativa* and *T. nelsoni* do not take any part in the propagation of trichinellosis among pigs and consequently cannot hinder the elimination of trichinellosis in settled areas.

Summary

Three species of *Trichinella* exist in nature. They do not interbreed (genetically isolated) and they are specific in relation to a definite number of hosts. *Trichinella nativa* and *T. nelsoni* parasitize wild carnivores, but they are not specific in relation to swine. *Trichinella spiralis* is the true agent of trichinellosis in swine. The identification of *Trichinella* species may contribute to the general scheme of trichinellosis control.

References

Britov, V. A. (1971a). Results of interbreeding of *Trichinella spiralis* from wild animals with *T. spiralis* from pigs. *Dokl. Vses. Ordena Lenina Akad. Selsko-q khoz. Nauk Imeni V. I. Lenina* (2), 40–41.

Britov, V. A. (1971b). Biological methods of determination of *Trichinella spiralis* (Owen, 1835) varieties, *Wiad. Parazytol.* **17,** 477–480.

Britov, V. A., and Boev, S. N. (1972). Taxonomic rank of different strains of *Trichinella spiralis* and the characteristics of its circulation. *Vest. Akad. Nauk Kazakhskoi SSR* (4), 27–32.

Kruger, S. V., Collins, M. H., van Niekerk, J. W., McCully, R. M., and Basson, P. A. (1969). Experimental observations on the South African strain of *Trichinella spiralis Wiad. Parasitol.* **15,** 546–554.

Nelson, G. S., Guggisberg, C. W. A., Mukundi, J. (1963). Animal host of *Trichinella spiralis* in East Africa. *Ann. Trop. Med. Parasitol.* **57,** 332–346.

Zimoroi, I. Y. (1963). The changes in the virulence of *Trichinella spiralis* during their passages from carnivores into rodents. *In: "Gelminty Tcheloveka, Zhivotnykh i Rastenii i Borba s Nimi,"* 71–74.

Trichinellosis in California: A 52-Year Review

Donald O. Lyman

Center for Disease Control
Health Services and Mental Health Administration
Public Health Service, USPHEW
State of California Department of Public Health
Berkeley, California

Introduction

The State of California Department of Public Health has been collecting case reports on human trichinellosis since 1920. It became a reportable disease in 1930. This paper reviews the collected data for the past 52 years (1920–1971). Reliability in this circumstance is as questionable as any semivoluntary reporting system. But several new patterns found are of note.

Materials and Methods

Case report forms submitted to the State of California Department of Public Health from 1920 through 1971 were reviewed. Two different case report forms were used during the interval studied. From 1920 through 1954 a postcard form for reporting "an infectious disease" was used. It requested limited information: name, address, age, sex, date of clinical onset, date of diagnosis or first doctor visit. From 1955 through 1971 a specific trichinellosis case history form was used. It included the same general questions as the card but added specific space for clinical description, serologic tests, biopsy reports, skin test, and remarks.

Results

Table I lists the number of reported cases in 5-year intervals since 1920. In 1930–1934 we find the greatest number of cases. Before 1930

Table I Reported Trichinellosis Cases, California,
1920–1971

Year of onset	Number of cases
1920–1924	24
1925–1929	155
1930–1934	341
1935–1939	278
1940–1944	215
1945–1949	131
1950–1954	166
1955–1959	38
1960–1964	63
1965–1969	40
1970–1971	41
TOTAL	1492

reporting was voluntary; there are fewer cases in those years. Following 1930 the number of cases drops off year by year with some variation. In the first 2 years of this decade (1970–1971) only 41 cases are known to us. The distribution of cases by age has changed in the last 20 years (Fig. 1). In the 1920–1949 period, the mean age reported was 31 years; from 1950–

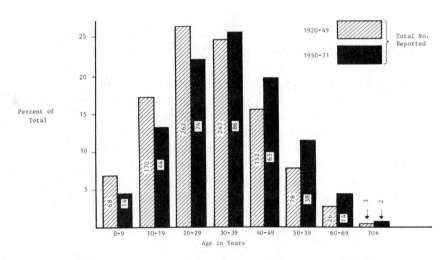

AGE DISTRIBUTION OF REPORTED TRICHINOSIS CASES
IN CALIFORNIA, 1920-49 AND 1950-71

Age Not Recorded in 118 (8%) of Reported Cases

Figure 1 Age distribution of reported trichinellosis cases in California, 1920–1949 (hatched column) and 1950–1971 (solid black bar). Age not recorded in 118 (8%) of reported cases.

1971 the mean age reported was 35 years. This difference is the reverse of the changing age pattern of the state as a whole. Census data show a slightly lower average age in California in 1950 as compared to 1940 (Brunsman, 1952; Truesdell, 1943). The sex ratio of 53% males was fairly constant throughout the 52-year period surveyed.

A definite seasonal pattern was present from 1920 through 1944 which was reversed in the period 1945 through 1971 (Fig. 2). More than 66% (613/919) of cases reported in 1920–1944 had clinical onset during the fall and winter months, September through February. Forty-two percent occurred in winter alone. From 1945–1971, 62% (188/467) had onset during the spring or summer months, March through August.

The source of infection was recorded for 730 cases (49% of total) and of that number 572 noted the location of preparation of the food item (Table II). Whole meat in the form of pork or ham accounted for 37% (273/731) of the total; 72% infected by whole meat ate home prepared food. Pork products in the form of sausage, salami, and bacon accounted for 54% (394/731) of the total; 50% of these were reportedly infected by commercially prepared pork products. Home cured bear meat was responsible for 44 cases; 12 of those occurred in 1971 in connection with two separate outbreaks. The pattern of high infection and outbreak rates for eaters of home prepared whole meats and eaters of commercially prepared pork products is constant through each decade of this survey.

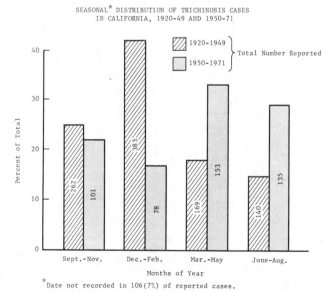

SEASONAL* DISTRIBUTION OF TRICHINOSIS CASES
IN CALIFORNIA, 1920–49 AND 1950–71

*Date not recorded in 106(7%) of reported cases.

Figure 2 Seasonal distribution of trichinellosis cases in California, 1920–1944 (hatched column) and 1945–1971 (gray column). Date not recorded in 106 (7%) of reported cases.

Table II Food Sources of Trichinellosis Cases and Outbreaks[a] in California, 1920–1971

Year of disease onset	Cases	Outbreaks	Home prepared						Commercially prepared						Preparation site unknown					
			Pork[b]		Pork products[c]		Other[d]		Pork		Pork product		Other		Pork		Pork product		Other	
			C[e]	OB[f]	C	OB	C	OB	C	OB	C	OB	C	OB	C	OB	C	OB	C	OB
1920–1929	49	11	31	3	12	2	4	1	2	0	0	0	0	0	0	0	0	5	0	0
1930–1939	351	55	94	13	36	5	22	3	6	0	99	21	0	0	24	2	66	11	4	0
1940–1949	127	22	12	3	12	1	0	0	3	0	36	6	0	0	30	4	32	8	2	0
1950–1959	66	8	20	2	10	1	5	2	5	1	22	2	4	0	0	0	0	0	0	0
1960–1969	99	13	36	6	17	2	0	0	5	1	36	4	5	0	0	0	0	0	0	0
1970–1971	38	4	4	0	11	1	16	3	1	0	5	0	1	0	0	0	0	0	6	0
TOTAL											198	33	10	0	54	6	98	24	6	0
TOTAL by source			C = 342; OB = 48						C = 230; OB = 35						C = 158; OB = 30					
TOTAL	730	113																		

[a] Two or more persons infected by same food items.
[b] Pork or ham.
[c] Sausage, salami, bacon.
[d] Bear, hamburger, chow mein.
[e] C, Individual cases.
[f] OB, Number outbreaks involving all or some of individual cases

For 115 histories reporting incubation period the mean was 13.4 days, the median 8 days, and the range 0–72 days. Elevation of the percentage of eosinophils in the peripheral blood count, positive skin test, the presence of larvae in a muscle biopsy, and the finding of antibodies by serologic methods all support a diagnosis of trichinellosis. Ninety-three percent of cases reported after 1955 had at least one of these four tests reported. Of the total cases in this period, 27% had only one of the four tests performed as part of the diagnostic procedure; 43% had two; 18% had three; 5% had all four. Table III lists the reported results of these four tests. Unfortunately, no criteria are stated for positivity of skin test and muscle biopsy on the forms used. Three different serologic tests have been reported: complement fixation, latex agglutination, and flocculation. Few reports ststed that acute and convalescent sera had been drawn.

Discussion

The 1930s was the period of the Great Depression in this country when pork was an inexpensive food item, the population was largely rural, garbage feeding of pigs was commonplace, and much of the meat was home prepared. During the 1945–1949 period economic conditions were markedly improved, the population was shifting from rural to urban with greater reliance on commercially prepared meats. The decrease in human trichinellosis may reflect the changing demographic and economic conditions. During this period as well, more and more California pig raisers were feeding only cooked garbage or grains to the animals as protection against the pig disease vessicular erythema; human benefit from decreased numbers of trichinous pigs may be regarded as a "spinoff" (or incidental) benefit.

There was a change in seasonal incidence. We should like to think the lower fall–winter numbers represent decreased reliance on home-grown meat sources for winter foodstuffs. After all, individuals who slaughter and prepare their own meats are not as reliably careful as large inspected commercial concerns. But we are at a loss to explain the new spring–summer pattern. Perhaps city folks are picnicking more with inadequately cooked pork on open campfires.

Of particular interest is the present importance of wild bear meat as a source of human trichinellosis. In 1970–1971 this source accounted for 39% (16/41) of cases reported.

Since 1920, 44 deaths have been reported as due to trichinellosis. Only 5 of the 44 have occurred since 1950. The food source of 80% was home prepared food, usually whole meat in the form of pork, ham, or wild bear meat.

Table III Diagnostic Test Results of Trichinelosis Cases Reported in California

Test	Period during which test was reported	Number of cases for whom test was performed	Percent reported as positive	Comments
Eosinophilia	1929–1971	196	100	Mean reported value: 32% Range of reported values: 4–90%
Skin test	1935–1971	135	78	1% reported as "done"
Muscle biopsy	1925–1971	97	74	
Complement fixation serology	1946–1971	51	75[a]	Acute/convalescent sera drawn for 6 cases of whom 5 had diagnostic titer rise.[b] Titer range 1:4–1:160
Latex fixation serology	1962–1971	42	86[a]	Acute/convalescent sera drawn for 4 cases all of whom had diagnostic titer rises.[b] Titer range 1:5–1:10, 240
Flocculation serology	1955–1971	91	90*	Acute?/convalescent sera drawn for 12 cases of whom 8 had diagnostic titer rise.[b] Highest median titer per case 1:80

[a] Demonstrable antibody present.
[b] Fourfold rise in titer or "negative to positive" reported.

Summary

Trichinellosis is now a rare disease in California. During the past 20 years the disease pattern has changed to spring–summer predominance among persons in their 30s. In the last 2 years meat from wild bears has become a major disease source in California.

References

Brunsman, H. G. (1952). 1950 U.S. Census of Population, Vol. II, General Characteristics, California, 1950 Population Report P-B5. U.S. Government Printing Office, Washington D.C.

Truesdell, L. E. (1943). 16th Census of the United States: 1940, Population Volume, II. U.S. Government Printing Office, Washington D.C.

Physical Methods for Rapid On-Line Detection of *Trichinella* in Pork

John D. Seagrave and Dale M. Holm

Los Alamos Scientific Laboratory,
University of California
Los Alamos, New Mexico

Introduction

A pilot study has been initiated to evaluate the feasibility of applying new technology and instrumentation toward ultimate development of rapid on-line screening for the presence of *Trichinella spiralis* in pork. The style of presentation of this paper is intended to illuminate some stimulating activity at an interdisciplinary interface, and to illustrate some solorful new methods of looking at an old problem.[1]

Digestion

Figure 1 shows what might be involved in automating the digestion process. We will not describe this scheme in detail except for the final stages. One needs the stages shown: excystment, filtration, staining, further filtration, identification of the stained larvae, sorting, and verification. Since the several stages differ in amount of time required, they are shown as process loops on discs. These would be synchronized so that sample identity can be maintained. The filtrate containing larvae stained with a fluorescent dye passes into a tube system. When a larva passes through a blue laser or mercury lamp beam, the fluorescence is detected by a photocell, and after a suitable delay, the slug of fluid containing the larva is diverted by a fast-acting fluid switch into a jar or onto filter paper, where the count and identification can be recorded after operator verification. A suitable fluid switch is under development, and carbol fuchsin has been found to be a specific, rather weakly fluorescent stain.

---

[1] In the original presentation a number of color slides were shown which have been replaced here by monochrome photographs.

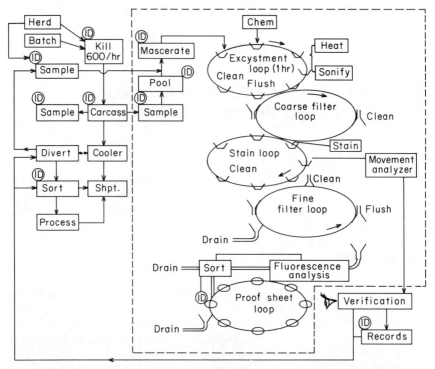

Figure 1 Schematic diagram of a system for automation of the digestion process.

Before leaving this illustration, we wish to point out a box marked Movement Analyzer at an intermediate stage. This idea will later be described in detail, but note that if active larvae are present in the digestate, even before staining, their motion will be communicated to the more visible tissue debris. Motion sensing at this point could either serve to shorten the process, or its absence could be used to preclude processing of inactive samples. We have found, however, that excystment can be greatly accelerated *if* the larvae may be killed in the process. In this case, either formic acid or sodium hypochlorite works better than more concentrated artificial gastric juice. Also, pepsin does not seem to be necessary. Sonification and introduction of the fluid in fine jets are useful techniques. The flow-fluorimeter stage is a scaled-up version of the flow microfluorimeter technique developed at Los Alamos (Van Dilla *et al.,* 1969) and elsewhere for rapid monitoring of cell suspensions.

Figure 2 shows an excysted larva amid the tissue debris, stained with carbol fuchsin. It is quite possible that the larvae in a flow system could be distinguished from debris of this contrast in character, *without staining,* by analysis of the electronic pulse shape of the light scattered or absorbed when the material flows past a laser beam. In that case an inexpensive red

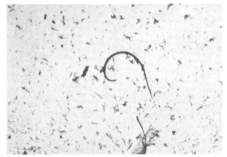

Figure 2   Excysted larva in digestate, stained with carbol fuchsin.

laser could be used. Although the debris has taken up some of the stain, it does not fluoresce at the excitation wavelength optimal for the larval fluorescence. Figure 3 shows the dark-field fluorescence of the stained larva. This is not the same field, but it serves to illustrate the absence of fluorescent debris.

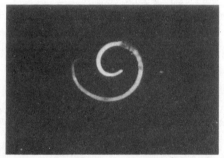

Figure 3   Dark-field fluorescence of a larva stained with carbol fuchsin. Exciting wavelength has been chosen to suppress fluorescence of the tissue debris.

Motion Sensing

Figure 4 is a diagram of the basic idea of motion sensing using television techniques. A single frame is *stored*—either by videotape, videodisc, or storage tube—and at a later time the stored picture signal is mixed in a subtractive mode with a new frame. The circuit shown as a comparator then provides an output which contains information only where the two frames differ, namely, where something has moved. This scheme is widely used industrially for intruder surveillance. A stored picture of a shop is compared with the continous "live" picture. If a thief or animal enters or even if a bottle of pop explodes, the monitor will immediately reveal the

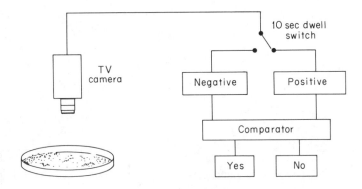

Movement analyzer

Figure 4 Schematic diagram of motion sensing using television techniques.

action. The idea is the electronic equivalent of superimposing an altered film negative over a positive film print.

Figures 5–8 illustrate this concept. Figure 5 shows a bottle with a number of particles in suspension being magnetically stirred. When this picture and another taken a moment later are run through the comparator, the output is Fig. 6: the bottle has vanished but the moving contents remain. In Fig. 7 the bottle is back, but the fluid is now loaded with only a few

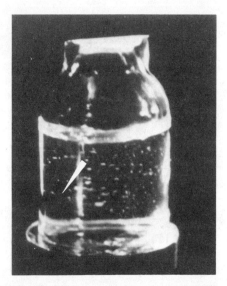

Figure 5 Live T.V. image of a bottle showing heavy concentration of moving particles in the contained fluid. (Courtesy of W. M. Herbener, Princeton Electronic Products, Box 101, Princeton, New Jersey.)

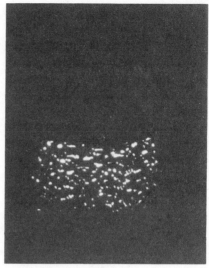

Figure 6 Image of Fig. 5 processed to delete nonmoving background of bottle. (Courtesy of W. M. Herbener, Princeton Electronic Products, Box 101, Princeton, New Jersey.)

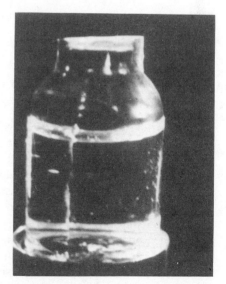

Figure 7 Bottle with low-level particle concentration. (Courtesy of W. M. Herbener, Princeton Electronic Products, Box 101, Princeton, New Jersey.)

particles, which are not readily seen in the normal picture. With the same
magic, Fig. 8 now reveals the moving bits. We do not need to belabor the
many possible applications of this technique not only in parasitology, but

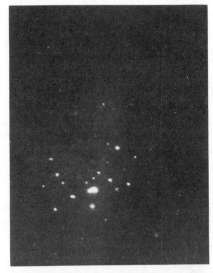

Figure 8 Figure 7 processed to reveal particles. (Courtesy of W. M.
Herbener, Princeton Electronic Products, Box 101, Princeton, New Jersey.)

to the dynamic physiology and pathology of any living subject scanned in
a television-raster format.

Scanning

Let us next consider how we might automate the compression method
(Fig. 9). As before, we want a sample-handling system with provision for
identification and feedback, but we need discuss only the components of
the monitoring station. We may see illustrated schematically a compressed
specimen scanned in a television-raster format by a laser beam. The light
transmitted is detected by a photocell, and the electrical signal passes
through a Scan Converter which prepares it for display as a television picture. When an anomaly of interest is detected, an alarm alerts the operator; he may study either the image on the screen or the tissue itself through
a microscope. The sample would be automatically repositioned for examination of the fields of interest selected by the system.

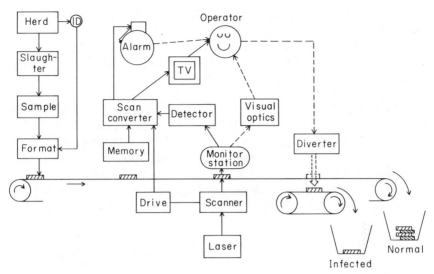

Figure 9 Schematic diagram of a system for automation of the compression method.

Laser Scanning

Before explaining the formation of the Scan Converter, let us first show why a laser beam offers more than a bright light source. In Figure 10, a piece of trichinellous tissue has been clarified with Oil of Clove, which approximately matches the optical index of refraction of the muscle tissue but not that of the capsule wall or the larval cuticle. A phase-contrast microscope would make these discontinuities much more distinctive, but these are also places where a *ray* of light would be refracted (bent away

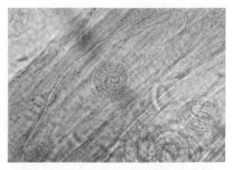

Figure 10 Trichinous tissue clarified with Oil of Clove. Ordinary illumination.

from the incident direction). This point is further illustrated in Figure 11. A laser beam is naturally highly collimated, and the beam may be optically compressed to a diameter of a few microns (μm) if desired. A light detector may be similarly collimated with lenses and diaphragms. For simplicity, the laser and collimated detector are shown fixed in space, and the sample is to be imagined as being translated across the beam. An inclusion which absorbs part of the beam will have the effect of reducing the detector signal by an amount which is nearly independent of the depth of the inclusion (exactly so if the bulk tissue is uniformly absorbing). Because of the high degree of of collimation a refractive index discontinuity may refract the beam entirely out of the detector. For discontinuities sufficiently marked to do this, the effect is also independent of depth. Thus such a scan has *a*

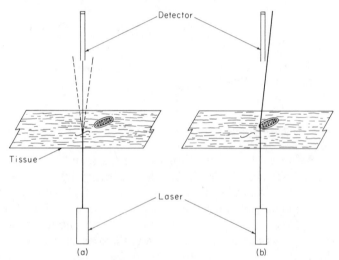

Figure 11 Diagram of laser-beam transmission through compressed tissue detected by a collimated detector. (a) Absorption and scattering; (b) refraction at a discontinuity in optical index.

large depth of field, limited only by the bulk tissue absorption, just as for an X-ray. A centimeter thickness of tongue or diaphragm can be compressed to 2 mm without crushing cysts and remain sufficiently translucent, at least for red laser beams. With ordinary illumination, scattered light appears elsewhere in the field of the retina or television camera and washes out contrast. The laser beam is readily polarized (naturally so in some lasers) to take advantage of any birefringence present in the tissues. It may be noted that laser light is *coherent* and thus capable of revealing interference between a portion of the incident light and the transmitted light. Moreover, if a portion of the optical path (*viz.,* the larva) *moves,* the Doppler effect in the interfering beams is capable of the most exquisite sensitivity to the velocity of the motion—5μm/sec motion in the direction of the laser beam would give an audible pitch. If the beam were stopped on a suspicious anomaly, the heat input might serve to induce motion of a larva. Very much simpler techniques are expected to suffice in a practical field instrument.

Scan Conversion

In order to store a T.V. picture for the motion-sensing application one needs some sorm of memory. Video tape loops or a videodisc could serve, but standard units have more capacity (and a corresponding price) than is required. For a mechanically scanned laser, the scanning rate would have to be much slower than the T.V. image rate and the image would have to be built up at the scanning rate for subsequent repetitive readout at the T.V. rate. Storage-tube devices would be suitable for this purpose, though they have a limited signal-to-noise ratio. A special form of storage tube called a Moving Target Indicator provides internal cancellation of identical portions of two input frames, and thus serves to combine the functions of two Scan Converters and Comparator.

Color Enhancement

A well-known application of artificial color enhancement is in medical infrared thermography for differential diagnosis of mammary tumors or disturbed blood supply patterns. Similar use of such enhancement is helpful in interpreting infrared aerial photographs. With this type of equipment the intensity or "gray-scale" seen by the television camera is divided into a number of bands which are assigned contrasting colors on a display monitor. We are planning to use a densitometric T.V. camera[2] and a flexible image analyzer[3] to study the effect of tissue treatment and scanning arrangements to optimize recognition of *Trichinella* in tissue. The following series of figures were obtained with such equipment; these are based on normally illuminated speciments.

Figure 12 shows several larvae "developed" by the silver iodide technique (Gould, 1970). If such natural contrast were practicable we would not need much help in finding the cysts, but the process is too slow and fussy for on-line automation. It will serve to introduce a color-enhanced image of the same field, shown in Fig. 13. The strip across the top indicates

[2] Camera model 201/C supplied by Antech, Inc., Box 297, Harwood Station, Littleton, Mass.

[3] Color-enhanced illustrations for this paper courtesy of M. D. Buchanan, Interpretation Systems Incorporated, Box 1007, Lawrence, Kansas.

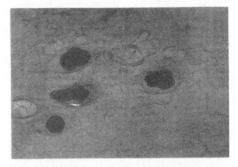

Figure 12 Larvae stained with the silver iodide technique. Note the empty cysts at the left and at the center.

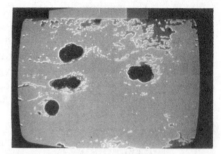

Figure 13 Enhanced image of Fig. 12. In the color original the background was dark blue, the cysts bright red, and the borders and other details yellow.

the coloration of the optical density bands on a scale from light at the left to dark at the right. Figure 14 illustrates yet another type of presentation, an isometric or pseudo-three-dimensional array of the actual T.V. signals. One of the 525 lines has been brightened and we may follow the trace up over the dark stained cyst and down in the region of an empty cyst. This type of presentation is more effective if one can manipulate the controls to rotate and skew the display in real time. The selected line shown brightened is available for more detailed examination on a separate display oscilloscope.

Figure 15 is a conventionally fixed and stained thin section of trichinous tissue which shows the characteristic eosinophillic infiltration. In the corresponding enhanced image (Fig. 16) the controls have been set to color the larval turns yellow, the eosinophils green, and to drop out everything else. The yellow blob in the middle is an artifact corresponding to an extraneous dark blemish on the slide. Figure 17 is a sample stained with a red-on-red Delafield stain of only moderate contrast. In the enhanced image (Fig. 18) we have colored most of the cyst areas red but retained in green a low-contrast version of the rest of the normal field for

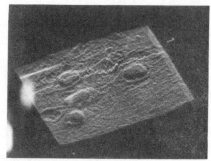

Figure 14 Pseudo-three-dimensional image of the field of Fig. 12 created by skewing the T.V. video line signals. A selected line has been intensified for study.

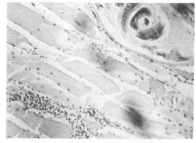

Figure 15 Thin, fixed section of trichinous tissue with conventional hematoxylin and eosin staining, showing sectioned cyst at the upper right, and characteristic eosinophilic infiltration.

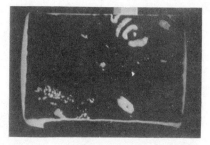

Figure 16 Enhanced image of Fig. 15. In the original the larval turns were yellow and eosinophils green. The blob at lower right is an artifact present in Fig. 15.

better orientation. Finally, the last example (Fig. 19) is a specimen stained with a combination of iodine and carbol fushsin; in Fig. 20 this appears as a distinctive group of red cysts with yellow fringes on a black field, and in Fig. 21, as red cysts with blue background and the intermediate shade *suppressed,* as indicated by the band at the top of the picture.

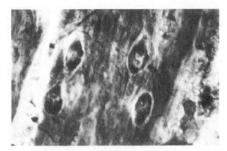

Figure 17 Thick section of tissue with Delafield stain.

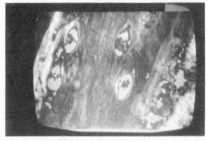

Figure 18 Enchanced image of Fig. 17. In the original the darkest cyst areas were colored bright red, with a low-contrast image of Fig. 17 retained in green.

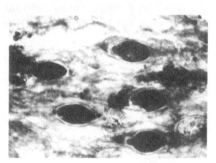

Figure 19 Thick section stained with iodine and carbol fuchsin.

Costs

All of the equipment described is commercially available. A complete color-enhancement system of camera, analyzer, and display can be obtained for between $8000 and $9000. Suitable lasers would cost between $100 and $1000; scanners between $500 and $4000, depending on speed; detectors and optics, $200–$1000; scan converters, $2500–$3500; and a

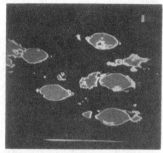

Figure 20 Enhanced version of Fig. 19 with background suppressed. In the original the cyst areas were bright red, with edge details in yellow.

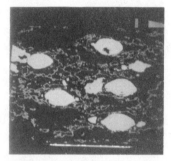

Figure 21 Enhanced version of Fig. 19 with intermediate edge areas suppressed. In the original the cysts were bright red and the tissue background was dark blue.

comparator, $1000. A complete system with all the features described can be assembled for under $20,000. A simplified field station with simplified electronics, but *including* sample preparation and handling, might also cost about $20,000.

Summary

With the long-range goal of development of instrumentation for auto-mated on-line screening of pork for the presence of *T. spiralis* larvae at a level of one larva per gram and at a testing rate of one hog every 10 sec, a pilot study is in progress to apply modern physical technology toward achieving this goal.

For automation of the digestion method, an accelerated excystment technique followed by specific fluorescent staining of the larvae is planned to prepare the filtrate for processing by a liquid flow fluorimeter system which will electronically recognize fluorescent flashes from the larval fragments as they flow past the exciting lamp, and subsequently divert the material giving such signals to a proof sheet by means of an electronically controlled fluid switch for visual confirmation.

For automation of the compression method, the compressed clarified samples are to be scanned past a laser beam while the absorption or scattering of the light is recorded by an electronic Scan Converter for T.V.-screen presentation. Gray-scale image enhancement by contrasting color contouring (electronic staining) will be applied to facilitate recognition. When a significant location is encountered, the scan can be repositioned to fix on that location for operator visual confirmation.

In both basic approaches, an additional technique of motion sensing will be investigated using the "intruder-surveillance" concept where two television scans separated in time are compared in such a manner that only the differences are presented on the screeen.

Acknowledgment

Work was performed under the auspices of the U.S. Department of Agriculture and the U.S. Atomic Energy Commission.

References

Van Dilla, M. A., Trujillo, T. T., Mullaney, P. F., and Coulter, J. R. (1969). Cell microfluorometry: A method for rapid fluorescence measurement. *Science* **163**, 1213.

Gould, S. E. (1970). "Trichinosis in Man and Animals." Thomas, Springfield, Illinois, p. 174.

Trichinellosis Surveillance in the United States

Myron G. Schultz and Dennis D. Juranek

Center for Disease Control
U.S. Public Health Service,
Atlanta, Georgia

Prior to 1965 cases of human trichinellosis were reported on an annual basis to the Center for Disease Control (CDC) by individual state and territorial health departments. In 1965 trichinellosis was included among the notifiable diseases that are reported weekly to CDC through the National Morbidity Reporting System (NMRS). Reports of fatal cases were obtained from the National Center for Health Statistics, Vital Statistics Division, U.S. Public Health Service.

In 1967, a comprehensive surveillance system for trichinellosis was initiated to supplement the NMRS report and to gather detailed epidemiologic information on each case. A Trichinosis Surveillance Case Report Form was developed to standardize this data. This form is completed by state and territorial health department personnel and submitted to the Parasitic Diseases Branch. Bureau of Epidemiology, CDC. In addition to the Trichinosis Case Reports, new cases of trichinellosis are disclosed through continuous reviews of Trichinosis Serology Reports from the Parasitology Section, Laboratory Division, CDC.

We recognize that surveillance for trichinellosis is far from perfect. Many infections are mild or asymptomatic and frank disease may be misdiagnosed or unreported. Nevertheless, this crude index is the best means available for determining the incidence of trichinellosis in the United States and would, we believe, detect any significant outbreak in this country. Table I shows the number of cases and deaths due to trichinellosis that have been reported to CDC from 1947 to 1971.

It is readily apparent that there has been a substantial decline in the incidence of trichinellosis in the United States during the past two decades. This finding is supported by a comparable decline in the prevalence of trichinellosis in humans as reported by Zimmerman *et al.* (1973). The majority of trichinellosis cases reported in the United States comes from two adjacent geographic areas, the New England states and Middle Atlantic

Table I Reported Trichinellosis in the United States, 1947–1971

Year	Cases	Deaths
1947	451	14
1948	487	15
1949	353	9
1950	327	9
1951	393	10
1952	367	10
1953	395	7
1954	277	1
1955	264	4
1956	262	5
1957	178	4
1958	176	4
1959	227	3
1960	160	3
1961	306	7
1962	194	1
1963	208	5
1964	198	1
1965	199	3
1966	115	3
1967	67	0
1968	84	1
1969	192	0
1970	109	3
1971	115	3

states. No seasonal trend in the incidence of trichinellosis has been apparent. The mean age of patients has been 34.8 years and the sex distribution of cases has been essentially equal.

Our surveillance data indicate that pork products account for 78% of the cases of trichinellosis reported in the United States. In those cases where a food product was specifically implicated, 63% were associated with improperly prepared sausage. Recently trichinellosis acquired from the consumption of wildlife has increased; 7.8% of the cases reported to CDC during the past 5 years were attributed to the ingestion of bear meat. Only a minority of cases (6.9%) were attributed to pork products prepared and consumed on farms. The majority of cases (85.3%) have been attributed to pork products purchased from commercial sources.

A summary of the diagnostic information from 567 cases of trichinellosis reported to CDC during the past 5 years is as follows:

A total of 462 (81.5%) cases underwent serologic testing, 172 (30.3%) received muscle biopsies, and 119 (21.0%) received both a serologic examination and a muscle biopsy.

Serologic tests were positive on 394 (85.3%) of the 462 specimens submitted. The variable which has not been accounted for is time. Sufficient time for antibody development may not have elapsed before blood was drawn on the 68 individuals who did not demonstrate antibody to *T. spiralis*. False positives may result from previous infections.

Muscle biopsies were positive in 131 (76.2%) of 172 instances. Biopsies may be negative when: (1) they are performed too early in the course of infection, (2) infection is mild, or (3) an inadequate number of microscopic serial sections are examined. Positive biopsies require careful interpretation since they may indicate either recent or past infection.

Of the 119 persons who received both a serologic examination and a muscle biopsy, 70 (58.8%) were positive by both tests; 31 (26.0%) were serologically positive but had negative biopsies; 14 (11.8%) were biopsy positive but serologically negative; and 4 (3.4%) were both biopsy and serologically negative.

The dates of consumption of trichinous meat and onset of illness were available for 316 of the 567 cases. The mean incubation period was 12.3 days. In 352 cases the mean period between the date of onset of illness and a serologic diagnosis was 27 days.

References

Zimmermann, W. J., Steele, J. H., and Kagan, I. G. (1973). Trichiniasis in the U.S. population. 1966–70, prevalence epidemiologic factors. *Health Serv. Rep.* **88,** 606–623.

Prevalence and Distribution of *Trichinella spiralis* in Carnivorous Mammals in the United States Northern Rocky Mountain Region

David E. Worley, J. Carl Fox, John B. Winters

Montana State University

Kenneth R. Greer

Montana Fish and Game Department
Montana

Introduction

The occurrence of *Trichinella spiralis* in the human population and in swine in the United States has been studied periodically since the latter part of the nineteenth century. However, the existence of wildlife reservoirs of the infection and their relationship to the disease in man in North America are poorly understood. Surveys in Iowa (Zimmermann and Hubbard, 1969), Colorado (Olsen, 1960), and Alaska (Rausch *et al.,* 1956) have indicated that a sylvatic cycle exists in a variety of wild mammals which in some cases have little or no contact with domestic sources of infection. The present study was designed to determine the prevalence of *T. spiralis* in native carnivores from rural or wilderness areas in Montana, Idaho, and Wyoming where swine, rats, and domestic garbage generally are absent.

Materials and Methods

Efforts were made to obtain tissue samples from the major carnivorous species native to the survey area. This includes the region extending from Yellowstone National Park, Wyoming north along the Rocky Mountain chain to Glacier National Park in northwestern Montana, and west to the Salmon River drainage in central Idaho. Carcasses of grizzly and black bears were made available by the Montana Fish and Game Department, the National Park Service, and the Fish and Wildlife Service. Various fur-bearing and predatory mamals were provided by biologists and commercial trappers. Many of the mountain lions were collected in central Idaho by

Dr. Maurice Hornocker of the Idaho Cooperative Wildlife Research Unit. Specimens collected between 1966 and 1972 form the basis for this paper.

Tissues were removed from many of the hosts shortly after death. In some instances, carcasses were refrigerated or frozen for several months before the tissues were removed and processed. Samples of tongue, masseter, diaphragm, and femoral muscle were examined routinely when the entire carcass was available. If only the head was submitted, tongue and masseter were examined. Approximately 25 gm of each tissue were digested when available. Samples were cut into small pieces with scissors and in most instances were comminuted with an Omnimixer before they were digested in a solution of 0.7% HCl and 0.8% pepsin. After 12–20 hr. at 37° C under constant agitation, the digested material was washed on a 150- or 200-mesh screen to remove fine debris. The retained material was examined for *Trichinella* with a dissecting microscope; results were expressed as larvae per gram of host tissue (LPG).

Results

The prevalence and intensity of *T. spiralis* infections in 371 individuals representing 15 species of mammals is shown in Table I. The grizzly bear *(Ursus arctos)* was the most commonly infected host, followed in order of prevalence by the mountain lion *(Felis concolor)*, wolverine *(Gulo gulo)*, fisher *(Martes pennanti)*, coyote *(Canis latrans)*, bobcat *(Lynx rufus)*, striped skunk *(Mephitis mephitis)*, black bear *(Ursus americanus)*, marten

Table I Prevalence and Intensity of *Trichinella spiralis* in Wild Mammals from Montana, Idaho, and Wyoming

Host	% Infected	Av. Intensity of Infection (Range)[a]
Grizzly bear	57.7 (75/130)	46.6 (0–708)
Black bear	11.9 (5/42)	18.1 (0–26)
Mountain lion	54.5 (36/66)	3.1 (0–21)
Bobcat	17.2 (5/29)	36.4 (0–351)
Marten	8.3 (2/24)	23.5 (0–46)[b]
Fisher	40.0 (2/5)	1.16 (0–4)
Wolverine	50.0 (3/6)	11.2 (0–31)
Striped skunk	16.6 (1/6)	0.07 (0–1)
Badger	0 (0/2)	–
Long-tailed weasel	0 (0/2)	–
Mink	0 (0/14)	–
River otter	0 (0/1)	–
Red fox	7.1 (2/28)	43.4 (0–67)
Coyote	25.0 (2/8)	0.05 (0–0.1)
Raccoon	0 (0/8)	–

[a] Based on larvae per gram of tongue except as noted.
[b] Based on larval concentrations in diaphragm and thigh.

(Martes americana), and red fox *(Vulpes vulpes)*. No infections were found in the badger *(Taxidea taxus)*, long-tailed weasel *(Mustela frenata)*, mink *(Mustela vison)*, river otter *(Lutra canadensis)*, or raccoon *(Procyon lotor)*, although limited numbers of these species were examined.

In relation to food habits and ecological relationships of the host, trichinellosis was most prevalent in bears (46.5%). Of the infected grizzly bears, approximately half originated in Yellowstone or Glacier National Park or environs. In both parks, the presence of open-pit garbage dumps for disposal of food scraps and other domestic refuse from lodges and campgrounds created a quasi-urban situation within the bears' habitat where artificial sources of food were readily available. Prior to 1968, no attempts were made to prevent bears from using these dumps as summer foraging areas, with the result that domestic garbage provided a significant portion of the diet of many bears within the parks (Craighead and Craighead, 1971). For this reason, garbage-fed bears could be considered an ecological equivalent of garbage-fed swine so far as transmission of *T. spiralis* is concerned. This analogy, may be reflected in the frequency with which grizzly bears taken in park areas were infected: 45.1%. However, the prevalence of *T. spiralis* in bears collected in wilderness areas in north-central and western Montana, where contact with man or domestic animals is at a minimum, was 58.4%. Furthermore, the average concentration of larvae in the tissues of wilderness bears was 59.02 LPG, compared with 32.01 LPG in park bears. These trends strongly suggest that the availability to bears of infected sources of food was inversely proportional to their degree of association with "civilization." In Alaska, Rausch *et al.* (1956) found 10 of 20 grizzly (brown) bears from widely scattered localities to be infected.

The composite percentage of infection in the mountain lion, fisher, marten, and wolverine was 42.5%. Thus, infections occurred almost as frequently in species from remote wilderness areas which subsist primarily by scavenging or predation on other wildlife as in bears in national parks, where access to domestic garbage was widespread. In farm and rangeland mammals, including the red fox, coyote, bobcat, striped skunk, badger, raccoon, and mink, the composite prevalence of infection was 10.5%.

Based upon the concentration of encysted larvae in the tongue, grizzly bears harbored the most intensive infections of the 10 positive species: 46.6 LPG (Table I). Next in order of larval concentration were the red fox, bobcat, marten, black bear, wolverine, mountain lion, fisher, striped skunk, and coyote, respectively. Using both prevalence and intensity of tissue infections as indices of exposure and/or susceptibility, the grizzly bear ranked highest among the positive hosts. Wolverine and bobcat also ranked high according to these criteria. Infections in the fisher, coyote, and skunk were relatively common but of low intensity, based on limited evidence.

A comparison was made of predilection sites of *Trichinella* larvae in a

series of 42 grizzly bears in which two or more tissues were examined from
each animal. In order of larval density, tongue ranked first (46.1 LPG),
followed by femoral muscle (17.1 LPG), masseter (14.2 LPG), and diaphragm (10.3 LPG). In the black bear, mountain lion, and wolverine,
tongue also had the highest concentration of *Trichinella* larvae among the
tissues examined, whereas in the bobcat, masseter was the preferred site. In
other host species, the data were inadequate to determine areas of maximum larval concentration.

Discussion

The widespread distribution of trichinellosis in wild carnivores from
a variety of ecosystems (rangeland, farms, river valleys, public parks, and
high mountains) suggests that some commonly occurring and generally
available food source(s) is involved in the epidemiology of the infection in
the study area. The high prevalence of *T. spiralis* in grizzly bears and
mountain lions from wilderness areas suggests that prey species such as
rodents or lagomorphs might be involved in the cycle as maintenance
hosts. Domestic rats (*Rattus* spp.) are absent in most of the survey area,
but voles (*Microtus* spp.), deer mice (*Peromyscus* spp.) ground squirrels
(*Spermophilus* spp.), pine squirrels (*Eutamiasciurus* sp.), and pocket
gophers (*Thomomys* sp.) occur throughout the region at most altitudes
where infected carnivores were collected. In Alaska, Rausch *et al.* (1956)
found natural infections in a variety of native rodents, including voles,
lemmings, ground squirrels, and pine squirrels. In addition, infected snow-
shoe hares were found in one locality (Rausch *et al.,* 1956). The latter species is an important food item for the mountain lion in Idaho (Hornocker,
1970), where a third of the animals sampled harbored *Trichinella*.

The high percentage of *T. spiralis* infection in mountain lions from
various other localities scattered throughout the study area indicates that
lions are one of the important hosts for this nematode in the northern
Rocky Mountain region. Most of the infected animals originated from
locations west of the Continental Divide in Montana and in Idaho. Previous
observations on the occurrence of trichinellosis in *Felis concolor* were
reported by Winters (1969).

The wide distribution and moderately high prevalence of *T. spiralis* in
black bears in western Montana and Wyoming (11.9%) contrasts with the
sporadic occurrence of *Trichinella* in *Ursus americanus* from other areas
of the UnitedStates. Harbottle *et al.* (1971) reported *Trichinella* in 1.3%
of 372 black bears from Maine, New Hampshire, New York, Pennsylvania,
Vermont, and West Virginia during the period 1967–1969. Babbott and
Day (1968) found no positives among 35 bears taken in Vermont in 1964–
1965, although they did refer to an outbreak of human trichinellosis traced
to a black bear shot in Vermont in 1963. In New York, three of 45 black

bears were found infected (King *et al.*, 1960). Two and one-half percent of 364 bears from Arizona, California, Colorado, Idaho, Michigan, Minnesota, New Mexico, Oregon, Wisconsin, and Wyoming were positive (Zimmermann, 1972, personal communication).

The possibility exists that the unusually high level of *T. spiralis* infection in black bears in the present study was a result of the rather unique situation in Yellowstone and Glacier Parks where grizzly and black bears inhabit the same territory. All black bear infections were in Park animals, where the prevalence of the infection in grizzly bears was approximately 45%. Bears are known to feed on carrion, including carcasses of other bears when available (Rausch *et al.*, 1956). The frequency of trichinellosis in bears as well as coyotes and wolverines in this study points to the probability that scavenging is an important factor in the transmission of the parasite in Rocky Mountain carnivores. The role of scavenging in the epidemiology of the infection in European mammals has been pointed out by Madsen (1961).

Although direct infection of humans with *T. spiralis* from wild sources seldom occurs in the United States, one recent outbreak involving 23 persons which resulted in 12 clinical cases was traced to the consumption of trichinous meat from a black bear taken in northern Idaho (Gnaedinger *et al.*, 1971). The public health significance of the sylvatic form of the infection appears to lie largely in the inability to eradicate the etiologic agent from the environment in areas where diversified populations of wild carnivores occur.

Acknowledgments

The cooperation of the Montana Fish and Game Department, the National Park Service, Montana and Idaho Cooperative Wildlife Research Units, and the Division of Wildlife Services of the Bureau of Sport Fisheries and Wildlife in supplying animals for examination is gratefully acknowledged. We are also indebted to Marvin Donahue, Bob Savage, and Dr. W. L. Jellison for providing animal carcasses or tissues, and to Richard H. Jacobson and Nelson Samuel for technical assistance during the laboratory phase of the study.
This study was a joint contribution from the Veterinary Research Laboratory, Agricultural Experiment Station, Bozeman, Montana, and Federal Aid in Wildlife Restoration, Montana Project W-83-R, Paper No. 395, Journal Series.

References

Babbott, F. L., Jr., and Day, B. W., Jr. (1968). A survey of trichinosis among black bears in Vermont, *Arch. Environ. Health* **16**, 900–902.
Craighead, J. J., and Craighead, F. C., Jr. (1971). Grizzly bear-man relationships in Yellowstone National Park. *BioScience* **21**, 845–857.
Gnaedinger, E. E. *et al.* (1971). Epidemiologic notes and reports. Trichinosis—

Idaho and California. *Cent. Dis. Control Morbidity Mortality Weekly Rep. Jan. 9*, p. 8.

Harbottle, J. E., English, D. K., and Schultz, M. G. (1971). Trichinosis in bears in northeastern United States. *Health Serv. Mental Health Admin. Health Rep.* **86**, 473–476.

Hornocker, M. G. (1970). An analysis of mountain lion predation upon mule deer and elk in the Idaho Primitive Area. *Wildl. Monogr.* (21), 39.

King, J. M., Black, H. C., and Hewitt, O. H. (1960). Pathology, parasitology and hematology of the black bear in New York. *N.Y. Fish Game J.* **7**, 99–111.

Madsen, H. (1961). The distribution of *Trichinella spiralis* in sledge dogs and wild mammals in Greenland. *Medd. Gronland* **159**, 1–124.

Olsen, O. W. (1960). Sylvatic trichinosis in carnivorous mammals in the Rocky Mountain region of Colorado. *J. Parasitol.* **46** (Suppl.) 22.

Rausch, R. L., Babero, B. B., Rausch, R. V. and Schiller, E. L. (1956). Studies on the helminth fauna of Alaska. XXVII. The occurrence of larvae of *Trichinella spiralis* in Alaskan mammals. *J. Parasitol.* **42**, 259–271.

Winters, J. B. (1969). Trichiniasis in Montana mountain lions. *Bull. Wildl. Dis. Ass.* **5**, 400.

Zimmermann, W. J. and Hubbard, E. D. (1969). Trichiniasis in wildlife of Iowa. *Amer. J. Epidemiol.* **90**, 84–92.

The Current Status of Trichinellosis in the United States

W. J. Zimmermann

Veterinary Medical Research Institute
Iowa State University
Ames, Iowa

Introduction

The trichinellosis problem long has been a major blemish on the pork industry and public health image of the United States. Nearly a century ago, many countries placed embargoes on the importation of United States pork because of the trichinellosis problem in swine. Most of these embargoes still persist. Stoll (1947) estimated that the United States had three times the number of human cases as the rest of the world together. In light of the relatively advanced public health and technologic progress in this country it is surprising that such occurrences failed to stimulate development of specific control or eradication program. Only recently has consideration been given to the possible development of such a program with implementation still pending.

Even with this inattention, the trichinellosis problem has decreased markedly in recent decades. This report, based on recently completed national human and swine trichinellosis studies, will briefly review these changes.

Human Beings

The changing problem can best be exemplified by the downward trend in human prevalence. Numerous studies carried out during the 1930s and 1940s indicated an overall prevalence of about 16% in cadavers examined at autopsy. A major study by the National Institutes of Health (Wright *et al.*, 1943, 1944) during 1936–1941, included 5313 human diaphragms

603

from 37 states and the District of Columbia. Trichinellae were detected in 16.1%. The prevalence by geographic areas varied from 18.5% in the Pacific region to 10.0% in the Mountain region. Other significant epidemiologic findings included: (a) relatively high infection rates for all age groups, 18.3% for those 45 years and older and 12.6% for those under 45 years; (b) 45% of the infected diaphragm samples contained live trichinellae, an indication of "recent" infections; and (c) the infection rates for those of Italian (29.7%) and German ancestry (28.3%) were nearly double the overall rate while the 2.1% prevalence for those who are Jewish reflected their general abstinence from pork.

The above findings of three decades ago contrast markedly with the results obtained in a recent, statistically designed national study carried out at the Veterinary Medical Research Institute (VMRI), Iowa State University, during 1966–1970 (Zimmermann *et al.,* 1968; 1973). Diaphragm samples were obtained from 48 states and the District of Columbia. Trichinellae were detected in only 4.1% of 8071 diaphragms examined, a reduction of nearly 75% in three decades. Regionally, the problem is now centered in the Middle Atlantic (5.5%), Pacific (5.5%), and New England (5.2%) areas. Prevalences in other regions ranged from 3.0% to 3.8%. States with prevalences of 6% or more include: Oregon, 8.3%, New Jersey, 7.7%; Maine, 6.9%; and Washington, 6.1%.

An age differential was noted with an infection rate of 4.8% for individuals 45 years and older and 1.8% for those under 45 years. Only 14% of the infected diaphragms contained live trichinellae, which are indicative of "recent" infections.

Any study based on deaths has an inherent bias in regard to age. Therefore, in order to obtain a truer estimate of the current problem, the prevalences for each 10 year age-grouping was multiplied by the actual population for this group. This yielded an estimate that 4,400,000 individuals or 2.2% of the current population has detectable *Trichinella* infections. Similar estimates for prevalences with live trichinellae indicates that 1,490,000 individuals, or 0.73% of the population, are infected with live trichinellae. If the average life span of trichinellae in the musculature is estimated at 5–10 years, 150,000 to 300,000 individuals are infected yearly.

By comparison, similar estimates for the 1936–1941 National Institues of Health study would indicate that 12% of the 1940 population, or 15,900,000 individuals, was infected with trichinellae. Of these, 9,675,000 individuals, or 7.3% of the population had live trichinellae in their diaphragms. Again based on an estimated 5–10 year life span for trichinellae, between 1 and 2 million infections were being acquired each year.

The infections detected in the Veterinary Medical Research Institute (1966–1970) study were generally of light intensity; 37.9% of the positive diaphragms contained less than one *Trichinella* per gram while another 5.19% contained 1–10/gm. Only 2.1% contained more than 50/gm. Prevalence again was related to national extraction with rates of 10.7% for Italian ancestry and 9.2% for Germans. In contrast to marked decreases for other characteristics, the prevalence for Jewish sample declined only slightly to 1.6%.

The trend in clinical cases has paralleled findings in prevalence studies (Schultz and Juranek in Part VI, this volume). A yearly average of 404.5 cases was reported during 1947–1950, 339.2 during 1951–1955, 200.6 for 1956–1960, 221 for 1961–1965, and only 113.4 for 1966–1970. In 1971, 115 cases were reported.

Swine

The downward trends in prevalence cited for humans are a reflection of parallel changes in the disease problem of swine. Farm-raised swine, which comprise 98.5% of the nation's swine production, had an infection rate of 0.95% in the 1930s (Schwartz, 1962). This decreased to 0.63% in 1948–1952. Studies during 1961–1965 revealed a prevalence of 0.12% in farm-raised butcher weight pigs and 0.22% in breeder swine (Zimmermann and Brandly, 1965). An apportioned study by Zimmermann and Zinter (1971) during 1966–1970 yielded a prevalence of 0.125%, indicating that the prevalence rates may have leveled off. Although the rates were similar for 1961–1965 and 1966–1970 studies, certain other differences were noted. The latter study indicated increased intensity of infection, greater herd involvement, and increased concentration of the problem in the major hog-producing regions. These findings, along with the highest yearly prevalence of the decade in 1970, may possibly indicate a potential increase in the problem.

Garbage-fed swine, long considered the primary reservoir for the disease, present an even more dramatic decrease. Studies on raw garbage-fed swine by Schwartz (1962), during the 1930s, had a prevalence rate of 5.7%; this increased to 11.0% in 1950. A nationwide outbreak of vesicular exanthema, a viral disease of swine, during 1952 resulted in legislation requiring the cooking of garbage before feeding to swine. The prevalence then decreased to 2.2% during 1954–1959. After eradication of vesicular exanthema, Zimmermann and Brandly (1965) noted an upswing in prevalence to over 5%. However, a national hog cholera eradication program initiated in 1962 placed further emphasis on cooking of garbage. The prevalence then decreased to 0.5% in 1964–1966 and 1966-1970 studies (Jefferies *et al.* 1967; Zimmermann and Zinter, 1971).

Current Problem

Based on current production and prevalence data, about 105,000 farm-raised and 6000 garbage-fed pigs are marketed yearly with *Trichinella* infections, giving about 40 million potential human exposures. Federal regulations requiring the destruction of trichinellae in ready-to-eat pork products in conjunction with home cooking or freezing reduce the public health hazard markedly, resulting in an estimated 150,000–300,000 human infections per year. Most of these are nonclinical, although some may be misdiagnosed, resulting in about 115 reported clinical cases.

Wildlife

Comparatively few studies have been made to determine the trichinellosis problem in wildlife. In an Alaskan study by Rausch *et al.* (1956) involving 2433 animals, trichinellae were isolated from 23 of 42 species examined. Species with high prevalence rates included polar bear, 52.9%; grizzly bear, 50.0%; wolverine, 50.0%; red fox, 40.8%; ermine, 35.3%; wolf, 33.1%; lynx, 23.5%; and black bear, 21.7%.

A 1953–1968 study of 11,162 wildlife specimens in Iowa, by Zimmermann and Hubbard (1969), revealed trichinellae in 15 native species. Prevalences of over 5% were reported for fox, dump rat, and mink. Infected species were found throughout the state. Since Iowa produces nearly 25% of the nation's swine, this natural reservoir presents an important potential source of trichinellosis for swine if poor management practices are utilized.

Although wildlife studies from other parts of the United States are limited and often involve only a single species, they do indicate that the wildlife trichinellosis problem persists throughout the country.

With decline of trichinellosis in swine, bear meat is gaining increased significance as a direct source of human trichinellosis; 7.8% of the clinical cases in humans reported during the past 5 years were attributable to ingestion of bear meat (Schultz and Juranek, in Part VI, this volume). A recent study by Worley *et al.* (Part VI, this volume) in Montana and neighboring states revealed a prevalence of 58% in grizzly bear and 12.6% in black bear. A prevalence of 1.3% has been reported for bears from Northeastern United States (Harbottle *et al.,* 1971). A study in progress by the author involving bears from 10 states indicates reservoirs in California and Wisconsin.

Discussion

Although it is recognized that the trichinellosis problem is still of major importance in the United States and that control and eradication must still be accomplished, much of the stigma attached to this country by the trichinellosis problem has now been removed. A decrease in prevalence of more than 75% has been noted for swine and human beings in recent decades; clinical cases have similarly decreased. Although the prevalence in swine, the primary indicator of the problem, is still higher than that reported from most countries of the world, in some cases this may be attributable to methodology. The digestion procedure, used as the primary diagnostic tool in the studies cited, may detect many infections that are missed by routine trichinoscopic methods, as indicated by the findings in the Netherlands (Ruitenberg and Sluiters, in Part VI, this volume).

It is noteworthy that the reductions in the problem have occurred without the benefit of a specific control program. The reductions reflect the side benefits on nontrichinellae oriented programs and developments in recent decades. The primary change would be in swine management. Swine production is now a major agricultural industry. Life-span feeding programs are the rule, often carried out under complete confinement. Commercial garbage feeding has sharply decreased while the feeding of unofficial garbage occurs only occasionally. The vesicular exanthema and hog cholera eradication programs, with emphasis of proper cooking of garbage, sharply reduced the problem. The use of freezers, both domestically and commercially, has rapidly expanded. The Wholesome Meat Act enacted in 1967 as an amendment to the Federal Meat Inspection Act, greatly increased the number of establishments under Federal or equivalent regulations. Home or nonregulated processing of pork products has decreased sharply.

There is evidence that the influences of the above programs and developments have now waned, indicating the problem will not disappear by itself. The prevalence in swine has remained stable during the past decade; in fact, the high prevalence in swine during 1970, along with increased intensity of infection may be the forewarning of a potential upswing in the problem. Therefore, immediate attention must be given to the development and implementation of a control program with a goal of eventual eradication. The pork industry is now cognizant of the problem and supports the need for a control program such as developed for consideration by the USDA. Slaughterhouse diagnosis, followed by destruction of trichinellae in infected carcasses, provides the base for the proposed program. Epidemiologic traceback of infected swine to farm of origin also would be a key feature. The pooled sample method (Zimmermann, 1968; Andrews et al., 1970) has been the diagnostic procedure incorporated in the proposed program, but if serologic or physical tests prove safe and economical, these could be readily utilized.

Summary

During the 1930s and 1940s, trichinellosis was of major health significance in the United States. Prevalences of about 16% were obtained at human autopsy, while rates for swine approximated 1% in farm-raised and

5.0% in garbage-fed. Recently completed national studies for humans and swine indicate that the problem has decreased markedly in recent decades.

The examination of 8071 human diaphragms, obtained in a statistically designed study during 1966–1970, revealed a prevalence of 4.2%. Weighting of the observed prevalence by population within age groups indicates that approximately 2.2% of the current population has detectable trichinellae infections; 0.73% is estimated to have live trichinellae, indicative of "recent" infections.

A similar reduction in the problem has been noted for swine. A 1966–1970 study revealed a prevalence of 0.125% in 20,003 farm-raised butcher swine and 0.5% in garbage-fed swine. Although these prevalences represent a decrease from three decades previously, comparison with a 1961–1965 study indicates a leveling off in prevalence rates. The 1966–1970 study also indicates an increase in intensity of infection, more herd involvement, and increased concentration of the disease in farm-raised swine of the North Central regions.

An estimated 111,000 swine are infected each year in the United States, resulting in at least 40 million potential meal exposures. Meat inspection regulations, home cooking, and freezing reduce this potential to 150,000–300,000 human infections and about 110 reported clinical cases per year.

Acknowledgment

These studies were supported in part by grants E606 and AI06658 from the Public Health Service, and Cooperative Agreement No. 12-14-100-5259(93) with the Meat and Poultry Inspection Service, United States Department of Agriculture.

References

Andrews, J. S., Zinter, D. E., and Schulz, N. E. (1970). Evaluation of the trichinosis pilot project. *Proc. 73rd Annu. Meet. U.S. Animal Health Ass., Millwaukee, Wisconsin,* pp. 332–353.

Harbottle, J. E., English, D. K., and Schultz, M. G. (1971). Trichinosis in bears in northeastern United States. *Health Serv. Mental Health Admin. Health Rep.* **86,** 473–476.

Jefferies, J. C., Beal, V., Jr., Murtishaw, T. R., and Zimmermann, W. J. (1967). Trichinae in garbage-fed swine. *Proc. 70th Annu. Meet. U.S. Livestock Sanit. Ass. Buffalo N.Y.* pp. 349–357.

Rausch, R. L., Babero, B. B., Rausch, R. V., and Schiller, E. L. (1956). Studies on the helminth fauna of Alaska. XXVII. The occurrence of larvae of *Trichinella spiralis* in Alaskan mammals. *J. Parasitol.* **42,** 259–271.

Schwartz, B. (1962). Trichinosis in the United States. *In:* Z. Kozar (ed) "Trichinellosis," *Proc. 1st Int. Conf. Trichinellosis,* Warsaw, pp. 68–75.

Stoll, N. R. (1947). This wormy world. *J. Parasitol.* **33,** 1–18.

Wright, W. H., Kerr, K. B., and Jacobs, L. (1943). Studies on trichinosis. XV. Summary of the findings of *Trichinella spiralis* in a random sampling and other sampling of the population of the United States. *Pub. Health Rep.* **58**, 1293–1313.

Wright, W. H., Jacobs, L., and Walton, A. C. (1944). Studies on trichinosis. XVI. Epidemiological considerations based on the examination for trichinae of 5,313 diaphragms from 189 hospitals in 37 states and the District of Columbia. *Pub. Health Rep.* **58**, 669–681.

Zimmermann, W. J. (1968). A pooled sample method for post-slaughter detection of trichiniasis in swine. *Proc. 71st Annu. Meet. U.S. Livestock Sanit. Ass. Phoenix, Arizona, pp.* 358–366.

Zimmermann, W. J., and Brandly, P. J. (1965). The current status of trichiniasis in U.S. Swine. *Pub. Health Rep.* **80**, 1061–1066.

Zimmermann, W. J., and Hubbard, E. D. (1969). Trichiniasis in wildlife of Iowa. *Amer. J. Epidemiol.* **90**, 84–92.

Zimmermann, W. J., and Zinter, D. E. (1971). The prevalence of trichiniasis in swine in the United States, 1966–70. *Health Serv. Mental Health Admin. Health Rep.* **86**, 937–945.

Zimmermann, W. J., Steele, J. H., and Kagan, I. G. (1968). The changing status of trichiniasis in the U.S. population. *Pub. Health Rep.* **83**, 957–966.

Zimmermann, W. J., Steele, J. H., and Kagan, I. G. (1973). Trichiniasis in the U.S. population, 1966–70, prevalance epidemologic factors. *Health Serv. Rep.* **88**, 606–623.

The Modified Pooled Sample Method for Post-Slaughter Detection of Trichinellosis in Swine

W. J. Zimmermann

Veterinary Medical Research Institute
Iowa State University
Ames, Iowa

Introduction

After long ignoring the trichinellosis problem, the pork industry of the United States in 1966·abruptly requested the development of a *Trichinella* eradication program. Before any program could be developed, there was a need for a diagnostic procedure which was effective, economically feasible, and adaptable to slaughterhouse operations. The trichinoscopic method, which is routinely used in many countries of the world, was considered too costly to adapt to a yearly slaughter of approximately 85,000,000 swine. Therefore, the pooled sample method was proposed as a possible procedure (Zimmermann, 1968). The procedure underwent a 32-week pilot study involving 482,392 swine (Andrews *et al.*, 1970). With the experience gained in the pilot study and subsequent laboratory evaluations, various modifications have been made in the proposed procedure. The revised procedure will be presented in this report.

The Pooled Sample Method

1. The procedure is initiated by dividing the slaughter into lots of 20–25 consecutive carcasses with each carcass identified as to lot. The 25-carcass lot is recommended except in endemic areas such as commercial garbage feeding areas.
2. A portion of a pillar (crus) of the diaphragm is removed from each pig in the lot. The diaphragm is taken to the laboratory for processing.

611

3. The pillars are trimmed to weigh 5–6 gm for 25-pig lot or 7–8 gm for a 20-pig lot. As experience is gained in estimating sample size during step 2, step 3 may be minimal. The total capacity of the system is 150–160 gm. (Optional: lot size can be decreased and individual sample size proportionately increased in plants with limited slaughter.)

4. The pooled sample is finely ground by a mechanical food chopper with 3-mm plate openings. A separate grinder is used for each pooled sample.

5. The ground pooled sample is placed in a 3-liter beaker which is identified as to lot. The beaker is filled with a digestive fluid containing 1.0% pepsin (NF 1:3000) and 1.0% hydrochloric acid. The digestive fluid is prewarmed to 43.3° C. The beaker is placed in an incubator where the sample undergoes digestion at 43.3° C for 4–6 hr with constant agitation.

6. Optional: after digestion, the residue is allowed to settle for 45 min after which the upper two-thirds of the supernatant is siphoned off and discarded. This gives greater clarity at examination.

7. The supernatant and debris is poured through a 60-mesh screen fitted into a 3-liter capacity (250 mm or 175 mm Buchner shaped) funnel closed at bottom with rubber tubing and clamp. Water prewarmed to 43.3° C is added to cover screen. The debris is allowed to settle for 45 min. Steps 7 step 8 can be carried out either in incubator or at room temperature with little change in efficacy.

8. The clamp is then opened to allow fluid from the large funnel to fill a 125-mm funnel which is similarly clamped off. This fluid is again allowed to settle for 45 min.

9. A portion of the fluid is then drained into a ruled Syracuse watch glass or a ruled Petri dish for microscopic examination at $\times$ 25–30.

10. The finding of a *Trichinella* larvae indicates a positive lot. The carcasses in the lot are retained for further examination. A 50-gm portion of the pillars from each pig in lot is collected and examined individually by the digestive procedure. Any infected swine carcass is then processed to kill *Trichinella* by methods prescribed in Federal meat inspection regulations. Negative carcasses in lot are released for routine processing.

Discussion

The pooled sample method has been proposed as a safe, relatively low cost diagnostic method adaptable to swine slaughter procedures as utilized in the United States. The procedure has a distant advantage in safety when compared to the trichinoscopic method. The use of a 5–8 gm diaphragm sample gives increased efficacy, and therefore safety, when contrasted to the maximum 1-gm sample used for trichinoscopic examination. The pooled sample method would not detect all infections, but the intensity of the infections not detected would be such that they would not cause clinical infection in man, and it is unlikely in most cases that infection would be established. The minimal theoretical limit of efficacy is one larva per 5 gm of diaphragm. Since the concentration of *Trichinella* in the diaphragm is generally two to five times higher than in other muscles excepting the tongue (Zimmermann, 1970), the margin of safety would be even greater.

The pooled sample procedure underwent a 32-week pilot study during 1968–1969 at the George Hormel and Company swine slaughter plant in Fort Dodge, Iowa (Andrews *et al.,* 1970). The study was a cooperative project between the Hormel Company, the United States Department of Agriculture, and various segments of the pork industry. A total of 482,392 swine carcasses was examined, with daily slaughter exceeding 4000 swine on various occasions. Eight employees, excluding the veterinary supervisor, were required for the study. The day shift, including five personnel, collected the diaphragm samples and processed these for the digestion procedure (steps 1–5). A night shift of three individuals carried out concentration procedures and made microscopic examinations (steps 6–10). The two-shift employee schedule was made possible by overnight cooling of all carcasses before cutting. A reduction in time needed for the complete process, from about 13 hr as used in pilot study to 7 hr as currently recommended, would allow distribution of employees in a more efficacious, overlapping three-shift schedule. In Europe, swine carcasses are generally cut warm. The almost immediate loss of animal identification would therefore preclude routine usage of the pooled sample method.

The cost per animal for examinations during the pilot study was 9.35 cents including labor, chemicals, other supplies, and equipment amortized over a 10-year period. Trichinoscopic examinations for the same plant, based on German regulations limiting examinations to 60 per employee per day (Lehmensick, 1970), would have necessitated nearly 70 employees with an estimated cost exceeding 50 cents per animal.

Only 42 (0.0087%) of the 482,392 carcasses were found infected. The marked difference in prevalence between this study and the 0.125% reported nationally (Zimmermann and Zinter, 1971) is more a reflection of swine management procedures than in methodology. Nearly all swine originated from farms where swine production was a major industry. Swine were bought on a grade and yield basis, thereby excluding poor producing animals. Twenty-four of the 42 positive samples contained less than one *Trichinella* per gram, thus demonstrating increased efficacy over the trichinoscopic method; 16 of these contained less than 0.2 per gram which is the theoretical limit of efficacy for the pooled sample method.

The procedure did not interfere with normal plant operation. Samples

W. J. ZIMMERMANN

were readily obtained even with a slaughter rate of about 500 pigs/hr. The detection of positive lots accompanied by the extra 24 hr retainment did not affect plant operation.

The pooled sample method is the basic diagnostic method included in a proposed *Trichinella* eradication program developed by the USDA. Epidemiologic tracebacks are also included. The program is currently under study and may or may not be implemented in the future.

Summary

The modified pooled sample method for detection of *Trichinella* in swine at slaughter is an adaptation of the artificial digestion–Baermann procedure. The use of pooled diaphragm samples from 20–25 swine as a single digestive unit enables the procedure to be adaptable to the high-speed, large-scale slaughter methods as carried out in the United States.

References

Andrews, J. S., Zinter, D. E., and Schulz, N. E. (1970). Evaluation of the trichinosis pilot project. *Proc. 73rd Annu. Meet. U.S. Anim. Health Ass.* pp. 332–353.

Lehmensick, R. (1970). Inspection of pork and control of trichinosis in Germany. *In:* S. E. Gould (Ed.), "Trichinosis in Man and Animals." Thomas, Springfield, Illinois, pp. 437–448.

Zimmermann, W. J. (1968). A pooled sample method for post-slaughter detection of trichiniasis in swine. *Proc. 71st Ann. Meet. U.S. Livestock Sanit. Ass. Phoenix, Arizona,* pp. 358–366.

Zimmermann, W. J. (1970). Reproductive potential and muscle distribution of *Trichinella spiralis* in swine. *J. Amer. Vet. Med. Ass.* **156,** 770–774.

Zimmermann, W. J., and Zinter, D. E. (1971). The prevalence of trichiniasis in swine in the United States, 1966–70. *Health Serv. Mental Health Admin. Health Rep.* **68,** 937–945.

The Principles of the Epidemiology of Trichinelliasis with a New View on the Life Cycle

Holger Madsen

Zoological Laboratory
University of Copenhagen
Copenhagen

Introduction

When studying the literature on the epidemiology (transmission and dispersion) of the anthropozoonosis trichinelliasis (Sprent, 1969), it appears that in several respects confusion in concepts flourish. For instance, .the "normal" condition of infection is very often not kept clearly apart from the disease connected with the intake of high dosages of *Trichinella* larvae. Without question, the disease (trichinellosis) has often been seen in man, although many cases also have been overlooked. Nevertheless, compared with the incidence of infection (trichinelliasis) in man, as in other parasitic infections, the disease is a rare phenomenon. In animals, the disease has been observed only in astonishingly few cases of domestic animals like cats and pigs, sometimes in zoo animals like the polar bear (recent examples are given by Kroneberger *et al.,* 1970), and, of course, in experimental infections. The endings "-osis" and "-iasis" are used in the sense suggested by Whitlock (1949).

Confusion also prevails because up the present day, consequences of actual epidemiological knowledge have not always been drawn. Commonly and to a significant degree, what may happen and what actually happens are often not clearly kept apart; the literature on *Trichinella* epidemiology is simply plagued by this (Madsen, 1970). It appears to be obvious, particularly when it comes to comprehensive measures of control, that only the significant phenomena count. At most others play only a certain role locally. First of all, the life cycle must be known and understood comprehensively. I had the opportunity of going into considerable

615

detail on several of these points some years ago (Madsen, 1961). In regard
to trichinelliasis, Zimmerman (1970a) makes the following statement: "The
key to any eradication program in swine and man is a thorough understanding of the epizootiologic aspects of disease in the wildlife reservoir."

Taxonomic Considerations

The starting point for any study of epidemiology is the question of
taxonomy. It may sound incredible that there could be taxonomic problems in respect to *T. spiralis* nowadays. Nevertheless, two such problems
have again turned up in recent years after a century.

The first of the taxonomic problems is the alleged occurrence of *T.
spiralis* in sectivores. The larvae called trichinae have turned out to be
ascaridoid or spiruroid nematode larvae. Nevertheless, the matter goes on
until recent years (Iaremenko, 1963). Misidentification has been known
for more than a century, particularly regarding the nematode larvae frequently found in moles (Pagenstecher, 1865, Gerlach, 1866). In more
recent years Kotlán (1952) was the first to demonstrate the error, and
quite recently Kulikova (1967) again stressed the same thing. Further
references in this respect can be found in my monograph (Madsen, 1961)
and in Gould (1970). In this connection it is of particular interest that
Rauhut and Skoczen (1971) were not able to establish an infection in 67
moles with dosages of 1000-3000 *Trichinella* larvae. One consequence
of all this is that any report of occurrence of trichinae in insectivores,
and also in small nonsynanthropic rodents, not to mention birds (Merkushev, 1960; Nemeseri, 1968; Nenov, 1962; Zimmerman, 1971) can be dis-
regarded unless it specifically demonstrates that the larvae have been
properly determined, either morphologically (which is a fairly easy thing
to do) or experimentally.

It cannot be completely excluded that *Trichinella* may be found in
insectivores under special circumstances, but it will not be of any epidemiological significance. In spite of this, insectivores are on their way into
the textbooks with diagrams of their life cycles, probably to stay there
and confuse concepts for the following century. The insectivores also
haunt many of the quite recent comprehensive papers (Nelson, 1968;
Merkushev, 1970; Lukashenko *et al.,* 1971a).

The second point in regard to taxonomy is that Britov (1969, 1971,
and his chapter in Part VI, this volume), and Britov *et al.* (1971) threaten
to describe a new species for the genus *Trichinella.* Until recently only
strains or varieties have been named. Now a new synonym, *I. pseudo-
spiralis* has been published (Garkavi, 1972). It is of some interest in this
context that Britov and Smirnova (1966) were in the situation of not being
able to demonstrate strains. Much literature has accumulated around the

problem of strains (Gould, 1970); however, the phenomena observed thus far were to be expected. The occurrence of strains with minor genetic differences, which, as in the case of *T. spiralis,* do not express themselves morphologically, is known in innumerable numbers of animal species. Furthermore, as might be expected, several of the observed differences are evidently phenotypic in nature. Several of the strains described have been shown to change their faculties during passages through experimental animals (Gretillat, 1970b, 1971a,b; Gretillat and Vassiliades, 1968b). Arakawa and Todd (1971) in demonstrating the same thing, used the expression "isolates," rather than "strains." Arctic and African isolates, in particular, have been used in experimental work. Several studies quoted in Gould (1970), recent papers by Baldelli and Frescura (1963) using trichinae from foxes in Sicily, and Pawlowski and Rauhut (1971) finding differences between a human and pig isolate suggest that isolates with various and varying faculties might be found in many places.

Many authors stress the epidemiological significance of all these findings for the establishment of trichinelliasis. However, as they themselves describe the situation, in regard to the natural (sylvatic) cycle (see below), and considering the lability of the differences found, the whole phenomenon is bound to be of only restricted local importance, particularly in regard to the interplay between man-made and natural cycles. When it comes to the question of human trichinellosis, the condition for it must be as for trichinelliasis, i.e., the dispersion of the trichinae. As in any infection versus disease, further epidemiological factors to be considered are the faculties of the involved species, including strains, and of the parasite and of the host, and the ecological interplay between them. In the end, whether disease occurs or not depends upon the physiological state of the host in an interplay with the number of viable larvae taken in. Ozeretskovskaya (1968), and Ozeretskovskaya *et al.* (1969) stress differences in the clinical course of trichinellosis according to the different strains of larvae ingested.

Problems of the Life Cycle

Although there have been three international conferences on trichinellosis, one may pose the question as to what is meant by meat or flesh. Everyone would agree that it is part of a carcass, in varying degrees of decomposition. It is important in this respect that it has been known, again for more than a century, that the larvae are exceptionally tolerant against putrefaction. In some older textbooks, e.g., Neumann, 1905, this is mentioned as a well-known fact, but it has since been largely forgotten. I have mentioned it briefly (Madsen, 1961). The larvae have been found to be alive and also often infective up to at least 4 months in extremely rotten meat. Most references are from before the turn of the century (Bischoff, 1840; Luschka, 1851; Claus, 1860; Davaine, 1863; Pagenstecher, 1865; Piana, 1887; Petropavlovskij, 1899, 1905; Ifland, 1924). The matter has been taken up again only in quite recent time, by Dykova (1964, 1967), with the same result, and she suggests that the phenomenon must be of epidemiological significance. The encapsulated larvae are also very resistant to several other external "stresses." Hemmert-Halswick and Bugge (1934) were able to demonstrate living larvae in meat kept in a refrigerator at 2–4 °C, protected against desiccation, for 300 days. The free larvae were still hardy. Levin (1940) observed that they survived for 4 months at 5 °C in Tyrode solution and for 11 days at 38 °C, whereas according to Shaver and Mizelle (1955) they only survived for 30 days at 3 °C in physiological saline solution. The encapsulated larvae are fairly resistant to desiccation (Zimoroi, 1963). The remarkable resistance of the encapsulated larvae against salt concentrations of up to 4% has been known. (Ifland, 1924; Hemmert-Halswick and Bugge, 1934; Lörincs and Nemesëri, 1954; Sachs, 1954; Strobl, 1954; Anon., 1955; Varges, 1955; Allen and Goldberg, 1962; Pódhajecký, 1962a); this feature must play a role in the natural cycle in regard to the occurrence in marine mammals. There is also information on the high resistance to temperatures below 0 °C (Pódhajecký, 1962b; and others). Shaver and Mizelle (1955) demonstrated that the larvae cannot withstand very low temperatures although it depends upon the freezing state. They made the interesting observation that the resistance to freezing may vary according to host species. Another interesting study was presented by Marazza (1960), which was of practical as well as of epidemiological interest. Inspired by the fact that many organisms and even tissues of animals may become acclimatized to increased resistance to very low temperatures by initial exposure to fairly high freezing temperatures. Marazza attempted to determine if a similar phenomenon would occur with encapsulated *T. spiralis*. However, he was unable to demonstrate it in his experiments.

Recently, there has been an extremely interesting report which presents a kind of a model for a situation, which plays a great role epidemiologically in the natural cycle (Clark *et al.,* 1972). After 81 days under permanent frost (even if the time as indicated at −18 °C is questionable) living larvae could be demonstrated although their infectivity was not tested. It should be extremely interesting to find out if, say, the African and Arctic strains differ in respect to resistance to freezing temperatures. It will be seen that the encapsulated larvae are in some respects, e.g., putrefaction, just as or even more resistant than many nematode eggs and many encysted helminths such as metacercariae.

It is indeed astonishing that nobody as yet has studied these phenomena with modern methods, particularly in regard to the role the capsule may play. It is however known that decapsulated larvae are fairly resistant to low O_2 and high CO_2 pressure (Castro et al., 1973). All the studies on the action of salt and temperatures have been made for practical purposes. According to the literature, other substances seem hardly to have been investigated. Only Riedler (1863) and Erb (Pagenstecher, 1865) found the larvae in the capsules fairly resistant to salts of picric acid. All this demonstrates that the resistance of the encapsulated larvae matches the resistance of helminth eggs very well.

Ultrastructural studies in recent years have shown that the larvae live under quite special circumstances, since they are really intracellular, living in the changed muscle cell, without any necrosis ever having been observed. This means that they are protected against antibodies. There is a complete "symbiosis" between the parasite and the cell, the larvae feeding on dissolved low-molecular subst nce, which may even be taken up through the cuticle via the cell (Themann, 1960; Beckett and Boothroyd, 1961; Gould, 1970; Bruce, 1970; Ribas-Mujal and Rivera-Pomar, 1968; Ribas-Mujal, 1971; Kozek, 1971a, b; Purkerson and Despommier, Part I in this volume; Backwinkel and Themann, 1972; Berezantsev, 1963 and Part II in this volume; Teppema et al., 1973). Intracellular hematode larvae are also known to occur in probably all filarioid species, in the arthropod intermediate hosts, except that they leave the cell in order to continue their life cycle, which results in the death of the cell (Hawking and Worms, 1961). Furthermore, in the organization of the cell, the host organism is busy in establishing this symbiosis, as was demonstrated by Pagenstecher (1865), and by others later, by the structural changes in regard to capillaries and nerves around the invaded muscle cell, which assist in building up the surrounding capsule. The main substance in this capsule is collagen (Ritterson, 1966; Bruce, 1970), but glycoproteins (Lewert and Lee, 1954), mucopolysaccharides, hyaluronic acid (Zarzycki, 1963), and cystine (Bruce, 1970) are also present. The "quality," so to speak, of the capsule naturally depends upon conditions in the host. Saowakontha (1972) demonstrated an earlier capsule formation in rats on a high protein diet. As a consequence of the fact that the cell in which the larva lives is alive, there is a layer of lipoid substance around the larva. It should be interesting to know if this layer may still afford some protection to the larva in the carcass, as it does to the merozoites in the case of *Toxoplasma* (Jacobs, 1967).

Until the present time it has been generally assumed that there was an intermediate host in the life cycle of *T. spiralis,* although of a special kind (Holmes and Bethel, 1972). When the life cycle was discovered in the early 1860s, the concept of an intermediate host was quite new, and it is understandable why the phenomenon was put into that category. However, when drawing the consequences of the considerations above on the hardiness of the trichinae in the carcass, the phenomenon must be interpreted otherwise. What we are actually observing is that *T. spiralis* is dispersed in a way analogous to many nematodes which have hardy eggs or a free-living stage in water or soil. *Trichinella spiralis* has a similar free-living stage, with populations of larvae in the capsules in the special biotope, the carcass, which may even rot. These populations are maintained in a way analogous to helminth egg populations with new carcasses becoming available all the time.

Kozek (1971a) in connection with his studies of the molting patterns of *T. spiralis* came to the same conclusion: "the extraintestinal (tissue) phase, consisting of the muscle-infecting and intestine-infecting larvae stages, corresponds to the external phase of other nematodes." Kozak did not touch upon any epidemiological consequence of his conclusion. It is indeed fascinating to observe the great difficulties we are facing in a seemingly simple matter like the number of stages. The muscle larva is without a doubt the first-stage larva (Ali Khan, 1966; Shanta and Meerovitch, 1967b; Harley, 1972). Shanta and Meerovitch (1967a) were only able to consider the intestinal *Trichinella* to be neotenic larvae, whereas Ali Khan and Harley found four molts, the most probable situation being in agreement with the development of other trichuroids (Kozek, 1971a).

The new concept of a free-living stage in the carcass is of high significance, epidemiologically, since the intermediate host concept has always led to an extreme overstressing of the importance of predation (e.g., Nelson, 1968; Zimmerman, 1970a,b, 1971). All this of course does not mean that a transmission cannot occur via predation, but on a broad scale it is of no epidemiological importance.

An Interlude: *n*th Attempt of Conjuring Down the "Rat Theory"

Here we come to a sore point in the history of studies on and concepts of the epidemiology of trichinelliasis; in fact, it is more a question of psychology rather than of biology. Already more than a century ago Zenker (1871), very explicitly, put the epidemiological kernel of the matter, in regard to infections in pigs this way: "I consider the trichinous rats as a symptom of the presence of trichinois pigs." Here he referred to Leuckart's "rat theory," a term he coined in this paper, and implied that a population of trichinae cannot be maintained within a population of rats and that the source of infection in pigs was the pig carcass. Incidentally, domestic dogs and cats can become "symptoms," too, as Zenker of course also realized. He also showed evidence of his statement. It is a pure pleasure to follow his clear and cogent argumentation, and he is not without a certain dry humor. After having summarized the various arguments in favor of the rat theory he observes: "We have here the situation that the painter imaginatively depicts the possibilities in detail.

Afterward he scrutinizes the very good picture he has succeeded in producing until he believes in its reality, and then even gets other people to believe the same thing. This appears to be a questionable procedure in a matter of such practical importance." And he concludes his paper by saying,

> The general war against the rats seems to me to lie outside the limits of the trichina problem. That is, indeed, a consolation, because I cannot deny that I feel a kind of acrid humor in the sentence: "Destroy the rats, and we shall destroy the trichinae.." As long as the rats are that forceful in the struggle for existence as they are still today, the prospect would appear to be gloomy.

Zenker's epidemiological view was understood by some investigators through the years, again and again. Moreover, all evidence ever since justifies his views on an overall scale. In regard to the pig-to-pig cycle a particularly impressive phenomenon is the decline of the incidence of trichinelliasis in human beings in the United States after cooking of garbage became compulsory (Zimmermann *et al.,* 1968).

The factual basis for Leuckart's rat theory is simply that he was stubborn, which he admits himself (Madsen, 1961). One may therefore wonder how it is possible that the theory survives in broad circles up to the present day, in spite of three international conferences on trichinellosis, and two international congresses of parasitology. My only explanation is that Leuckart wrote textbooks while Zenker did not. And it may be that the intermediate-host theory, with the the belief that the main transmission is by predation, plays a role, too.

A few curious examples of recent influences of the rat theory are cited. Gerzanits (1964) had a patient with trichinellosis. Presumably he had only eaten fish. Therefore, Gerzanits assumed that fish eating had been the source of infection because he had read about a salmon which had swallowed a mouse. One could hardly invent a better joke if one should want to ridicule the rat theory. It must be said that Barriga (1964), in the same journal pointed out the absurdity of the case. Although realizing the natural cycle in carnivores in Germany, and even the rare occurrence there in pigs that can be traced back to carcasses of carnivores, Schoop and Lamina (1962) still wrote that "the circulation pig–rat–pig is interrupted" as a result of the trichina inspection. The following quotation also demonstrates how persistent the concepts are once they are acquired: "As Madsen (1961) pointed out, the role of rats in the transmission cycle of *T. spiralis* has been greatly exaggerated"; furthermore, "It is only in urban areas where rats are highly susceptible to local strains of *T. spiralis,* e.g., in Europe and America, that they are of significance in transmission" (Beck and Beverley-Burton, 1968). Romanov (1970) propounds his creed in the rat theory.

Similar to Grétillat and Vassiliadès (1968a), Sachs (1970) in a study
on trichinae in wild carnivores in Africa still feels compelled to assure
us that pigs and rats there play a minor role, in spite of the fact that his
own observations clearly demonstrate the role played by carrion, and he
is aware of the old knowledge of the resistance ot the larvae to putrefaction
tion. A kind of peak of, shall we say, misunderstanding, can be found in
a paper by Steiniger (1969). In the most irresponsible way the author
recommends the use of excess of pesticides against rats as a control measure against trichinelliasis in pigs. In a paper by Schenone *et al.* (1967)
the authors are of the opinion that they present some cases where rats have
played a decisive role in connection with a warfaring campaign against
rats. In two pig-breeding centers near Santiago where for a long period
no or almost no trichinae had been found, trichinae suddenly appeared
in high frequency a couple of months after the said campaign. In one of
the centers 43.6% of 71 pigs, and in another 12.3% of 480 pigs, proved
to be lightly or moderately infected. In the first place it was observed
that the young pigs in an enclosure consumed parts of rats lying dead or
moving slowly around due to intoxication. Here the food was garbage
from a restaurant and remnants from a bakery. It was not investigated
whether the garbage had been infectious for a brief period. The authors
argue that because of the low protein content of the feed the pigs might
have been particularly eager for scavenging on the rats, a reasonable argument. In the other center the feed was fundamentally grain, and here the
rats were found to be highly infected. This is a marginal situation, which
is emphasized in the slums in many cities of South America, where pigs
are produced under access to all kinds of offal, including human carcasses.
Regarding the rat theory on a broader scale this paper does not say much
because the carcasses available to rats in most cases are also available
to pigs.

Development of the Knowledge of the Natural (Sylvatic) Cycle of Trichinelliasis

Particularly after the stir aroused by Zenker's (1860) demonstration
of a case of trichinellosis, and by the subsequent large outbreaks in various
regions of Germany in the 1860s, quite a number of variety of animals
was investigated, and several "trichinae" were found, many of them being
anything but *Trichinella*. However, *T. spiralis* was demonstrated in many
wild carnivores and in wild boar, starting with Virchow (1866), and
throughout the next 60 years many, mostly isolated findings were reported,
mainly from Germany. Little attention was paid to these reports. Reports
of outbreaks of human trichinellosis were reported in many parts of the
world; outbreaks stemming from eating flesh of various wildlife species,

even foxes (Pampiglione and Doglioni, 1971). The first to realize the epidemiological significance of all this on a broader scale was Kotlán (1927).

There was some astonishment in Germany, particularly in the 1930s when it was eventually understood that trichinelliasis was widespread in foxes and badgers. On the assumption that predation was the main epidemiological factor, great numbers of small rodents, particularly voles, were examined, but in vain. Reluctantly the conclusion was drawn that the source of the infection must be carrion of the said carnivores. Still, the more comprehensive significance of this was not grasped. About the same time the occurrence of trichinelliasis in polar bear and arctic fox in the arctic was demonstrated. However, no special notice was taken of this. In the 1940s, trichinelliasis was found to occur particularly in foxes and several other carnivores in parts of Central Europe beyond Germany, and in the Scandinavian Peninsula.

The great turning point in our knowledge of trichinelliasis in nature was inaugurated by the now classical studies by the German-Danish parasitologist, Hans Roth (1949, 1950). The most famous result of his work was the now well-known presence of *T. spiralis* in various marine mammals in the Arctic, regularly in walrus *(Odobenus rosmarus)* and bearded seal *(Erignathus barbatus)*, more exceptionally in ringed seal *(Phoca hispida)* and more recently also in spotted seal *(Phoca vitulina)* (Merkushev, 1963) and white whale *(Delphinapterus leucas)*. These studies inspired an outburst of investigations on trichinelliasis in wildlife all over the world. One of the most outstanding of these is the study by Rausch *et al.* (1956) from Alaska. The consequences of this excellent study appears not yet to have been drawn in full, a point to which I shall refer later.

Owing to Dr. Hans Roth's premature death in 1951, I had the privilege of finishing up the extensive material collected on the initiative of Hans Roth. He was able to publish results based on only parts of the material. A preliminary report on the total material was given in 1953 (Roth and Madsen, 1956). The final report was published in 1961. In this latter paper, I took the world literature on trichinelliasis in wildlife into account, and thus was able to predict an almost worldwide occurrence. The numerous papers which have appeared since (Gould, 1970) have brought profuse verification of this prediction. Also, the main point of the epidemiological role of even the decaying carcass was verified in every respect.

I should like to go into a little detail on a few points. I predicted the occurrence of trichinelliasis in the wildlife in New Zealand. This has been verified in recent years (Cairns, 1966). Besides, trichinae were found in feral cats. Considering the widespread occurrence of mustelids, and feral cats and pigs (Wodzicki, 1950; Marshall, 1963), and the history of these animals in New Zealand, there can be no doubt that trichinelliasis is widespread in these animals. Although there are no reports of trichinelliasis in Australia, considering the widespread occurrence there of foxes, feral cats (Serventy, 1966), and feral pigs (Pullar, 1950), I venture to predict a widespread occurrence in these mammalian populations, too. Furthermore, New Zealand and Australia have a special feature in common which will tend to increase the spread of trichinelliasis in the host populations mentioned. This feature is the widespread use of poisons in the control of the said "pest" species, with the result that still more carrion will be available. Trichinae were established in feral pigs in the Hawaiian Islands where they are maintained up to the present. They occur also in the mongoose (Alicata, 1970). In regard to elucidating particulars of the epidemiology, it should be of interest if it were possible to correlate differences in frequency of trichinelliasis in the various islands to varying degrees of contact between populations of mongoose and feral pigs. Such a correlation would be of consequence also in regard to the apparent lack of trichinelliasis in the Indian mongoose in Jamaica, from where the mongoose was introduced to Hawaii (Alicata and Amiel, 1971). In Hawaii, like in many similar places, more or less feral populations of dogs and cats must play a role epidemiologically, too. These animals have been investigated for trichinae only in New Zealand (Tomich, 1969).

Trichinelliasis had been known to occur in man and pigs in all South American countries, with the exception of Brazil (Neghme and Schenone, 1970). Recently, the first investigation comprising wildlife was published in Argentina (Minoprio and Abdon, 1967). They quote reports of human outbreaks from meat of wild boars *(Sus scrofa)* which have established a population in the investigated region close to the Chilean border; they point out that it has partly been mixed up with domestic pigs. In five investigated boars they did not happen to find trichinae, however. On the other hand, trichinae were found in one of four foxes *(Pseudolopex gracilis)*, one old specimen of an omnivorous species of edentate *(Chaetophractus villosus)*, and finally in one of eight partly synanthropic rat-like rodents *(Graomys griseoflavus)*. The people in the region of investigation live under fairly primitive conditions. In a similar study, comprising 2063 mammals from Chile (Alvarez *et al.,* 1970) no trichinae were found, thus appearing to be an exception in regard to the world-wide occurrence of trichinelliasis in wildlife. However, taking a closer view of which mammals were investigated, of the most promising species reaching a fairly old age, only five specimens of the puma *(Felis concolor)* were examined and proved to be negative. The same was the case with two specimens of a smaller cat, *Felis guigna.* Of other carnivores, more short-lived species have been examined: 274 foxes (222 *Dusicyon culpaeus,* 52 *D. griseus),* and 27 mustelides (24 *Grison cufa* and three skunks, *Conepatus chingua).* The rest consists of 1585 rodents, the majority of which was a small rat-like species (1396 *Octodon degus),* and 70 lagomorphs (20 European hares, *Lepus capensis europaeus* and 50 rabbits, *Oryctolagus cuniculus).* The two latter groups demonstrate the common finding in most places that they do not play any role epidemiologically. Still, the material of carnivores is not negligible. However, no particulars are given of the biotopes on which the foxes and mustelids were collected, and there is also no indication of the age of the animals. Neghme and Schenone (1970) indicate that the digestion method (without indicating the amount of meat used) and trichinoscopy have been used on 656 and 1407 animals, respectively, unfortunately without stating the species. Thus various uncertainties are involved which do not exclude the possibility that the negative result may be due to chance. This notion is supported by the fact that a sylvatic cycle as outlined above has been demonstrated close to the Chilean border at about the same latitude. It can be mentioned that the rat theory partly, and the predation theory particularly, are rampant in this paper, which can be seen by the choice of animals examined. Finally, I shall again venture a prediction: if someone would examine the larger carnivores in the wilderness areas in Brazil and in other regions of South America, he or she should have a very good chance of finding *T. spiralis*.

Concluding Observations on the Epidemiology

The various facets of the epidemiology of trichinelliasis and trichinellosis are dependent upon four main cycles, each of which requires to some extent different approaches when it comes to measures of control. As in several parasitic infections, the matter of disease is simple in principle. If the larvae in the flesh consumed are killed nothing more happens. However, that is exactly what will not always be. The four cycles are:

1. The natural (sylvatic) cycle, from carcasses of carnivores in most parts of the world, with very little influence of significance by man, perhaps with the exception of the senseless slaughtering of polar bears in the Arctic, by "civilized" European and Americans. One of its central points is populations of fairly long-lived host species. Here large omnivores and scavengers like species of wild boars and bears are of special importance because of the large amounts of flesh that are available.
2. The man-made cycle, from pig flesh (carcass) to pig, all over the world where flesh of swine is eaten. There are offshoots to domestic carnivores and synanthropic rodents of minimal epidemiological consequence. Some input from the natural cycle may occur.
3. The man-made cycle, from dog carcass to dog, in the Arctic, with offshoots to the natural cycle, and to some degree also input from there.
4. The man-made cycle mainly in farm fur-animals, in various parts of the world, with internal circulation and/or input from the natural cycle.

Some Comments

The natural cycle is the original one, from which the three others stem. It is in many regions of the world a not negligible problem of public hygiene, causing outbreaks of disease in human beings directly by consumption of inadequately prepared meat of wildlife, one recent example being that reported by Doege *et al.* (1969) from a bear in Thailand.

The thorough understanding of the significance of the natural cycle has been impaired mainly because of psychological reasons, the main "culprits" being the rat theory and the predation theory, which have blurred the understanding of the decisive epidemiological factor, i.e., the extent of availability of carcasses in the various situations.

Most pronouncedly in wilderness areas, as well as in many other regions, one cannot, as is often done, particularly in papers from East European countries, speak of "focal" or "nidal" infections in the sense of Pavlovsky (1966) but rather of a "natural diffusion infection" (Boev *et al.*, 1966), a concept which Horning (1968) and Zimmermann (1970a,b) have also adopted. To what extent a "focal" distribution may occur in some marginal regions, still remains to be elucidated.

I should like to go a little into detail on a few points, first choosing two geographically extreme regions, which present very different situations, Africa and the Arctic–Subarctic region, respectively.

Grétillat and Chevalier (1969) and Grétillat (1971c) were astonished that warthogs, in spite of their high susceptibility, were less frequently infected than jackals. They even speculated that putrefaction and drying of carcasses might be the cause, evidently unaware of the remarkable resistance of the encapsulated larvae. They demonstrated infectious larvae in parts of a warthog after 12 hr of drying in the sun at temperatures above 30 °C. It is not quite clear why the supposed cause should be active in the case of warthogs only, and not in that of the jackals. They ask for some other as yet unknown ecological or ethological factor. This factor is so far known as the low frequency of infection is habitual for wild boars. The explanation is that the boars as omnivores are less active than carnivores in regard to eating carrion, although this varies according to the availability of other foods. Merkushev (1970) observed differences in frequency of infection in *Sus scrofa* in Siberia depending upon types of vegetation in the biotopes of the boars. Gretillat (1970a) stated that "ecological and ethological factors prevent the normal life cycle of the parasite in West Africa."

In the Arctic some special features are obvious, the most outstanding and disputed being the occurrence of *Trichinella* in various marine mammals (Rausch, 1970). In this special field of dispersion the rat theory eventually has no chance at all, but the predation theory is rampant in the discussions. A most curious example is that of Ass (1968), who, because of the predation theory, goes as far as to deny the occurrence of *Trichinella* in walrus.

Fay (1960) discards a walrus-polar bear cycle proposed by some workers, and suggests that polar bear and walrus contract trichinellosis primarily from the flesh of ringed and bearded seals. "I do not necessarily dispute this, but I do suggest that Fay unduly discounts other sources of infection," writes Manning (1961) in his most refreshing comments on Fay's paper. He points to carcasses as the most probable source of infection, and is aware of the epidemiological significance of the long-lived carnivores, as in the case of polar bear where there is evidence for a higher frequency in older than in younger bears (Madsen, 1961). Man may have some influence through the habit of discarding dead dogs by throwing them into the sea. The occurrence in marine mammals is a purely arctic phenomenon, closely connected with carrion exchanged between the few terrestrial mammals and the sea mammals (Kozlov, 1971). Polar bear and Arctic fox, the main species in the first category both have a strong affinity for the sea via the icecover along the High Arctic coasts. In the second category the main species are the walrus and the bearded seal.

In the continental parts of the Arctic no clear delimitation is possible between the high- and subarctic regions, not even the temperate regions, which in the border regions, are wilderness areas. The multiplicity of mammalian species gives these regions their special stamp. In the numerous surveys of trichinelliasis in temperate, even warm-temperate zones, thousands and thousands of rodents have been found to be negative, and numerous indications of trichinelliasis are at least highly doubtful, or of no consequence in an epidemiological respect; they are at most "symptoms," in the sense of Zenker, extended to the natural cycle. This is somewhat different in the Arctic-Subarctic regions of the continents.

The most comprehensive survey has been reported by Rausch *et al.* (1956) from Alaska; and only a few records are available from the arctic USSR (Merkushev, 1970; Lukashenko *et al.,* 1971 a,b,). Here *Trichinella* evidently occurs in rodents with a certain regularity, which of course means that they will enter into the natural cycle, but still of restricted epidemiological avail. Also in these papers the predation theory exerts a certain influence, whereas Rausch (1970) accepts the importance of scavenging almost in full. The comparatively high frequency in this arctic region can be explained by the well-known fact that rodents and hares in this region are forced into scavenging for food due to its scarcity and inaccessibility; and of course they come across carnivore carcasses, too. That carnivores scavenge under any circumstances, although to varying degrees and probably ethologically determined, is also a well-known fact. This is so even to a higher degree than is generally acknowledged. One reason why there are great difficulties in understanding this is that one consequence of host population dynamics is not sufficiently realized, namely, the enormous numbers of carcasses that are bound to lie around in nature. And if specific scent should play a role, it is certainly not present in the rotten carcass, besides that the scavengers also come across carrion of other species.

In more or less marginal situations man may have a finger in the pie of the natural cycle:

1. Under war conditions, special burial customs like that of the Massais in Africa (Nelson, 1972), or the many accidents among the Eskimos in the Arctic, human infections may not be a blind alley for the larvae as is often assumed. This may, if only for periods, increase the chance of infection for wildlife species.

2. Trichinous offal can become available to wildlife through carcasses produced by human hunting, and in some regions, such as Germany, carcasses may be even purposely laid out as part of a measure of control of carnivores *(Luderplatze)*. In the latter case, "domestic" trichinae may also enter the picture, as is the case in some of the National Parks in the United States with the bears, and in innumerable places, at least until recently, with raccoons (Zimmermann, 1970a,b, 1971). There is a similar situation all over the world in the case of rats, which some people curiously enough consider as belonging to "wildlife." The epidemiological significance will at most be of a local kind, and in many regions there may be a decline with the decline of infections in pigs.

3. Inadvertently, wildlife carcasses can become available to domestic animals. It may happen with pigs which is of considerable importance in Germany and Poland where there is a highly developed trichina inspection. In Germany, it appears that the very few trichinous pigs found have acquired their infection this way. Similar cases have been reported from the United States (Zimmerman, 1970a,b, 1971). In Norway, particularly during the Second World War, wildliving carnivores played a role in fur-animal farms. The source of infection was partly their "own" carcasses, and partly those of wildliving foxes. The latter was in fact the main reason for the discovery that the natural cycle occurs in Norway. In Arctic regions like Greenland and Arctic Siberia, the natural cycle plays a role in fur-animal farms.

4. The inadvertent intake of improperly cooked flesh of wildlife by man under more or less "primitive" conditions is in many regions of considerable epidemiological significance. The source in most places are wild boars and bears, and in the Arctic the walrus; but badgers and even foxes might be involved. Often the regular intake of small dosages of larvae in all probability offers some degree of protection against trichinellosis due to the development of immunity.

But what about the many theories of various aspects of epidemiology? Of course infections can spread in nature in several other ways than directly by carcasses of carnivores (Madsen, 1961):

1. Intake of flesh of any infected animal, including rats, may cause infection, be it by predation or even by tail chewing in pigs. (Schultz, 1970; Visnjakov and Georgiev, 1972).
2. Pieces of carcasses spread by or, for brief periods, taken up by scavenging animals, like birds, insects, and gammarids (Britov, 1962; Fay, 1968; Kullmann and Nawabi, 1971).
3. By larvae (or even adults?) voided in the feces of recently infected scavenging animals (Schnurrenberger *et al.,* 1964; Trommer, 1970; Zimmermann, 1970a,b).

However, it is often forgotten that without carcasses available in one or another form the above modes of spread would not occur, not even by caudophagy. Therefore, they are bound to be insignificant compared to the direct transmission by consumption of carcasses. It appears evident that under no circumstance can the natural cycle from carnivore to carnivore be maintained by predation. In the end the case is the same with the man-made cycles. When taking a comprehensive view of the epidemiology of *T. spiralis* all over the world, it is obvious that we are facing extremely complex phenomena in all of the four above-mentioned main cycles. In the natural cycle particularly, on an overall scale, the population dynamic processes are the most important since they determine the amount of carrion being available at a certain time. Population dynamics are again dependent upon ecological and ethological phenomena. In the available information there is a tendency for the frequency of infection to be higher as more wilderness conditions prevail. An ethological factor is expressed in the partly perplexing differences in the infection rates in the different species of hosts, where availability of carcasses alone does not seem to be the explanation, but rather the differences in regard to the degree to which the single species utilizes the carrion. When it comes to the man-made cycles, varying living conditions and therefore habits are bound to produce differences in the infection rates in the animals. Regarding the frequency of human infections, eating habits are all decisive.

The cause of the differences in epidemiology in different man-made cycles is fairly easy to determine, and an enormous amount of knowledge has been collected. Our knowledge in regard to the natural cycle is however still imperfect. An impressive paper by Zimmermann and Hubbard (1969) on trichinelliasis in wildlife in Iowa deserves to be mentioned. In this context we can disregard the rats. No less than 8743 carnivores from a number of different regions were investigated over a period of 15 years with most interesting results.

In the case of foxes (2511 adult specimens comprised of mostly red fox, *Vulpes fulva,* and some gray fox, *Urocyon cinereoargenteus*) and mink, *Mustela vison* (2124 specimens) the material was large enough to determine differences in frequency from year to year and from area to area. The overall frequency was 6.4% and 5.0%, respectively [χ^2 (chi square) = 4.01* $P <$ .025], a most curious difference when considering that in regard to intensity of infection only 1.2% of the 160 positive foxes contained more than 51 larvae/gm and no less than 53.8% of the 106 infected minks did. Here probably some ethological factor is working. It should be interesting if this phenomenon somehow could be correlated with the differences according to year and/or area. During the years 1953–1954, to 1967–1968, the frequencies in foxes present a two-peaked curve, the highest years being 1953–1954 and 1960–1961, and the low years being 1958–1959 and 1966–1968. The minks present for the same period a seemingly three-peaked curve, with the highest figures in 1953–1954, 1959–1960 and 1963–1965, and the corresponding lowest figures in 1957–1958, 1961–1963 and 1966–1968. When comparing 7 high years with 7 low years, χ^2 is 23.63*** and 16.75*** in foxes and minks, respectively. Can these differences be correlated to population dynamic phenomena in the two species? The differences between the areas investigated also seem to be significant. Unfortunately the number of investigated specimens is not indicated. Can these differences be correlated to specific characteristics of the areas?

Some other interesting things can be interpreted from the material presented. There is again evidence that old animals are more frequently infected than young ones. When comparing foxes with fox cubs, χ^2 is 5.74* ($P >$ .025). The frequencies of 6.4% in foxes and 4.3% in 207 coyotes, *Canis latrans,* are not significantly different. The low frequency of 0.6% in no less than 1362 raccoons, *Procyon lotor,* does not speak in favor of any epidemiological influence of offal from pigs. And the 3.1% frequency of infection in 65 badgers, *Taxidon taxus,* is probably on the same level as in foxes and minks, although, because of the small number available there is no significant difference from the frequencies in either skunks. *Mephites mephites* and *Spilogale interrupta,* or foxes. On the other hand, the frequencies between skunks (1.5%) and raccoons (0.6%) are significantly different (χ^2 = 4.74*, $P <$ .02), and those between minks and skunks are significantly different to a higher degree (χ^2 = 31.78*).

The ideal condition in this kind of study is a close cooperation between wildlife biologists and parasitologists. As already suggested it might be possible in this way to extract still more information from the extremely valuable material presented.

Finally, I should like to briefly comment on the frequently assumed epidemiological importance of chemotherapy (Leiper, 1970). It has been overstressed in an overwhelming number of cases. In the case of trichinellosis, not to speak of trichinelliasis, according to the prevailing situation, it appears evident that chemotheraphy cannot be of any significance. Nevertheless, two papers suggest that it may (Lamina, 1963; Larsh *et al.,* 1962); and the latter paper approaches irresponsibility in suggesting treatment of pigs with cadmium oxide as an epidemiological measure.

Summary

For more than a century five decisive epidemiological points in the biology of *T. spiralis* have been known, without the consequences having yet been drawn in full:

1. Transmission occurs when host species of mammals eat meat containing viable larvae.
2. The larvae can survive in the flesh (pieces of carcasses in varying degrees of decomposition) for a long time, even in rotten carcasses.
3. The older an animal, the greater is its chance of harboring an infection.
4. Trichineae occur in wildliving carnivores and some wildliving omnivores, all of which scavenge.
5. The falseness of Leuckart's "rat theory" was established by Zenker. Nevertheless, it has confused concepts until now.

Consequence: for the establishment and maintenance of *T. spiralis* in a host population, infected carcasses must be available.

It is demonstrated that in the life cycle of *T. spiralis* there is a free-living stage analogous to the eggs in many helminths—the very resistant encapsulated larvae in the special biotope, the carcass. Since this has not been understood thoroughly as yet, the "predation theory" has caused much confusion.

Four cycles of *T. spiralis* transmission occur. The original one is the natural (sylvatic) cycle, from carcasses of carnivores and certain other scavengers like wild boars and in many regions feral pigs, to carnivores and scavengers, with minimal human influence. Then there are three man-made cycles in existence: (1) the pig-to-pig cycle all over the world; (2) the dog-to-dog cycle in the Arctic; and (3) the farm fur-animal to farm fur-animal in various regions. The natural cycle may penetrate into all of these latter cycles to varying degrees, depending upon varying circumstances.

References

Anonymous. (1955). Temperature control and salt treatment of meat containing trichinae or cysticerci. *WHO Tech. Rep. Ser. 99,* 44–47.

Alicata, J. E. (1970). *In:* S. E. Gould (ed), "Trichinosis in Man and Animals." Thomas, Springfield, Illinois, pp. 465–472.

Alicata, J. E., and Amiel, D. K. (1971). On the absence of *Trichinella spiralis* in mongooses and rodents in Jamaica, West Indies. *J. Parasitol.* **57,** 807.

Ali Khan, Z. (1966). The postembryonic development of *Trichinella spiralis* with special reference to ecdysis. *J. Parasitol.* **52,** 248–259.

Allen, R. W., and Goldberg, A. (1962). The effect of various salt concentrations on encysted *Trichinella spiralis* larvae. *Amer. J. Vet. Res.* **23,** 580–586.

Alvarez, V., Rivera, G., Neghme, A., and Schenone, H. (1970). Triquinosis em animales. *Bol. Chil. Parasitol.* **25,** 83–86.

Arakawa, A., and Todd, A. C. (1971). Comparative development of temperate zone and arctic isolates of *Trichinella spiralis* in the white mouse. *J. Parasitol.* **57,** 526–530.

Ass, M. J. (1968). Bemerkungen uber die Helminthen von *Erignathus barbatus. Angew. Parasitol.* **9,** 33–35.

Bäckwinkel, K. P., and Themann, H. (1972). Electronenmikroskopische Untersuchungen uber die Pathomorphologie der Trichinellose. *Beitr. Pathol. Anat. Allg.* **146,** 259–271.

Baldelli, B., and Frescura, T. (1963). Ulteriori osservazioni sulla trichinosi silvestre in Umbria. *Parassitologia* **5,** 145–155.

Barriga, O. (1964). Triquinosis transmitida por peces. *Bol. Chil. Parasitol.* **19,** 134.

Beck, J. W., and Beverly-Burton, M. (1968). The pathology of *Trichuris, Capillaria* and *Trichinella* infections. *Helminthol. Abstr.* **37,** 1–26.

Beckett, E. B., and Boothroyd, B. (1961). Some observations on the fine structure of the mature larva of the nematode *Trichinella spiralis. Ann. Trop. Med. Parasitol.* **55,** 116–124.

Berezantsev, Y. A. (1963). Advances in the study of migration and encapsulation of *Trichinella* larvae in the host organism (in Russian). *Med. Parazitol. Parazit. Bol.* **32,** 171–176.

Bischoff, T. L. W. (1840). Ein Fall von *Trichina spiralis. Med. Ann. Heidelberg* **6,** 232–250, 485–494.

Boev, S. N., Bondareva, V. J., Sokolova, J. B. and Tazeva, Z. H. (1966). Trichinellosis in Kazakhstan. *Wiad. Parazytol.* **12,** 519–525.

Britov, V. A. (1962). On the role of fishes and crustaceans in the transmission of trichinellosis to marine mammals. *Zool. Zh.* **41,** 776–777.

Britov, V. A. (1969). Some differences between natural and synanthropic strains of *Trichinella* (in Russian). *Wiad. Parazytol.* **15,** 555–560.

Britov, V. A. (1971). Biological methods of determining *Trichinella spiralis* Owen, 1835 varieties. *Wiad. Parazytol.* **17,** 477–480.

Britov, V. A., and Smirnova, M. L. (1966). About *Trichinella spiralis* strains. *Wiad. Parazytol.* **12,** 527–530.

Britov, V. A., Ermolin, G. A., Tarakanov, V. I., and Nikitina, T. L. (1971). Genetic isolation of two variants of *Trichinella* (in Russian). *Med. Parazitol. Parazit. Bol.* **40,** 515–521.

Bruce, R. G. (1970). The structure and composition of the capsule of *Trichinella spiralis* in host muscle. *Parasitology* **60,** 223–227.

Cairns, G. C. (1966). The occurrence of *Trichinella spiralis* in New Zealand pigs, rats and cats. *N. Zeal. Vet. J.* **14,** 84–88.

Castro, G. A., Cotter, M. V., Ferguson, J. D. and Gorden, C. W. (1973). Trichinosis: physiological factors possibly altering the course of infection. *J. Parasitol.* **59,** 268–276.

Clark, P. S., Brownsberger, K. M., Saslow, A. R., Kagan, I. G., Noble, G. R., and Maynard, J. E. (1972). Bear meat trichinosis: Epidemiologic, serologic, and clinical observations from two Alaskan outbreaks. *Ann. Intern. Med.* **76**, 951–956.

Claus, C. F. W. (1860). Fütterungsversuche mit *Trichina spiralis. Wuerzburg. Naturwissenschaftl. Z.* **1**, 155–157.

Davaine, C. J. (1863). Faits et considerations sur la trichine *(Pseudalius trichina). Gaz. Med. France* **34**, 58–59, 75–78, 130–131, 174–177.

Doege, T. C., Thienprasit, P., Headington, J. T., Pongprot, B., and Tarawanich, B. (1969). Trichinosis and raw bear meat in Thailand. *Lancet* **1**, 459–461.

Dykova, I. (1964). The ability of invasion of larval *Trichinella spiralis* obtained from decaying flesh. *Sb. Vys. Sk. Zemed. Brne, Rada B* **12**, 495–497.

Dykova, I. (1967). The invasion ability of *Trichinella* larvae from putrifying muscles of *Felis silvestris* and artificially infected *Felis domestica. Acta Univ. Agr. Brno Fac. Vet.* **36**, 255–258.

Fay, F. H. (1960). Carnivorous walrus and some arctic zoonoses. *Arctic* **13**, 111–122.

Fay, F. H. (1968). Experimental transmission of *Trichinella spiralis* via marine amphipods. *Can. J. Zool.* **46**, 597–599.

Fiedler, C. L. A. (1863). Versuche uber die Einwirkung des Natrum und Kali picronitricum auf die Trichinen. *Virchows Arch. Pathol. Anat. Physiol. Klin. Med.* **26**, 573–579.

Garkavi, B. L. (1972). Species of *Trichinella* from wild carnivores. *Vet. Mosk.* **49**, 90–91.

Gerlach, A. C. (1866). "Die Trichinen." Hannover, Schmorl und von Seefeld, pp. 1–90.

Gerzanits, P. (1964). Triquinosis transmitida por peces. *Bol. Chil. Parasitol.* **19**, 134.

Gould, S. E. (ed.) (1970). "Trichinosis in Man and Animals." Thomas, Springfield, Illinois, 540 pp.

Grétillat, S. (1970a). Epidemiology of trichinosis of wild animals in West Africa. Wart-hog receptivity of the West African strain of *Trichinella spiralis. J. Parasitol.* **56** (Suppl.), 124.

Grétillat, S. (1970b). Épidémiologie de la trichinellose sauvage au Sénégal. *Wiad. Parazytol.* **16**, 109–110.

Grétillat, S. (1971a). Studies on variations in adaptation and ubiquity of West African strain of *Trichinella spiralis* (in French). *Bull. WHO* **45**, 520–524.

Grétillat, S. (1971b). La trichinose des animaux sauvages en Afrique doit être considérée comme une zoonose d'avenir. *Écon. Méd. Anim.* **12**, 113–116.

Grétillat, S. (1971c). Trichinelliasis, a zoonosis with an unusual epidemiology conditioned by the nature and importance of the reservoir hosts (in French). *Cah. Med. Vet.* **40**, 130–138.

Grétillat, S., and Chevalier, J. L. (1969). Réceptivité du phacochère *(Phacochoerus aethiopicus)* a la souche ouest-africaine de *Trichinella spiralis. C. R. Acad. Sci., Ser. D* **269**, 2381–2383.

Grétillat, S., and Vassiliades, G. (1968a). Particularités biologiques de la souche ouest-africaine de *Trichinella spiralis.* Réceptivité et sensibilité de quelques mammifères domestiques et sauvages. *Rev. Élevage Méd. Vét. Pays Trop.* **21**, 85–89.

Grétillat, S., and Vassiliadès, G. (1968b). Réceptivités compareés du chat et du porc domestiques à la souche ouest-africaine de *Trichinella spiralis. C. R. Acad. Sci. Ser. D* **226**, 1134–1141.

Harley, J. P. (1972). Clarification of *Trichinella spiralis* (Nematoda) life cycle terminology. *Acta Parasitol. Pol.* **20**, 463–467.

Hawking, F. and Worms, M. (1961). Transmission of filarioid nematodes. *Annu. Rev. Entomol.* **6**, 413–432.

Hemmert-Halswick, A. and Bugge, G. (1934). Trichinen und Trichinose. *Ergeb. Allg. Pathol. Pathol. Anat.* **28**, 313–392.

Hörning, B. (1968). Zur Naturherd-Problematik der Trichinellose in der Schweiz. *Rev. Suisse Zool.* **75**, 1063–1066.

Holmes, J. C. and Bethel, W. M. (1972). Modification of intermediate host behavior by parasites. *In:* E. U. Canning and C. A. Wright (eds.), "Behavioral Aspects of Parasitic Transmission." Academic Press, New York, pp. 123–143.

Iaremenko, I. I. (1963). Trichinelliasis among moles of the Termopol region. *Med. Parazitol. Parazit. Bol.* **32**, 226–227.

Ifland, R. (1924). Uber die bisherigen Beobachtungen des Abtotens der Trichinen. *Z. Fleisch- Milchhygiene* **34**, 294–296.

Jacobs, L. (1967). *Toxoplasma* and toxoplasmosis. *Adva. Parasitol.* **5**, 1–45.

Kotlán, A. (1927). Die Bedeutung der fleischfressenden Tiere bei der bertragung der Trichinose. *Prager Arch. Tiermed.* **7**, 142.

Kotlán, A. (1952). Ergebnisse der 1. ungarischen parasitologischen Inlandexpedition. *Acta Vet. Acad. Sci. Hungar.* **2**, 337–341.

Kozek, W. J. (1971a). The molting pattern in *Trichinella spiralis*. I. A light microscope study. *J. Parasitol.* **57**, 1015–1028.

Kozek, W. J. (1971b). The molting pattern in *Trichinella spiralis*. II. An electron-microscope study. *J. Parasitol.* **57**, 1029–1038.

Kozlov, D. P. (1971). The ways in which pinnipeds become infected with *Trichinella. Tr. Gelmintol. Lab. Vopr. Biol. Fiziol. Biokh. Gelmintol. Zhivotn, Rast.* **21**, 36–40.

Kroneberger, H., Schuppel, K. F., and Seifert. (1970). Trichinose als Lahmheitsursache. *In:* D. Mathias (ed.), *Verh. Ber. XII Int. Symp. Erkrank, Zootiere, Akad. Verl. Berlin,* pp. 139–140.

Kulikova, N. A. (1967). On the role of moles in the distribution of trichinosis. *Zool. Zh.* **46**, 962–964.

Kullmann, E., and Nawabi, S. (1971). Studies on the role of carrion-eating beetles (Silphidae, Carabidae) as carriers of *Trichinella spiralis* (in German). *Z. Parasitenk.* **35**, 234–240.

Lamina, J. (1963). The world distribution of trichinae and the possibilities of chemotherapeutic control (in German). *Wiener Tieraerzl. Monatsschr.* **50**, 981–995.

Larsh, J. E., Jr., Goulson, H. T., and West, A. I. (1962). The effect of cadmium oxide against *Trichinella spiralis* in mice given only a brief exposure to medicated feed. *J. Parasitol.* **48**, 772–777.

Leiper, J. W. G. (1970). The possibilities of eradication of helminths by chemotherapy. *J. Parasitol.* **56**, 206.

Leisering, A. G. T. (1866). Untersuchungen von Ratten auf Trichinen betreffend. *Ber. Vet. Königsr. Sachs.* 1865. **10**, 97–100, 101–104.

Levin, A. J. (1940). Culturing *Trichinella spiralis* in vitro. 1. Preliminary experiment: A basic medium to sustain larvae unchanged for long periods in vitro. *J. Parasitol.* **26** (Suppl.), 31.

Lewert, R. M., and Lee, C. L. (1954). Studies on the passage of helminth larvae through host tissues. I. Histochemical studies on the extracellular changes caused by penetrating larvae. II. Enzymatic activity of larvae in vitro and in vivo. *J. Infec. Dis.* **95,** 13–51.

Lörincs, F., and Nemeséri, L. (1954). Die Konservierungsverfahren der Fleischwarenindustrie als Präventionsmethoden gegen Trichinellose. *Acta Vet. Acad. Sci. Hungar.* **4,** 71–92.

Lukashenko, N. P. (1961). On the location of larval *Trichinella spiralis. Acta Vet. Acad. Sci. Hungar.* **12,** 269–278.

Lukashenko, N. P. (1962). On elective dissemination of larvae of *Trichinella spiralis* in the organism of mammals. *Wiad. Parazytol.* **8,** 603–612.

Lukashenko, N. P., Volfson, A. G., Istomin, V. A., and Chernov, V. Y. (1971a). Trichinellosis of animals of Chukotka Peninsula. *Acta Parasitol. Pol.* **19,** 151–161.

Lukashenko, N. P., Volfson, A. G., Istomin, V. A., and Chernov, V. Y. (1971b). Trichinellosis of animals in Chukotka, USSR: A general review. *Int. J. Parasitol.* **1,** 287–296.

Luschka, H. V. (1851). Zur Naturgeschichte der *Trichina spiralis. Z. Wissenschaftl. Zool.* 3, 69–80.

Machnicka-Roguska, B. (1969). *Trichinella spiralis* larval distribution in muscles of albino rat. *Abstr. Papers 2nd Int. Conf. Trichinellosis Wroclaw,* pp. 15–16.

Madsen, H. (1961). The distribution of *Trichinella spiralis* in sledge dogs and wild mammals in Greenland, under a global aspect. *Medd. Gronland* **159,** 1–124.

Madsen, H. (1970). The influence of life histories on the epidemiological patterns of helminth infections. *J. Parasitol.* **56** (Suppl.), 222–223.

Manning, T. H. (1961). Comment on carnivorous walrus and some arctic zoonoses. Arctic **14,** 76–77.

Marazza, V. (1960). Ändert sich die Wiederstandsfahigkeit der Muskel-Trichinen, wenn die Gefriertemperatur während der prophylaktischen Desinfektions-Behandlung des Fleisches herabgedrückt wird? *Wiad. Parazytol.* **6,** 311–312.

Marshall, W. H. (1963). The ecology of mustelids in New Zealand. *Inform. Ser. 38 (N. Zeal. Dep. Sci. Indust. Res.),* 32 pp.

Merkushev, A. V. (1960). The role of birds in *Trichinella spiralis* circulation in nature. *Zool. Zh.* **39,** 161–164.

Merkushev, A. V. (1963). Trichinelliasis in the Soviet Arctic. *Wiad. Parazytol.* **9,** 493–495.

Merkushev, A. V. (1970). *In:* S. E. Gould (ed.), "Trichinosis in Man and Animals." Thomas, Springfield, Illinois, pp. 449–456.

Minoprio, J. L. and Abdon, H. D. (1967). Factores ecologicos que determinan la trichiniasis silvestre en el Oeeste de San Luis y Este de Mendoza. *An. Soc. Cie. Argen.* **183,** 19–30.

Neghme, A. and Schenone, H. (1970). In S. E. Gould (ed.), "Trichinosis in Man and Animals." Thomas, Springfield, Illinois, pp. 407–411.

Nelson, G. S. (1968). The transmission of *Trichinella spiralis* from wild animals to man and domestic animals. *In:* "Some Diseases of Animals Communicable to Man in Britain," Pergamon Press, New York, pp. 77–89.

Nelson, G. S. (1972). Human behaviour in the transmission of parasitic diseases. *In:* E. U. Canning and C. A. Wright (eds.), "Behavioural Aspects of Parasite Transmission." Academic Press, London. pp. 109–122.

Nemeseri, L. (1968). Invasionsversuche beim Geflügel mit *Trichinella spiralis*. *Helminthologia* **8–9,** 417–420.

Nenov, S. (1962). Trichinellosis in Bulgaria. *Proc. 1st Int. Conf. Trichinellosis Warsaw 1960,* pp. 108–121.

Neumann, L. G. (1905). "A Treatise on the Parasites and Parasitic Diseases of the Domesticated Animals," London, 697 pp.

Ozeretskovskaya, N. N. (1968). Clinical and epidemiological features of trichinelliasis in different geographical regions of the USSR. *Med. Parazitol. Parazit. Bol.* **37,** 387–397.

Ozeretskovskaya, N. N., Tumolskaya, N. I., Tschernyaeva, A. I., Pereverzeva, E. V., Uspenskiy, S. M., Romanowa, V. I., and Bronshtein, A. M. (1969). Characteristics of human trichinellosis caused by natural (Arctic) and several synanthropic strains of *Trichinella spiralis* in the USSR. *Abstr. Papers 2nd Int. Conf. Trichinellosis Wrocław,* pp. 18–22.

Pagenstecher, H. A. (1865). "Die Trichinen. Nach Versuchen im Auftrage des grossherzoglich Badischen Handelsministerium ausgefuhrt am Zoologischen Institute in Heidelberg." W. Engelmann, Leipzig, 116 pp.

Pampiglione, S., and Doglioni, L. (1971). Osservazioni e ricerche su di episodio epidemico di trichinosi verificatosi in Provincia di Trento. *Parassitologia* **13,** 241–255.

Pavlovsky, E. N. (1966). "Natural nidality of transmissible diseases, with special reference to the landscape epidemiology of zooanthroponoses." University of Illinois Press, Urbana, Illinois.

Pawłowski, Z., and Rauhut, W. (1971). Comparative observations on three strains of *Trichinella spiralis*. *Wiad. Parazytol.* **17,** 481–486.

Petropavlovskij, N. N. (1899). On the problem of trichinellae and trichinellosis. *Arch. Vet. Sci.* **7,** 118–124.

Petropavlovskij, N. N. (1905). On the problem of trichinellae and trichinellosis. *Arch. Vet. Sci.* **7,** 595–653; **8,** 714–743; **9,** 841–879.

Piana, G. P. (1887). Studio sulla trichina spirale e sulla trichinosi. *Clin. Vet.* **10,** 17–28, 69–71, 108–117, 197–200, 304–312, 383–390, 438–442, 502–505.

Pódhajecký, K. (1962a). Resistance of muscle trichinae to NaCl. *Proc. 1st Int. Conf. on Trichinellosis Warsaw,* pp. 163–165.

Pódhajecký, K. (1962b). Resistance of muscle trichinae to higher and low temperature. *Proc. 1st Int. Conf. Trichinellosis Warsaw,* pp. 166–168.

Pullar, E. M. (1950). The wild (feral) pigs of Australia and their role in the spread of infectious disease. *Austr. Vet. J.* **26,** 99–110.

Rauhut, W., and Skoczen, S. (1971). Studies on experimental trichinellosis in the mole (*Talpa europaea* L.). *Wiad. Parazytol.* **17,** 487–495.

Rausch, R. L. (1970). *In:* S. E. Gould, "Trichinosis in Man and Animals." Thomas, Springfield, Illinois, pp. 348–373.

Rausch, R. L. (1972). Observations on some natural-focal zoonoses in Alaska. *Arch. Environ. Health* **25,** 246–252.

Rausch, R. L., Babero, B. B., Rausch, R. V., and Schiller, E. L. (1956). Studies on the helminth fauna of Alaska. XXVII. The occurrence of larvae of *Trichinella spiralis* in Alaskan mammals. *J. Parasitol.* **42,** 259–271.

Ribas-Mujal, D. (1971). Trichinosis. *In:* R. A. Marcial-Rojas (ed.), "Pathology of Protozoal and Helminthic Diseases," Williams & Wilkins, Baltimore, pp. 677–710.

Ribas-Mujal, D., and Rivera-Pomar, J. M. (1968). Biological significance of the early structural alterations in skeletal muscle fibers infected by *Trichinella spiralis. Virchows Arch. Abt. Pathol. Anat.* **345,** 154–168.

Ritterson, A. L. (1966). Nature of the cyst of *Trichinella spiralis. J. Parasitol.* **52,** 157–161.

Romanov, I. V. (1970). The role of the brown rat in the distribution of trichinelliasis in the USSR. *Zool. Zh.* **49,** 1391–1397.

Roth, H. (1949). Trichinosis in arctic animals. *Nature London* **163,** 805. [Reprinted in *Can. J. Comp. Med.* (1949) **13,** 227–228].

Roth, H. (1950). Nouvelles expériences sur la trichinose avec considérations spéciales sur son existence dans les régions arctiques. *Bull. Office Int. Épizootol.* **34,** 197–220.

Roth, H. and Madsen, H. (1956). Die Trichinose in Gronland, abschliessender Bericht der Jahre 1948–1953. *Proc. 14th Int. Congr. Zool. Copenhagen,* pp. 340–341.

Sachs, R. (1954). "Uber die Lebensfahigkeit von Trichinen in Hartwürsten von verschiedenem Kochsalzgehalt." Dissertation, Justus Leibig University, Giessen, 28 pp.

Sachs, R. (1970). Zur Epidemiologie der Trichinellose in Africa. *Z. Tropenmed. Parasitol.* **21,** 117–126.

Saowakontha, S. (1972). Pathohistological study of the intestinal and muscular stages of trichinosis in rats fed on low (ND_pCal %5) and high (ND_pCal %10) protein diets. *Southeast Asian J. Trop. Med. Pub. Health* **3,** 242–248.

Schenone, H., Carrasco, J., Villarroel, F., Chinchou, R., and Urriola, J. (1967). Epizootics of trichinosis in pigs and its relation with anti-rat procedures using Warfarin. *Bol. Chil. Parasitol.* **22,** 138–143.

Schnurrenberger, P. R., Masterson, R. A., Suessenguth, H., and Bashe, W. J., Jr. (1964). Swine trichinosis. I. Fecal transmission under simulated field conditions. *Amer. J. Vet. Res.* **25,** 174–178.

Schoop, G., and Lamina, J. (1962). Die Rolle des Fuchses in der Epidemiologie der Trichinose. *Deut. Med. Wochenschr.* **87,** 335–339.

Schultz, M. G. (1970). Reservoirs of *Trichinella spiralis* in nature and its routes of transmission to man. *J. Parasitol.* **56** (Suppl.), 309.

Serventy, V. (1966). "A Continent in Danger. A Survival Special." Andre Deutsch., London, 240 pp.

Shanta, C. S., and Meerovitch, E. (1967a). The life cycle of *Trichinella spiralis.* I. The intestinal phase of development. *Can. J. Zool.* **45,** 1255–1260.

Shanta, C. S., and Meerovitch, E. (1967b). The life cycle of *Trichinella spiralis.* II. The muscle phase of development and its possible evolution. *Can. J. Zool.* **45,** 1261–1267.

Shaver, R. J., and Mizelle, J. D. (1955). Effects of rapid and ultra rapid freezing on *Trichinella spiralis* larvae from guinea pigs and rats. *Amer. Midland Natural.* **54,** 65–77.

Sprent, J. F. A. (1969). Helminth "Zoonoses": An Analysis. *Helminthol. Abstr.* **38,** 333–351.

Steiniger, F. (1969). Trichinose und Rattensicherung mit Bekämpfungsmittelreserven. *Deut. Tieraerztl. Wochenschr.* **76,** 404–406.

Strobl, F. (1954). Versuche über das Gefrieren vön trichinösemSchweinefleisch als Grundlage für eine Gefriervorschrift. Dissertation, Univ. Munich, 50 pp.

Teppema, J. S., Robinson, J. E., and Ruitenberg, E. J. (1973). Ultra structural aspects of capsule formation in *Trichinella spiralis* infection in rats. *Parasitology* **66,** 291–296.

Themann, H. (1960). Eletronenmikroskopischer Beitrag zur Entwicklung und zum Aufbau der Trichinenkapsel. *Wiad. Parazytol.* **6,** 352–354.

Tomich, P. Q. (1969). "Mammals in Hawaii." Bishop Museum Press, Honolulu, pp. 1–238.

Trommer, G. (1970). Fleischfressende Vögel als Überträger von Trichinen. *Prakt. Tierarzt* **51,** 46–47.

Varges, W. (1958). Versuche über das Abtöten der Trichinen durch Kälteeinwirkung. *Monatsh. Vet. Med.* **13,** 365–369.

Virchow, R. 1866. Trichinen beim Iltis, beim Fuchs und bei der Ratte. *Arch. Pathol. Anat. Physiol. Klin. Med.* **36,** 149–152.

Visnjakov, J. I., and Georgiev, M. (1972). Swine caudophagy, a new epizootiological link of trichinellosis in the industrial swine farms. *Acta Parasitol. Pol.* **20,** 597–604.

Whitlock, J. H. (1949). The relationship of nutrition to the development of the trichostrongylidoses. *Cornell Vet.* **39,** 146–182.

Wodzicki, K. A. (1950). Introduced mammals of New Zealand. An ecological and economic survey. *Res. Bull. 98, Dep. Sci. Indust. Res. 250 pp.*

Zarzycki, J. (1963). Histochemical studies on capsules of Trichinella. *Wiad. Parazytol.* **9,** 453–458.

Zenker, F. A. (1860). Ueber die Trichinen-Krankheit des Menschen. *Virchow Arch. Pathol. Anat.* **18,** 561–572.

Zenker, F. A. (1871). Zur Lehre von der Trichinenkrankheit. *Deut. Arch. Klin. Med.* **8,** 387–421.

Zimmermann, W. J. (1970a). The epizootiology of trichiniasis in wildlife. *J. Wildl. Dis.* **6,** 329–334.

Zimmermann, W. J. (1970b). Reservoirs of *Trichinella spiralis* in nature and possible routes of transmission from one host to another. *J. Parasitol.* **56** (Suppl.), 378.

Zimmermann, W. J. (1971). Trichinosis. *In:* J. W. Davis (ed.), "Parasitic Diseases of Wild Mammals." Iowa State Univ. Press, pp. 127–139.

Zimmermann, W. J., and Hubbard, E. D. (1969). Trichiniasis in wildlife of Iowa. *Amer. J. Epidemiol.* **90,** 84–92.

Zimmermann, W. J., Steele, J. H., and Kagan, I. G. (1968). The changing status of trichiniasis in the U.S. population. *Pub. Health Rep.* **83,** 957–966.

Zimoroi, I. Y. (1963). The effects of desiccation and of ultra-sound on the viability of *Trichinella. Med. Parazitol. Parazit. Bol.* **32,** 603–606.

Author Index

The numbers in italics refer to pages on which complete references appear.

Subject Index